Physician Assistant

Acute Care Protocols and Disease Management

For Family Practice, Urgent Care, and Emergency Medicine

SIXTH EDITION

Donald C. Correll, M.D., FACEP

Acute Care Horizons

Cocoa, FL

Physician Assistant Acute Care Protocols and Disease Management
SIXTH EDITION: For Emergency Departments, Urgent Care Centers, and Family Practices

Acute Care Horizons, LLC
Cocoa, FL
acutecarehorizons.com

Printed in the United States of America.

Library of Congress Control Number: 2012940144

HARDCOVER
ISBN: 978-1-7377389-5-4 (Hardcover)
Version: COV – 9781737738954_cov(1) TXT – 9781737738954_txt(3)

SOFTCOVER
ISBN: 978-1-7377389-4-7 (Softcover / Paperback)
Version: COV – 9781737738947_cov(1) TXT – 9781737738947_txt(3)

DEDICATION

To the reviewers of this work.

To my brother John for his creativity and work to make this book possible.

To my mother Glenna who worked two jobs to put me through college.

To my father-in-law Joe Keller for his wisdom over the past 45 years.

To my wife Christina for her steadfast love and devotion.

To my children Joanna, Donny and Diana for bringing more meaning into my life.

CONTENTS

REVIEWERS

(Since beginning)

John Howard, PA-C
Emergency Department Physician Assistant
Jackson-Madison County General Hospital; Jackson, Tennessee

Ron Hoffmeyer, PA-C
Past President – Tennessee Academy of Physician Assistants

Robert E. Turner III, M.D., FACEP
Emergency Physician
Jackson-Madison County General Hospital
Volunteer Clinical Instructor, University of Tennessee Family Medicine; Jackson, Tennessee

Sharai C Amaya, M.D.
Obstetrics and Gynecology
Women's Advanced Care of Self Regional Healthcare
Greenwood, SC

Neil Wangstrom, M.D.
Otolaryngology
La Porte, Indiana

Karl E. Misulis, M.D., PhD
West Tennessee Neurosciences
Jackson-Madison County General Hospital
Jackson, Tennessee
Associate Clinical Professor of Neurology, Vanderbilt University School of Medicine; Nashville, Tennessee

Frederick (Rick) E. Barr, M.D.,MSCI
Professor of Pediatrics and Anesthesiology

Timothy F. Linder, M.D., FAAFP
Family Physician Selmer, Tennessee
Volunteer Clinical Instructor, University of Tennessee Family Medicine; Jackson, Tennessee
Past President – Tennessee Academy of Family Physicians

David Roberts, M.D., FAAFP
Medical Director Jackson-Madison County General Hospital
Family and Geriatric Medicine
Past Director of University of Tennessee Family Medicine Residency Program

E. Scott Yarbro, M.D.
Jackson Urological Associates PC
Volunteer Clinical Instructor, University of Tennessee Family Medicine; Jackson, Tennessee

Gregg Mitchell, M.D.
Program Director – University of Tennessee Family Medicine Program Director
Jackson, Tennessee

Thomas Ellis, M.D., FCCP
The Jackson Clinic
Pulmonary and Critical Care

Robert Gilroy, M.D., FCCP
The Jackson Clinic
Pulmonary and Critical Care

E. Lee Murray, M.D.
Clinical Assistant Professor of Neurology, University of Tennessee Health Science Center
Memphis, TN
Attending Neurologist
West Tennessee Neuroscience
Jackson, TN

John Baker, M.D., FACC
The Jackson Clinic
Cardiology
Jackson, Tennessee

Robert Daggett, M.D.
Rheumatology
Brentwood, Tennessee

Jacob A Aelion, M.D., FACR, CCD
Arthritis Clinic, Jackson, TN
Clinical Professor of Medicine
The University of Tennessee Health Science Center
Memphis, Tennessee

John Guidi, M.D.
Past District Health Officer, State of Tennessee Dept of Health
Medical Director of the CDC Clinics for the West TN Region

Lucius Wright, M.D.
The Jackson Clinic
Nephrology
Jackson, TN

Steven Williams, D.O., MBA
Staff Hospitalist
Jackson-Madison County General Hospital
Jackson, Tennessee

PURPOSE

This book of protocols has been created to assist physician assistants and the physicians they work with. It focuses on acute care medicine as practiced in emergency departments, urgent care centers, and family practices.

These protocols are intended to be concise and yet reasonably comprehensive, and to have parameters that determine physician interaction with the physician assistant, where applicable, while permitting flexibility in patient care by the physician assistant.

NOTICE

~ Read This ~

The protocols presented in this book are *model guidelines.* Accordingly, they should be used — and, when necessary, modified — per any agreement that may exist between the supervising physician and physician assistant. In states, regions, or institutions where a supervisory model is in place, this agreement should be established *prior to use* of these protocols.

In writing these protocols the author has checked with sources believed to be reliable. However, medicine is an ever-changing science and art. As new research and clinical experience expand the knowledge base, changes in these protocols are required.

Further, there is a possibility of human error or of changes in medical science. Neither the author nor any party involved in the preparation or publication of this work warrants that the information contained herein is in every respect accurate or complete, and they disclaim all responsibility for any errors or omissions, or for results obtained from use of the information contained in these protocols or this publication.

Users are recommended and encouraged to confirm the information contained herein with other sources and by their own experience and knowledge. This recommendation is of particular importance with new or infrequently used drugs and therapies.

GUIDELINES OF PROPER USE

It is recommended that the protocols and other information provided in this book are to be used in accordance with the following understandings, concepts, and guidelines:

1. The protocols presented herein are *model guidelines.* Accordingly, they only should be used per written agreement between any supervising physician and physician assistant where applicable. Any agreement should be established *prior to use* of any of the protocols by the physician assistant.

2. When deemed appropriate, any protocol should be modified to reflect any authorized policies, procedures, or practices at a particular medical facility.

3. Not all patient presentations can be covered in these protocols. Those presentations not covered in protocols should be evaluated and managed according to the physician assistant's training and experience, and according to the usual scope of practice of any supervising physician where applicable.

4. The physician assistant should perform only those tasks that are within the physician assistant's skills and competence, and that are within the usual scope of practice of any supervising physician, if applicable, and that are consistent with the protection and safety of the health and well-being of the patient.

5. Any perceived potential conflict between patient safety and the Protocols book should be resolved by consultation with a physician, if applicable, and in favor of patient safely.

6. Specific protocols override the General Patient Criteria Protocol if there is a disparity between the specific protocol and the General Patient Criteria Protocol.

7. Sanford Guide to Antimicrobial Therapy or other databases can be used for infections in lieu of protocol-specified antimicrobial treatments.

8. "Consult criteria" usually means to discuss the patient with a physician, or given the appropriate context, to refer to a physician.

9. Life-saving care should not be withheld because of protocol instructions.

10. The physician assistant should discuss with a physician any patient care and safety concerns regardless of protocols.

11. Deviations from protocols should be reviewed by a supervising physician where applicable, feasible and appropriate.

12. Read the Notice (page 11) before applying the protocols contained herein. If you do not accept the limitations and disclaimers contained in the Notice you should refrain from using this book and the information and protocols contained herein.

SHARED DECISION-MAKING (SDM)

- Information transfer is two-way, with clinician providing medical information needed for decision-making, the patient providing information about preferences, and clinician and patient deciding together on the best evaluation and treatment to implement

Criteria that must be met for an interaction between a clinician and a patient to be classified as SDM:

- It must involve at least two participants, the clinician and the patient (or the patient's designated representative)
- Both parties must share information
- Both parties must take steps to build consensus on the preferred treatment
- Agreement on which treatment to implement must be reached
- Highly desirable model in certain circumstances
- Not appropriate for all clinical situations
- STEMI, surgical emergencies, respiratory failure, organ failure, etc. would be areas not amenable in most cases to shared decision making

The patient, family or guardian need to have "Capacity" as determined by the physician or provider to be able to understand decisions regarding evaluation, treatment, risks and disposition. The word Capacity may be documented within a statement of decisions in the medical record as indicated.

REFERENCES:

Hess EP, Grudzen CR, Thomson R, Raja AS, Carpenter CR. Shared decision-making in the emergency department: respecting patient autonomy when seconds count. Acad Emerg Med 2015 Jul;22(7):856-64

PROTOCOL GUIDELINE AGREEMENT

(Where needed for State regulations or institutional policies only)

By signing this Protocol Guideline Agreement each party acknowledges that he or she has read both the Notice section and the Guidelines of Proper Use section.

____
Provider's signature Date

____
Provider's signature Date

____
Provider's signature Date

____
Provider's signature Date

____
Provider's signature Date

____
Provider's signature Date

____
Provider's signature Date

____
Provider's signature Date

____
Provider's signature Date

____
Provider's signature Date

____
Provider's signature Date

____
Provider's signature Date

____
Provider's signature Date

General

Section Contents — one protocol

General Patient Criteria Protocol

When using any protocol, always follow the Guidelines of Proper Use (page 12).

GENERAL PATIENT CRITERIA PROTOCOL

Notify physician promptly during or after physician assistant initial assessment

- Acute myocardial infarction (AMI) or symptoms consistent with AMI — notify physician when AMI identified
- Acute central nervous system deficits
- Severe CHF
- Severe respiratory distress
- O_2 Saturation < 90% on room air, if acute
- Hypotension
- Acute altered mental status unless intoxicated
- Adult heart rate ≥ 140
- Malignant hypertension
- Age ≤ 28 days

Consult physician when:

- Age ≤ 28 days
- Age > 28 days and < 3 months (unless experienced with this age group)
- Moderate CHF
- SBP ≥ 240 or DBP ≥ 140 at presentation (that is asymptomatic) with preexisting hypertension history
- Adult heart rate ≥ 110 at time of disposition
- Patients sent to the ED or clinic from an outlying hospital, clinic, or from home by a medical provider
- Age ≥ 70 with systemic symptoms
- Patient receives more than one pain injection
- Patient returns ≤ 14 days for same acute complaint (Does not apply to chronic recurrent complaints unless a change in the complaint.)
- Elevated BP in pregnancy or ≤ 6 weeks postpartum
- Pregnancy complications
- Chest pain (potentially consistent with angina or anginal equivalent symptoms)
- Nonspecific chest pain age ≥ 30 with history of
  - Hypertension
  - Diabetes
  - Smoking
  - Coronary artery disease history
  - Hyperlipidemia
  - Family history of coronary artery disease by age of 60

  OR
  - Age ≥ 50 without risk factors
- Abdominal pain
  - Requiring narcotics
  - Age ≥ 70
  - Diabetic
  - Uncertain diagnosis

Lab consult criteria

- Adult WBC ≥ 18,000 or < 1,000 neutrophils
- Pediatric WBC ≥ 18,000 or < 1,000 neutrophils
- Bandemia ≥ 15%
- Acute thrombocytopenia
- Hemoglobin 8–10 gms (unless chronic and stable)
- Hemoglobin < 8 gms even if chronic
- O_2 Sat ≤ 93% on room air if acute (or moderate dyspnea)
- O_2 Sat 2% less than chronic levels

Vital sign and age consult criteria

Fever

- Adult ≥ 104°F or 40°C
- Pediatric ≥ 104.5°F or 40.3°C

Hypothermia

- Temperature ≤ 95°F or 35°C

Heart rate/minute

- Adult heart rate ≥ 115
- Pediatric heart rate:
  - 0–4 months ≥ 180
  - 5–7 months ≥ 175
  - 8–12 months ≥ 170
  - 1–3 years ≥ 160
  - 4–5 years ≥ 145
  - 6–8 years ≥ 130
  - 9–11 years ≥ 125
  - 12–15 years ≥ 120
  - 16 years or older ≥ 115

Inappropriate sinus tachycardia (no clinical explanation)

Hypertension

- Adult asymptomatic hypertension of SBP > 220 or DBP > 120 at time of disposition with history of hypertension
- Adult asymptomatic SBP > 195 or DBP > 115 at discharge without history of hypertension
- Pediatric hypertension — age < 14 years

NOTE: Specific protocols override this General Patient Criteria Protocol

Cardiovascular

Section Contents

Chest Pain Protocol

Cardiac Dysrhythmia Protocol

Hypertension Protocol

Congestive Heart Failure Protocol

Syncope/Near Syncope Protocol

When using any protocol, always follow the Guidelines of Proper Use (page 12).

Chest Pain Protocol

Definition

- Patient perception of discomfort in anterior chest or upper half of back

Differential Diagnosis

Pneumonia

- Cough
- Fever
- Chills
- Dyspnea
- Sweats
- Tachycardia

Pulmonary embolism

- Dyspnea
- Tachycardia
- Biphasic ST–T wave changes in V1–3 mimicking acute coronary syndrome and other EKG changes
- Hypoxia
- Pleuritic chest pain
- Well's criteria moderate-to-high probability
- Troponin may be elevated in moderate to massive pulmonary embolism

Chest wall pain

- Chest wall tenderness
- Pleuritic chest pain
- Pain with movement

Angina/AMI

- Anterior chest pressure or tightness
- **EKG changes**
    - Acute ST elevation in 2 or more contiguous leads or acute ST elevation in AVR even if isolated— ≥ 2mm in men and ≥ 1.5 mm in women
        - **AVR acute ST elevation** with multilead ST depression may indicate left main disease, proximal LAD or left main equivalent stenosis, though can be seen with massive PE, hemorrhagic shock, severe LVH, type A thoracic dissection and SVT
    - ST depression in V1–4 may indicate a posterior MI
    - Hyperacute T waves with reciprocal changes

    - Broad-based, symmetrical, and tall compared with the preceding R–wave
    - Most apparent in the precordial leads
  - **Sgarbossa AMI criteria for LBBB and pacemaker (repolarization of ST segment normally is opposite direction of QRS complex)**
    - Concordant repolarization, same direction as QRS, ≥ 1 ST mm elevation
    - ST disconcordant elevation or depression (opposite direction as QRS) ≥ 25% height of QRS
    - ST disconcordant changes ≥ 5 mm
  - New T wave inversion or ST depression may indicate NSTEMI
- Left or right arm pain
- Jaw pain
- Right arm pain only with chest pain highly specific for cardiac ischemia
- Approximately 50% of patients with angina pectoris have normal findings on a resting EKG
- Dyspnea (may be only presenting complaint in very elderly: age ≥ 80 years)
- Nausea and/or vomiting
- Diaphoresis
- Indigestion
- Angina may be exertional only
- Levine sign (characterized by the patient's fist clenched over the sternum when describing the discomfort) is suggestive of angina pectoris
- Angina decubitus is a variant of angina pectoris that occurs at night while the patient is recumbent
  - May be from an increase in myocardial oxygen demand caused by expansion of the blood volume from increased venous return during recumbency

Considerations

- All NSAIDs increase the risk of MI and death from CV disease, even with short-term use (7–10 days)
  - Celecoxib (Celebrex) causes the least amount of CV side effects it is thought, along with diclofenac for patients taking prophylactic low-dose aspirin
    - Take aspirin 30 minutes to 2 hours before single dose NSAID
- Medium-size coronary plaques (30%–40% stenosis) may be vulnerable to cause occlusion because they are less mature, with a large lipid core and a thin cap prone to rupture or erosion, exposing the thrombogenic subendothelial components causing thrombosis
- Cocaine metabolites which persist in circulation up to 24 hours can cause delayed or recurrent coronary vasospasm

Pleurisy

- Pain occurs or worsens with breathing
- No other comorbid symptoms or signs

Pericarditis

- Pleuritic pain
- Fever
- Worse lying down
- Better sitting and leaning forward
- Diffuse ST segment elevation
- Diffuse PR segment depression
- Pericardial effusion
- Elevated C-reactive protein
- Echocardiogram for pericardial effusion

Pericarditis treatment

- Pericarditis: NSAID's and/or colchicine (if uncomplicated)
  - Colchicine 1.2 mg qday for 3 months
  - Dexamethasone 6 mg qday for 2–4 weeks then slow taper if failure of NSAID's and/or colchicine

Myopericarditis

- Elevated troponin
- Similar symptoms and findings as Pericarditis

Herpes zoster

- Vesicular dermatomal rash
- May have pain 4 days prior to rash

Aortic dissection

- Caused by separation of aorta wall layers
- Ascending aorta most common location of thoracic dissection
- Mortality ~ 30% in hospital
- The mediastinum is considered widened on an AP radiograph if its width is > 8 cm at the level of aortic knob
  - This is not an absolute number and in general the more the width, the higher the probability of underlying aortic dissection
- Three variants
  - Intimal Flap tear – ~70-80% of cases
    Intramural hematoma – ~10–15% (believed to start from rupture of the vasa vasorum)
  - Penetrating atherosclerotic ulcer – ~10-15%

Risk Factors

- Hypertension – 72%
- Collagen disorders – Marfan's, Ehlers-Danlos
- Vasculitis disorders – Giant cell arteritis, Takayasu arteritis or rheumatoid arthritis
- Instrumentation or structural abnormalities
  - Cardiac catheterization
  - CABG
  - Bicuspid aortic valve
  - Aortic coarctation
  - Aortic valve replacement

Classification

- Stanford
  - Type **A** – **A**scending and **A**rch
    - Higher Mortality
    - Surgical Management
  - Type **B** – descending; **B**elow the left subclavian
    - Lower Mortality
    - Medical management usually

Symptoms or findings that may occur

- Chest pain
- Neck or jaw pain
- Tearing or ripping intrascapular pain: May indicate dissection involving the descending aorta
- May be mild pain
  - No pain in 10% of patients
- Hypertension or hypotension
- New diastolic murmur
- Located or radiates to back
- Signs and symptoms above and below diaphragm frequently
- CVA, AMS, Horner's syndrome, syncope, dyspnea, hemoptysis, abdominal pain (with abdominal involvement), dysphagia and fever are possible

Tests

- Chest x-ray
- EKG
- CT chest with contrast (inform radiology what you are looking for)
  - CTA for PE may miss aortic dissection
- Echocardiography (TEE)
- Troponin
- D–dimer in the first 24 hours if negative is helpful in ruling out dissection with negative likelihood ratio of 0.07 (not 100% accurate)

Treatment

- **Control pain**
- Lower systolic blood pressure to 100–120 mmHg
- **Type A**
  - Treated with surgery
  - Hypertension control
- **Type B**
  - Medical management possible

- Hypertension control
- May need surgery
- Stent with thoracic endovascular aortic repair used ~ 50%

Medications

- **Beta–blocker** (select one)
  - Esmolol initial bolus: 80 mg (~0.5–1 mg/kg) IVP over 30 seconds then 0.15-0.3 mg/kg/min IV infusion prn
  - Labetalol 20mg IVP
    - Repeat 20–40 mg IVP q10–15 minutes prn
    - Alternative start drip at 1–2mg/ minute after initial bolus prn
    - NMT 300mg
- **Vasodilators** if blood pressure still elevated **after** beta–blocker
  - Nitroprusside start at 0.3 mg/minute IV and titrate to SBP 100–120 mmHg
- **Calcium channel blocker** (if beta–blocker cannot be given or further BP control needed after beta–blocker)
  - Nicardipine 5 mg/hr. and titrate as needed 2.5 mg/hr. every 5 minutes with maximum of 15 mg/hr.
- **Analgesics**
  - Morphine 2–5 mg IVP q5minutes prn
  - Dilaudid (hydromorphone) 0.5–2 mg IVP q5minutes prn

Consult criteria

- All patients promptly

Chest Pain with Respiratory (Pleuritic) or Movement Exacerbation

- May need no further testing if vital signs and O_2 Sat are normal and clinical suspicion is low for cardiac or serious pulmonary disease
- Consider chest x-ray and D-dimer
- Consider EKG and troponin if diagnosis is uncertain for a non-cardiac etiology
- Consider CTA chest to evaluate for pulmonary embolism
- Apply Well's criteria

Evaluation options

- Chest x-ray
- CBC if febrile or tachycardic
- BMP if diabetic or tachycardic
- D-dimer (if negative with Well's criteria 0–1 makes PE unlikely)
- CT chest (see below)
- Apply Well's pulmonary embolism and DVT criteria and chart Well's score as indicated
- Record positive or negative calf tenderness and Homan's sign (Homan's sign if negative useful for malpractice considerations to avoid litigation but has no clinical usefulness)

Evaluation with D-dimer

- Useful if negative at cutoff value to rule out DVT or PE
- Negative D-dimer with low to moderate probability Well's DVT or PE score largely excludes venous thromboembolic disease
- Well's DVT criteria high probability: order ultrasound scan regardless of D-dimer result
- If positive — not as useful as a negative result which usually rules out VTE (venous thromboembolic) disease
- Frequently positive with
  - Hospitalization in past month
  - Chronic bedridden or low activity state
  - Increasingly positive with age without significant acute disease process
    - D-dimer increases 10 mcg/L for every year over 50 years of age if the upper cutoff is 500 mcg/L (80 year old with d-dimer 700 mcg/L would be in the normal range)
    - If another assay used, then 2% increase/year over age 50 may be used to adjust upper limit for age

- CHF
- Chronic disease processes
- Edematous states

Well's DVT criteria

- One point each:
  - Active cancer
  - Paralysis/recent cast immobilization
  - Recently bedridden > 3 days or surgery < 4 weeks ago
  - Deep vein tenderness
  - Entire leg edema
  - Calf swelling > 3 cm over other leg
  - Pitting edema > other calf
  - Collateral superficial veins
- Two points — alternative diagnosis less likely

High probability: ≥ 3 points

Moderate probability: 1–2 points

Low probability: 0 points

Testing and imaging for DVT

Well's DVT criteria ≥ 1–2 with painful or swollen extremity

- Order D-dimer test (unless patient likely to have positive result regardless of DVT potential)
- Venous Doppler ultrasound of extremity (unless D-dimer negative)
  - May be falsely negative with calf DVT
- Venography if needed
- MRI if needed
- Coumadin (warfarin) therapy can cause falsely negative D-dimer
- Ultrasound may be repeated if negative, and DVT suspicion persists, in 5–7 days

Well's PE criteria score 3 or greater consider D-dimer and CT chest PE protocol

- Suspected DVT = 3
- Alternative diagnosis less likely than PE = 3
- Heart rate > 100 = 1.5
- Immobilization/surgery past 4 wks. = 1.5
- Previous DVT/PE = 1.5
- Hemoptysis = 1
- Cancer past 6 months = 1

Well's score ≥ 6: order CTA chest PE protocol

Document positive or negative Homan's sign and calf tenderness regardless of Well's scores

Document PERC and/or Well's scores when appropriate

Pulmonary Embolism Rule-out Criteria (PERC Rule)

(Reportedly decreases significantly the likelihood of pulmonary embolism if all 8 criteria met — recent studies state not superior to clinical gestalt)

- Age < 50
- Pulse oximetry > 94%
- Heart rate < 100
- No history of DVT or VTE
- No hemoptysis
- No estrogen use
- No unilateral leg swelling
- No recent surgery or trauma hospitalization past 4 weeks

Treatment for chest wall pain or pleuritic chest pain that is not PE

- Treat pneumonia/bronchitis per current recommendations and Sanford Guide or database
- Pericarditis: NSAID's and/or colchicine (if uncomplicated)
  - Colchicine 1–1.2 mg qday for 3 months
  - Dexamethasone 6 mg qday for 2–4 weeks then slow taper if failure of NSAID's and/or colchicine
- NSAID or hydrocodone, or other narcotics as needed
- Treat chest pain from abdominal causes or other causes as per

training, experience, and Protocols

Chest Pain that Could Represent Acute Coronary Syndrome (ACS) or Stable Angina

Evaluation

- EKG
- CBC
- BMP
- Chest x-ray
- Troponin

Acute Coronary Syndrome treatment (STEMI, NSTEMI and Unstable Angina) — consult physician promptly

- **Aspirin** 160–325 mg chew and swallow
- **Clodidogrel** with aspirin
  - **NSTEMI** give Clopidogrel 300 mg PO age <75 years
  - Clopidogrel 75 mg PO age ≥75
  - **STEMI**
    - 300 mg PO if thrombolytics given age <75 years
    - 600 mg PO if no thrombolytics given
    - Clopidogrel 75 mg PO age ≥75
- **Nitrates** prn (See nitrate contraindications and side-effects below)
- Oxygen — maintain O_2 Saturation > 90%
  - Monitor O_2 saturation
- Morphine 2–5 mg or Dilaudid 0.5–1 mg q5–15 minutes prn IV q5–15 minutes prn (caution if SBP < 105 mm Hg)
- Atrial fibrillation with rapid ventricular rate and ACS, beta–blocker preferred over calcium channel blocker (diltiazem) or amiodarone

Short-acting nitrates

- NTG 0.3–0.6 SL prn — may repeat × 2 q5minutes prn continued ischemic cardiac pain (caution if SBP < 105–110 mm Hg)
- May use before anginal provoking activities
  - Comes in tablets or spray
  - Tablets need refrigeration and last 3–6 months, and should tingle tongue when used
  - NTG spray lasts 2–3 years

NTG paste if needed

- 0.5–2 inch — caution if SBP < 105 mm Hg (if SBP ≥170 mm Hg may use the higher dose range)
- Antianginal effects start at 30 minutes
- Hemodynamic effects lasts 3–6 hours
- Peak plasma time 3–4 hours

NTG drip if needed

- Start at 10–50 mcg/minute IV (depending on BP and severity of chest pain and findings) and titrate for chest pain and limit SBP decrease to 10% if normotensive and 30% if hypertensive
  - NTG 0.4 mg SL is 400 mcg which reaches peak blood levels in 2 minutes and falls to 50% of peak at 7.5 minutes by comparison, and is gone by 20 minutes, so more vigorous IV dosing can be considered for angina or hypertensive CHF when indicated
- Keep SBP ≥ 90 mm Hg
- See nitrate contraindications and side-effects below

Heparin if needed (for STEMI or NSTEMI)

- Bolus 60 units/kg IV — NMT 4,000 units
- 12 mg/kg/hour IV drip — initially NMT 1,000 units/hour to be adjusted to PTT 1.5–2.5 times normal (50–75 seconds)

OR

Enoxaparin if needed

- 1 mg/kg SQ q12hr

- May give first dose as 30 mg IV along with the SQ dose for STEMI
  - Age > 75 years give 0.75 mg/kg SQ and no IV dose for STEMI
- Dose 30 mg SQ qday for creatinine clearance < 30 ml/minute

STEMI reperfusion treatment

- Ischemic symptoms < 12 hours
- Cardiogenic shock or acute heart failure regardless of time from AMI onset
- Clinical or EKG evidence of ongoing ischemia between 12–24 hours from symptom onset

PCI capable hospital

- **Oxygen** only if hypoxic (≤90% O_2 Sat) or having dyspnea, respiratory distress or in heart failure
  - Monitor O_2 Saturation
- **Aspirin (ASA)** 162–325 mg chewed before PCI
- **Clodidogrel** with aspirin
  - 300 mg PO if thrombolytics given age <75 years
  - 600 mg PO if no thrombolytics given age <75 years
  - Clopidogrel 75 mg PO age ≥75 years
- **Heparin (UFH)** 60 units/kg IV load — NMT 4,000 units then 12–15 units/kg/hr. IV infusion titrated to PTT 1.5–2.5 times normal (50–75 seconds)

  OR
- **Bivalirudin** 0.75 mg/kg bolus then 1.75 mg/kg/hour infusion as alternative to heparin or high risk of bleeding or history of heparin induced thrombocytopenia (Creatinine clearance < 30 ml/minute give 1 mg/kg/hour)
- FMC (**first medical contact**) to needle time of ≤30 minutes
- Diagnostic angiogram ≤ 90 minutes

PCI non–capable hospital

- Transfer to PCI capable hospital if FMC to cardiac catherization ≤ 120 minutes
- Thrombolytics within 30 minutes if ongoing ischemia 12 hours from symptom onset present and PCI cannot be performed in 120 minutes from FMC (first medical contact) to device deployment — see STEMI reperfusion treatment criteria above

Thrombolytics

- **Tenecteplase (TNK–tPA)** single weight based bolus over 5 seconds
  - < 60 kg give 30 mg
  - 60–70 kg give 35 mg
  - 70–80 kg give 40 mg
  - 80–90 kg give 45 mg
  - > 90 kg give 50 mg (NMT 50 mg)
- **Altepase (tPA)** 90 minute infusion
  - > 67 kg give 100 mg total dose
    - 15 mg IV over 1–2 minutes
    - 50 mg over next 30 minutes
    - 35 mg over remaining 60 minutes
  - ≤ 67 kg
    - Give 15 mg IV over 1–2 minutes
    - Then 0.75 mg/kg IV infusion over 30 minutes (not to exceed 50 mg)
    - Then 0.5 mg/kg IV over next 60 minutes (not to exceed 35 mg over 1 hr.)

PLUS

- **Oxygen** only if hypoxic (≤92% O_2 Sat) or having dyspnea, respiratory distress or in heart failure
  - Monitor O_2 saturation
- **Aspirin (ASA)** 162–325 mg chewed before PCI
- **Clopidogrel** with aspirin

  - 300 mg if thrombolytics given age <75 years
  - 600 mg PO if no thrombolytics given age <75 years
  - Clopidogrel 75 mg PO age ≥75 years
- **Heparin (UFH)** 60 U/kg IV load — NMT 4,000 units then 12–15 U/kg/hr. IV infusion titrated to PTT 1.5–2.5 times normal (50–75 seconds)

  OR
- **Enoxaparin** 30 mg IV bolus then 1mg/kg SQ bid if age <75 years
  - Age ≥75 years give no bolus and give 0.75 mg/kg SQ bid

  OR
- **Bivalirudin** 0.75 mg/kg bolus then 1.75 mg/kg/hour infusion as alternative to heparin or high risk of bleeding or history of heparin induced thrombocytopenia (Creatinine clearance < 30 ml/minute give 1 mg/kg/hour)

Thrombolytic contraindications

- Do not administer for treatment of AMI in the following situations in which the risk of bleeding is greater than the potential benefit
- Active internal bleeding
- History of recent stroke within 3 months (except within 4.5 hours)
- Recent (within 3 months) intracranial or intraspinal surgery or serious head trauma
  - Caution with history of recent major surgery (past 2 weeks)
  - Caution with acute pericarditis or subacute endocarditis
- Presence of intracranial conditions that may increase the risk of bleeding (e.g., some neoplasms, AV malformations, aneurysms)
- Bleeding diathesis
- Current severe uncontrolled hypertension: SBP ≥180 mm/Hg, DBP ≥ 115 mm/Hg
- Suspected aortic dissection
- Platelet count < 100,000 cu/mm
- Warfarin treated patients

Stable angina treatment

Short-acting nitrates

- NTG 0.3–0.6 SL prn — may repeat x 2 q5minutes prn continued ischemic cardiac pain (caution if SBP < 105–110 mm Hg)
- May use before anginal provoking activities
  - Comes in tablets or spray
  - Tablets need refrigeration and last 3–6 months, and should tingle tongue when used
  - NTG spray lasts 2–3 years

Long-acting nitrates for stable angina

- Timing — taken at time of day that anginal symptoms or anginal equivalent symptoms (e.g., dyspnea) are most prevalent
- NTG 2.5 mg or 6.5 mg PO bid
- Isosorbide mononitrate
  - Standard dose — 20 mg PO bid given 7 hours apart
  - Smaller patients start 5 mg PO bid given 7 hours apart and increase to 10–20 mg PO bid given 7 hours apart over 2–3 days
  - Take on empty stomach 30 minutes prior to a meal or 1 hour after a meal
- Isosorbide mononitrate ER (extended release)
  - 30–120 mg PO qday
- Transdermal nitroglycerin (Nitro-Dur)
  - 0.2–0.4 mg/hr. qday — remove for 10–12 hours each day

- Max dose 0.4–0.8 mg/hr. qday
- Starts acting in 30 minutes and lasts 8–14 hours

Nitrate side–effects (some)

- Headache
- Hypotension
- Tachycardia
- Nausea

Nitrates contraindications and cautions

- Shock or hypotension
- SBP < 90 m Hg or ≥ 30 mm Hg below baseline SBP in ACS
- Bradycardia < 50 beats per minute
- Tachycardia in absence of heart failure (>100 beats per minute)
- Acute right ventricular myocardial infarction
    - Caution in inferior myocardial infarction
- Use of erectile dysfunction medications (sildenafil, tadalafil, or vardenafil)
- Severe anemia

Beta-blockers for stable angina

- Reduce heart rate, blood pressure and cardiac contractility which decreases cardiac work and oxygen needs
- First choice usually with stable angina
- Prolongs survival and decreases second AMI incidence

Selective beta–1 blocker

- Metoprolol tartrate initially 50 mg PO bid and may be increased to 200 mg PO bid
- Metoprolol (Toprol XL) 100 mg PO qday — NMT 400 mg PO qday
- Atenolol (Tenormin) 50 mg PO qday — NMT 200 mg PO qday

Beta–blocker side effects

- Bradycardia
- Hypotension
- Worsening of asthma and COPD
- Heart failure
- Exacerbation of angina and hypertension on abrupt withdrawal (Black Box Warning)
- Worsening of peripheral arterial disease symptoms

Contraindications

- Pre-existing sinus bradycardia (< 60 beats/minutes)
- Moderate to severe left ventricle failure and pulmonary edema
- SBP < 100 mm Hg
- Signs of poor peripheral perfusion
- 2nd and 3rd degree heart block
- Asthma and COPD
- Sick sinus syndrome without pacemaker
- Untreated pheochromocytoma

ACEI or ARB added to a beta-blocker if needed in stable angina

Consult criteria

- Consult cardiology or medicine for ACS or worsening anginal pattern
- Notify physician promptly for ACS (STEMI, NSTEMI and Unstable angina
- Consult physician for suspected stable angina

Heart score (point system)

May not be too useful in patients with previous ischemic cardiac events and multiple risk factors and with an atypical or nonsuspicious acute history (i.e., all patients would be scored 4 or higher despite low suspicion for the current visit). Not useful with cocaine induced chest pain.

History

- Highly suspicious = 2
- Moderately suspicious = 1
- Slightly suspicious = 0

EKG

- Significant ST deviation = 2

- Nonspecific ST repolarization abn = 1
- Normal = 0

Age

- ≥ 65 years = 2
- 45–65 years = 1
- ≤ 45 years = 0

Risk factors

- ≥ 3 risk factors or history of atherosclerotic disease = 2
- 1 or 2 risk factors = 1
- No risk factors known = 0

Troponin

- ≥ 3 times normal limit = 2
- 1–3 times normal limit = 1
- ≤ normal limit = 0

Risk factors for atherosclerotic disease

- Hypercholesterolemia
- Hypertension
- Diabetes mellitus
- Cigarette smoking
- Positive family history for CAD
- Obesity

Interpretation

- 0–3 points indicates low risk of MACE (0.9–1.7%)
  - Usually discharged
- 4–7 points indicates moderate risk of MACE (12–16.6%)
  - Usually admitted
- 8–10 points indicates high risk of MACE (50–65%)
  - Admit

MACE defined as Major Adverse Cardiac Event within 6 weeks

- Acute MI
- Requires PCI
- Requires CABG
- Death
- If troponin is normal in low risk patient then incidence of MACE at 6 weeks is 1%

Author recommendations

- Do not discharge chest pain patients with acute onset of elevated troponin usually
  - Chronic myocardial injury from conditions such as LVH, LV dysfunction, diabetes, or chronic kidney disease may have elevated troponins, commonly or chronically, that if stable and not increasing or decreasing significantly on repeat draw 3 hours later, <u>might be</u> considered not significant and not represent an acute coronary syndrome
- Follow-up for cardiac stress testing in 3 days
- 2 negative troponins 3 hours apart and 2 negative EKG's helpful for disposition and discharge purposes considering parameters of lower risk and chest pain timing
  - ACS pain ≤ 20 minutes or so frequently may have negative troponins and nonacute EKG's that cannot be relied on fully for disposition purposes

2015 American College of Cardiology/American Heart Association (ACC/AHA) guideline recommendations on the workup of non-ST-elevation ACSs to assist in maximizing patient outcomes

- Patients with chest pain or other symptoms suggesting acute coronary syndromes (ACS) should have 12-lead electrocardiography (ECG) performed and evaluated within 10 min of arrival at an emergency facility, and serial ECGs should be performed to detect ischemic changes.
- Serial cardiac troponin I or T levels (using a contemporary assay) should be obtained at presentation and at 3-6 hours after symptom onset. Risk scores can help assess prognosis
- In patients with a normal EKG and symptoms suggestive of

acute coronary syndrome that started at least 3 hours before arrival, a single hs-cTn (high sensitive troponin) below the limit of detection on initial measurement may be reasonable to exclude myocardial injury
- In patients with symptoms consistent with ACS without objective evidence of myocardial ischemia (nonischemic ECG and normal cardiac troponin levels), noninvasive imaging is reasonable before emergency department discharge or within 72 hours after discharge

General Discharge Criteria for Chest Pain

- Benign noncardiac chest pain
- Chest wall pain
- Pleurisy or pleurodynia
- Adult heart rate < 110
- Herpes zoster
- O_2 Saturation on room air or chronic home oxygen concentration ≥ 94% or at baseline for chronic hypoxic patients and in no respiratory distress
- Normal cardiac marker lab tests (see exception above)
  - Chest pain that is continuous for ≥1–2 hours, and has 2 troponins that are 3 hours apart, usually is not from ischemic cardiac disease ≥ 8 hours out from start of chest pain
  - If chest pain episode was ≥ 8–10 hours prior to evaluation, and was sometime in the past 5–7 days and was continuous for ≥ 2 hours, then 1 normal troponin usually is not consistent with an ischemic cardiac cause
- Stable and nonacute CBC, BMP and chest x-ray

Discharge instructions

- Chest pain aftercare instructions
- Follow up with primary care provider or cardiologist within 1–3 days as indicated

Consult criteria recommendation

- Suspected angina or acute coronary syndrome
- Suspected anginal equivalent — arm, neck, jaw or epigastric pain, or dyspnea
- Acute chest x-ray abnormalities
- Pulmonary embolism (see Hestia criteria)
- Aortic dissection/aneurysm (stable aneurysm does not usually need a consult)
- Pericarditis
- Severe pain in practitioner's clinical judgment
- Chest pain of uncertain etiology in medium to high risk patient

Suggested consult criteria

- Suspicious chest pain for ACS age ≥ 30 with or without history of
  - Hypertension
  - Diabetes
  - Smoking
  - Coronary artery disease history
  - Hyperlipidemia
  - Family history of coronary artery disease by age of 60

Suggested vital signs and lab consult criteria

- Elevated troponin
- New and significantly elevated BNP in patient with no explanation for the rise otherwise (can be from PE)
- Hyperglycemia with metabolic acidosis (decreased serum CO_2 or elevated anion gap)
- Chest pain with O_2 saturation on room air < 94% in non-COPD or non-bronchospasm presentation or with acute respiratory distress or complaints(see Dyspnea Guide)
- Adult heart rate ≥ 110
- Developing hypotension or relative hypotension (SBP < 105 with history of hypertension)

Notes

REFERENCES:

Circulation 2010;122:S787–S817

CHEST October 2011;140(4_MeetingAbstracts):594A-594A. doi:10.1378/chest.1112163

CHEST August 2011;140(2):509–518. doi:10.1378/chest.10–2468

Angina Pectoris Author: Jamshid Alaeddini, MD, FACC, FHRS; Chief Editor: Eric H Yang, MD emedicine.medscape.com/article/150215

Amsterdam EA, Wenger NK. The 2014 American College of Cardiology ACC/American Heart Association guideline for the management of patients with non-ST-elevation acute coronary syndromes: ten contemporary recommendations to aid clinicians in optimizing patient outcomes. *Clin Cardiol*. 2015 Feb. 38(2):121-3

Acute Coronary Syndrome; Author: David L Coven, MD, PhD; Chief Editor: Eric H Yang, MD emedicine.medscape.com/article/1910735

Circulation. 1979 Mar;59(3):585-8; Blood levels after sublingual nitroglycerin. Armstrong PW, Armstrong JA, Marks GS

Age-Adjusted D-Dimer Cutoff Levels to Rule Out Pulmonary Embolism: The ADJUST-PE Study *JAMA.* 2014;311(11):1117-1124. doi:10.1001/jama.2014.2135

JEM, epub, 7/29/16

CCJM;81:233

Emerg Radiology, 2016;23:405

Circulation, Vol. 117, pg. 1897

Harhash AA, et al. *Am J Med.* 2019 Jan 8. [Epub ahead of print]

PT O'Gara, et al. *Circulation.* 2013;127: e362-e425

DJ Engelen, et al. *J Am Coll Cardiol.* 1999;34: 389-395

Tamura A. *World J Cardiol.* 2014;6: 630

Celecoxib Associated With Lower MACE Risk Than Naproxen and Ibuprofen; Brandon May; thecardiologyadvisor.com May 21, 2018

CARDIAC DYSRHYTHMIA PROTOCOL

Definition

- Disorders of cardiac rhythm

Differential Diagnosis

- Sinus tachycardia
- Atrial tachycardia
- Multifocal atrial tachycardia
- Atrial fibrillation
- Atrial flutter
- Sinus bradycardia
- Junctional bradycardia
- Atrioventricular blocks
- Premature atrial contractions
- Premature ventricular contractions

Considerations

- Unifocal premature ventricular contractions (PVCs) without associated symptoms of acute ischemic disease are usually benign acutely and typically do not warrant treatment
- Premature atrial contractions (PACs) are usually benign

- Sinus bradycardia ≥ 40 beats/minute, without hypotension or presyncope/syncope, or other concerning complaints, usually does not warrant acute treatment
- Prolonged QTc interval on the EKG can lead to a serious or life threatening arrhythmia
- PVCs with R wave on the T wave of preceding beat on the EKG or monitor can lead to ventricular tachycardia

General evaluation options

- Cardiac history
- Complete physical exam
- Associated symptoms
- Medication history
- EKG; consider monitor if heart rate ≥ 130 (adults) or ≤ 50
- CBC (depending on clinical situation)
- BMP (depending on clinical situation)
- Chest x-ray (depending on clinical situation)
- Troponin for anginal complaints or dyspnea
- BNP for dyspnea if needed (chest x-ray usually suffices)
- Consider D-dimer if PE suspected

Atrial Dysrhythmias

Sinus tachycardia

Definition

- Tachycardia in adults arising from the sinus node with a rate in adults > 100 beats/minute. Sinus tachycardia rates in pediatrics dependent on age

Considerations

- Significant sinus tachycardia (ST) that is unexplained can represent a high risk disease process
- Sinus tachycardia context is important: ST of 120 with influenza may be less concerning than ST at 105 with GI bleeding

Causes

Physiologic

- Pain or exertion

Pharmacologic

- Sympathetic agents; caffeine; bronchodilators

Pathologic

- Fever
- Dehydration
- Anemia
- Hemorrhage
- Pulmonary embolism
- Hypoxemia
- Infarction
- Ischemia
- Hyperthyroidism

Evaluation and treatment are aimed at underlying condition

Discharge instructions

- Sinus tachycardia aftercare instructions
- Follow up within 1–2 days if tachycardia persists
- Return if no improvement or worsening

Consult criteria recommendation

- Consult for unexplained adult ST ≥ 120 unless otherwise specified in other Protocols

Premature atrial contractions

- Commonly benign; can be anxiety provoking
- Fatigue, stress or high adrenergic state can be the cause
- Evaluation is for associated disorders and not for PACs per se
- Usually no treatment needed
- If treatment desired, atenolol 50 mg PO qday or metoprolol 50–100 mg PO qday can be used (follow up recommended to evaluate response and side effects)

- Metoprolol tartrate is bid dosing and metoprolol succinate is qday dosing

Discharge instructions

- Premature atrial contractions aftercare instructions

Atrial fibrillation

Definition

- Lack of organized atrial electrical activity and contractions — an irregularly irregular rhythm on EKG and cardiac auscultation or pulse palpation
- Atrial flutter with atrial flutter waves

Differential diagnosis

- Multifocal atrial tachycardia
- Wolf-Parkinson-White Syndrome (WPW)
- Atrial flutter
- Atrial tachycardia
- Supraventricular tachycardia

Considerations

- Most common sustained adult tachyarrhythmia
- Up to 9% of patients ≥ 80 years of age are affected
- CVA risk increased (do not acutely convert if present > 48 hours without therapeutic anticoagulation)
- BNP usually elevated even without overt CHF
- Recent onset of atrial fibrillation converts spontaneously to normal sinus rhythm in 2–3 days in 2/3 of patients
- Increases mortality 1.5–2 times more than general population without atrial fibrillation
- Risk of stroke 1.5% in age 50–59 years and nearly 30% in age 80–89 years
- Commonly heart rates are 110–140 per minute
- No treatment may be needed if heart rate ≤ 110 per minute and patient is on appropriate stroke prophylaxis
- Standing the patient up may reveal degree of tachycardia
- Loss of up to 20% of stroke volume

Causes

- Hypertension
- CHF
- Coronary artery disease
- Carditis
- Sick sinus syndrome
- Alcohol
- Pulmonary embolism
- Hyperthyroidism
- Sympathetic drugs
- Pneumonia
- Hyperthermia
- Hypothermia
- Postoperative
- Hypokalemia, hypomagnesemia and hypocalcemia

Management options

- Medication management to maintain normal sinus rhythm
- Medication management to achieve rate control of atrial fibrillation
- Catheter ablation
- Anticoagulation to prevent thromboembolic disease

Signs and symptoms

- Altered mental status
- Weakness
- Hypotension
- Syncope
- Angina
- CHF
- Emboli
- Digit ischemia
- Neurologic deficits
- Mesenteric ischemia

Evaluation options

- EKG
- CBC
- BMP
- Chest x-ray
- Troponin for anginal complaints or dyspnea
- BNP for dyspnea or suspected CHF (chest x-ray alone may suffice)

- Thyroid function tests if hyperthyroidism suspected
- D-dimer if pulmonary embolism suspected
- Digoxin (digitalis) level if currently prescribed

Treatment options

- IV NS KVO
- Oxygen if dyspneic; O_2 saturation < 92% on room air
- Treatment of fever or hypovolemia if contributing to rapid ventricular response > 110
- Treat medical cause of rapid ventricular response if tachycardia is compensatory or driven by another condition
  - May not need initial atrial fibrillation direct treatment, unless rate is ≥ 150–160, if underlying medical condition treatment ameliorates tachycardia to a satisfactory level

Oral rate control medications may be considered if rate not too high or needed for chronic rate control as outpatient (increased interactions with any of PO medications listed below when used in combination)

Beta-blockers PO to choose from

- Metoprolol 25–200 mg PO
  - Metoprolol tartrate is bid dosing and metoprolol succinate is qday dosing
- Atenolol 25–100 mg PO qday
- Avoid in acute heart failure

Calcium channel blocker PO

- Cardizem CD 180–360 mg PO qday
- Avoid in heart failure

Amiodarone 200–600 mg PO qday

IV treatment for rapid ventricular response

- May need emergent cardioversion if unstable (see below)
- **Cardizem** (diltiazem) 0.25 mg/kg IV over 2 minutes (usually 20 mg initial dose) for rate ≥ 130/min
  - May be repeated at 0.35 mg/kg IV over 2 minutes after 15 minutes of initial dose if needed (usually 25 mg)
  - Lower dose 0.2 mg/kg may be effective with less hypotension
    - Maintenance is 5–15 mg/hour IV
  - Exercise caution in patients with a pre-existing low ejection fraction **(systolic heart failure)** or low preload — may cause hypotension
    - Probably should use different medication
  - Avoid with wide QRS unless it is a preexisting bundle branch block
  - If high atrial fibrillation rate is from systemic condition, address that condition also (increased rate, if not very excessive, may be needed to compensate for underlying systemic condition)
- **Amiodarone** 150 mg IV over 10 minutes and then drip at 1 mg/minute for 6 hours, followed by 0.5 mg/minute next 18 hours — may repeat bolus if needed
- **Metoprolol** 5 mg IV, may repeat q5 minutes prn × 2 up to 3 doses total
  - **May be best choice for atrial fibrillation with angina (ACS)**
  - AHA/ACC guidelines recommend IV beta-blocker s over non-dihydropyridine calcium channel blockers for acute rate control of hemodynamically stable patients in the setting of ACS

  - Do not use if patient hypotensive or acute heart failure
  - Do not use in atrial fibrillation wide complex WPW QRS unless it is a preexisting bundle branch block
- **Digoxin** 0.25 mg may be used as adjunct to other medications (slows rate on onset)
  - Repeat dose 0.25 mg IV q2hr. as needed (do not exceed 1.5 mg over 24 hr.)
  - Do not use in atrial fibrillation WPW (wide QRS complex)

Unstable patients

- Cardioversion with 120-200J with biphasic waveform device for hypotension with rapid ventricular response
- May repeat up to 2 times if needed with increasing joules
- If there is difficulty with synchronization, change leads to choose larger R wave and smaller T wave
- If unable to synchronize, cardioversion without synchronization may be attempted, with knowledge that ventricular fibrillation may result, requiring ventricular defibrillation and resuscitation
- If cardioversion unsuccessful and patient still unstable, then amiodarone 300 mg IV over 10-20 minutes may be given
  - If still unstable, another shock may be given, then give amiodarone 900 mg IV over 24 hours

Wide complex atrial fibrillation

- Is potentially a life threatening rhythm with preexcitation or antidromic WPW
- Be prepared to perform defibrillation if needed
- Procainamide 10–18 mg/kg IV and infusion of 1–4 mg/min. may be considered
- Ibutilide 1 mg IV if weight > 60kg, may repeat in 10 minutes prn, if procainamide not available
  - < 60kg give 0.01/kg IVP, may repeat in 10 minutes prn
  - For atrial fibrillation < 90 days
  - May need anticoagulation prior to use
  - Be prepared for lethal arrhythmias
- Amiodarone 150 mg IV over 10 minutes and then drip at 1 mg/minute for 6 hours, followed by 0.5 mg/minute next 18 hours — may repeat bolus if needed **(use if no preexcitation present, e.g., WPW antidromic conduction)**
  - **Atrial fibrillation with wide QRS with rates ≥250 beats per minute usually is WPW and amiodarone should not be used usually**
  - Characteristic findings with atrial fibrillation and WPW is QRS morphology changes beat to beat
  - Having an old EKG showing a bundle branch block that has same QRS width and morphology as current EKG, and no preexcitation is helpful in making a judgment call whether to use beta–blockers, calcium channel blockers, digoxin, amiodarone or adenosine
- **Potentially dangerous to use digoxin, beta–blockers, calcium channel blockers or adenosine if WPW is antidromic conduction present (wide QRS complex)**
  - WPW is uncommon
  - May have rhythm deterioration to ventricular fibrillation with antidromic WPW, especially with digoxin or verapamil

Anticoagulation

- Aspirin 325 mg PO qday in low risk patients if direct thrombin or factor Xa inhibitors cannot be used or are not indicated

- Age 60–74 years
- Female
- CHA_2DS_2VASc score 0–1
- High risk of bleeding

- Coumadin (warfarin) 5–10 mg PO qday — (INR target of 2–3) with moderate or high risk factors
  - Age > 75 years
  - CAD
  - CHF
  - Hypertension
  - Diabetes mellitus
  - Mitral stenosis
  - Prior TIA/CVA
  - **Mechanical valve**
- Lovenox 1 mg/kg SQ q12hr

Stroke prevention in atrial fibrillation

- Should be screened for at age > 65 years
- Aspirin 325 mg PO daily may be used for low risk for stroke — CHA_2DS_2VASc score 0–1
- Treatment with warfarin in post–AMI patients with left ventricular thrombus or akinetic segment is reasonable

Anticoagulation recommendations in patients with nonvalvular atrial fibrillation per American Academy of Neurology

- Inform patients of the benefits of anticoagulation vs. the risks of major bleeding
- TIA/CVA patients with atrial fibrillation should be offered anticoagulation therapy
- Dabigatran, Rivaroxaban or Apixaban, which have a lower risk of intracranial bleeding than warfarin, may be offered to patients who have a higher risk of intracranial bleeding
- Dabigatran, Rivaroxaban or Apixaban may be used in patients unable to undergo frequent INR testing for warfarin therapy
- Dementia patient families or those that fall occasionally should be informed that the risk–benefit ratio is uncertain

CHA_2 DS_2 –VASc score

- Used to quantify risk of stroke in atrial fibrillation patients
- 2014 AHA/ACC/HRS Guideline for the Management of Patients With Atrial Fibrillation deemphasizes aspirin or use of platelet agents if warfarin (Coumadin), dabigatran (Pradaxa), rivaroxaban (Xarelto) or apixaban can be safely used and are indicated
- Stands for heart failure, hypertension, age ≥ 75 years , diabetes mellitus and prior stroke/TIA, vascular disease (MI, PAD or aortic plaque), age ≥ 65 with sex category (female)
- 1 point each for heart failure, hypertension, diabetes mellitus, age ≥ 65 and sex category (female)
- 2 points for prior stroke/TIA and age ≥ 75 years
  - Low risk = 0 points
  - Moderate risk = 1–2 points
  - High risk = 3–6 points

Long–term anticoagulation for nonvalvular atrial fibrillation recommended with score of ≥ 2, if no significant risk of hemorrhage

- Warfarin, dabigatran, rivaroxaban or apixaban
- With warfarin determine INR weekly initially, then monthly when stable
- Direct thrombin or factor Xa inhibitor recommended if unable to maintain therapeutic INR
- Evaluate renal function prior to direct thrombin inhibitors or factor Xa inhibitors and annually
- Adjust dosage per creatinine clearance for each specific drug (warfarin

adjusted per INR) per PDR or other references

Warfarin prophylaxis

- CHA_2DS_2VASc score ≥ 2
- Age > 75 years
- Target INR 2.0–3.0
- May be lower (1.8–2) in high risk bleeding patients, or 2.5–3.5 in mechanical artificial valve, rheumatic heart, or recurrent stroke patients
- May be used age 65–75 years at discretion of clinician based on underlying disorders such as valvular disease etc.
- No heparin bridging therapy needed

Dabigatran (Pradaxa)

- CHA_2DS_2VASc score ≥ 2
- 150 mg PO bid for stroke prevention in nonvalvular atrial fibrillation is indicated in patients > 30 mL/min
- 75 mg PO bid CrCl 15–30 mL/min
- Not recommended if CrCl < 15 mL/min
- Less bleeding risk than warfarin
- Read Physician Desk Reference (PDR) drug or database information

Rivaroxaban (Xarelto)

- CHA_2DS_2VASc score ≥ 2
- 20 mg PO qday for stroke prevention in nonvalvular atrial fibrillation/min for CrCl > 50 mL/min
- 15 mg PO qHS if creatinine clearance (CrCl) 15–50 mL/minute
- Not recommended for CrCl ≤ 15
- Less bleeding risk than warfarin
- Andexxa for significant bleeding
  - Consider PCC (Kcentra prothrombin complex concentrate or recombinant activated factor VII — not a specific antidote) if Andexxa not available for life threatening bleeding
- Read Physician Desk Reference (PDR) drug or database information

Apixaban (Eliquis)

- CHA_2DS_2VASc score ≥ 2
- 5 mg PO bid for CrCl ≥ 30 mL/min
- 2.5 mg PO bid for age > 80 years, weight < 60 kg, creatinine ≥ 1.5 mg/dL
- Not recommended in severe liver disease
- Less bleeding risk than warfarin
- Andexxa for significant bleeding
  - Consider PCC (Kcentra prothrombin complex concentrate or recombinant activated factor VII — not a specific antidote) if Andexxa not available for life threatening bleeding
  - Andexxa
  - — Coagulation factor Xa recombinant, inactivated-zhzo (for life threatening bleeding or uncontrolled bleeding)
    - Very expensive — hospital pharmacies may not stock
    - Half-life of Andexxa is far shorter than the FXa inhibitors (onset of action within 2 minutes)
    - Anti-FXa activity starts to resume to baseline after the 2-hour infusion and goes back to the baseline by 4 hours after drug initiation, so further bleeding may resume
    - Prothrombotic
      - Arterial and venous thromboembolic events
      - Ischemic events, including AMI and stroke
      - Cardiac arrest
      - Sudden death
- Read Physician Desk Reference (PDR) drug or database information

Dabigatran, rivaroxaban, apixaban or warfarin should not be used in the following patients — aspirin safer

- Poor compliance
- Uncontrollable hypertension
- Aortic dissection
- Bacterial endocarditis
- Alcohol dependency
- Liver disease
- Bleeding lesions
- Malignant tumor
- Retinopathy with bleeding risk
- Advanced microvascular changes in the brain
- Known aneurysm of a cerebral artery
- Previous spontaneous cerebral hemorrhage
- Bleeding diathesis (e.g., coagulopathies, thrombocytopenia)
- Benefit/risk is uncertain in patients with frequent falls

Bleeding risk with warfarin (2 points for history of bleeding, 1 point for the rest)

HEMORR$_2$HAGES 100 patient years of warfarin

- Hepatic or renal disease
- Ethanol abuse
- Malignancy
- Old age (>75 y)
- History of bleeding
- Low platelet counts or platelet dysfunction
- Hypertension that is uncontrolled
- Anemia
- Genetic factors
- Elevated fall risk
- Stroke

HEMORR$_2$HAGES data

Score	Bleeding risk 100 pt. yr.
0	1.9%
1	2.5%
2	5.3%
3	8.4%
4	10.4%
>5	12.3%
Any score	4.9%

Monitor routinely for bleeding

Discharge criteria recommendation

- Stable chronic atrial fibrillation with rate ≤ 110 and pre-existing history of atrial fibrillation
  - Standing the patient may clarify degree of tachycardia
- Appropriate stroke prevention treatment in place or initiated
- No other concerning symptoms

Discharge instructions

- Atrial fibrillation aftercare instructions
- See treatment options above
- Adjust Digoxin (digitalis) if needed
- Follow up within 7 days

Consult criteria recommendation

- Adult heart rate ≥ 110
- Chest discomfort
- Dyspnea
- Hypotension
- Suspected hyperthyroidism
- Acute neurologic complaints or findings
- New onset atrial fibrillation
- Age > 55
- Digoxin (digitalis) toxicity
- PT/INR not therapeutic on warfarin and not experienced in adjusting dosage
- Anticoagulation therapy

- Antiarrhythmia therapy

Supraventricular tachycardia (SVT)

Definition

- Tachycardia not involving the sinus node that is maintained by the atria or atrioventricular node
- Regular rhythm

Differential diagnosis

- Atrial fibrillation
- Atrial flutter
- Multifocal atrial tachycardia (commonly in COPD patients)
- Ventricular tachycardia
- Sinus tachycardia
- Wolf-Parkinson-White Syndrome (WPW)

Considerations

- Usually narrow complexes on EKG with rapid and regular rhythm
- Paroxysmal most common
- Can have wide complexes with aberrant or retrograde conduction
- Heart rate usually 150–200/minute in adults
- Higher rates may be present in WPW
- Wide complex SVT can be ventricular tachycardia
- Treatment of wide complex SVT with calcium channel blockers, beta–blockers or Digoxin (digitalis) may result in deterioration of rhythm to ventricular fibrillation if antidromic (retrograde conduction) WPW is present
- Caffeine may block adenosine effectiveness

Presenting complaints

- Palpitations
- Dizziness
- Chest pain
- Shortness of breath
- Diaphoresis

Evaluation options

- EKG (may be all that is needed in young healthy patient without concerning complaints or comorbidities)
- CBC
- BMP
- Chest x-ray if respiratory complaints or findings present
- Troponin for anginal complaints
- BNP or NT–ProBNP for dyspnea or suspected CHF (chest x-ray may suffice)
- Digoxin (digitalis) level if taking digoxin
- Drug screen as indicated

Treatment options

- IV NS KVO or INT
- Oxygen if dyspneic or O_2 saturation < 92% on room air (unless stable and chronic)
- **Vagal maneuvers in stable patient**
  - Breath holding
  - Bearing down like in having a bowel movement
  - Unilateral nondominant carotid artery massage for 10 seconds at a time in young healthy patients
  - Face immersion in cold water
- Cardioversion 50–100 Joules initially **if unstable**

Medication treatment options for stable patients

Narrow complex options

- Adenosine 6 mg rapid IVP followed by 10–20 ml of saline — may repeat with 12 mg if needed
  - Half the dose if using central line or PICC line or taking dipyridamole or carbamazepine
  - Caution with asthma
  - May need higher dose if patient drinking/taking caffeine products
- Diltiazem 0.25 mg/kg over 2 minutes (usually 20 mg in adults — may be repeated with 0.35 mg/kg IV over 2 minutes (usually 25 mg in adults)
  - Caution if CHF present

- Metoprolol 5 mg slow IV, may repeat q5min up to total of 15 mg
- Esmolol 300–500 mcg/kg IV over 1 minute, may repeat in 2–5 minutes prn, then IV drip 50 mcg/kg/minute

Outpatient PO medications for PSVT prevention with narrow QRS only (select one)

- Metoprolol tartrate 25 mg PO bid or propranolol 10–30 mg tid PO
- Verapamil 240–480 mg/day PO divided tid–qid or diltiazem PO
- Digoxin 0.125–0.25 mg qd–q.o.d depending on age and renal function (for patients intolerant of beta–blockers or CCB)
- Recommend cardiology consult

Discharge criteria recommendation

- SVT conversion in stable patient without cardiac or other concerning comorbidities

Discharge instructions

- Supraventricular tachycardia aftercare instructions
- Follow up with PCP or cardiologist within 1–7 days

Consult criteria recommendation

- New onset or concerning associated symptoms such as chest pain, hypotension etc.

Wide complex tachycardia (regular rhythm)

Ventricular tachycardia

Definition

- Tachycardia originating from the ventricles that is ≥ 120/minute and is wide complexed of ≥ 140 msec on EKG (typically have structural heart disease)
- AV dissociation (faster V rate than A rate) is diagnostic of VT, surface ECG findings (dissociated P waves, fusion or capture beats) are present in only about 20% of cases
- Same QRS polarity or deflection in anterior leads suggests monomorphic ventricular tachycardia, especially if negative concordance
- Nonsustained ventricular tachycardia is 3 ventricular beats in a row lasting up to 30 seconds
- Sustained ventricular tachycardia > 30 seconds
- Torsades de Pointes is rapidly changing polarity and amplitude of QRS complexes around isoelectric line associated with prolonged QTc interval (may be from electrolyte abnormalities, drug effects, ischemia, or a genetic cardiac channelopathy)

Differential diagnosis

- Ventricular fibrillation
- PSVT with aberrancy
- Artifact
- PVC's
- Multifocal atrial tachycardia
- Wolff–Parkinson–White syndrome
- Accelerated idioventricular rhythm

Causes

- Cardiac ischemia
- Hypokalemia, hypomagnesemia, or hypocalcemia
- QTc prolonging drugs
- Digoxin (digitalis) toxicity

Symptoms or findings

- May be asymptomatic, especially in nonsustained ventricular tachycardia (30 beat run or less)
- Chest pain
- CHF
- Dyspnea

- Diaphoresis
- Hypotension
- Syncope
- Altered mental status

Evaluation

- Order EKG; CBC; BMP; chest x-ray; troponin
- Cardiac monitor
- Magnesium and phosphorus levels
- Digoxin level if taking
- Urine drug screen as indicated

Treatment see below

- IV NS KVO
- Oxygen to keep O_2 saturation > 90%
- **PSVT with aberrancy treatment is same as narrow complex PSVT**

Stable ventricular tachycardia

- Blood pressure normotensive (may use MAP) and no related acute coronary syndrome or acute heart failure
- Amiodarone 150 mg IV over 10 minutes followed by drip of 1 mg/min

  OR
- Procainamide 100-200 mg/dose or 15–18 mg/kg, no faster than 50 mg/minute IV (if available), then 1–4 mg/min by continuous IV

  OR
- Lidocaine 1 mg/kg IV up to 100mg — may repeat × 2 up to 3 mg/kg followed by drip of 2–4 mg/min IV (if left ventricular function is impaired use instead of procainamide)
- Phenytoin can be considered if other medications fail or digoxin toxic ventricular tachycardia present and digibind not immediately available or effect delayed
- If tricyclic antidepressant overdose suspected give $NaHCO_3^-$ (sodium bicarbonate) 1–2 amps IVP, target is pH 7.50–7.55, give further bolus treatment and/or $NaHCO_3^-$ 0.5 mEq/kg/hour drip as needed
- Have nurse deploy cardiac defibrillation pads on patient
- Synchronized cardioversion if needed and if pulse present is biphasic shock 100–200 joules
  - If time permits, pretreat with midazolam (Versed) 0.5–2 mg IVP, and fentanyl 1 mcg/kg IVP or morphine 2–4 mg IVP

Unstable ventricular tachycardia

- Hypotension
- Acute coronary syndrome
- Acute heart failure
- Acute altered mental status
- Synchronized cardioversion biphasic shock 100–200 joules
  - If time permits, pretreat with midazolam (Versed) 0.5–2 mg IVP, and fentanyl 1 mcg/kg IVP or morphine 2–4 mg IVP

Pulseless ventricular tachycardia

- Biphasic defibrillation 150–200 joules
- Activate cardiac code and start CPR and ACLS if no pulse present and patient unconscious

Torsades de Pointes

Stable

- Magnesium 1–2 gms IV over 30–60 seconds, repeat in 5–15 minutes prn or continuous infusion can be started at a rate of 3–10 mg/min
- Isoproterenol 2–10 mcg/minute IV with heart rate goal > 90/minute — if magnesium unsuccessful
- Phenytoin (Cerebyx: fosphenytoin) PE) 15–20 mg/kg IV at up to 150 mg/minutes can be considered if other medications ineffective

- Amiodarone, procainamide, and lidocaine (some anecdotal reports of success with lidocaine) are best avoided
- If needed, transvenous overdrive pacing
- Usually brief and recurring, so cardioversion used if unstable or sustained

Unstable

- Biphasic defibrillation 150–200 joules if ventricular fibrillation occurs
- Biphasic cardioversion 100 joules for sustained ventricular tachycardia with hypotension

Consult criteria recommendation

- All ventricular tachycardia and torsades de pointes patients
- Most wide complex tachycardia

Junctional rhythm

Definition

- Heart rhythm arising from AV node

Differential diagnosis

- Second and third degree AV block
- Digoxin (digitalis) toxicity
- Sinus node dysfunction
- AV nodal reentry tachycardia
- Idioventricular rhythm

Evaluation options

- EKG
- CBC
- BMP
- Chest x-ray
- Troponin for anginal complaints
- BNP or NT Pro–BNP for dyspnea or suspected CHF

Treatment options

- IV NS KVO or INT
- Oxygen if dyspneic or O_2 saturation < 92% on room air unless chronic and stable
- Dependent on cause of the rhythm

Recommended consult criteria

- Discuss all cases with physician

Sinus bradycardia

Definition

- Sinus rhythm < 50 beats per minute

Causes

Physiologic

- Vagal tone

Pharmacologic

- Calcium channel blockers; beta–blockers; Digoxin (digitalis)

Pathologic

- AMI
- Hypothyroidism
- Sick sinus syndrome
- Carotid hypersensitivity
- High intracranial pressure
- Hypoglycemia

Evaluation

- EKG
- Per other complaints or findings

Treatment

- Usually no treatment needed if heart rate ≥ 40 in healthy patient with normal BP
- IV NS bolus if hypotensive and not in CHF
- Atropine 0.5–1 mg IV if SBP < 90 mmHg and heart rate < 50/minute

Discharge criteria recommendation

- Asymptomatic sinus bradycardia ≥ 45 beats/minute and chronic

Discharge instructions

- Sinus bradycardia aftercare instructions
- Follow up with PCP or cardiologist within 7 days if new onset

Consult criteria recommendation

- Heart rate < 50 unless chronic and stable or healthy athlete
- Hypotension
- Dyspnea
- Anginal complaints

Second and third degree AV block

Definition

- Second degree heart block has some of the atrial electrical impulses not conducted to the ventricles through AV node
- Third degree heart block has no atrial electrical impulses conducted to the ventricles

Considerations

- Can be caused by AMI or myocarditis
- Can be seen with Lyme disease
- Can occur with structural heart disease

Mobitz type 1 second degree heart block (Wenkebach)

- PR interval progressively lengthens before dropping a ventricular beat
- Can be seen in healthy athletes
- Usually asymptomatic
- May have chest pain if ischemia or myocarditis present
- Rarely have syncope
- May be drug induced — beta–blocker, calcium channel blockers, Digoxin (digitalis), amiodarone

Mobitz type 2 second degree heart block

- Intermittent dropped ventricular beats without progressive lengthening of the PR interval
- Syncope may occur
- AMI or myocarditis more common than with mobitz type 1
- May be drug induced
- More serious type of heart block than mobitz type 1
- Frequently treated with pacemaker

Third degree heart block

- Most patients are asymptomatic
- May be hypotensive or have syncope
- Sudden death can occur
- May be caused by AMI
- Confusion can occur in elderly

Evaluation

- Cardiac monitor
- EKG
- CBC
- BMP
- Chest x-ray
- Troponin
- BNP or NT Pro–BNP for dyspnea or suspected CHF

Treatment

- IV NS KVO
- Oxygen if dyspneic; O_2 saturation < 92% on room air
- External pacing if hypotensive and heart rate < 60 (apply external pacing pads to mobitz type 2 and third degree heart block)
- Atropine 0.3–1 mg IV

Consult criteria

- Notify physician promptly on all heart block patients

Ventricular Dysrhythmias

Premature ventricular contractions

Definition

- A premature ventricular contraction caused by an ectopic cardiac pacemaker in the ventricle usually > 120 msec on EKG

Consideration

- Usually benign and stable acutely
- Usually unifocal and needs no acute treatment
- There is some statically increase long term mortality from underlying causes

Causes

- Frequently normal finding
- Digoxin (digitalis) toxicity
- Cardiac ischemia
- Cardiomyopathy
- Hypoxemia
- Mitral valve prolapse
- Myocarditis
- Cardiac contusion
- Stimulant medications or drugs (caffeine, cocaine, methamphetamines, tobacco)
- Hypokalemia
- Hypomagnesemia
- Hypercalcemia
- CHF
- Alkalosis

Evaluation

- EKG
- BMP if comorbid conditions present or on diuretics
- Other tests as dictated by symptoms or other findings

Treatment options

- Consult physician
- Usually none
- Correction of potassium and magnesium levels if checked
- Treat underlying condition causing PVCs if present
- If antiarrhythmic treatment desired, atenolol 50 mg PO qday or metoprolol (Lopressor) 50–100 mg PO qday can be used (follow up with primary care provider)

Discharge criteria recommendation

- If it is a benign finding without concerning comorbid conditions

Discharge instructions

- PVC aftercare instructions
- Follow up with primary care provider or cardiologist as needed

Consult criteria recommendation

- EKG shows R on T phenomenon
- Comorbid conditions of concern: chest pain; dyspnea; syncope; etc.
- Potassium ≤ 2.5 mEq/L
- Digoxin (digitalis) toxicity
- Prolonged QTc interval
- New onset renal insufficiency

PVC couplets or multifocal PVCs

- Usually needs no treatment
- Treating the cause may be indicated unless benign
- If antiarrhythmic treatment desired, atenolol 50 mg PO qday or metoprolol (Lopressor) 50–100 mg PO qday can be used (follow up with primary care provider)

Accelerated idioventricular rhythm (AIVR)

Definition

- Wide complex ventricular rhythm
- Rate 40–120 per minute

Considerations

- Associated with reperfusion in AMI

Treatment

- Observe
- Treating with antiarrhythmia drugs can cause asystole — do not treat patient with these drugs

Consult criteria recommendation

- Discuss all cases of AIVR with physician promptly

Warning

- Treating **"slow ventricular tachycardia"** (rate ≤120 beats/minute) with an antiarrhythmia drug, may actually be treating accelerated idioventricular rhythm (a life sustaining ventricular escape rhythm), resulting in asystole and death

Notes

REFERENCES:

Guidelines for the Primary Prevention of Stroke

A Guideline for Healthcare Professionals from the American Heart Association/American Stroke Association

ACC/AHA/ESC Practice Guidelines

ACC/AHA/ESC 2006 Guideline for the Management of Patients with Atrial Fibrillation

2014 AHA/ACC/HRS Guideline for the Management of Patients with Atrial Fibrillation

Am J Emerg Med. 2011 Oct;29(8):849–54. doi: 10.1016/j.ajem.2010.03.021

Anticoagulation After Cardioembolic Stroke: To Bridge or Not to Bridge? www.ncbi.nlm.nih.gov/pmc/articles/PMC2678170/

[Guideline] January CT, Wann LS, Alpert JS, Calkins H, Cigarroa JE, Cleveland JC Jr, et al. 2014 AHA/ACC/HRS guideline for the management of patients with atrial fibrillation: executive summary: a report of the American College of Cardiology/American Heart Association Task Force on practice guidelines and the Heart Rhythm Society. *Circulation*. 2014 Dec 2. 130 (23):2071-104

medscape.com/viewarticle/858839

Danon A, et al. *Am J Emerg Med.* 2019 Aug;37(8):1539-1543

Kaufmann MR, et al. *Tex Heart Inst J.* 2018;45: 39-.

HYPERTENSION PROTOCOL

Definition

- Adult SBP ≥ 140 or DBP ≥ 90
- Age 1 ≥ 104/58
- Age 6 ≥ 115/75
- Age 12 ≥ 125/82
- Age 17 ≥ 138/87

Considerations (acute care settings)

- Most hypertension is acutely asymptomatic
- Care should be exercised in too aggressively over-treating asymptomatic hypertension acutely
- Blood pressure usually comes down with repeated measurements only. Repeat q15 min. prn
- Poor outcomes possible from acutely lowering asymptomatic blood pressure too much
- In ED patients with asymptomatic markedly elevated blood pressure, routine screening for acute target organ injury (e.g., serum creatinine, urinalysis, EKG) is not required
- In certain patient populations (poor follow-up, etc.), checking for an elevated serum creatinine level may identify kidney injury that affects disposition
- In patients with asymptomatic markedly elevated blood pressure, routine ED medical intervention is usually not required.
- In select patient populations (such as poor follow-up), providers may treat markedly elevated blood pressure and/or initiate therapy for long-term control

- Patients with asymptomatic markedly elevated blood pressure should be referred for outpatient follow-up
- 70% ED patients with BP ≥ 140/90 with no prior history of HTN will continue to have elevated BP on follow up

Hypertensive categories

- Hypertensive urgency*:* SBP ≥ 180 or DBP ≥ 115 with cardiac risk factors
- Severe uncontrolled hypertension: SBP ≥ 180 or DBP ≥ 115 without cardiac risk factors
- Hypertensive emergency*:* elevated blood pressure with acute end organ compromise or injury

Evaluation

- Complete history and physical exam
- Detailed cardiopulmonary exam
- Check for peripheral edema
- Asymptomatic hypertension in above hypertensive categories, excluding hypertensive emergency, by itself may require no further acute tests
- BMP and U/A (for protein/blood) can be considered, especially if starting new hypertensive medications or in pregnancy
- Add CBC if pregnant to check platelet count
- EKG, CXR, BNP or NT Pro–BNP and troponin for acute signs/symptoms of cardiac disease
- Hypertensive urgency — lab appropriate to address existing risk factor screening

Treatment Options

- Hypertensive urgency — begin treatment within 24–48 hours per primary care provider
- Severe asymptomatic hypertension — begin treatment within 1–7 days per primary care provider
- SBP > 200 or DBP > 120 at discharge can begin treatment as indicated; May need 2 medications or combination medication
- Hypertensive emergency consult physician for treatment options
- Hypertensive emergency blood pressure should not be lowered more than 25% acutely
- IV therapy safer in hypertensive emergency: better control
- See CVA/TIA Protocol for CVA/TIA presentation

Discharge Criteria

- Asymptomatic SBP < 220 or DBP < 120 mm Hg
- No concerning comorbidities

Discharge instructions

- Hypertension aftercare instructions
- Follow up with PCP within 1–2 days if SBP ≥ 200 mm Hg or DBP ≥ 110
- Patient to notify PCP of visit and blood pressure readings within 1–2 days if markedly elevated

Consult Criteria

- SBP ≥ 240 or DBP ≥ 140 at presentation (asymptomatic) with preexisting hypertension history
- Asymptomatic SBP > 220 or DBP > 120 at time of disposition with history of hypertension
- Asymptomatic SBP > 195 or DBP > 115 at time of disposition without history of hypertension
- Hypertension in pregnancy or within 6 weeks postpartum
- Hypertensive emergency
- Acute cardiac, neurologic or renal disorder suspected
  - Intracranial hemorrhage, TIA, CVA, CHF, angina, MI, acute renal failure
- New onset renal insufficiency or worsening renal insufficiency
- See General Patient Criteria Protocol (page 15)

Acute care initiation of outpatient treatment options (if desired)

JNC 8 Goals of Therapy

- Age < 60 years initiate treatment for a SBP ≥ 140 mm Hg or DBP ≥ 90 mm Hg to achieve a target SBP of < 140 mm Hg and DBP < 90 mm Hg in patients without diabetes or chronic kidney disease
- Age ≥ 60 years treat SBP ≥ 150 mm Hg or DBP ≥ 90 mm Hg to achieve SBP < 150 mm Hg and DBP < 90 mm Hg
  - If SBP < 140 mm Hg is well tolerated and without adverse effects on quality of life, then medications do not need to be adjusted
- Age ≥ 18 years with diabetes or chronic kidney disease (CKD), initiate treatment if SBP ≥ 140 mm Hg DBP ≥ 90 mm Hg to achieve SBP < 140 mm Hg and DBP < 90 mm Hg
- General nonblack population initiate treatment with either a thiazide diuretic, CCB, ACEI or ARB
- General black population
  - Initial therapy with either a thiazide diuretic or CCB
    - More effective than beta–blockers, ACEIs or ARBs
  - ACEI induced angioedema occurs 2–4 times more frequently than in other groups
    - Treat with FFP (fresh frozen plasma) if needed
    - Tranexamic acid 1 gm IV over 10 minutes may be effective (no faster than 100 mg/minute)
- Age ≥ 18 years with CKD, initial or add-on therapy should include an ACEI or ARB regardless of ethnic background, either as first-line therapy or in addition to first-line therapy
  - Improves renal outcomes
- CCBs and thiazide-type diuretics should be used instead of ACE inhibitors and ARBs in patients over the age of 75 years with impaired kidney function due to the risk of hyperkalemia, increased creatinine, and further renal impairment
- If blood pressure goal cannot be achieved in 1 month, increase or add a second drug from the list of thiazide diuretic, CCB, ACEI or ARB. If blood pressure control cannot be achieved with 2 drugs from the above list, add and titrate a third drug. If 3 drugs do not control blood pressure, a drug from another class can be added.
  - Do not use an ACEI with an ARB

Stable angina

- Atenolol 50 mg PO qday

Congestive heart failure

- Lisinopril 5–10 mg PO qday
- Lasix (furosemide) 20–40 mg PO qday

Other medications than listed above are acceptable as indicated

Notes

______

______

______

REFERENCES:

www.nhlbi.nih.gov/guidelines/hypertension/express.pdf

JNC 7 — The Seventh Report of the Joint National Committee on Prevention, Detection, Evaluation and Treatment of High Blood Pressure

Hypertension Treatment & Management Author: Meena S Madhur, MD, PhD; Chief Editor: David J Maron, MD, FACC, FAHA

2014 Evidence-Based Guideline for the Management of High Blood Pressure in Adults
Report From the Panel Members Appointed to the Eighth Joint National Committee (JNC 8)

ACEP Clinical policy: critical issues in the evaluation and management of adult patients in the emergency department with asymptomatic elevated blood pressure (revised 2013)

Wolf SJ, Lo B, Shih RD, Smith MD, Fesmire FM, American College of Emergency Physicians Clinical Policies Committee. Clinical policy: critical issues in the evaluation and management of adult patients in the emergency department with asymptomatic elevated blood pressure. Ann Emerg Med. 2013 Jul;62(1):59–68

Current Hypertension Reports, April 2016, 18:37

Preston RA, et al. *J Hypertens.* 2018 Dec 4. [Epub ahead of print]

Whelton PK, et al. *Hypertension.* 2018; 71:e13-e115. Clinical pearl

Congestive Heart Failure Protocol

This protocol is for acute heart failure decompensation

Definition

- Cardiac dysfunction secondary to decreased ability of the left ventricle (LV) to eject or fill with blood

Systolic dysfunction

- Decreased left ventricular ejection fraction (LVEF) < 50%

Diastolic dysfunction

- Abnormal left ventricular filling
- LVEF > 50%

Differential Diagnosis

- Pneumonia
- COPD
- Bronchitis
- Pulmonary embolism
- Noncardiac pulmonary edema
- Adult respiratory distress syndrome

Considerations

- Main treatment is vasodilatation in nonhypotensive patients
- Isolated right heart failure is without dyspnea or pulmonary congestion
- Troponin can be mildly elevated with CHF alone

BNP or NT–ProBNP

- BNP < 100pg/mL rules out CHF if not obese (lower in obese patients: < 50 is cutoff)
  - NT–ProBNP < 300 pg/mL is normal
- Elevated in renal insufficiency, renal failure or atrial fibrillation (sometimes markedly)
- BNP > 200 CHF likely
- BNP > 500 : acute exacerbation likely

BNP level cutoffs dependent on the assay used

Classification of heart failure

- Class 1 – no limitation of normal physical activity
- Class 2 – slight limitation of activity (fatigue, dyspnea)
- Class 3 – marked limitation of activity
- Class 4 – symptoms at rest

Findings

- Fatigue
- Malaise
- Dyspnea
- Peripheral pitting edema

- Orthopnea and paroxysmal nocturnal dyspnea
- Rales
- Cough
- Hepatomegaly
- Ascites
- Jugular venous distension
- Hypotension
- Cardiac gallop sounds

Chest x-ray

- Cephalization of flow
- Pulmonary vascular congestion
- Cardiomegaly
- Pleural effusion
- Accurate in diagnosis
- Can have delayed findings

Evaluation

- EKG
- Chest x-ray (upright if possible)
  - Chest x–ray may alone suffice for diagnosis
- CBC
- BMP
- Troponin
- BNP or NT–ProBNP

Treatment Options (Non-hypotensive Patients)

- Oxygen — avoid high flow oxygen
  - Causes coronary and systemic vasoconstriction
  - Avoid high O_2 saturations caused by supplemental oxygen
- IV KVO
- Nitroglycerin (NTG) 0.4 mg SL — may repeat to decrease SBP 15–30% (if initial SBP ≥ 140 mmHg)
  - Keep SBP ≥ 90 mmHg
- IV NTG for refractory significant hypertension (SBP ≥ 180 mmHg) in CHF
  - Nitroglycerin IV > 250 mcg/minute useful in heart failure with hypertension
- Nitroglycerin IV > 250 mcg/minute dilates arterioles lowering blood pressure and afterload. Lower doses dilate venules decreasing preload
- NTG 0.4 mg SL is 400 mcg which reaches peak blood levels in 2 minutes and falls to 50% of peak at 7.5 minutes by comparison, and is gone by 20 minutes, so more vigorous IV dosing can be considered for angina or hypertensive heart failure when indicated
- Nitroglycerin paste ½–2 inch (if SBP ≥ 110)
- Captopril 25 mg PO (or SL) if NTG not decreasing SBP adequately
  - If SBP ≥ 110 (effects start in 10 minutes and peaks in 30–40 minutes)
  - Chronic ACE inhibitors prolong survival
- Lasix (furosemide) 40–80 mg IV bolus (match home single dose)
- **Preferable to use vasodilators initially if possible**
  - NTG and/or ACEI then Lasix (furosemide) 15 or more minutes later
- Avoid morphine
- Avoid NSAID's and calcium channel blockers

Discharge Criteria

- Good response to treatment for mild chronic CHF
- Back to baseline respiratory function

Discharge instructions

- CHF aftercare instructions
- Follow up with PCP or cardiologist within 1 day
- Return immediately if worse

Outpatient medications for heart failure reduced ejection fraction (HFrEF)

- Metoprolol tartrate 6.25–75 mg PO bid or carvedilol 3.125–25 mg PO bid
- Enalapril (ACEI) 2.5–20 mg PO qday (start at 2.5 mg) or lisinopril 2.5-5 mg PO qday NMT 40 mg qday, or other ACE inhibitors or angiotension

receptors blockers ARB (do not combine ARB with patients taking beta –blockers and ACEI

- ARB candesartan (Atacand) 4 mg PO qday titrated up to 32 mg PO qday as needed, or other angiotensin receptor blockers, if ACEI not tolerated (do not use with ACEI)
  - ARB's may be used for diastolic heart failure (HFpEF—heart failure preserved ejection fraction)
- Spironolactone 25 mg PO qday (if potassium ≤ 5mEq/L and creatinine ≤ 2.5mg/dL) for treatment of NYHA class III–IV with standard therapy
- Canagliflozin, dapagliflozin (Farxiga) and empagliflozin may be used in systolic heart failure NYHA class II–IV (They are selective sodium-glucose transporter-2 (SGLT-2) inhibitors used in Type 2 diabetes)
- Furosemide (Lasix) 20–80 mg PO qday if needed (may also be used for HFpEF) for volume overload
- African–American patients may take Bidil (isosorbide/ hydralazine dinitrate) 1 tab tid PO up to 2 tabs PO tid
- Digoxin 0.125–2.5 mg PO qday may be added if needed to decrease hospitalizations (adjust for renal function) — not first line
- Avoid calcium channel blockers in HFrEF (heart failure reduced ejection fraction)
  - CCB be used in HFpEF with hypertension

Consult Criteria

- CHF exacerbation including
  - Inadequate response to treatment
  - New onset congestive heart failure
  - Preferable to discuss all cases with physician prior to discharge
- Normotensive (contact physician for treatment options if SBP < 120)
- Hypotension (notify physician)
- Elevated troponin
- Chest pain or anginal symptoms
- Near syncope or syncope

Notes

REFERENCES:

Cornet AD, et al. *Crit Care* 2013 Apr 18;17:313

emedicine.medscape.com/article/16306 2

Circulation. 1979 Mar;59(3):585-8; Blood levels after sublingual nitroglycerin. Armstrong PW, Armstrong JA, Marks GS.

Am J Emerg Med, epub, 6/25/19

SYNCOPE/NEAR SYNCOPE PROTOCOL

Definitions

- Transient loss of consciousness or near loss of consciousness secondary to decreased perfusion of the brain

Differential Diagnosis

- Cardiac arrhythmia
- Pulmonary embolism
- TIA
- CVA
- Seizures
- Dehydration

- Aortic stenosis
- Hypoglycemia
- Subarachnoid hemorrhage
- Intracranial hemorrhage
- Hemorrhage
  - GI bleeding
  - Ectopic pregnancy
- Adrenal insufficiency
- Sepsis

Causes

Neurally mediated

- Vasodepressor type — loss of upright vasoconstrictor tone
- Cardioinhibitory type — bradycardia
- Mixed type — both occur together

Examples

- Vasovagal
- Situational
- Carotid sinus

Orthostatic vital signs (assuming upright from recumbent position)

- Definition
  - SBP drop 20 mm Hg or DBP 10 mm Hg with assumption of upright posture
  - Sustained HR increase 30 bpm within 10 min of moving from recumbent to nonexertional standing position (or 40 bpm if 12-19 yrs. of age)
  - Orthostatic vital signs are present in up to 40% of asymptomatic patients older than 70 years, and 23% of those younger than 60 years

Causes

- Volume depletion or hemorrhage
- Advanced age
- Autonomic dysfunction
- Vasodepressor drugs
- Sepsis (distributive shock)
- Vasovagal

Cardiac causes

- Dysrhythmias
- Heart block — 2nd and 3rd degree types
- Atrial fibrillation/flutter
- Ventricular tachycardia
- Sick sinus syndrome
- Brugada syndrome (precordial pseudo appearing right bundle branch block with > 2 mm ST coved elevation and negative T wave
  - May have normal EKG in 1/3 patients when initially seen
  - Cause of sudden cardiac death in younger adults from ventricular fibrillation
  - Admit to ICU/CCU and needs AICD (implantable defibrillator is treatment)
- Valvular heart disease
  - Aortic stenosis
  - Mitral stenosis
- Cardiomyopathy
- Cardiac tamponade
- Aortic dissection
- Severe heart failure

Other causes

- Unknown etiology
- Psychiatric
- Medications
- Neurologic
- Pulmonary embolism
- Pulmonary hypertension

Considerations

- EKG recommended in all patients
- Testing for unexplained syncope is based on risk factors
- Near syncope patients experience nearly the same amount of interventions and adverse events as syncope patients
- Vasovagal episode is the most common cause
- Postural blood pressure changes can occur after standing for 10 minutes and so blood pressure should be checked again at 10–15 minutes if low orthostatic blood pressure is suspected as cause of the fall

- Orthostatic measurements do not, in isolation, reliably diagnose or exclude orthostatic syncope, nor do they exclude life-threatening causes of syncope
- Medication can cause syncope or near syncope
- Sharp increase in age > 70 years
- All-cause mortality after an ED visit for syncope
  - 30 days — 1.4%
  - 6 months — 4.3%
  - 1 year — 7.6%

Clinical important features suggestive of specific cause

Exertion

- Aortic stenosis
- Mitral stenosis
- Coronary artery disease

Head rotation

- Carotid-sinus syncope

Arm exercise

- Subclavian steal

Mimics

- Seizures (post-ictal and lateral tongue bite helpful, as is prolactin level)
- Vertebrobasilar TIA
- Subarachnoid hemorrhage
- Subdural/epidural hematoma
- Hypoglycemia
- Hypoxia
- Hyperventilation
- Intoxication
- Chemical/drug exposure
- Anxiety/somatization/conversion disorder

Red Flags

- Exertional onset: ischemic coronary disease or aortic stenosis
- Chest pain: ischemic coronary disease
- Severe headache: subarachnoid or cerebral hemorrhage
- Back pain: aortic dissection or aneurysm
- Dyspnea: pulmonary embolism or CHF
- Palpitations: symptomatic arrhythmia
- Neurologic deficits

Evaluation

- Syncope/Near syncope lasting < 20 seconds in healthy patients get an EKG, but may not need further testing if all the following exist:
  - Age < 50
  - Normal physical exam
  - Normal vital signs and O_2 sat on room air
  - No comorbidities
  - Clinically had a vasovagal episode
  - No other complaints
- Perform orthostatic vital signs
- Blood pressure measurements in both arms for comparison (not to be greater than 20 mm Hg difference)
- Record positive or negative calf tenderness and Homan's sign

Apply Well's pulmonary embolism and DVT criteria and Pulmonary Embolism Rule-out Criteria (PERC Rule) as indicated

- Review in Chest Pain or Dyspnea sections
- Document PERC and/or Well's scores when appropriate

All other patients testing options

- CBC
- BMP
- Chest x-ray
- EKG
- UCG if pregnancy possible
- Check stool hemoccult if any of the following
  - Acutely anemic
  - Tachycardic
  - Orthostatic vital signs
  - Melena or rectal bleeding history
  - BUN elevated out of proportion to creatinine level

- Chest pain: order troponin (angina) and D-dimer
- Consider CT head for neurologic complaints, findings or headache (low yield otherwise)

Pulmonary Embolism Rule-out Criteria (PERC Rule)

(Reportedly decreases significantly the likelihood of pulmonary embolism if all 8 criteria met — clinical gestalt as effective in identifying PE)

- Age < 50
- Pulse oximetry > 94%
- Heart rate < 100
- No history of DVT or VTE
- No hemoptysis
- No estrogen use
- No unilateral leg swelling
- No recent surgery or trauma hospitalization past 4 weeks

Treatment Options

- Dehydration — give oral rehydration in nontoxic pediatric or adult patients if appropriate (see Gastroenteritis protocols)
- IV NS or LR rehydration in all others as needed
- Blood transfusion for symptomatic anemia or hemorrhage prn
- Anti-emetics prn
- Treatment aimed at cause of syncope or near syncope

Discharge Criteria

- Benign cause of syncope or near syncope in healthy patient age < 50 years

Discharge instructions

- Syncope or near syncope aftercare instructions
- Follow up with PCP within 1–2 days
- Consider ambulatory holter monitor
- Return if symptoms recur

Consult Criteria

- Syncope or near syncope > 30 seconds
- Age ≥ 50 (elderly will usually need hospital admission)
- GI bleeding
- Acute anemia, or chronic anemia with hemoglobin < 10 gms or a decrease in hemoglobin > 1 gm from previous levels
- Hypotension or tachycardia
- O_2 sat < 95% on room air (less than patient's baseline) or acute dyspnea
- Relative hypotension (SBP < 105 with history of hypertension or age ≥ 50 years)
- Abnormal EKG
- Cardiac dysrhythmia
- Positive orthostatics (a normal finding occasionally in elderly)
- Unclear cause of syncope or near syncope
- Chest pain or arrhythmia

Comorbid conditions present

- Hypertension
- Diabetes
- Cardiac
- Pulmonary disease
- Pregnancy
- Pulmonary embolism
- DVT
- Neurologic complaints or findings
- Toxic ingestion
- Dehydration
- Fever

ACEP Critical Issues in the Evaluation and Management of Adult Patients Presenting to the Emergency Department with Syncope (April 2007)

Admission to hospital recommended

- Older age and associated comorbidities
- Abnormal EKG
    - EKG abnormalities include acute ischemia,

dysrhythmias, or significant conduction abnormalities

- Hct < 30% (if obtained)
- History or presence of heart failure, coronary artery disease, or structural heart disease

Low risk for adverse events

- Younger patients with nonexertional syncope, who have no history or signs of cardiovascular disease, no family history of sudden death and no comorbidities

Lab and x-ray consult criteria

- New onset renal insufficiency or worsening chronic renal insufficiency
- Metabolic acidosis (increased anion gap)
- Hemoglobin decrease > 1 gm or creatinine increased > 0.5 from baseline
- Newly elevated LFT's
- Elevated amylase or lipase
- WBC ≥ 15,000
- Bandemia ≥ 15%
- Significant electrolyte abnormally
- Glucose ≥ 400 mg/dL in diabetic patient
- Glucose ≥ 300 mg/dL in non-diabetic patient
- Hyperglycemia with metabolic acidosis (decreased serum CO_2 or elevated anion gap)
- Acute thrombocytopenia
- New chest x–ray infiltrate(s) or increased interstitial changes

Notes

REFERENCES:

CHEST August 2011;140(2):509–518. doi:10.1378/chest.10–2468

Grossman SA, Babineau M, Burke, L et al. Do outcomes of near syncope parallel syncope? Am J Emerg Med. 2012;30(1):203–206

Quinn J, McDermott D, Kramer N, et al. Death after emergency department visits for syncope: how common and can it be predicted? Ann Emerg Med. 2008;51(5):585–590

Roos M, Sarkozy A, Brodbeck J, et al. The importance of class-I antiarrhythmic drug test in the evaluation of patients with syncope: unmasking Brugada syndrome. J Cardiovasc Electrophysiol. 2012;23(3):290–295

ACEP Critical Issues in the Evaluation and Management of Adult Patients Presenting to the Emergency Department with Syncope (April 2007)

Circulation, epub, 3/9/17

Ann of EM, Vol.655:622

JEM. 2018;55:780

Annals of EM, Vol. 49, pg. 431

Respiratory

Section Contents

When using any protocol, always follow the Guidelines of Proper Use (page 12).

DYSPNEA PROTOCOL

Definition

- Subjective perception of shortness of breath

Differential Diagnosis

- COPD
- Asthma
- Bronchitis
- Pneumonia
- CHF
- Angina
- Pulmonary embolism
- Pleural effusion
- Cardiac tamponade
- Pulmonary hypertension
- Panic attack (disorder)
- DKA or metabolic acidosis
- Salicylate toxicity/overdose

Dyspnea of Uncertain Cause

Evaluation options

If CHF suspected order:

- Chest x-ray
- BNP or NT–ProBNP (chest x-ray alone may suffice if CHF findings seen in lieu of BNP in patient with prior heart failure)
- BMP
- CBC
- Troponin
- EKG

Consider pulmonary embolism if Well's PE criteria score 3 or greater

- Order D-dimer (can be frequently positive without DVT/PE in elderly, with history of hospitalization within past month, cancer history, edematous conditions, bedridden — see Chest Pain or Syncope Practice Guides)

Well's Pulmonary Embolism Criteria

- Suspected DVT = 3
- Alternate diagnosis less likely than pulmonary embolism = 3
- Heart rate > 100 = 1.5
- Immobilization/surgery past 4 wks. = 1.5
- Previous DVT = 1.5
- Hemoptysis = 1

- Cancer past 6 months = 1

Well's PE score > 6

- Order CTA chest PE protocol
- Document positive/negative Homan's sign and calf tenderness (documented negative Homan's sign useful for malpractice considerations only)

- If anginal equivalent suspected as complaint in elderly, refer to Chest Pain Practice Guide

Discharge criteria

- Panic disorder or benign hyperventilation
- Benign cause of dyspnea (i.e., mild to moderate asthma or bronchitis or CODP responding well to treatment)

Consult physician

- If angina equivalent suspected
- CHF suspected or diagnosed
- Pulmonary embolism suspected
- Uncertain diagnosis as cause of symptoms
- Discuss with physician if D-dimer positive or Well's PE criteria ≥ 3 and DVT and/or PE is considered as possible cause of dyspnea

Pulmonary Embolism (PE)

Definition

- Blockage of pulmonary artery usually by a migrating blood clot from legs (most commonly) or pelvic veins

Differential diagnosis

- Acute coronary syndrome
- Acute pericarditis
- ARDS
- Panic disorder
- Aortic stenosis
- Atrial fibrillation
- Cardiogenic shock
- Cor pulmonale
- Cardiomyopathy
- COPD
- Fat embolism
- Mitral stenosis
- Acute MI
- Pneumothorax
- Pulmonary hypertension
- Sudden cardiac death
- Superior vena cava syndrome
- Syncope or near syncope

Considerations

- Can be asymptomatic , minimally or moderately symptomatic, up to catastrophic
- Occurs 1 person per 1,000/year
- Commonly a missed diagnosis on initial evaluation
- Present in 60–80% of DVT patients even though one half have on PE symptoms
- More common cause of hospitalized patient death
- One year mortality is 24%
    - Mainly due to cardiac disease, recurrent PE, infection or cancer
- NT-proBNP >500 ng/L associated with central PE and possible predictor of increased risk of death (pre–existing conditions such renal failure and atrial fibrillation that have chronic increased NT-proBNP would make this assumption not as useful)
- Elevated troponin is an increased severity risk marker — 19% probability of death during hospitalization
- Massive PE second only to sudden cardiac death as a cause of sudden death
- Majority of deaths from PE occur in the first 1–2 hours of care
- Submassive PE has 15% mortality (PE causing right ventricular dysfunction demonstrable by echocardiography, computed tomography or elevated cardiac biomarkers)
    - May be treated with thrombolytics or direct intervention
- Nonmassive PE defined as a systolic BP ≥ 90 mmHG and

accounts for 95.5–96% of patients
  - No elevated biomarkers or right heart strain
- See Well's Pulmonary Embolism Criteria in above section

Pulmonary Embolism Rule-out Criteria (PERC Rule)

(Reportedly decreases significantly the likelihood of pulmonary embolism if all 8 criteria met — not superior to clinical gestalt)

- Age < 50
- Pulse oximetry > 94%
- Heart rate < 100
- No history of DVT or VTE
- No hemoptysis
- No estrogen use
- No unilateral leg swelling
- No recent surgery or trauma hospitalization past 4 weeks

American College of Physicians (ACP) evaluation of suspected pulmonary embolism guidelines 2015

- Plasma D-dimer tests are more appropriate for those at intermediate risk for a PE, and no testing may be necessary for some patients at low risk
- Use either the Wells or Geneva rules to choose tests based on a patient's risk for PE
- Low risk patients should use the 8 Pulmonary Embolism Rule-Out Criteria (PERC) and if negative for all 8 criteria then no testing is needed
- Intermediate risk patients or for those at low risk who do not meet all of the rule-out criteria, use a high-sensitivity plasma D-dimer test initially
- In patients >50 years use an age-adjusted threshold age × 10 ng/mL
  - Normal D-dimer levels increase with age
  - D-dimer increases 10 mcg/L for every year over 50 years of age if the upper cutoff is 500 mcg/L (for example an 80 year old with d-dimer 700 mcg/L would be in the normal range)
    - If another assay used, then 2% increase/year over age 50 may be used to adjust upper limit for age
- D-dimer level below the age-adjusted cutoff should not receive any imaging studies
  - Patients with elevated D-dimer levels should receive imaging
- Patients at high risk skip the D-dimer test and proceed to CT pulmonary angiography
  - Negative D-dimer test does not eliminate the need for imaging in these patients
- Obtain ventilation-perfusion scans in patients with a contraindication to CT pulmonary angiography or if CT pulmonary angiography is unavailable
- Use validated clinical prediction rules to estimate pretest probability in patients in whom acute PE is being considered

American College of Emergency Physicians (ACEP) 2011

- Negative quantitative D-dimer assay results can be used to exclude PE in patients with a low pretest probability for PE
- Negative quantitative D-dimer assay results may be used to exclude PE in patients with an intermediate pretest probability for PE
- Low or PE unlikely patients (with Wells score 4) pretest probability for PE who require additional diagnostic testing (positive D-dimer result or highly sensitive D–dimer not available), a negative multidetector CT pulmonary angiogram alone can be used to exclude PE
- Intermediate or high pretest probability for PE and a negative

CT pulmonary angiogram result in whom a clinical concern for PE still exists and CT venogram has not already been performed, consider additional diagnostic testing (e.g., D-dimer, lower extremity imaging, VQ scanning, traditional pulmonary arteriography) prior to exclusion of VTE disease

- Venous ultrasound
  - May be considered as initial imaging in patients with obvious signs of DVT for whom venous ultrasound is readily available
  - Patients with relative contraindications for CT scan (e.g., renal insufficiency, CT contrast agent allergy)
  - Pregnant patients
  - A positive finding in a patient with symptoms consistent with PE can be considered evidence for diagnosis of VTE disease and may preclude the need for additional diagnostic imaging

Risk factors

Virchow triad

- Endothelial injury
- Stasis or turbulence of blood flow
- Blood hypercoagulability

- Immobilization
- Malignancy
- Inherited or acquired thrombophilia states (hypercoagulable states)
- Acute medical illness
- Surgery past 3 months
- Trauma (mostly lower extremities or pelvis) past 3 months
- Oral contraceptives or estrogen
- Pregnancy
- Prior pulmonary embolism
- COPD
- Heart failure
- Stroke, hemiplegia or paralysis
- Central venous lines within past 3 months

Signs and symptoms

- Tachypnea (respiratory rate >16/min) — 96%
- Rales — 58%
- Accentuated second heart sound — 53%
- Tachycardia (heart rate >100/min) — 44%
- Fever>37.8°C (100.04°F) — 43%
- Diaphoresis — 36%
- S_3 or S_4 gallop — 34%
- Clinical signs and symptoms suggesting thrombophlebitis — 32%
- Lower extremity edema: 24%
- Cardiac murmur — 23%
- Cyanosis — 19%

Presenting complaints and findings

- Dyspnea — 73%
- Pleuritic chest pain — 66%
- Cough — 37%
- Hemoptysis — 13%
- Hypoxia
- Delirium in elderly
- Wheezing
- Productive cough
- Syncope or near syncope
- Hypotension or relative hypotension (for the patient with hypertension history)
- Lung infarction
- New onset atrial fibrillation
- Ventricular arrhythmia
- Pleural effusion
- Pulseless electrical activity

Testing options

- Chest x–ray (may be normal or nonspecific)
  - Westermark sign — decreased vascularity
  - Hampton hump — pleural based triangular density from pulmonary infarction (rare)
- CBC
- EKG
  - Sinus tachycardia most common

  - Nonspecific STT wave changes or with ischemic appearing biphasic T waves in V2 and V3
  - New right bundle branch block
  - S1Q3T3 pattern in 20%
  - Right axis deviation in 5%
  - Left axis deviation in 10%
  - New onset atrial fibrillation
- D–dimer (do not use in high clinical PE probability — scan instead)
  - More useful in eliminating younger healthy patients if negative
- ABG (may be normal or have increased A–a gradient or hypoxemia)
- BNP or NT-proBNP
- Troponin
- Echocardiogram with RV strain have ≥10% mortality, 0% mortality with normal RV function
- Chemistries
- CTA chest pulmonary embolism protocol
- V/Q lung scan if CTA chest not available or contraindicated
  - May be performed in healthy low risk patients (if normal then very useful)
  - Low probability scans can have PE from 4–20% depending whether clinical suspicion is low or high respectively
- Leg venous ultrasound

Treatment guidelines

American College of Chest Physicians (ACCP)

- Dabigatran, rivaroxaban, apixaban, or edoxaban are preferred over vitamin K antagonist (VKA) therapy as long-term (first 3 months) anticoagulant therapy for noncancer patients
- Low-molecular-weight heparin (LMWH) is recommended over VKA therapy, dabigatran, rivaroxaban, apixaban, or edoxaban as long-term (first 3 months) anticoagulant therapy for patients with cancer-associated thrombosis
- Aspirin is recommended over no aspirin to prevent recurrent venous thromboembolism (VTE) in patients who are stopping anticoagulant therapy and do not have a contraindication to aspirin
- In most patients with acute PE not associated with hypotension, systemically administered thrombolytic therapy is not recommended
- Selected patients with acute PE who deteriorate after starting anticoagulant therapy but have yet to develop hypotension and who have a low bleeding risk, systemically administered thrombolytic therapy is preferred over no such therapy
- Thrombolytic therapy is suggested in select patients with acute PE not associated with hypotension and with a low bleeding risk whose initial clinical presentation or clinical course after starting anticoagulation suggests a high risk of developing hypotension
- Thrombolytic therapy is not recommended for most patients with acute PE not associated with hypotension
- First episode of VTE and with a low or moderate risk of bleeding should have extended anticoagulant therapy
- First episode of VTE with a high bleeding risk should have therapy limited to 3 months
- Patients who have PE and preexisting irreversible risk factors, such as deficiency of antithrombin III, proteins S and C, factor V Leiden mutation, or the presence of antiphospholipid antibodies, should be placed on long-term anticoagulation

Treatments

- **Embolectomy** in very unstable patients in centers with CV surgery available and thrombolytics thought not to be adequate therapy or contraindicated
  - Nitric oxide 10ppm inhalation may be tried to temporize condition prior to surgery or thrombolytics

Anticoagulation

- Is a passive anticoagulation—prevents new thrombus formation while body breaks down existing thrombus
- **Enoxaparin** (LMWH) 1mg/kg q12hour SQ or 1.5 mg/kg q24hours SQ
  - Do not use with creatinine clearance <30
  - Do not use with history of heparin induced thrombocytopenia (HIT)
  - No PTT monitoring
- **Heparin** (unfractionated) load 80units/kg IV and 18 units/kg/hour IV
  - Goal is PTT 1.5–2.5 times normal
  - Creatinine clearance <30 increased bleeding risk

  Do not use with history of heparin induced thrombocytopenia Stop all heparins if platelet count drops to 100,000, or a 50% decrease in baseline platelet count occurs, or 30% decrease in platelet count with new thrombus formation development (heparin induced thrombocytopenia — a life threatening immune process)
- **Warfarin** 15 mg PO load
  - Overlap with heparin until INR 2–3
  - 2–10mg PO daily (start >6 hours after LMWH)
  - **Contraindicated in pregnancy**

Direct oral anticoagulants (DOACs)

- **Apixaban (Eliquis)** 10 mg PO BID x 7 days, then 5 mg BID
  - Not recommended in severe liver disease
- **Rivaroxaban (Xarelto)** 15 mg PO q12hr for 21 days with food, then 20 mg PO qday

Thrombolytics

- **TPA** 100mg IV over 2 hours
- May give 100mg IVP during CPR in PE or suspected PE coding patients and code for 1 hour
- Heparin bolus and drip near end to TPA infusion or immediately following

Disposition

Consult criteria

- Discuss all patients with a physician

Admission

- Unstable or severe PE admit to ICU
- Patients not meeting Hestia criteria
- New elevation of troponin and/or NT-proBNP
- Clinical judgment that overrides Hestia criteria

Discharge

- Hestia criteria for outpatient PE therapy — A "No" answer to all questions needed to treat as outpatient
- Clinical judgment that outpatient therapy is safe for patient
- No tachycardia

Principles of Asthma and COPD Management

- Recognizing severity of exacerbation
- Using correct therapy
- Identify and treat any precipitants

- Make correct disposition

COPD Exacerbation

Evaluation options

- Monitor cardiac and pulse oximetry
- EKG
- Troponin
- CBC
- BMP
- Chest x-ray (check radiology report if and when available)) and view x-ray and compare to prior films
- Consider ABG if severe dyspnea or significant respiratory fatigue
- BNP or NT–ProBNP if CHF is a consideration

Initial Treatment options

- Albuterol with or without atrovent, up to 3 treatments prn 10–20 minutes apart
- Oxygen therapy to keep O_2 Sat ≥ 90%
- Use titrated oxygen instead of high flow oxygen
  - Mortality was significantly lower with titrated oxygen
- BiPAP if patient is in severe respiratory distress and/or fatigue (consult physician)

Steroid treatment options useful for moderate to severe exacerbations (caution with diabetes)

- Course 5 days (no taper needed) — evidence B

Methylprednisolone, prednisolone and prednisone

- 40 mg PO qday x 5–7 days

Other steroids that can be used instead

- Depomedrol (methylprednisolone acetate) 80–160 mg IM

OR

- Decadron (dexamethasone) 10 mg IV/PO
  - Onset of action IV is 1 hour. PO onset of action is 1–2 hours
  - Duration of action is 36–54 hours
  - Dexamethasone 6mg =prednisone 40 mg PO qday x 5–7 days

OR

- Solumedrol (methylprednisolone) 80–125 mg IV (if being admitted)

Discharge treatment options

- Albuterol or Combivent inhaler with or without spacer q4hr prn

Antibiotic outpatient choices

Mild COPD exacerbation

- Rx PO Zithromax or doxycycline × 5 days for purulent sputum or increase sputum (limit antibiotics to 5 days preferably)
- Septra DS PO bid for 5 days
- Levaquin 500 mg PO for 5 days

- Sanford Guide or other drug databases
- Depomedrol (methylprednisolone acetate) 80–120 IM

OR

- Decadron (dexamethasone) 6 mg PO x 5–7 days

Inhaled steroid treatment options for COPD

- Consider inhaled steroid Rx to start only after acute exacerbation has resolved
  - Prescribe double dose if already on single strength dose

  OR

  - Advair diskus bid (combination of long acting beta–agonist and steroid) to be used only after acute exacerbation has resolved

Discharge criteria

- If patient returns to near baseline function with

respiratory effort and O_2 saturation level

Discharge instructions

- Follow up in 1–5 days depending on severity of illness and response to treatments
- Provide COPD exacerbation aftercare instructions
- Return if worse

Consult physician on

- Work of breathing is moderate to severe post-treatment
- Wheezing not resolving satisfactorily
- Patient feels they are too dyspneic to go home
- WBC ≥ 18,000 or < 3,000; Neutrophil count < 1,000
- Acute thrombocytopenia
- Bandemia ≥ 15%
- Anion gap > 18
- Significant electrolyte abnormality
- Glucose ≥ 400 mg/dL in diabetic patient
- Glucose ≥ 300 mg/dL new onset diabetic patient
- Hyperglycemia with metabolic acidosis (decreased serum CO_2 or elevated anion gap)
- Heart rate ≥ 110 after all treatment are completed

Acute Asthma and Bronchitis

Peak flow % of predicted

- Mild disease > 70%
- Moderate disease 40–69%
- Severe disease < 40%

Initial Treatment Options

- Albuterol with or without atrovent up to 3 treatments prn: 15–20 minutes apart
  - Nebulized lidocaine 1cc of a 1% solution in 4mL of saline to give 0.25% solution after albuterol treatment for intractable cough may be tried
- Oxygen therapy to keep O_2 Sat ≥ 92%
- Monitor pulse oximetry
- **Be careful to not suppress respiratory effort with benzodiazepines or sedating medications**

Steroid treatment options useful for moderate to severe exacerbations (caution with diabetes)

- Prednisolone or prednisone 0.5–1 mg/kg PO (NMT 60 mg)

  OR
- Decadron (dexamethasone) 0.6 mg/kg IV/IM/PO (NMT 16 mg) — preferred in children (see Pediatric Asthma section)
  - Onset of action IV is 1 hour. PO onset of action is 1–2 hours
  - Duration of action is 36–54 hours
- Dexamethasone 6mg =prednisone 40 mg PO qday x 5–7 days

Additional treatment options for severe exacerbations

- Terbutaline 0.25 mg SQ prn q15–20 minutes up to 3 as needed for age ≥ 12 years
  - Caution if history of coronary artery disease
- Terbutaline 0.005–0.01 mg/kg SQ q15–20 minutes up to 3 — age < 12 years (NMT 0.4 mg per dose)
- Epinephrine 0.3 mg SQ for adults
  - Caution if history of coronary artery disease
- Epinephrine 0.01 mg/kg in children not to exceed adult dose
- $MgSO_4$ (magnesium sulfate) 1–2 gms IV over 20 minutes in adults per physician
- $MgSO_4$ (magnesium sulfate) 25–50 mg/kg IV over 10–20 minutes per physician (NMT 2 gm) for children

- $MgSO_4$ (magnesium sulfate) 125–250 mg in 0.3 ml NS aerosol q 20 minutes up to 4 doses as needed (off label use)
  - May combine with albuterol
- Heliox 70:30 — do not use if > 30% oxygen needed to maintain O_2 saturation

Discharge treatment options

- Albuterol or Combivent inhaler with or without spacer q4hr prn
- Montelukast (Singulair) 10 mg PO qHs
- If bacterial infection suspected: Rx PO Zithromax (azithromycin) or doxycycline (age > 8 years) × 5 days, or per Sanford Guide or other drug databases
- Viral infection (most healthy patients) = no antibiotics

Discharge systemic steroid treatment options (caution with diabetes)

- Prednisone 20–60 mg qday for 5–7 days (no taper needed) age ≥ 12 yrs.

  OR

- Depomedrol (methylprednisolone acetate) 80–120 mg IM age ≥ 12 yrs.

  OR

- Decadron (dexamethasone) 10 mg IV/IM for adults (or 6 mg PO qday for 5–7 days)
- IV/IM for children not to exceed 10 mg/dose — recommended in children over prednisolone or prednisone (see Pediatric Asthma section)

  OR

- Pediatrics: prednisolone 1–2 mg/kg PO qday for 5 days (NMT 60 mg per day)

  OR

- Pediatric dexamethasone 0.15–0.3 mg/kg PO qday for 5 days or day 1 and day 3 (NMT 6 mg/dose usually)

Discharge inhaled steroid options

- Consider inhaled steroid Rx to start only after acute exacerbation has resolved
  - Prescribe double dose if already on single strength dose

    OR

  - Advair discus bid – age > 3 years (combination of long acting beta–agonist and steroid) to be used only after acute exacerbation has resolved

Discharge Criteria

- Good response to therapy
- If patient returns to near baseline function with respiratory effort and O_2 saturation level
- Wheezing resolution or significant improvement, and no significant respiratory distress
- Peak flow ≥ 70% predicted if checked
- O_2 saturation > 93% on room air
- Good follow up and compliance

Discharge instructions

- Follow up in 1–5 days depending on severity of illness and response to treatments
- Provide asthma or bronchitis aftercare instructions

Consult Criteria

- Severe respiratory distress on presentation (notify physician immediately)
- Insufficient response to treatment
- Wheezing not resolving adequately
- Patient or family feels they are too dyspneic to go home
- Cardiac cause of dyspnea suspected or confirmed
- Immunosuppression

- Peak flow < 70% predicted if measured after treatment is finished
- O_2 saturation < 94% on room air post treatments
- O_2 Sat < 92% in COPD patient on room air or lower than baseline O_2 Sat concentrations
- Significant comorbid conditions
- Heart rate ≥ 110 post treatment in adults
- Hypotension develops or relative hypotension SBP < 105 with history of hypertension
- Return visit for same acute dyspnea episode
- Immunosuppression
- Age ≥ 60

Vital signs and age consult criteria

- Age < 6 months
- Adult heart rate ≥ 110
- Pediatric heart rate
  - 0–4 months ≥ 180
  - 5–7 months ≥ 175
  - 6–12 months ≥ 170
  - 1–3 years ≥ 160
  - 4–5 years ≥ 145
  - 6–8 years ≥ 130
  - 9–11 years ≥ 125
  - 12–15 years ≥ 120
  - 16 years or older ≥ 110
- Developing hypotension or relative hypotension (SBP < 105 with history of hypertension)
- O_2 Sat < 94% on room air in non-COPD patient

Acute Respiratory Distress Syndrome

Definition

- Rapidly progressive dyspnea, tachypnea and hypoxemia within 1 week
- Bilateral infiltrates on chest x–ray not caused by cardiogenic pulmonary edema
  - Diffuse alveolar damage from structural changes in the alveolocapillary unit with injury causing non–cardiac pulmonary edema
  - Alveolar spaces fill with plasma fluid and proteins causing shunting
  - Hypoxemia must be present ($PO_2/FiO_2 \leq 300$ on ventilator with PEEP≥5)

Differential diagnosis

- Cardiogenic pulmonary edema
- Bilateral pneumonia
- Acute interstitial pneumonia
- Acute eosinophilic pneumonia
- Diffuse alveolar hemorrhage
- Neurogenic pulmonary edema
- Exacerbation of an interstitial lung disease
- Transfusion associated acute lung injury
- Pulmonary lymphangitic spread of malignancy
- Fat embolism syndrome
- Amniotic fluid embolism syndrome
- COPD
- CHF
- Sepsis
  - Multiple organ dysfunction syndrome in sepsis
- Salicylate toxicity
- Viral pneumonia
- Heroin toxicity
- Toxic shock syndrome
- Pneumocystis jiroveci pneumonia
- Transfusion reaction
- Hemorrhagic shock

Causes

Pulmonary

- Pulmonary sepsis
- COVID–19 or related viruses
- Aspiration lung injury
- Viral and bacterial pneumonia
- Lung contusion
- Inhalational or burn injury
- Near drowning
- Fat embolism

Nonpulmonary

- Sepsis

- Acute pancreatitis
- Trauma
- Multiple transfusion
- Bacteremia
- Fractures, particularly multiple fractures and long bone fractures
- Burns
- Massive transfusion
- Drug overdose
- Postperfusion injury after cardiopulmonary bypass
- Pancreatitis

COVID–19 signs and symptoms (not all inclusive)

- Cough
- Myalgias
- Fever
- Dyspnea
- Repeated shaking chills
- Headache
- Sore throat
- New loss of taste or smell
- Diarrhea
- Nausea and vomiting

Findings

- Respiratory failure
- Multiorgan dysfunction syndrome
- DVT and VTE
  - Pulmonary embolism
- Stroke
- AMI
- Distal extremity rash
- Antibody production 11–12 days after COVID symptom onset (clinical utility questionable)

Testing

- Chest x–ray
- CT chest if needed
- ABG
- CBC, CMP, lactic acid, LDH, d–dimer, blood cultures, sputum cultures, U/A, troponin, BNP or NT–ProBNP, ferritin
- COVID testing

Echocardiography (TEE if prone position)

- Determine RV strain and LV function
- IVC dynamics and CVP estimates

Chest ultrasound findings in COVID patients

- Pleural irregularity and thickening (early finding)
- Subpleural consolidations
- B lines may be seen, often derived from areas of irregular pleura; these become more confluent and diffuse as the disease progresses
- Spared areas (a pattern of normal lung interspersed between focal B lines) are usually present early in the disease
- Nonlobar and translobar consolidation with air bronchograms
- Small localized pleural effusions may be seen

Outpatient treatment and observation (may change)

- Return to work 10 days after symptom onset and no fever for 3 days with improved symptoms
- Close COVID–19 contact
  - No isolation and return to work after 7 days with negative COVID test and no symptoms, or 10 days without COVID test and no symptoms
- Vaccination
  - All ages without comorbidities are being lowered to receive vaccine over time
  - Ages 12-17 years greater than 40 kg
    - Sickle cell disease
    - Congenital or acquired heart disease
    - Neurodevelopmental disorder (e.g. cerebral palsy)
    - Asthma, reactive airway or other chronic respiratory disease requiring daily medication
    - A medical-related technological dependence (e.g. tracheostomy,

gastrostomy, or positive pressure ventilation not related to COVID–19)
    - BMI ≥ 85th percentile for age
- Ages 18–54 years
    - Chronic Kidney Disease
    - Diabetes (type 1 or 2)
    - Immunosuppressive disease (HIV/AIDS, etc.)
    - Receiving Immunosuppressive treatment (chemotherapy, etc.)
    - Body Mass Index (BMI) ≥ 35
- Ages 55–64 years
    - Cardiovascular disease
    - Hypertension
    - Chronic obstructive pulmonary disease (COPD) or other chronic respiratory
    - disease
- Age ≥ 65 years

Treatment (various treatments subject to changes over time)

- Supportive
- Oxygen if needed
    - High flow mask
    - Noninvasive positive-pressure ventilation (NIPPV)
    - High-flow nasal cannula
        - System of heated humidification and large-bore nasal prongs to deliver oxygen at flows of up to 50-60 L/min
    - Intubation and mechanical ventilation with ARDSNet strategies +/- proning as needed for severe ARDS (PO_2/FiO_2 < 150)
        - Tidal volume 4–6 mL/kg predicted body weight initially recommended
        - Inspiratory plateau pressure to 30 cm water or less
        - PEEP 5–10 to maintain O_2 saturation 88–95%
        - Proning (prone position) if needed
        - Any COVID-19 or ARDS patient with respiratory insult severe enough to be admitted to the hospital should be considered for rotation and proning
        - 30-120 minutes in prone position, followed by 30-120 minutes in left lateral decubitus, right lateral decubitus, and upright sitting position
        - Guided by patient wishes
        - Salutary effects are generally noticed within 5-10 minutes in a new position
        - Do not maintain a position that does not improve the patient's breathing and comfort

Panic disorder or attack

- State of hyperventilation causing decreased pCO2 measurement on blood gas (respiratory alkalosis), elevated pH, resulting in feeling short of breath, acute calcium shifts into cells (can cause carpospasm), hypokalemia, paresthesias, and a sense of impending doom when more severe

Tests if needed

- Serum electrolytes to exclude hypokalemia and acidosis
- Serum glucose to exclude hypoglycemia
- Cardiac enzymes in patients suspected of acute coronary syndromes
- Serum hemoglobin in patients with near-syncope
- Thyroid-stimulating hormone (TSH) in patients suspected of hyperthyroidism
- Urine toxicology screen for amphetamines, cannabis, cocaine, and phencyclidine in patients suspected of intoxication
- D-dimer assay to exclude pulmonary embolism
- Salicylate level if appropriate

- Imaging as indicated

Treatment

- Pharmacotherapy, cognitive-behavioral therapy (CBT), and other psychological treatment modalities
- Alprazolam (Xanax) 0.5 mg PO q8hr; may increase q3-4 days by ≤1 mg/day

REFERENCES:

CHEST August 2011;140(2):509–518. doi:10.1378/chest.10–2468

Austin MA, et al. *BMJ* 2010, 341:c5462

Chronic Obstructive Pulmonary Disease Author: Zab Mosenifar, MD; Chief Editor: Zab Mosenifar, MD
emedicine.medscape.com/article/297664

Vestbo J, et al. *Am J Respir Crit Care Med* 2013;187(4):347–65

Pediatr Emerg Care. 2018 Jan:34:53

Unlabeled Uses of Nebulized Medications
Mary Beth Shirk; Kevin R. Donahue; Jill Shirvani
Am J Health Syst Pharm. 2006;63(18):1704-171
Medscape .com/viewarticle/545484 _8

Acute Respiratory Distress Syndrome (ARDS)
Updated: Mar 27, 2020 Author: Eloise M Harman, MD; Chief Editor: Michael R Pinsky, MD, CM, Dr(HC), FCCP, FAPS, MCCM

Caputo ND, et al. *Acad Emerg Med.* 2020 Apr 22

Ding L, et al. *Crit Care*. 2020 Jan 30;24(1):28

Biomarker-based strategy for screening right ventricular dysfunction in patients with non-massive pulmonary embolism pubmed.ncbi.nlm.nih.gov/17165016

Notes

PNEUMONIA PROTOCOL

Definition

- Infection of pulmonary parenchymal tissue

Differential Diagnosis

- Pulmonary embolism
- COPD
- Asthma
- CHF
- Bronchitis
- Adult Respiratory Distress Syndrome
- Fluid overload from ESRD
- Bronchopulmonary dysplasia in children with history of prematurity

Considerations

- Number one leading cause of death from infectious disease
- Community acquired causes
  - Strep pneumoniae
  - Mycoplasma pneumoniae
  - H. influenzae
  - Legionella pneumophilia
  - Klebsiella pneumoniae
  - Influenza
- Comorbid conditions
  - Advanced age
  - Smoking
  - COPD
  - Diabetes
  - Alcoholism
  - CHF

  - HIV
  - Immunosuppression
- Signs and Symptoms
  - Cough
  - Sputum production
  - Fever
  - Chills
  - Rigors
  - Dyspnea
  - Chest pain
- WBC ≥ 15,000 suggests bacterial infection
- Very high or very low WBC predicts increased mortality

Evaluation

- CBC
- Chest x-ray (may be negative up to 30% even if pneumonia is present)
- ABG if moderate to severe respiratory distress or fatigue
- See Dyspnea Protocol
- Blood cultures if toxic or hypotensive and/or patient is to be admitted

Treatment Options

- Oxygen for O_2 saturation < 93% (in COPD patient < 91%) or in respiratory distress
- Viral pneumonia needs no treatment unless immunosuppressed
- IV NS/LR or oral rehydration if dehydrated (see Gastroenteritis Protocol for rehydration therapy)

Nontoxic patient treatment that is to be discharged

No chronic cardiopulmonary disease or other serious comorbidities

- Zithromax PO

  OR

- Doxycycline 100 bid PO x 10 days

Chronic cardiac disease, pulmonary disease, diabetes, alcoholism, renal disease, malignancy or asplenia present

- Second or third generation cephalosporin PO x 10 days
  - Cefdinir (Omnicef) 300 mg PO bid

  OR

- Augmentin (amoxicillin/clavulanate) 875mg bid x 10 days PO

  PLUS

- Zithromax (azithromycin) PO

  OR

- Doxycycline 100 mg bid x 10 days PO

  OR

- Levaquin (levofloxacin) 750 mg qday PO as a single agent x 10 days
- May use Sanford Guide or antibiotic database

CURB-65 scoring system and estimated 30–day mortality (was not meant as an admission tool when created, but more of a mortality prediction tool)

Scoring system *(One point is given for each component)*

- **C**onfusion (change from baseline or less than alert and oriented x 3)
- **U**remia (BUN > 19 mg/dl)
- **R**espiratory rate ≥ 30
- **B**lood pressure (< 90 mm Hg systolic or ≤ 60 mm Hg diastolic) and
- Age ≥ **65** years
- One point is given for each component met by the patient and they are assigned a total score of 0–5 points

Estimated 30 day mortality

- 1 point: 3.2% mortality
- 2 points: 13.0% mortality
- 3 points: 17.0% mortality

- 4 points: 41.5% mortality
- 5 points: 57.0% mortality

CURB-65 points and suggested disposition

- 0 points: Outpatient
- 1 point: Outpatient
- 2 point: Observation as inpatient
- 3 points: inpatient; consider ICU
- 4 points: Strongly consider ICU
- 5 points: Strongly consider ICU

Pneumonia Severity Index for community acquired pneumonia

- **Demographic factors are scored as follows:**
  - Age, men – Starting point value is age in years
  - Age, women – Starting point value is age in years minus 10 points
  - Nursing home resident – add 10 points
- **Coexisting illnesses are scored as follows:**
  - Neoplasia – add 30 points
  - Liver disease – add 20 points
  - Congestive heart failure, cerebrovascular disease, renal disease – add 10 points for each
- **Physical examination findings are scored as follows:**
  - Altered mental status – add 20 points
  - Respiratory rate of 30 breaths or more per minute – add 20 points
  - Systolic blood pressure less than 90 mmHg – add 20 points
  - Temperature less than 35°C or that is 40°C or higher – add 15 points
  - Pulse greater than 125 bpm – add 10 points
- **Laboratory and radiographic findings are scored as follows:**
  - Arterial pH less than 7.35 – add 30 points
  - BUN value of 30 mg/dL or greater – add 20 points
  - Sodium level less than 130 mmol/L – add 20 points
  - Glucose level of 250 mg/dL or greater – add 10 points
  - Hematocrit value less than 30% – add 10 points
  - Partial arterial pressure (PaO_2) less than 60 mm Hg or peripheral oxygen saturation (SpO_2) less than 90% while breathing room air – add 10 points
  - Pleural effusion – add 10 points
- **The combined total points make up the risk score, which stratifies patients into 5 PSI mortality risk classes, as follows:**
  - 0-50 points = Class I (0.1% mortality)
  - 51-70 points = Class II (0.6% mortality)
  - 71-90 points = Class III (0.9% mortality)
  - 91-130 points = Class IV (9.3% mortality)
  - More than 130 points = Class V (27% mortality)
- **Current guidelines suggest that patients may be treated in an outpatient setting or may require hospitalization depending on their PSI risk class, as follows:**
  - Classes I and II – Outpatient management
  - Class III – Admission to an observation unit or for short hospital stay
  - Classes IV and V – Treatment in inpatient setting

For patients with significant respiratory distress, hypoxemia, toxicity, or are to be admitted treatment options:

- IV NS
- IV Zithromax and Rocephin (ceftriaxone) or levofloxacin
- IV piperacillin/tazobactam (Zosyn) 4.5 gms q6hr IV or

meropenem 1 gm IV q8hr plus vancomycin weight based — ICU or nursing home patient

Aspiration pneumonia

- Admit

Antibiotic options

- Ampicillin/sulbactam (Unasyn) 1.5–3 gm IV q6hr. adjust for renal insufficiency if present
- Amoxicillin/clavulanate (Augmentin) 875 PO bid for those not severely ill and can tolerate PO medications as an alternative regimen
- Limited clinical data for metronidazole (Flagyl) 500 mg PO or IV q8hr. with amoxicillin 500 mg PO q8hr. or penicillin G 1–2 million units IV q4–6hr.
- Penicillin allergic patients may give clindamycin 450–900 mg IV q8hr. or if able to take cephalosporins then ceftriaxone 1–2 gms IV qday
- Levofloxacin 750 mg PO/IV qday
- Ertapenem 1 gm IV qday
- If anaerobes suspected (lung abscess or severe periodontal disease) then may use Zosyn 4.5 Gms q6hr IV or meropenem 1 gm IV q8hr.
  - Can add clindamycin 450 mg PO qid or 600 mg IV tid
- Adjust all antibiotic dosing for renal insufficiency

Discharge criteria recommendation

- Nontoxic patient
- No respiratory distress
- O_2 saturation ≥94%
- CURB–65 discharge criteria above

Discharge instructions

- Pneumonia aftercare instructions
- Follow up with primary care provider within 1–3 days
- Return if worse

Consult criteria recommendation

Clinical judgment may override any decision rules

- See CURB–65 points and suggested disposition (was not meant as an admission tool when created, more of a mortality tool)
- Significant pneumonia
- Patients that the Provider feels need admission
- Significant respiratory distress
- High fever ≥ 104°F (40°C)
- Temperature < 96°F (35.5°C)
- Appears ill or toxic
- Metabolic or respiratory acidosis
- Immunosuppression
- See Dyspnea Protocol
- Cavitary pulmonary disease
- **Pneumonia severity index Class 4 or higher**

Vital signs and age consult recommendations

- Age < 2 months
- Adult heart rate ≥ 125
- Pediatric heart rate
  - 0–4 months ≥ 180
  - 5–7 months ≥ 175
- Developing hypotension or relative hypotension (SBP < 105 with history of hypertension)
- O_2 Sat < 94% on room air in non-COPD patient; O_2 Sat < 90% in COPD patient on room air or home O_2 Rx

Lab and x-ray consult criteria recommendation

- New onset renal insufficiency or worsening renal insufficiency
- Acute thrombocytopenia
- Anion gap > 18
- Significant electrolyte abnormally
- Hyperglycemia with metabolic acidosis (decreased serum CO_2 or elevated anion gap)
- New or worsening pleural effusion
- Cavitary changes on chest x-ray

Notes

REFERENCES:

Aujesky D, Auble TE, Yealy DM, et al. Prospective comparison of three validated prediction rules for prognosis in community-acquired pneumonia. *Am J Med* 2005; 118:384–92

Mandell LA, Wunderink RG, Anzueto A, et al. Infectious disease society of America/American Thoracic Society consensus guidelines on the management of community-acquired pneumonia. *Clin Infect Dis* 2007: 44(2):S27–72

Bacterial Pneumonia Author: Nader Kamangar, MD, FACP, FCCP, FCCM, FAASM; Chief Editor: Zab Mosenifar, MD emedicine.medscape.com/article/300157

Am J Respir Crit Care Med. 2019;200:e45

Bacterial Pneumonia Updated: Sep 30, 2020 Author: Justina Gamache, MD; Chief Editor: Guy W Soo Hoo, MD, MPH; emedicine.medscape.com/article/300157

INFLUENZA PROTOCOL

Definition

- Infection by a single–stranded RNA virus

Differential diagnosis

- Viral URI
- Mononucleosis
- SARS
- Pneumonia
- Encephalitis
- Meningitis
- HIV infection
- Dengue
- Hantavirus Pulmonary Syndrome

Considerations

- One of the most common infectious diseases
- Airborne spread
- Incubation period usually 2 days, but can range from 1–4 days
- Usual infectious period from 1 day before symptom onset up to 5–7 days after symptom onset
- During peak flu season, clinical judgement may be as good as rapid testing, making rapid testing less necessary
- Rapid testing may be more beneficial in times of lower disease prevalence
- Empiric treatment of critically ill patients should be considered even if rapid testing is negative
- Baloxavir marboxil (Xofluza) is a new single-dose antiviral agent and is effective for treatment of influenza type A and type B strains
  - 40 to < 80 kg — 40 mg PO once
  - ≥ 80 kg — 80 mg PO once
- In children, the most common presenting symptoms are fever, cough, and rhinitis
- Vomiting and diarrhea are more common in children than adults
- Early treatment of within 2 days of symptom onset was associated with a reduction in mortality risk when compared to later treatment in adults
- Neuraminidase inhibitor therapy in children aged < 12 years found that symptoms was reduced by 36 hours among previously healthy children taking oseltamivir and by 30 hours among those taking zanamivir
- >23,000 US deaths annually

- <u>Washing hands with soap and running water for 20 seconds helpful in preventing spread</u>
- <u>Facemask on patient helpful in preventing spread to health care workers</u>

Vaccination

- Children 6–59 months
- Pregnancy or postpartum, or who may become pregnant
- Immunocompromised
- Caregivers of high risk patients
- Age ≥ 65 years
- Chronic kidney disease
- COPD and chronic pulmonary disease patients
- Patients with egg allergy may be given any recommended influenza vaccine as appropriate for their health status

Signs and symptoms

- Fever (2–5 days duration)
- Sore throat (3–5 days duration)
- Myalgias
- Frontal or retro-orbital headache
- Nasal discharge
- Weakness and severe fatigue
- Cough and other respiratory symptoms
- Tachycardia
- Red, watery eyes

High risk patients

- Age ≥ 65 years
- Age < 2 years
- Chronic pulmonary disease — asthma or chronic obstructive lung disease
- Chronic cardiovascular, renal, and/or hepatic disease
- Hematologic disease (e.g., sickle cell disease)
- Metabolic disorders (e.g., diabetes mellitus)
- Immunosuppression secondary to either a disease or medication
- Compromised respiratory function or other conditions that increase risk of aspiration
- Pregnancy and up to 2 weeks post-partum
- Long-term aspirin therapy for chronic medical conditions in patients aged < 19 years
- Neuromuscular disorders, seizure disorders, or other cognitive dysfunction that may compromise handling of respiratory secretions

Complications

- Acute bronchitis
- Primary viral pneumonia (uncommon)
- Secondary bacterial pneumonia (occurs 4–5 days after onset of illness)
    - Staphylococcus aureus, Streptococcus pneumoniae or Hemophilus influenzae
- EKG abnormalities
- Otitis media

Testing

- In epidemics, healthy patients with typical symptoms, no testing may be indicated
- Testing is appropriate in times of low disease prevalence
- Nasopharyngeal swab
    - Depending on the test, generally accurate 60–80%
- Chest x–ray in high risk patients or when diagnosis is unclear
- CBC and chemistries may be ordered for toxic patients or with concerning comorbidities and signs/symptoms as needed

Treatment considerations

- Supportive care may suffice in healthy patients
- Prescribe antiviral medications for patients who are more severely ill or at high risk for a more severe disease course
- Medication may shorten symptoms by ~ 1 day
- Nursing homes, etc. the CDC further recommends that antiviral chemoprophylaxis should be given for a minimum of 2 weeks and should continue for at least 7 days

after the last known case was identified.

- May be considered or offered to healthcare personnel who care for patients at high risk for complications

Medications

Oseltamivir (Tamiflu)

- Oseltamivir 75 mg bid for adults x 5 days
- Pediatric dosing
  - ≤15 kg 30 mg PO bid x 5 days
  - 15.1–23 kg 45 mg PO bid x 5 days
  - 23.1–40 kg 60 mg PO bid x 5 days
  - >40 kg same as adult
- Currently approved for the treatment of influenza in patients of all ages
- For patients with influenza symptoms ≤ 48 hours if prescribed

Zanamivir (Relenza)

- Adult inhalation 5 mg bid x 5 days
- Pediatric >10 mg inhaled q12hr x 5 days
- For patients with influenza symptoms ≤ 48 hours if prescribed

Permivir (Rapivab)

- 600 mg IV as a single dose
- For patients aged ≥2 years with influenza symptoms ≤ 48 hours if prescribed
  - CrCl 30-49 mL/min: 200 mg IV as a single dose
  - CrCl 10-29 mL/min: 100 mg IV as a single dose

Baloxavir marboxil (Xofluza)

- 40 to <80 kg: 40 mg PO x 1
- ≥80 kg: 80 mg PO as a single dose
- For patients with influenza symptoms ≤ 48 hours if prescribed

Prophylaxis

- Oseltamivir and zanamivir one dose daily for 10 days
- May be extended to 2 weeks in high risk patients
- May be extended for community outbreaks to 6 weeks for oseltamivir and 28 days for zanamivir

Admission criteria recommendation

- Exacerbations of underlying disease
- Elderly with signs of pneumonia
- Elderly with dehydration
- Significant respiratory compromise

Discharge criteria recommendation

- Most healthy patients without concerning comorbidities or signs/symptoms

Notes

____

____

____

REFERENCES:

cdc.gov/flu/professionals/infectioncontrol/ltc-facilityguidance.htm

ebmedicine.net/topics.php?paction=showTopic&topic_id=591

emedicine.medscape.com/article/219557

Stein J, Louie J, Flanders S, et al. Performance characteristics of clinical diagnosis, a clinical decision rule, and a rapid influenza test in the detection of influenza infection in a community sample of adults. Ann Emerg Med. 2005;46(5):412-419

Prevention and Control of Seasonal Influenza with Vaccines: Recommendations of the Advisory Committee on Immunization Practices—United States, 2018–19 Influenza Season

Recommendations and Reports / August 24, 2018 / 67(3);1–20

ADULT ASTHMA/ACUTE BRONCHITIS PROTOCOL

This protocol is for acute exacerbations

Definition

- Reversible acute bronchospasm and airway resistance secondary to infectious, allergic, environmental or internal causes

Differential Diagnosis

- Panic disorder
- Pneumonia
- Bronchitis
- CHF
- COPD
- Pulmonary embolism
- Anaphylaxis
- URI
- Vocal cord dysfunction
- Laryngospasm
- Epiglottitis
- Croup
- Retropharyngeal abscess

Considerations

- Cough is commonly the first symptom
- Viral URI, allergens or environmental factors are frequently precipitants
- Severe episode may have decreased breath sounds without wheezing
- Inability to speak more than 2–3 words at a time indicates a severe episode
- Steroids very useful — both PO, IM/IV and inhaled (inhaled steroids are for prophylaxis)
  - Cochrane review found that inhaled corticosteroids are superior to anti-leukotrienes when used as monotherapy in adults and children with persistent asthma
- Usually there is pre-existing asthma or bronchitis history

Peak flow % of predicted

- Mild disease > 70%
- Moderate disease 40–69%
- Severe disease < 40%

Risk Factors

- Prior intubation
- Visit in the last month for asthma
- Hospitalization > 1 time
- Two emergency visits past year
- Current or recent systemic steroid use
- Concomitant disease
- Illicit drug use

Evaluation

- Complete history and physical exam
- Assess respiratory effort
- Monitor O_2 saturation
- Consider peak flows before and after aerosols
- CBC and/or BMP for significant tachycardia and fever
- Check radiology interpretations prior to discharge if available

Chest x-ray

- If pneumonia suspected
- Significant respiratory distress
- If CHF considered as possible cause of dyspnea
- Respiratory distress not responsive to aerosols
- Age ≥ 50

- Cardiac history

If CHF suspected

- BNP or NT–ProBNP may be ordered though chest x–xay usually suffices
- Troponin
- EKG

Treatment Options

- Supplemental oxygen for O_2 Sat < 92% room air or significant respiratory distress
- Albuterol with or without atrovent aerosol every 15–20 minutes prn — up to 3 treatments total

Steroid treatment options useful for moderate to severe exacerbations in adults (caution with diabetes)

- Prednisone 40–60 mg PO

  OR

- May give Decadron (dexamethasone) 0.6 mg/kg IM instead (NMT 10 mg) if PO route not usable (caution with diabetes)
  - Onset of action IV is 1 hour. PO onset of action is 1–2 hours
  - Duration of action is 36–54 hours
  - Dexamethasone 6mg =prednisone 40 mg

  OR

- Depomedrol (methylprednisolone acetate) 120–160 mg IM (caution with diabetes)

Additional treatment options if needed for severe exacerbations

- Epinephrine 0.3 mg SQ (caution with coronary artery disease history)
- Terbutaline 0.25 mg SQ prn q15–20 minutes up to 3 treatments as needed (caution with coronary artery disease history)
- $MgSO_4$ (magnesium sulfate) 1–2 gms IV over 20 minutes in adults per physician
- $MgSO_4$ (magnesium sulfate) 25–50 mg/kg IV over 10–20 minutes per physician (NMT 2 gm) for children
- $MgSO_4$ (magnesium sulfate) 125–250 mg in 0.3 ml NS aerosol q 20 minutes up to 4 doses as needed (off label use)
  - May combine with albuterol
- Heliox 70:30 — do not use if > 30% oxygen needed to maintain O_2 saturation

Discharge medications

- Albuterol MDI with or without spacer q4–6hr prn
  - May direct up to 6 puffs per treatment if needed
- Antibiotics are not usually needed
  - Consider antibiotics in smokers
  - If bacterial infection suspected, may use Sanford Guide or other drug databases
    - Zithromax Z–pak PO

Discharge systemic steroid treatment (caution with diabetes)

- Prednisone 40–60 mg PO × 5 –7 days (NMT 60 mg qday)

  OR

- Dexamethasone 6 mg qday for 5 –7 days

  OR

- Decadron (dexamethasone) 0.6 mg/kg IV/IM/PO (NMT 10 mg) — duration of effect is 36–54 hours

Discharge inhaled steroids for asthma only

- Consider inhaled steroid Rx only after the acute exacerbation has resolved
  - Prescribe double dose if already on single strength dose

  OR

- Advair diskus bid for asthma or COPD only (combination long acting beta–agonist and steroid) to be used only after acute exacerbation has resolved

Discharge Criteria

- Good response to therapy
- Wheezing resolution and no significant respiratory distress
- Peak flow ≥ 70% predicted if checked
- O_2 saturation > 93% on room air
- Good follow up and compliance
- Primary care provider to follow up within 1–3 days if symptoms persist

Discharge instructions

- Follow up with primary care provider in 1–5 days depending on severity of illness and response to treatments
- Provide asthma or bronchitis aftercare instructions

Consult Criteria

- Severe respiratory distress on presentation (notify physician immediately)
- Insufficient response to treatment
- Family or patient feels they are too ill to go home
- Peak flow < 70% predicted if measured after treatment is finished
- Moderate or severe respiratory distress post treatment
- O_2 saturation < 94% on room air post treatments if O_2 saturation normal on room air in past
- Significant comorbid conditions
- Heart rate ≥ 110 post treatment
- Hypotension develops or relative hypotension SBP < 105 with history of hypertension
- Return visit for same acute episode
- Immunosuppression
- Age ≥ 60

Lab and x-ray consult criteria

- New onset renal insufficiency or worsening renal insufficiency with creatinine increase ≥ 0.5
- WBC ≥ 15,000 or < 3,000; Neutrophil count < 1,000
- Bandemia ≥ 15%
- Acute thrombocytopenia
- Anion gap > 18
- Significant electrolyte abnormally
- Glucose ≥ 400 mg/dL in diabetic patient
- Glucose ≥ 300 mg/dL in new onset diabetic patient
- Hyperglycemia with metabolic acidosis (decreased serum CO_2 or elevated anion gap)
- Pleural effusion
- New chest x–ray infiltrate(s) or increased interstitial changes

Notes

____

____

____

REFERENCES:

Asthma Author: Michael J Morris, MD, FACP, FCCP; Chief Editor: Zab Mosenifar, MD
emedicine.medscape.com/article/296301

Chauhan BF, Ducharme FM. Anti-leukotriene agents compared to inhaled corticosteroids in the management of recurrent and/or chronic asthma in adults and children. Cochrane Database Syst Rev. May 16 2012;5:CD002314

Unlabeled Uses of Nebulized Medications
Mary Beth Shirk; Kevin R. Donahue; Jill Shirvani

Am J Health Syst
Pharm. 2006;63(18):1704-171
Medscape .com/viewarticle/545484 _8

ALLERGY PROTOCOL

This Protocol is for an acute episode

Definition

- Systemic reaction to mediator release secondary to IgE sensitization from allergen

Considerations

- Most reactions are minor with itching with localized or generalized urticaria
- Anaphylaxis is due to IgE antibody release of histamine and vasoactive mediators
- Most common causes of allergies are food allergy
  - Milk and egg allergies are seen more commonly in younger children, while allergies to shellfish and fin fish are more frequent in teens
  - Peanut allergy has a high incidence and is consistent across all ages
- Symptom presentation possibilities
  - Occurs within 30 minutes usually
  - Can be mild
  - Wheezing
  - Dyspnea
  - Shock
  - Airway obstruction
  - Death
  - Can occur on long-term medication
- Urticaria
  - Etiology unknown usually
  - Usually self-limited
- True opioid allergy rare — usually GI upset or pseudoallergy
- Anaphylactoid reactions to contrast
  - Direct stimulation of mast cells and basophils
  - Seafood allergic patients are not allergic to radiographic contrast material
  - Related to high osmolarity of contrast materials
  - Narcotics can also cause anaphylactoid reactions

    No link between seafood allergy and iodinated contrast allergy
    - There is an increase in nonallergic contrast reactions in any type of allergy history (small increase)
    - Iodine is not an allergen
    - Reactions almost always non–IgE mediated
- Angioedema (may appear with urticaria)
  - Bradykinin mediated usually
  - May be histamine mediated
  - Commonly from ACE inhibitors
    - Decreased metabolism of bradykinin
  - Hereditary C1 esterase deficiency
    - Leads to increased bradykinin
    - Positive family history
  - Caution using steroids in diabetic patients

Evaluation

- Vital signs
- Oropharyngeal and respiratory distress assessment
- Pulmonary and cardiac exam
- Skin examination
- Chest x-ray for significant respiratory distress or O_2 saturation < 93% on room air
- Soft tissue neck films for hoarseness or complaints/findings of throat swelling
- CBC and BMP for moderate to severe systemic reactions

Urticaria

- Vascular reaction of the skin with transient wheals, soft papules and plaques usually with pruritus

Treatment options

Benadryl (diphenhydramine)

- Adult: 25–50 mg PO/IM/IV
- Pediatrics: 1–2 mg/kg PO or IM (NMT 50 mg)
- May continue for 5–7 days PO qid prn

Pepcid (famotidine)

- Adult: 20 mg IV or 40 mg PO
- Pediatric: 0.25 mg/kg IV or 0.5 mg/kg PO (not to exceed maximum adult dose)

Epinephrine

- If urticaria part of anaphylaxis reaction (see below sections)

Consider steroids (caution if diabetic)

- Prednisone 40–60 mg PO qday for 5–7 days (> 40 kg)
  - Prednisone/prednisolone 1 mg/kg PO qday for 5–7 days (< 40 kg)

OR

- Dexamethasone 4–6 mg qday PO for 5–7 days or 0.6 mg/kg IM/IV instead (NMT 10 mg)

Discharge criteria

- Discharge with good resolution of rash and itching

Discharge instructions

- Follow up with primary care provider within 7 days
- Avoid offending agent if known
- Provide urticaria aftercare instructions

Angioedema

- Non-life threatening presentation treated same as urticaria
- Less responsive to treatment than urticaria
- Evaluate for airway compromise or significant oropharyngeal swelling
- Oxygen prn
- Consult promptly for posterior oropharyngeal angioedema, stridor or hoarseness
- Discharge mild lip or non-oropharyngeal angioedema with normal vital signs and no distress
- Stop ACE inhibitors if currently taking
  - 4 times more common in African–Americans
  - May develop years after taking current ACE inhibitors
- May involve GI tract mimicking acute abdomen

Types of angioedema

- Histamine mediated
  - Allergic/immunogenic
- Bradykinin mediated
  - ACE inhibitors
    - Incidence peaks within the first month of treatment, with the risk of angioedema decreasing significantly after 9-12 weeks. However, the risk of ACE inhibitor induced angioedema persists even after many years of use
  - Hereditary
    - Decreased C1 inhibitor (or poorly functioning C1 inhibitor) allowing overproduction of bradykinin
  - Acquired
  - Bradykinin metabolized mainly by angiotensin converting enzyme
- Physically induced
- Idiopathic

Additional treatments if needed

Histamine mediated angioedema (allergic)

- Epinephrine
  - Caution if history of coronary artery disease
  - Adult: 0.3 mg SQ; (if respiratory distress notify physician promptly)

- Pediatrics: 0.01 mg/kg SQ not to exceed adult dose; give IV or IM (anterior thigh) if significant respiratory distress (notify physician promptly)
- Antihistamines (diphenhydramine 50 mg IV/IM) helpful in IgE/histamine mediated (may have pruritus)
- Pepcid (famotidine) 20 mg IV or 40 mg PO
- Dexamethasone 10 mg IV
  - Onset of action IV is 1 hour. PO onset of action is 1–2 hours
  - Duration of action is 36–54 hours
  - Dexamethasone 6mg =prednisone 40 mg

Bradykinin mediated (ACE inhibitor induced most common)

- May respond to fresh frozen plasma or C1 esterase inhibitor concentrate
  - FFP occasionally can worsen angioedema and may need intubation if it occurs
- Tranexamic acid 1 gm IV over 10 minutes may be effective (no faster than 100 mg/minute)

Mild Anaphylaxis

- Urticaria/angioedema
- O_2 saturation > 94% room air
- No respiratory distress
- Normotensive
- No tachycardia

Treatment options

Benadryl (diphenhydramine)

- Adult: 50 mg PO or IM
- Pediatric: 1–2 mg/kg PO or IM (NMT 50 mg)
- Continue for 5–7 days PO qid prn

Pepcid (famotidine)

- Adult: 20 mg IV–40 mg PO
- Pediatric: 0.25 mg/kg IV/PO (NMT 40 mg)

Consider steroids

- Prednisone 40–60 mg PO qday for 5–7 days (> 40 kg)
  - Prednisone/prednisolone 1 mg/kg PO qday for 5–7 days (< 40 kg)

OR

- Dexamethasone 4–6 mg qday PO for 5–7 days or 0.6 mg/kg IM/IV instead (NMT 10 mg)

Additional treatment if needed

Epinephrine

- Caution if history of coronary artery disease
- Adult: 0.3 mg SQ
- Pediatrics: 0.01 mg/kg SQ not to exceed adult dose

Moderate Anaphylaxis

(Notify physician)

- Urticaria/angioedema
- Wheezing
- O_2 saturation 90–94% room air
- Moderate respiratory distress
- No hypotension

Treatment options

Oxygen: nasal or mask (≥ 5 liters/minute if mask used)

Epinephrine (drug of choice)

- Caution if history of coronary artery disease
- Adult: 0.3 mg SQ/IM (thigh) — notify physician promptly
- Pediatric: 0.01 mg/kg SQ/IM (thigh) not to exceed adult dose — notify physician promptly

Benadryl (diphenhydramine)

- Adult: 50 mg IV or IM
- Pediatric: 1–2 mg/kg IV or IM (NMT 50 mg)

Pepcid (famotidine))

- Adult: 20–40 mg IV
- Pediatric: 0.25 mg/kg IV (NMT 40 mg)

Albuterol aerosol

- With or without atrovent
- Repeat q15 min × 2 additional treatments prn
- Continuous prn (for severe dyspnea)

Additional treatments if needed

Glucagon

- 1–2 mg IV if on beta–blocker or resistant to epinephrine

Steroids

- Adult: Solumedrol (methylprednisolone) 125 mg IV
- Pediatric: 1–2 mg/kg IV
- Prednisone 40–60 mg PO qday for 5–7 days (> 40 kg) if discharged
- Prednisone/prednisolone 1 mg/kg (NMT 60 mg) PO qday for 5–7 days if discharged (pediatrics)
- May give Decadron (dexamethasone) 0.15–0.6 mg/kg IV/IM instead (NMT 10 mg) and continue PO up to 5–7 days if needed

Severe Anaphylaxis

(Notify physician immediately)

- Urticaria/angioedema
- Wheezing
- O_2 saturation < 90% room air
- Severe respiratory distress
- Oropharyngeal airway swelling or compromise
- Hypotension
- Intubation if impending respiratory failure — notify physician immediately
- Observation for 6 hours if to be discharged by physician
- Usually admitted

Treatment options

Oxygen: nasal or mask (> 5 liters/minute if mask used)

Epinephrine (drug of choice)

- Adult: 0.3–0.5 mg IV (if in shock) or IM anterior lateral thigh if no IV/IO access
  - 1 mg IV/IO if no pulse
    - Activate ACLS and call a code
- Pediatric: 0.01 mg/kg IV (if in shock) or IM anterior thigh (do not exceed adult doses)
- Caution with history of coronary artery disease

For shock

- IV NS 1–2 liters rapidly if hypotensive adult
- 20 cc/kg IV NS if hypotensive pediatric patient — may repeat × 2 prn

Benadryl (diphenhydramine)

- Adult: Benadryl (diphenhydramine) 50 mg IV (preferred) or IM
- Pediatric: 1–2 mg/kg IV (preferred) or IM (NMT 50 mg)

Pepcid (famotidine)

- Adult: 20–40 mg IV
- Pediatric: 0.25 mg/kg IV (NMT 40 mg)

Albuterol aerosol

- With or without atrovent
- Repeat q10–15 min × 2 prn
- Continuous aerosol prn for severe dyspnea

Steroid options

- Adult
  - Methylprednisolone 125 mg IV (Solumedrol)
  - Prednisone 40–60 mg PO qday for 5–7 days (> 40 kg) if discharged

    OR
  - Dexamethasone 6 mg PO qday for 5–7 days if discharged
- Pediatric

- Methylprednisolone 1–2 mg/kg IV (NMT 125 mg)

  OR
- May give Decadron (dexamethasone) 0.6 mg/kg IM/IV instead of PO (NMT 10 mg per dose)

  OR
- Prednisone/prednisolone 0.5–1 mg/kg PO qday for 5 days (NMT 60 mg qday)

  OR
- Dexamethasone dose 0.15–0.6mg/kg qday for 5–7 days (NMT 6 mg qday usually)

Additional treatment if needed

Glucagon

- 1–2 mg IV if on beta–blocker or resistant to epinephrine (consult physician if possible)

Discharge Criteria

- Good resolution of rash and itching in urticaria
- Discharge patients presenting with mild symptoms that have observation post-treatment for 2–4 hours without symptoms

Discharge medication options

- Epipen for moderate or more severe anaphylaxis
- Dexamethasone 6 mg qday for 5–7 days
- Benadryl 25–50 mg PO qid prn allergy symptoms
- Famotidine 40 mg PO qday prn allergy symptoms

Discharge instructions

- Follow up with primary care provider within 7 days
- Avoid offending agent if known
- Provide allergy aftercare instructions
- Return if worse

Consult Criteria

- Hypotension
- O_2 saturation < 95% on room air after treatments
- Moderate to severe anaphylaxis or respiratory distress on presentation or during stay
- Altered mental status
- Oropharyngeal or throat swelling, complaints of throat swelling, hoarseness or dyspnea
- Wheezing not resolved
- Adult heart rate ≥ 110 post treatment
- Pediatric heart rate post treatment
  - 0–4 months ≥ 180
  - 5–7 months ≥ 175
  - 8–12 months ≥ 170
  - 1–3 years ≥ 160
  - 4–5 years ≥ 145
  - 6–8 years ≥ 130
  - 9–11 years ≥ 125
  - 12–15 years ≥ 120
  - 16 years or older ≥ 110

Notes

____

____

____

REFERENCES:

Beaty AD, Lieberman PL, Slavin RG. Seafood allergy and radiocontrast media: are physicians propagating a myth? Am J Med 2008 Feb;121(2):158.e1–4.doi: 10.1016/J amjmed.2007.08.025

Seidmann MD. Christopher AL. Sarpa JR. Potesta E. Angioedema related to angiotensin converting enzyme inhibitors. Otolaryngology – Head & Neck Surgery. 102:727–31, 1990.

Brown NJ. Ray WA. Snowden M. Griffin MR. Black Americans have an increased rate of angiotensin converting enzyme inhibitor-associated angioedema. Clinical Pharmacology & Therapeutics. 60(1):8–13, 1996 Jul

World Allergy Organization Guidelines for the Assessment and Management of Anaphylaxis

World Allergy Organ J. Feb 2011; 4(2): 13–37

Am J Med, Vol. 127: S17World Allergy Organization

Wang K, et al. *Am J Emerg Med.* 2020 Oct 21. Online ahead of print.

Beauchene J, et al. *Rev Med Interne.* 2018;39(10): 772-776.

Cureus. 2021;13:e14021

Long BJ, et al. *West J Emerg Med.* 2019;20(4): 587-600.

Wang K, et al. *Am J Emerg Med.* 2020 Oct 21. Online ahead of print.

Beauchene J, et al. *Rev Med Interne.* 2018;39(10): 772-776.

Long BJ, et al. *West J Emerg Med.* 2019;20(4): 587-600

Acute Care Ultrasound

Section contents

Acute Care Ultrasound

When using any protocol, always follow the Guidelines of Proper Use (page 12).

ACUTE CARE ULTRASOUND

Definition

- Limited bedside point of care ultrasound performed by the medical provider directly performing patient care

This is a brief introduction

Ultrasound exams

FAST (trauma) — overlaps with RUSH exam

RUSH (shock)

FOCUS ON THE INFERIOR VENA CAVA (IVC)

PULMONARY (DYSPNEA)

PULMONARY EMBOLISM CASE

CARDIAC

GALLBLADDER

RENAL

DEEP VENOUS THROMBOSIS

SOFT TISSUE

Considerations

- Attend ultrasound course
- Practice needed to attain ultrasound pattern recognition
- Credentialing with 25+ exams with quality review in each area
- Limited bedside ultrasounds does not compete with or preclude complete ultrasounds performed and/or read by radiology, cardiology or specific specialties in their area of expertise
- Structures at the top of the image are closest to the probe
- B mode is most commonly used
- M mode is used for imaging over a time window
- PW (Doppler) is pulse wave to determine if vessel is a vein or artery or if there is any flow in a structure
- Orientation of probe — marker on side of probe corresponds to icon on upper side of screen

Types of probes

Curved (low frequency for deeper structures)

- Abdomen
  - Gallbladder
  - Renal – check for hydronephrosis and possibly stones
  - Shock (or hypotension) RUSH exam
  - FAST for trauma
  - Subcostal cardiac imaging

Linear (high frequency for superficial structures)

- Starting central lines (usually internal jugular or femoral)
- Skin abscess determination
- DVT exam
- Pneumothorax (pleura sliding determination)
- Ocular (do not perform if globe rupture present or suspected)
  - Select ophthalmology exam setting (and then reduce power to 25%)
    - May be safer to avoid prolonged scan times
  - Retinal detachment
  - Papilledema of optic nerve
  - Lens dislocation in trauma without globe rupture

Phased array (mid-lower frequency)

- Cardiac
- Abdomen
- Lung

FAST (Focused assessment with Sonography in Trauma)

Curved probe

- Orientation of probe (marker) to patient's right or toward head

Areas to scan

- **Epigastrium** to view heart for pericardial effusion
  - Phased array probe (if used) with marker pointed to right shoulder and probe in the 4-5th area intercostal space (long parasternal view)
- **Right lateral flank** with marker to head to view Morrison's pouch (potential space between right kidney and liver) for fluid (black area represents blood or fluid) – may see with ruptured ectopic pregnancy also
  - May detect as little as 200 mL
- **Left lateral flank** to view left kidney and spleen for bleeding (not as good as CT for extent of injury)
- **Bladder** for surrounding fluid in pelvis (marker pointed to right)
- Both costophrenic angles for pleural effusion

  Linear probe bilateral upper chest that detects presence of pleural movement and comet tail artifacts/B lines (lung fluid) = no pneumothorax

---

FAST Indications

- Hemodynamically unstable patients
- Patients who need an emergent bedside procedure and a rapid trauma exam needed
- Patients at a community hospital who require transfer to a trauma center
- Blunt trauma in unconscious or paralyzed patient, or who has altered mental status, or about to be anesthetized for other injuries
- Intoxicated patients who can be observed and re-examined
- Blunt trauma with suspected intraperitoneal injury
- Patients with penetrating trauma, especially with wounds in upper abdomen or lower chest
- Patients with a concerning mechanism of injury but no definite indication for CT
  - Consider a period of observation and serial FAST exams

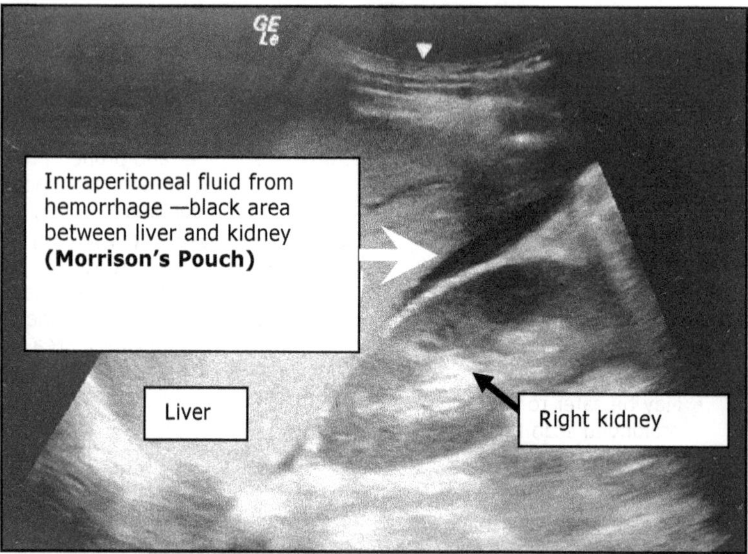

Rapid Ultrasound for Shock (RUSH) – undifferentiated shock (overlaps with FAST exam)

- **Use all probes**

HIMAP

- **H** – Heart for pericardial effusion (with phased array probe 4-5th ICS area with marker pointed to right shoulder)
  - LV contractility (ballpark guestimate)
  - RV size should be 2/3 LV size (if > 2/3 LV may indicate PE, COPD, pulmonary HTN etc.
- **I** – IVC for size and inspiratory collapse
  - > 50% inspiratory collapse and < 1.5 cm diameter may need IV fluid (epigastrium view)
  - Little respiratory phasicity and > 2.5 cm diameter may need pressor
  - See below
- **M** –Morrison's pouch for intraperitoneal bleeding
- **A** – Aortic aneurysm (> 3 cm diameter)
  - Aorta bifurcates at the umbilicus
  - Find spine and its shadow – IVC top right side and aorta top left side of spine
  - Use transverse and longitudinal views
- **P** – Pleural effusion and pneumothorax (linear probe for pneumothorax evaluation)
  - In pneumothorax there is no sliding of pleura and no B lines

Pericardial effusion

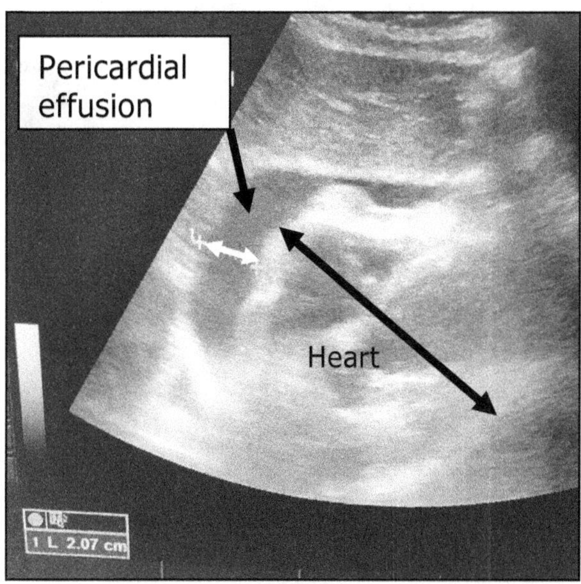

Abdominal aortic aneurysm

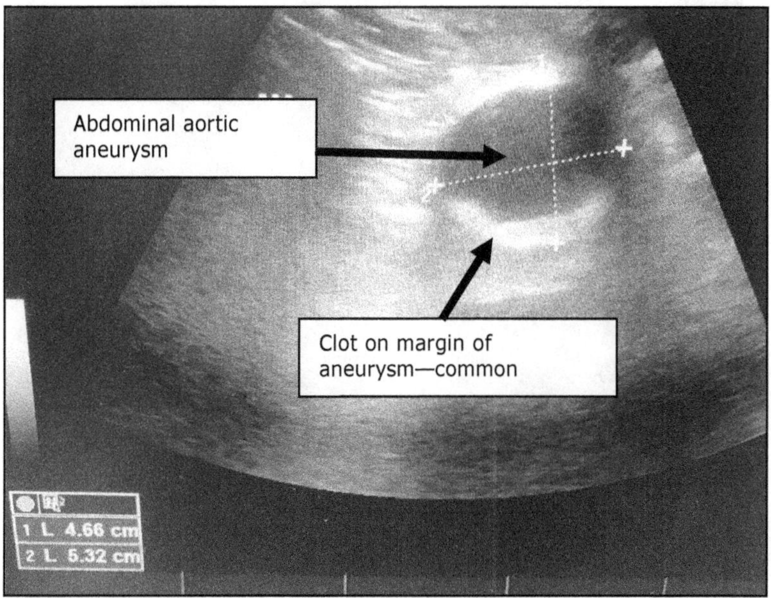

Systolic heart failure

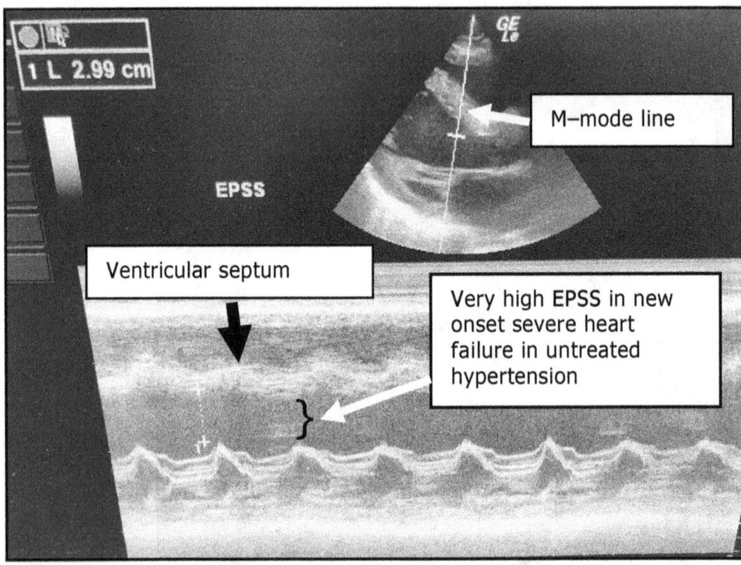

Hyperdynamic heart or high ejection fraction in sepsis, dehydration or high sympathetic state

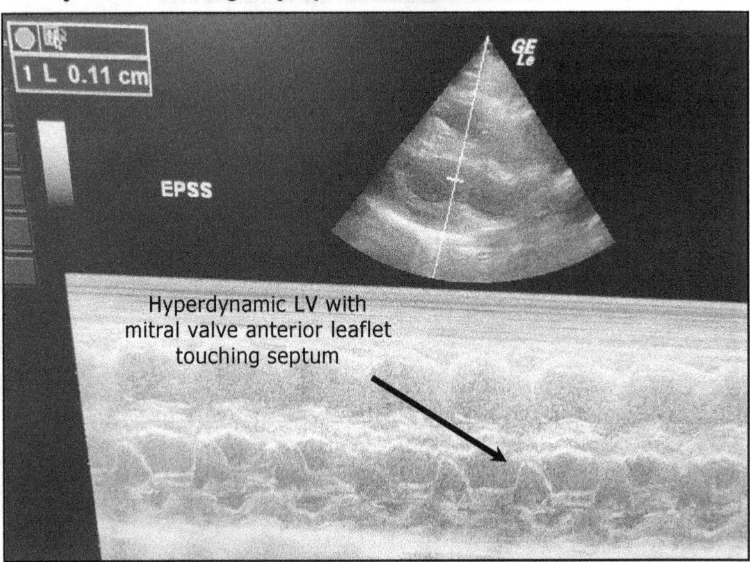

M–mode measures movement over time and is displayed as second image at above

Focus On Inferior Vena Cava (IVC)

- If dilated with little to no inspiratory change may have
  - Large pulmonary embolism burden
  - Heart failure

  - COPD
  - Pulmonary hypertension
  - Renal failure
  - Fluid overload
- If small size with near or total inspiratory collapse may have
  - Dehydration
  - Sepsis
  - Hemorrhage

Enlarged IVC (high CVP)

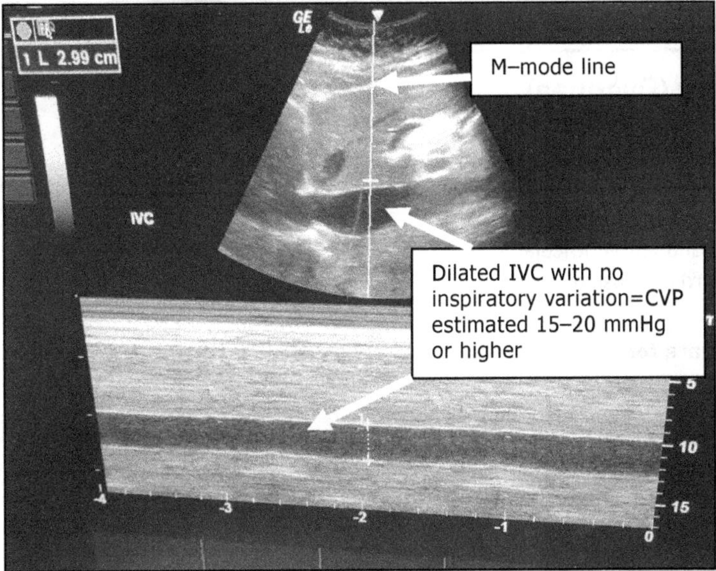

M–mode measures movement over time and is displayed in second image as below

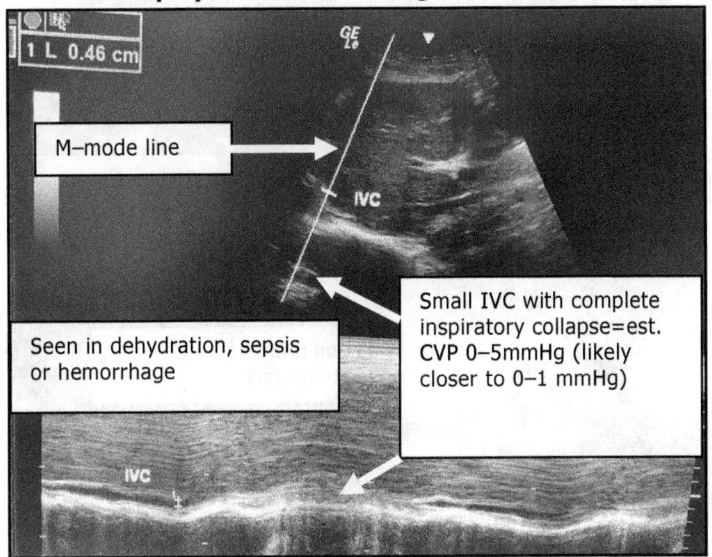

CVP (central venous pressure) estimation

IVC measured	% collapse during inspiration	CVP(mmHg)
< 1.5 cm	>50%	0–5
1.5–2.5 cm	>50%	5–10
1.5–2.5 cm	<50%	10–15
>2.5 cm	Little phasicity	15–20

Pulmonary (Dyspnea)

(see RUSH exam also)

- Evaluate for
- Systolic cardiac contractility (guestimate)
- Diastolic dysfunction if able
- Right and left ventricular size
- Pericardial effusion

Lungs

- **Evaluate for**
- Pleural effusion(s)
- Pulmonary parenchymal fluid (B lines)
- A lines
- Pneumothorax

Pleural effusion

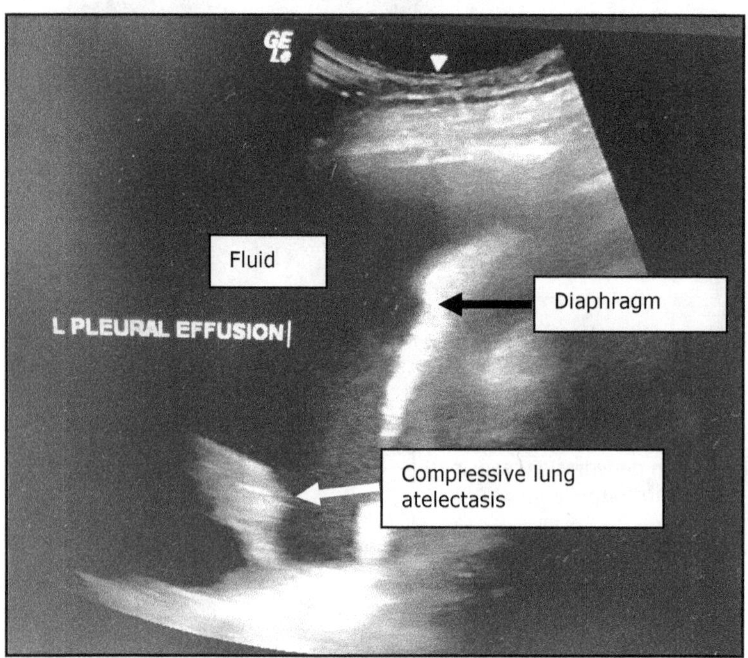

B Lines

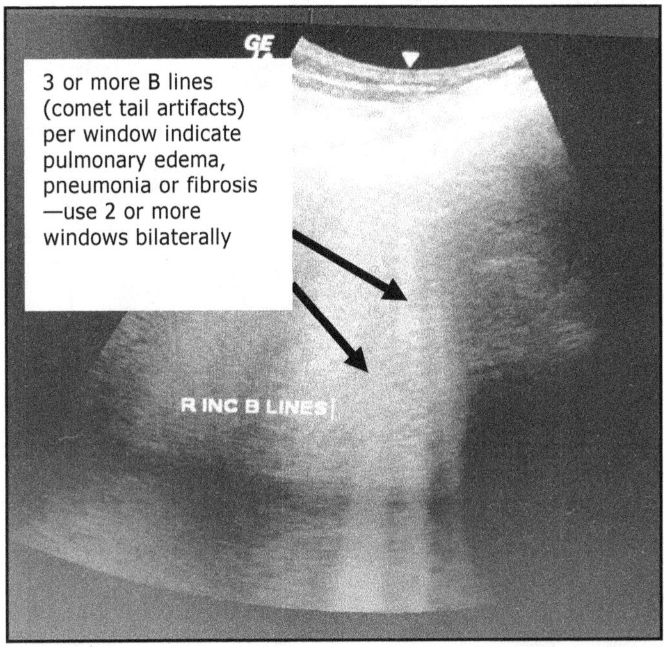

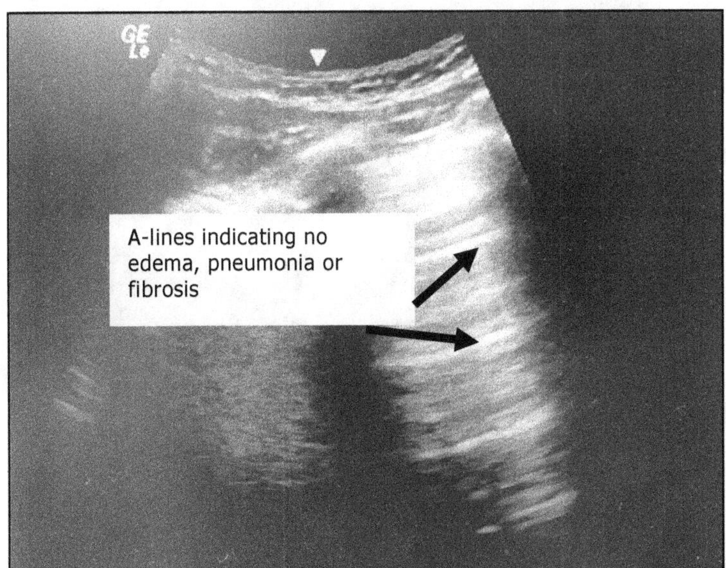

"A–Lines" above image when present are horizontal and indicate no pulmonary edema, and can be taken usually with other clinical indicators to infer that the patient is at least IV fluid tolerant. Does not establish fluid responsiveness. "B–Lines" indicate interstitial thickening — 94% sensitivity, 92 % specificity. No B lines and no pleura sliding or motion usually indicates pneumothorax

Pulmonary embolism case ultrasound

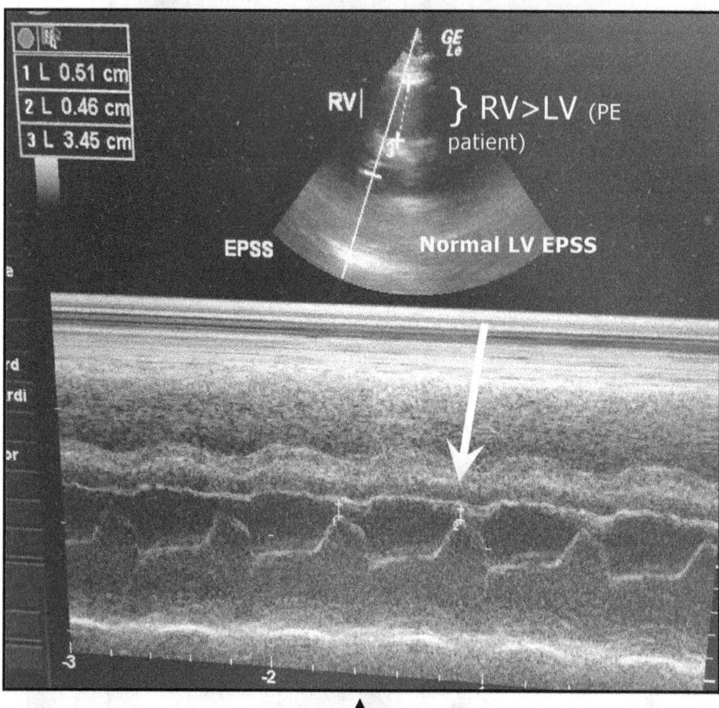

This patient required open embolectomy

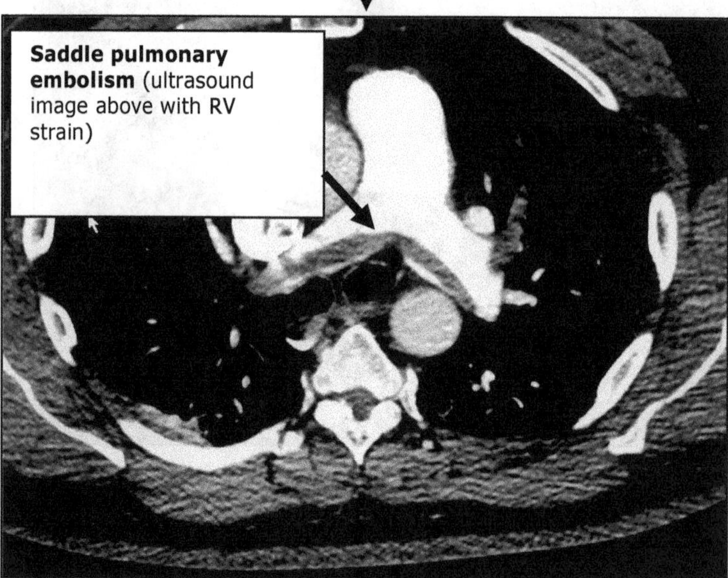

Right ventricular enlargement (Should normally be around 60% or 2/3 size of left ventricle)

Right ventricular enlargement

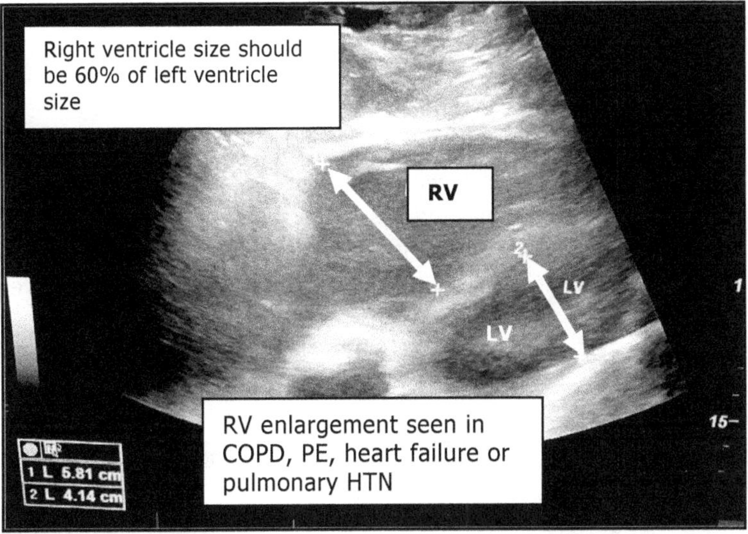

Cardiac Exam (see **FAST, RUSH and Pulmonary Exams for representative images)**

Windows

- **Subxiphoid (subcostal)** with phased array or curvilinear to view heart and IVC/aorta
  - Evaluate RV and LV size, contractility, wall thickness and for pericardial effusion
- **Apical** area with phased array probe and marker pointed to patient's left slightly angled cephalad 20 degrees
  - Visual inspection of heart function
  - Assess for diastolic dysfunction if able
- **Parasternal long axis** on left sternal border near 4th intercostal space with probe marker aimed at right shoulder
- **E Point Septal Separation** is the distance from the anterior leaflet of the mitral valve, (which is the first deflection of the mitral valve toward the interventricular septum), and the septum seen in parasternal long axis view
  - Elevated in systolic failure — usually > 0.6 cm
  - Decreased in hyperdynamic states such as dehydration, sepsis and high sympathetic states
- **Parasternal short axis** is long axis rotated 90° cephalad
  - Observe wall motion

Gallbladder

Curved probe

- Subcostal sweep with marker toward head
- RUQ – 7 cm medial to xiphoid
- Flatten probe as needed with transverse view
- Gallbladder wall normally is < 4 mm – measure in the short axis
- Gallstones or sludge have shadows
- If gallbladder difficult to visualize, try lateral view looking above the right kidney
- Pericholecystic fluid presence may indicate inflammation or cholecystitis

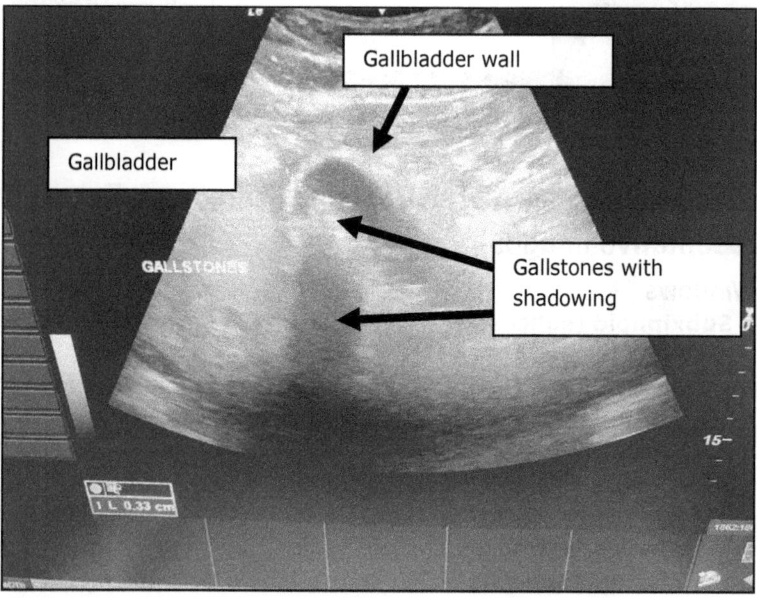

Renal

Curved probe

- Right kidney in midclavicular line inferior ribs
- Left kidney in posterior clavicular line inferior ribs
- Look for dilated collecting system and stones
- Marker probe pointed to head

Hydronephrosis

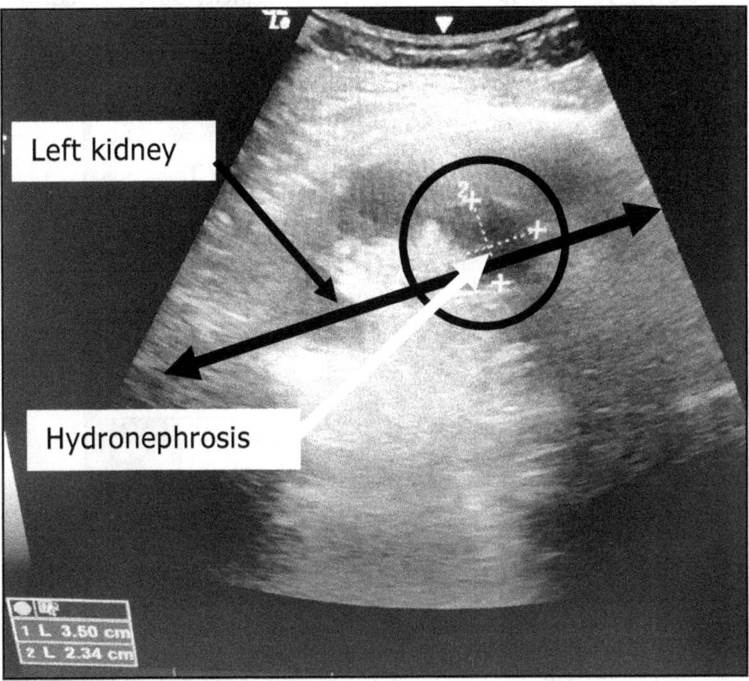

Definition

- Distention of the renal calyces and pelvis as a result of obstruction of the outflow of urine distally

Causes

- Pregnancy
- Bladder outlet obstruction
- Ureteral calculus
- Benign prostatic hypertrophy
- Post-surgical complication
- Vesicoureteral reflux

Considerations

- Permanent of loss renal function by 6 weeks of obstruction

DVT

- **Linear probe** with transverse orientation
- Position thigh externally rotated up to 30 degrees with knee flexed 10 degrees may help with exam
- Start at inguinal ligament and identify common femoral artery and vein
- Compress down anterior thigh 10–20 cm from inguinal ligament
- Blood clot prevents vein from being compressed fully
- Color flow is sometimes absent with DVT
- Popliteal fossa 12 cm above and 5 cm below is compressed

- If negative, then 98% have no DVT
- Sensitivity 95% (95% CI 87-99%) and specificity 96% (95%CI 87-99%)

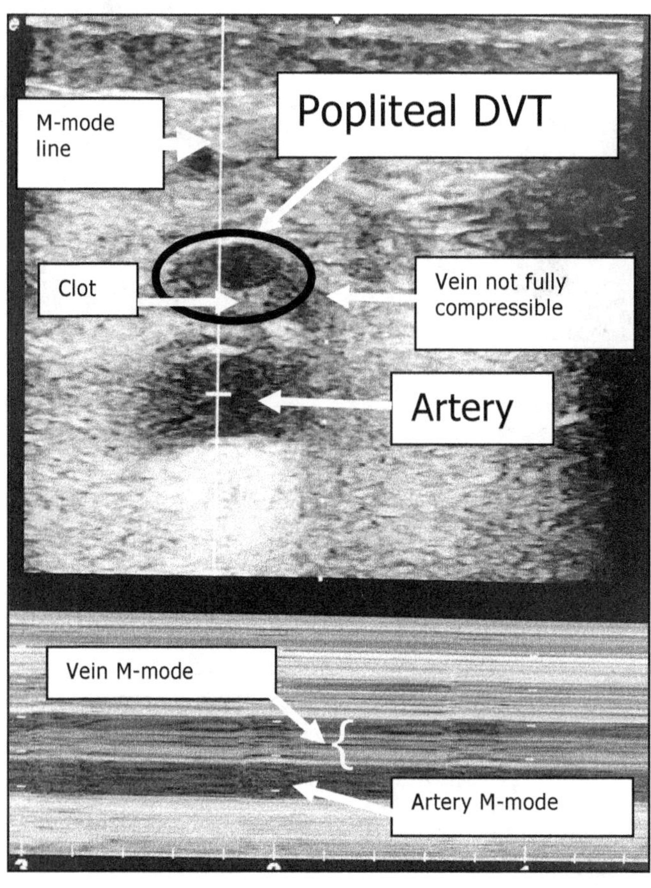

Soft tissue

- **Linear probe**
- Abscess is a black space with white scattered debris
- Cellulitis has cobblestone appearance of the fat globule

Abscess

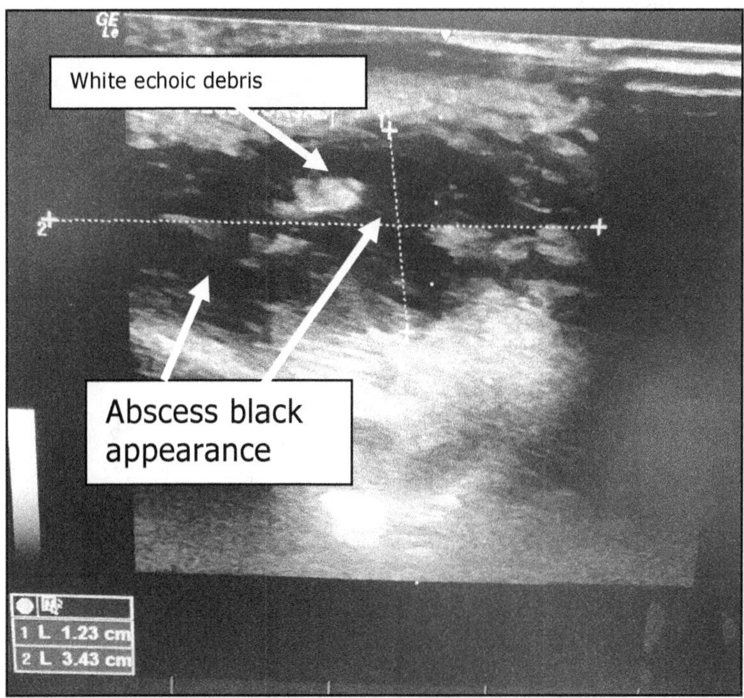

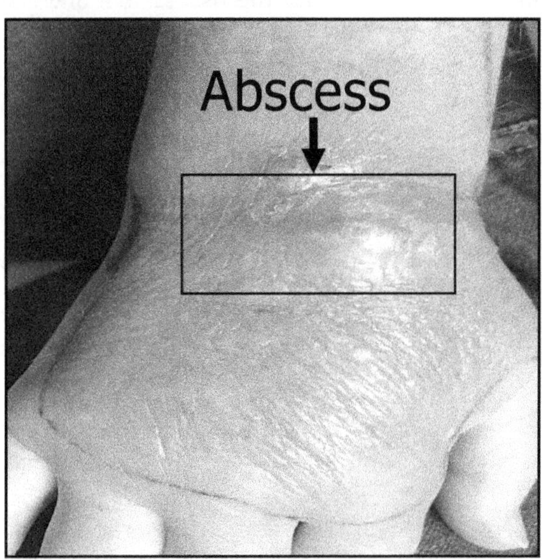

Conclusion

- Ultrasound provides important bedside point of care data that may assist in critical patient management
- Practice is critical in achieving competency
- Ultrasound is an important adjunct and needs to be combined with clinical evaluation and other data

Notes

REFERENCES:

Sonoguide.com

Ultrasound Volume Assessment
R. Starr Knight, MD

Emedhome.com feature article: Rapid Ultrasound for Shock and Hypotension (RUSH) Scott D Weingart, MD, RDMS
Assistant Professor of Emergency Medicine

emergencyultrasoundteaching.com/assets/us_billing_summary

ultrasonix.com/webfm

https://sinaiem.org/accuracy-of-bedside-dvt-study

World Allergy Organization Guidelines for the Assessment and Management of Anaphylaxis

Endocrine

Section Contents

When using any protocol, always follow the Guidelines of Proper Use (page 12).

DIABETES AND HYPOGLYCEMIA PROTOCOL

This Protocol is mostly for acute diabetic presentations

Definition

- Defect in glucose regulation secondary to inadequate secretion of insulin or resistance to insulin

Considerations

Types

- Type 1: dependent on exogenous insulin to live
- Type 2: does not need insulin to live (peripheral insulin resistance and insulin-secretory defect)
- Type 2 can present initially as DKA (diabetic ketoacidosis) in African-Americans or Hispanic descent patients
  - "Ketosis-prone type 2 diabetes mellitus (KPD)"
    - Usually obese, present with DKA as their first manifestation of diabetes but are subsequently found to have type 2 diabetes
    - African-Americans, or are of African, Hispanic or Caribbean descent
    - KPD has been reported to account for up to 60% of cases of new onset-diabetes with DKA in US African-American and Hispanic patients
- Hospital therapy for DKA in type 2 diabetes is the same as for type 1 diabetes.
- Gestational — appears with pregnancy only

Complications

- Increased infections
- Peripheral arterial insufficiency
- Skin ulcers and gangrene of lower legs and feet
- Hyperglycemic and hypoglycemic emergencies
- Pediatric cerebral edema with hyperglycemic emergencies

Vascular

- Retinopathy
- Renal insufficiency and failure
- Coronary arteries occlusion
- Aortic atherosclerosis
- Stroke

DKA

Definition

- Plasma glucose > 250 mg/dL (usually is > 350 mg/dL)
- Serum bicarbonate < 15 mEq/L
- Anion gap over 12
- Arterial pH <7.3 with moderate ketonemia
- Euglycemic diabetic ketoacidosis is associated with the use of SGLT–2 inhibitors, excessive alcohol intake, partial treated diabetes, and prolonged starvation

Common causes

- Secondary to stress
  - Infection most common
  - AMI
  - Pregnancy
  - Surgery

Differential Diagnoses

- Alcoholic ketoacidosis
- Appendicitis
- Hypophosphatemia
- Hypothermia
- Lactic acidosis
- Metabolic acidosis
- Myocardial infarction
- Pneumonia
- Salicylate toxicity
- Hyperosmolar Coma
- Pancreatitis
- Septic shock
- Sepsis
- UTI

Considerations

- Average adult fluid deficit is 6–10 liters (osmotic diuresis)
- Adjustment to serum Na^+ (sodium) levels — each additional 100 mg% over plasma glucose of 100 add 1.6 mEq/L to serum Na^+ levels to determine actual Na^+ serum level
- Potassium body deficit can be severe despite initial normal serum level (a decrease of 0.3–0.7 mEq/L for each decrease of pH of 0.1)
  - Total body potassium deficit may be 3–5 mEq/kg
- IV PO4 (phosphorous) may be needed if respiratory failure occurs
- Venous pH add 0.03 to estimate arterial pH — if used instead of ABG to measure pH
- Serum osmolarity > 320 mOsm/L
- The overall mortality rate for DKA is 2% or less
  - Presence of deep coma at the time of diagnosis, hypothermia, and oliguria are signs of poor prognosis
- Euglycemic diabetic ketoacidosis with normal or near normal blood glucose present in 3–9% of adults presenting with DKA
  - Associated with the use of SGLT–2 inhibitors, excessive alcohol intake, partial treated diabetes, and prolonged starvation
  - Treated with insulin and dextrose 5–10% is administered concurrently with IV insulin

Symptoms and findings (some or all)

- Polyuria
- Polydipsia (increased thirst)
- Weakness
- Weight loss
- Mental status changes
- Dry mucous membranes
- Tachycardia
- Nausea and vomiting
- Abdominal pain
- Kussmaul respirations (deep rapid breathing to partially compensate for metabolic acidosis)
- Peripheral vasodilatation can cause normothermia or hypothermia despite infection

Evaluation

- CBC
- BMP or CMP
- Accucheck
- Chest x-ray

- U/A
- ABG or venous pH (add 0.03 to adjust to arterial pH)
- Blood, urine or infected site cultures if infection suspected

Serum osmolality

- If < 320mOsm/L, look for another cause of altered mental status
- Osmolol gap > 10–20; suspect substance ingestion (normal < 10)
  - Gap = Osmolality measured – Osmolality calculated (Osmolality calculation equation: 2(Na^++K^+) + glucose/18 + BUN/2.8; normal 280–300mOsm/L)
  - Ethanol mg%/4.6 is added to osmolol gap equation if present
  - Gap > 50 carries high specificity for toxic alcohol such as methanol, ethylene glycol, or isopropyl alcohol (treatment for toxic alcohol is fomepizole and may need emergent hemodialysis — check lactic acid level)

Fluid therapy

Adult

- IV NS infused 15–20 cc/kg/hour (1–1.5 liters average)
  - Administer 1-3 liters during the first hour
  - Administer 1 liter during the second hour
  - Administer 1 liter during the following 2 hours
  - Administer 1 liter every 4 hours, depending on the degree of dehydration and central venous pressure readings if measured (may use bedside ultrasound—see Ultrasound chapter
- Continue NS if corrected Na^+ is low
- 0.45% NS at 4–14 cc/kg/hour after bolus infusion if "corrected" Na^+ is normal or high
- Add potassium 20–30 mEq/L when serum K^+ reaches < 5.3 mEq/L (if urine output 0.5–1 cc/kg/hour)

Pediatric (< 16 years of age)

- Initial fluid NS IV bolus 20 ml/kg
- May repeat IV fluid boluses if insufficient improvement in circulatory status
- Continued IV with 0.45% or NS after initial fluid therapy
- Replace estimated fluid deficit over 24 - 36 hours
- If altered mental status acutely or headache occurs, suspect cerebral edema (treatment 1–2 gms/kg mannitol IV — per physician) — cerebral edema should not occur with IV fluids within proper fluid ranges
  - CT brain scan

Insulin therapy

- Use short acting insulins
- Insulin should be started about an hour after IV fluid replacement is started to allow for checking potassium levels and because insulin may be more dangerous and less effective before some fluid replacement has been obtained
- If patient is on an insulin pump, it should be stopped
- Check K^+ level first (can cause K^+ to drop; can be dangerous if already low; should be at least 3.3 mEq/L)
- 2011 JBDS guideline recommends the intravenous infusion of insulin at a weight-based fixed rate until ketosis has subsided
  - Should blood glucose fall below 14 mmol/L (250 mg/dL), 10% glucose should be added to allow for the continuation of fixed-rate insulin infusion
- Euglycemic DKA is associated with the with the use of SGLT–2 inhibitors, excessive alcohol intake, partial treated diabetes, and prolonged starvation

- Adults
  - Bolus 0.15 units/kg IV and/or continuous infusion 0.1 unit/kg/hour (up to 5–7 units/hour)
  - Should decrease plasma glucose 50–75 mg%/hour (if not, check hydration status)

Pediatrics

- Insulin bolus not recommended
- Continuous infusion same as adult

Potassium

- Add potassium 20–40 mEq to each liter of IV fluids when serum K^+ < 5.3 if urine output 0.5–1 cc/kg/hour or initial potassium < 3.3 mEq/L
  - Serum K^+ 4.5–5.2 mEq/L give 10 mEq/hour IV
  - Serum K^+ 3.0–4.5 mEq/L give 20 mEq/hour IV
  - Serum K^+ initially < 3.0 mEq/L hold off starting insulin and give potassium IV

Consult criteria

- All DKA patients after initial assessment

Hyperglycemic Hyperosmolar Syndrome (HHS)

- Develops over days or weeks
- Plasma glucose > 600
- Serum osmolality > 320 mOsm
- Profound dehydration: adult 8–12 liters fluid deficit
- Small amount of ketonuria; small or absent ketonemia
- Serum bicarbonate > 15
- Arterial pH > 7.3
- Some alteration of consciousness
- Higher mortality than DKA

Associated medications contributing to HHS

- Diuretics
- Propranolol
- Calcium channel blockers
- Dilantin
- Cimetidine
- Corticosteroids

Evaluation

- Same as for DKA

Treatment options

- IV NS 10–20 cc/kg/hour; may repeat prn; should not exceed 50 cc/kg total over 4 hours
- Continued IV with $^1/_2$NS or NS at 5 cc/kg/hour after initial fluid therapy
- Add D5$^1/_2$NS or D5NS when plasma glucose reaches 300 mg/dL
- Start insulin infusion 0.1 unit/kg/hour (up to 5–7 units/hour) after first hour of IV fluid therapy
  - Insulin doses often lower than used in DKA

Potassium treatment

- Add potassium 20–40 mEq to each liter of IV fluids when serum K^+ < 5.3 mEq/L if urine output 0.5–1 cc/kg/hour or initial potassium < 3.3 mEq/L
  - Serum K^+ 4.5–5.2 mEq/L give 10 mEq/hour IV
  - Serum K^+ 3.0–4.5 mEq/L give 20 mEq/hour IV
  - Serum K^+ initially < 3.0 mEq/L hold off starting insulin and give potassium IV

Consult criteria

- Notify physician on all HHS patients

Hypoglycemia

Definition

- < 70 mg/dL in adults (usually symptoms < 50 mg/dL)
- < 45 mg/dL in infants and children

Differential diagnosis

- CVA
- TIA
- Epilepsy
- Multiple sclerosis

- Psychosis

Considerations

Caused by:

- Accidental or intentional overdose of diabetic medications
- Sepsis
- Alcohol use
- Decreased caloric intake

Symptoms

- Severity of symptoms depends on glucose level and rate of glucose decline
- Symptoms may be masked by beta–blockers
- Altered and decreased mental status
- Sweating
- Shaking
- Anxiety

Evaluation

- ABCs (Airway, breathing, circulation)
- IV
- Oxygen if hypoxic (avoid hyperoxia)
- Monitoring
- Accucheck
- History and physical exam
- Medication and food intake history

- Accucheck every 30 minutes × 2 hours or longer until stable glucose levels achieved
- BMP
- CBC if infection suspected
- Chest x-ray if pneumonia or aspiration suspected, or hypoxic
- U/A if infection suspected

Treatment options

- Awake and alert: complex calorie intake or fruit juice or dextrose gel or 1.5 tsp of jelly PO
- Altered mental status: IV D50W 1 amp adults (100 calories)
- D25W — 1 gm/kg in pediatrics not to exceed adult dose
- D12.5W for neonates (1 gm/kg)
- D10W drip at 75–100 cc/hour (adult) if repeat D50W boluses needed for recurrent hypoglycemia or hypoglycemic agent overdose
- Glucagon 1 mg IM if no IV access, may be repeated once only
  - May not work with depleted glycogen stores in malnutrition
    - Liver disease
    - Alcoholics
    - Neonates
- Octreotide can be used in sulfonylurea refractory hypoglycemia
- Hydrocortisone IV for adrenal insufficiency

Discharge criteria

- Stable glucose levels in diabetic patients on preexisting insulin therapy
- Good home support
- Reliable patient

Discharge instructions

- Hypoglycemia aftercare instructions
- Follow up with primary care provider within 12–24 hours

Consult criteria

- Oral hypoglycemia therapy (usually need admission)
- Fasting hypoglycemia not on diabetic medication
- Intentional insulin overdose
- Poor home situation
- Abnormal vital signs
- Continued altered mental status
- Significant comorbidities (cancer, hepatic disease, malnutrition, etc.)

Hyperglycemia without DKA or HHS

Considerations

- Most diabetic patients with elevated glucose levels are asymptomatic

- High glucose levels can affect body water balance
- Acute treatment for levels up to 400 mg/dL usually not needed unless there is a concurrent disease process

Common symptoms

- Polyuria
- Polydipsia (increased thirst)
- Weakness
- Blurred vision

Evaluation

- Glucose < 400 mg/dL without other disease processes or symptoms may not need further testing acutely in patient with history of poor control (if vital signs normal and mentation changes or comorbidities absent)
- Tests are directed to disease processes that may be elevating glucose levels
- BMP or CMP
- CBC if infection or inflammatory process suspected
- U/A if UTI suspected

Discharge criteria

- If new onset DM in obese adult patient without DKA or HHS and glucose ≤ 400
- Diabetic history with glucose ≤ 400 mg/dL
- No metabolic acidosis
- No dehydration
- Normal vital signs and no mentation changes

Discharge instructions

- Hyperglycemia aftercare instructions
- Follow up with primary care provider within 1–5 days
- Return if patient develops symptoms

Consult criteria

New onset

- New adult onset DM with glucose > 400 mg/dL
- New onset pediatric DM with glucose ≥ 200 mg/dL
- Hyperglycemia with metabolic acidosis (decreased serum CO_2 or elevated anion gap)

Diabetic patient with

- Significant comorbid symptoms
- Metabolic acidosis
- Vomiting
- Dehydration
- Tachycardia
- Hypotension
- Relative hypotension SBP < 105 with history of hypertension
- Orthostatic vital sign changes
- Progressive renal insufficiency creatinine increase > 1
- Adult heart rate ≥ 110
- Pediatric heart rate
  - 12–15 years ≥ 120
  - 16 years or older ≥ 115

Glucose > 400 mg/dL in asymptomatic diabetic patient

Treatment for Type 2 Adult Diabetes If desired at discharge from acute care facility

Obese

Monotherapy

- Metformin 500 mg PO bid with or after meals × 1 week, increase weekly by 500 mg to achieve 1000 mg PO bid
  - Decreases HbA1c approximated 1.5%

Second drug if needed

- Glipizide (Glucotrol) 5 mg PO qday with breakfast (elderly 2.5 mg PO)

OR

- Consider GLP-1 agonist such as Exenatide (Byetta) 5 mcg SQ bid x 1 month and then may increase as needed to 10 mcg SQ bid

  - Give 1 hr. before AM and PM meals

OR

- Consider SGLT–2 inhibitor such as Empagliflozin (Jardiance) 10 mg PO daily

Third drug if needed

- Insulin glargine 10 units SQ (or 0.2 units/kg) –adjust by 1 unit/day to achieve fasting glucose < 100 mg/dL

OR

- Sitagliptin (Januvia 50 or 100 mg qday

Non-obese

Monotherapy

- Metformin 500 mg PO bid with or after meals × 1 week, increase weekly by 500 mg to achieve 1000 mg PO bid

OR

- Glipizide (Glucotrol) 5mg PO qday (elderly 2.5 mg PO)

Second drug if needed

- Metformin 500 mg PO bid with or after meals × 1 week, increase weekly by 500 mg to achieve 1000 mg PO bid

OR

- Glipizide 5mg (Glucotrol) PO qday (elderly 2.5 mg PO)

Third drug if needed

- Consider DLP-1 Agonist such as Exenatide (Byetta) 5 mcg SQ bid x 1 month and then may increase as needed to 10 mcg SQ bid
  - Give 1 hr. before AM and PM meals

OR

- Insulin glargine 10 units SQ – adjust by 1 unit/day to achieve fasting glucose < 100 mg/dL

Elderly

Monotherapy

- Metformin 500 mg bid with or after meals x 1 week, increase weekly by 500 mg to achieve 1000 mg PO bid
- If unable to tolerate metformin, consider repaglinide (Prandin) 0.5–4 mg PO up to qid ac (not to exceed 16 mg daily)

Monotherapy failure

- Consider DPP–4 inhibitor such as Januvia (Sitagliptin) 50 mg PO daily

OR

- Consider switch to long acting insulin 10 units SQ bedtime

Asians

Monotherapy

- Pioglitazone (Actos) 30 mg PO qday — do not use in bladder cancer, history of bladder cancer, moderate or severe hepatic disease or symptomatic heart failure (NYHA class 3 or 4)

Second drug if needed

- Metformin 500 mg PO bid with or after meals × 1 week, increase weekly by 500 mg to achieve 1,000 mg PO bid

Third drug if needed

- Glipizide or glimepiride

OR

- Exenatide (Byetta) 5 mcg SQ bid x 1 month and then may increase as needed to 10 mcg SQ bid (not FDA approved with Actos)
  - Give 1 hr. before AM and PM meals

OR

- Insulin glargine 10 units SQ — adjust by 1 unit/day to achieve fasting glucose < 100 mg/dL

Symptomatic patients

- Repaglinide (Prandin) 0.5–4 mg PO up to qid ac (not to exceed 16 mg qday) or insulin to decrease glucose at start of monotherapy initiation

Diabetic medications, mechanism of actions and clinical effects

Biguanides

- Metformin is the only biguanide in clinical use
- Initial drug of choice
- Decreases hepatic gluconeogenesis production
- Decreases intestinal absorption of glucose
- Improves insulin sensitivity by increasing peripheral glucose uptake and utilization
- Unlike oral sulfonylureas, metformin rarely causes hypoglycemia
- Significant improvements in hemoglobin A1c and lipid profile
- Only oral diabetes drug that reliably facilitates modest weight loss
- Probably improves macrovascular risk
- Lactic acidosis during metformin use is very rare (CKD with IV contrast—GFR<30–45 mL/minute)

Sulfonylureas

- Glyburide, glipizide and glimepiride
- Stimulate insulin release from pancreatic beta cells
- Indicated for use as adjuncts to diet and exercise in adult patients with type 2 diabetes mellitus
- Generally well-tolerated, with hypoglycemia the most common side effect
- Glyburide had highest cardiovascular mortality (7.5%) compared with other sulfonylureas, such as gliclazide and glimepiride (2.7%) and raises question of whether it should be used

Meglitinide derivatives

- Repaglinide and nateglinide
- Much shorter-acting insulin secretagogues that stimulate insulin release more than the sulfonylureas
- Can be used as monotherapy
- If adequate glycemic control is not achieved, then metformin or a thiazolidinedione may be added

Alpha-glucosidase inhibitors

- Acarbose (Precose) and Miglitol (Glyset)
- Delay sugar absorption and help to prevent postprandial glucose surges
- Induction of flatulence greatly limits their use

Thiazolidinediones (TZDs)

- Pioglitazone (Actos) and rosiglitazone (Avandia)
- Insulin sensitizers and require presence of insulin to work
- May be used as monotherapy or in combination with sulfonylurea, metformin, meglitinide, DPP-4 inhibitors, GLP-1 receptor agonists, or insulin
- Only antidiabetic agents that have been shown to slow the progression of diabetes (particularly in early disease)
- Edema (including macular edema) and weight gain may be problematic adverse effects
- May induce or worsen heart failure in patients with left ventricular compromise and occasionally in patients with normal left ventricular function
- Food and Drug Administration (FDA) currently recommends not prescribing pioglitazone for patients with active bladder cancer and using it with caution in patients with a history of bladder cancer
- In women with type 2 diabetes, long-term (1 yr. or longer) use of TZDs doubles the risk of fracture

- Elevated risk of myocardial infarction in patients treated with rosiglitazone (FDA limits to patients already being successfully treated with this agent and to patients whose blood sugar cannot be controlled with other antidiabetic medicines and who do not wish to use pioglitazone)

Glucagonlike peptide–1 (GLP-1) agonists

- Exenatide, liraglutide, albiglutide and dulaglutide
- Stimulate glucose-dependent insulin release
- Reduce glucagon and slow gastric emptying
- GLP-1 in addition to metformin and/or a sulfonylurea may result in modest weight loss

Dipeptidyl peptidase IV (DPP-4) inhibitors

- Sitagliptin, saxagliptin and linagliptin
- Prolong the action of incretin hormones (stimulate insulin secretion)
- May be added, if inadequate diabetic control, to metformin and sulfonylurea combination improving glycemic control
- Saxagliptin and alogliptin may increase heart failure risk, especially in patients with preexisting heart or renal disease

Selective sodium-glucose transporter-2 (SGLT-2) inhibitors

- Canagliflozin, dapagliflozin (Farxiga) and empagliflozin
- Increased urinary glucose excretion
- Adjunct to diet and exercise to improve glycemic control
- Renal dosing adjustments and warnings
- Dapagliflozin is indicated as monotherapy, as initial therapy with metformin, or as an add-on to other oral glucose-lowering agents, including metformin, pioglitazone, glimepiride, sitagliptin, and insulin
- May be used in systolic heart failure NYHA class II–IV
- May result in weight loss

Insulins

- Many patients with type 2 diabetes mellitus become markedly insulinopenic
- Most patients are insulin resistant
- Small changes in insulin dosage may make no difference in glycemia in some patients
- Therapy must be individualized
- For lowering postprandial glucose, premixed insulin analogues are more effective than either long-acting insulin analogues alone or premixed neutral protamine Hagedorn (NPH)/regular human insulin 70/30
- For lowering HbA1c, premixed insulin analogues are as effective as premixed NPH/regular human insulin 70/30 and more effective than long-acting insulin analogues
- The frequency of hypoglycemia reported with premixed insulin analogues is similar to that with premixed human insulin and higher than that with oral antidiabetic agents

Amylinomimetics

- Pramlintide
- Mimics the effects of endogenous amylin, which is secreted by pancreatic beta cells
- Delays gastric emptying, decreases postprandial glucagon release, and modulates appetite

Bile acid sequestrants

- Colesevelam

- Developed as lipid-lowering agents for the treatment of hypercholesterolemia but were subsequently found to have a glucose-lowering effect
- Adjunctive therapy to improve glycemic control
- Favorable, but insignificant, impact on FPG and HbA1c levels

Dopamine agonists

- Bromocriptine mesylate (Cycloset)
- Adjunct to diet and exercise to improve glycemic control in adults with type 2 diabetes mellitus
- May be considered for obese patients who do not tolerate other diabetes medications or who need only a minimal reduction in HbA1c to reach their glycemic goal
- Can cause orthostatic hypotension and syncope

Agency for Healthcare Research and Quality

- AHRQ concluded that although the long-term benefits and harms of diabetes medications remain unclear, the evidence supports the use of metformin as a first-line agent
- On average, monotherapy with many of the oral diabetes drugs reduces HbA1c levels by 1 percentage point (although metformin has been found to be more efficacious than the DPP-4 inhibitors), and 2-drug combination therapies reduce HbA1c about 1 percentage point more than do monotherapies

Other AHRQ findings included the following:

- Metformin decreased LDL cholesterol levels more relative to pioglitazone, sulfonylureas, and DPP-4 inhibitors
- Unfavorable effects on weight were greater with TZDs and sulfonylureas than with metformin (mean difference of +2.6 kg)
- Risk of mild or moderate hypoglycemia was 4-fold higher with sulfonylureas than with metformin alone; this risk was more than 5-fold higher with sulfonylureas plus metformin than with a TZD plus metformin
- Risk of heart failure was higher with TZDs than with sulfonylureas
- Risk of bone fractures was higher with TZDs than with metformin

Notes

REFERENCES:

Umpierrez, GE, et al. Narrative review: ketosis-prone type 2 diabetes mellitus *Ann Intern Med* 2006;144: 350

Type 2 Diabetes Mellitus Treatment & Management Author: Romesh Khardori, MD, PhD, FACP; Chief Editor: George T Griffing
emedicine.medscape.com/article/117853

Type 1 Diabetes Mellitus Author: Romesh Khardori, MD, PhD, FACP; Chief Editor: George T Griffing, MD
emedicine.medscape.com/article/117739

Diabetic Ketoacidosis Author: Vasudevan A Raghavan, MBBS, MD, MRCP(UK); Chief Editor: Romesh Khardori, MD, PhD, FACP
emedicine.medscape.com/article/118361

Savage MW, Dhatariya KK, Kilvert A, Rayman G, Rees JA, Courtney CH, et al. Joint British Diabetes Societies guideline for the management of diabetic ketoacidosis. *Diabet Med.* May 2011;28(5):508–15

Acute Hypoglycemia Author: Frank C Smeeks III, MD; Chief Editor: Erik D Schraga, MD
emedicine.medscape.com/article/767359

Effectivehealthcare.ahrq.gov/ehc/products/155/644/CER27_OralDiabetesMeds_20110623.pdf

Ped Emerg Care;31:376

Diabetic ketoacidosis; Davie E. Trachtenbarg, M.D., *University of Illinois College of Medicine, Peoria, Illinois*
Am Fam Physician. 2005 May 1;71(9):1705-1714

Kuppermann N, et al. *N Engl J Med.* 2018;378(24): 2275-2287.

Glaser N, Kuppermann N. *Pediatr Diabetes.* 2018 Nov 11

Am J EM. 2021;44:157

Diabetic Ketoacidosis (DKA)
Updated: Jan 19, 2021 Author: Osama Hamdy, MD, PhD; Chief Editor: Romesh Khardori, MD, PhD, FACP
emedicine.medscape.com/article/118361

Hypothyroidism Protocol

Definition

- Deficiency or lack of thyroid hormone that causes slowing of metabolic processes

Differential Diagnosis

- Hypothermia
- Sepsis
- Depression
- Constipation
- Addison's disease
- Chronic fatigue syndrome
- Dysmenorrhea
- Goiter — lithium induced
- Nontoxic goiter
- Hypopituitarism
- Subacute thyroiditis
- Iodine deficiency
- Ovarian insufficiency
- Prolactin deficiency

Considerations

- Deficiency of thyroid hormone
- Develops over months to years
- Primary hypothyroidism 95% of cases
- Secondary hypothyroidism 5% of cases
- Postpartum thyroiditis is 5% and usually occurs 3–6 months after delivery
- Myxedema coma is a rare, life threatening condition usually of elderly women
  - Precipitated by environmental stress, infection and medications
  - Frequently a clinical diagnosis initially

Signs and symptoms

- Goiter
- Cold intolerance
- Hypothermia
- Bradycardia
- Lethargy
- Altered mental status
- Ataxia
- Coma
- Depression
- Hair loss
- Dry coarse skin
- Weight gain
- Constipation
- Headache
- Husky voice
- Deep tendon ankle jerk reflex with prolonged recovery phase
- Hypercarbia
- Hyponatremia

- Cardiomegaly, pericardial effusion, cardiogenic shock, and ascites may be present

Causes

- Idiopathic
- Iodine deficiency (most common cause worldwide)
- Hashimoto's thyroiditis (most common cause in U.S.)
- Radioiodine treatment for hyperthyroidism (Graves's disease)
- Thyroid resection
- Lithium
- Amiodarone
- Dilantin
- Carbamazepine
- Iodides
- Pituitary or hypothalamic disorders: tumor, radiation, surgery, sarcoidosis
- Postpartum

Evaluation

- Complete history and physical examination

Testing options depending on history and findings

- CBC (may be anemic)
- BMP (reversible increases in creatinine)
- Chest x-ray for pericardial effusions and cardiomegaly
- ABG if respiratory insufficiency present
- EKG
- U/A
- Thyroid stimulating hormone (TSH) is elevated with low FTI (free thyroxin index) or T4
  - Mild disease if FTI or T4 normal
  - Subclinical hypothyroidism with TSH 4.5-10 mIU/L with normal T4 and T3
- Thyroid function tests if available
- Routine screening at age 35 and every 5 years after that
  - Closer attention to pregnant females or females > age 60, type-1 diabetes or autoimmune disease, or with history of neck irradiation

Treatment Options

- Preferable for primary care provider to start thyroid hormone replacement
- Clinical benefits occur in 3–5 days
- Controversy exists on whether to treat subclinical hypothyroidism (asymptomatic), unless TSH > 10 mIU/L or pregnant
- Treat subclinical hypothyroidism patients with TSH levels of 5–10 mIU/L in conjunction with goiter or positive anti-TPO antibodies
- Adjust levothyroxine every 6–8 weeks until reference range of TSH achieved
- May take months to achieve target TSH reference range
  - Levothyroxin 0.1 mg PO qday — age ≤ 60 years
  - Levothyroxin 0.025–0.05 mg PO qday — age > 60 years (1/4–1/2 of this dose if there is history of heart disease)

Myxedema coma — notify physician immediately

- End of spectrum of hypothyroidism
- IV NS/LR as needed for hypotension
- Levothyroxine 400 mcg IV slow infusion
- May need intubation
- Hydrocortisone sodium succinate (Solu–Cortef) 100 mg IV
- Treat any infection
- Passive rewarming

Discharge Criteria

- Mild disease

Discharge instructions

- Hypothyroidism aftercare instructions
- Follow up with primary care provider within 7 days if seen in acute care facility
- Return if worse

Consult Criteria

- Unstable patient
- Altered mental status
- Hypothermia
- Metabolic or respiratory acidosis
- Respiratory insufficiency
- Refer to General Patient Criteria Protocol (page 15)

Notes

REFERENCES:

Kreisman SH, Hennessey JV. Consistent reversible elevations of serum creatinine levels in severe hypothyroidism.*Arch Intern Med.* Jan 11 1999;159(1):79–82

Ladenson PW, Singer PA, Ain KB, Bagchi N, Bigos ST, Levy EG, et al. American Thyroid Association guidelines for detection of thyroid dysfunction. *Arch Intern Med.* Jun 12 2000;160(11):1573–5

Hypothyroidism Treatment & Management; Updated: Mar 03, 2021
Author: Philip R Orlander, MD, FACP; Chief Editor: George T Griffing, MD
emedicine.medscape.com/article/122393

Hyperthyroidism Protocol

Definition

- Condition from excess thyroid hormone

Differential Diagnosis

- Panic disorder
- Septic shock
- Delirium tremens
- Neuroleptic malignant syndrome
- Serotonin syndrome
- Withdrawal syndromes
- Heat illness
- Cocaine toxicity
- Sympathomimetic drug overdose
- Congestive heart failure
- Pheochromocytoma
- Pregnancy

Considerations

- Graves' disease most common form — autoimmune disease
- 1–2% of patients progress to thyroid storm
- Thyroid storm is potentially fatal
- Normal TSH usually excludes hyperthyroidism
- Subclinical hyperthyroidism, defined as a low thyroid-stimulating hormone (TSH) level with normal free thyroxine (FT4) and free triiodothyronine (FT3) levels, is associated with no or minimal clinical symptoms of thyrotoxicosis
  - 3 fold increase of atrial fibrillation

Treatment considerations

- Counteracting the peripheral effects of thyroid hormones
- Inhibition of thyroid hormone synthesis
- Treatment of systemic complications
- These measures should bring about clinical improvement within 12–24 hours
- Cardiopulmonary failure most likely cause of death, particularly in the elderly
- Beta blockage can cause collapse

Signs and Symptoms

- Tachycardia
- Weight loss
- Heat intolerance
- Fever
- Diaphoresis

- Dehydration
- Diarrhea
- Goiter
- Hypotension
- Atrial fibrillation
- Exophthalmos and lid lag (Graves' disease only)
- Fine tremor

Causes

- Grave's disease — most common
- Idiopathic — second most common (toxic multinodular goiter)
- Subacute thyroiditis
- Postpartum thyroiditis
- Overdose of thyroid hormone
- Iodine induced
- Amiodarone (high iodine content or induces autoimmune thyroid disease)

Thyroid storm

- Normal TSH usually excludes thyroid storm
- Is a clinical diagnosis initially and start treatment early
- Thyroid function tests do not differentiate between thyrotoxicosis and thyroid storm
- LFT's elevated and hyperglycemia may be present

Severe symptoms

- Shock (use isotonic fluid resuscitation) — avoid norepinephrine as it can worsen symptoms
- Fever
- Altered mental status
- Psychosis
- CHF
- Jaundice

Precipitated by

- Stress
- Infection
- Surgery
- Cardiovascular events
- Preeclampsia
- DKA or HHS
- Stopping antithyroid medication
- Vigorous palpation of thyroid

Evaluation

- Complete history and physical examination

Testing

- CBC
- BMP
- Calcium
- LFT's
- EKG
- Thyroid function tests
- TSH

Treatment Options

- O_2 supplemental
- Tylenol for fever (no aspirin)

Mild hyperthyroidism

- Methimazole 15 mg/day PO divided q8hr initially (drug of choice)

Moderate thyrotoxicosis

- Methimazole 30–40 mg/day PO divided q8hr initially (drug of choice)
- PTU (propylthiouracil) 150–450 mg/day PO or NG tube (second-line drug to methimazole)
- Propranolol 20–40 mg PO q4hr until tachycardia controlled (also blocks conversion of T4 to T3)
- Dexamethasone 2 mg PO or IV q6h to q8hr in adults
- Dexamethasone 0.15 mg/kg/dose PO or IV q6hr in pediatrics (not to exceed adult dose)

Thyroid storm treatment options

- IV NS 100–200 cc/hr in adults or higher if needed for vital sign findings
- IV NS 1–3 times daily fluid maintenance prn for pediatrics
- IV LR/NS hydration usually needed for volume contraction

Propylthiouracil (PTU)

- Adult: 600–1,000 mg PO or 200–300 mg q4–6h PO/NG (preferred over methimazole in thyroid storm)
- Pediatric: 5–7 mg/kg/day

Methimazole

- 20–30 mg q6–12hr for short term, then reduce dosage to maintenance (5–15 mg/day) or reduce frequency to q12hr or q24hr

SSKI

- 1–5 drops PO 1–2 hours after PTU
    - Earlier than this can increase release of thyroid hormone from the thyroid

Decadron (dexamethasone)

- Adult: 2 mg IV q6hr
- Pediatric: Dexamethasone 0.15 mg/kg/dose PO or IV q6hr in pediatrics (not to exceed adult dose)

Propranolol

- 1–2 mg IV; repeat q 10–15 min. prn (caution with CHF and DKA)

Outpatient treatment (Graves' disease)

- Methimazole 10–20 mg/day PO (drug of choice)
    - After euthyroidism is achieved, reduce dosage by 50% and administer for 12–18 months
- PTU can be used if pregnant in 1st trimester or contraindications/allergy to methimazole
    - Initiate PTU 150 mg PO qday divided q8h (second–line drug to methimazole)
    - Taper and discontinue if euthyroidism restored (TSH) is normal

Discharge Criteria

- Mildly symptomatic patients that respond to therapy

Discharge instructions

- Hyperthyroidism aftercare instructions
- Follow up with primary care provider or endocrinologist within 1–2 days

Consult Criteria

- Moderate thyrotoxicosis
- Fever
- Thyroid storm — notify physician immediately
- Adult heart rate ≥ 110
- Pediatric heart rate
    - 0–4 months ≥ 180
    - 5–7 months ≥ 175
    - 8–12 months ≥ 170
    - 1–3 years ≥ 160
    - 4–5 years ≥ 145
    - 6–8 years ≥ 130
    - 9–11 years ≥ 125
    - 12–15 years ≥ 115
    - 16 years or older ≥ 110

Notes

____

____

____

REFERENCES:

Dtsch Med Wochenschr. 2008 Mar;133(10):479–84. doi: 10.1055/s-2008–1046737. Thyroid storm--thyrotoxic crisis: an update

Hyperthyroidism, Thyroid Storm, and Graves Disease
Author: Erik D Schraga, MD; Chief Editor: Romesh Khardori, MD, PhD, FACP
emedicine.medscape.com/article/767130

Hyperthyroidism and Thyrotoxicosis
Updated: Oct 19, 2020
Author: Stephanie L Lee, MD, PhD; Chief Editor: Romesh Khardori, MD, PhD, FACP
emedicine.medscape.com/article/121865

Toxic Ingestions

Section Contents — one protocol

Toxicology Protocol

When using any protocol, always follow the Guidelines of Proper Use (page 12).

Toxicology Protocol

Considerations

Principles of toxicology

- Reduce exposure (remove from skin and environment)
- Reduce absorption
- Increase elimination
- Supportive care
- Give specific therapy and antidotes when appropriate

Pearls

- Most pediatric accidental ingestions of common OTC medications are of low dose and may require only observation for 2–4 hours
- Intentional ingestions require acute psychiatric intervention
- Ascertain types and amount of ingestions

Syrup of Ipecac not usually recommended

Activated charcoal

- Usually of no benefit
- Can be used if no aspiration risk < 1 hour post ingestion with serious ingestions
- May be considered > 1 hour post serious ingestion with agents that delay absorption or GI transit

Orogastric lavage use indications

- Presentations approximately within one hour post-ingestion
- No known antidote
- Substance does not bind activated charcoal

Whole bowel irrigation indications and considerations

- With lithium and iron ingestion
- In "body stuffers"
- Beware of aspiration risk
- Avoid with decreased bowel sounds, surgical abdomen, or hypotension

Toxidromes (causes and symptoms)

Opioids

Agents

- Narcotics

Findings

- CNS depression
- Respiratory depression
- Miosis

Treatment options

- Narcan (Naloxone) 1–2 mg IV, may need to be repeated more than once or IV drip, 0.005 mg/kg load, 0.0025

mg/kg/hr. for opiate symptom recurrence
    - May use dose that achieved desired result as IV drip rate/hr.
    - Chronic opiate abuse use smallest doses and titrate prn respiratory depression
- Narcan (Naloxone) nasal spray 4 mg/spray, one nostril alternating q2–3 minutes prn
- Observe over 4 hours, admit if needed depending on clinical situation and substance used

Sympathomimetics

Agents

- Cocaine
- Amphetamine
- Methamphetamine

Findings

- Agitation
- Pupil dilation
- Diaphoresis
- Tachycardia
- Hypertension
- Hyperthermia

Treatment

- Agitation
    - Lorazepam or other benzodiazepines
    - Haloperidol or droperidol second line agent
- Seizure
    - Lorazepam 2–4 mg IV to start, increase or repeat as needed (see Seizure Protocol)
    - Cerebyx 15–20 mg PE IV at 100–150 mg/minute
    - Neuromuscular blockage for intractable seizure after intubation
- Hypertension and/or chest pain (AMI)
    - Labetalol 20 mg IV over 2 minutes, may repeat q10 minutes, increasing to 40–80 mg IV q10 minutes if needed (NMT 300mg)
        - Infusion 1–2 mg/minute if needed
    - Metoprolol 2.5–5 mg IV q5minutes prn (medical dogma concerned about unopposed alpha simulation though case reports are rare)
    - Nitroprusside for hypertension
- Arrhythmia — same as Hypertension or chest pain treatment above
- Hyperthermia
    - Ice packs to groin
    - Cooling measures
    - Neuromuscular paralysis after intubation if severe

Cholinergic

Agents

- Insecticides

Findings

- Salivation
- Lacrimation
- Diaphoresis
- Nausea
- Vomiting
- Urination
- Defecation
- Muscle fasciculations
- Weakness
- Bronchorrhea

Treatment options

- Atropine 2–4 mg IV (may need 20–40 mg IV total over time)
- Decontamination
- Pralidoxime

Anticholinergic

Agents

- Antihistamines
- Atropine
- Scopolamine

Findings

- Altered mental status
- Dilated pupils
- Dry/flushed skin and mucous membranes
- Urinary retention
- Decreased bowel sounds

- Hyperthermia

Treatment

- If acute wide QRS and tachycardia give sodium bicarbonate ($NaHCO_3^-$) 1–2 ampules, repeat prn
  - Bicarbonate drip 0.5–1 mEq/kg/hour IV
- Agitation or seizures
  - Lorazepam 2–4 mg IV to start, increase as needed (see Seizure Protocol)
- Physostigmine 0.5–2 mg IV over 5 minutes (controversial)

Salicylates

Agents

- Aspirin
- Oil of wintergreen (1 tsp lethal in child weighing < 10 kg; 1 cc has 14 gms of salicylate)

Findings

- Tachypnea
- Respiratory alkalosis
- Metabolic acidosis
- Altered mental status
- Tinnitus
- Tachycardia
- Nausea
- Vomiting
- Diaphoresis

Treatment

- See hemodialysis indications below
- If significant exposure and toxicity—IV NS or LR 10–20 mg/kg/hour to maintain urine output 1–1.5 ml/hour
- Sodium bicarbonate ($NaHCO_3^-$) 1meq/kg IV bolus
- 3 ampules of $NaHCO_3^-$ /D5W liter at 2 times maintenance
  - Goal is urine pH 7.5

Hypoglycemia

Agents

- Oral hypoglycemia agents
- Insulin

Findings

- Altered mental status
- Diaphoresis
- Tachycardia
- Hypertension

Treatment

- Glucose IV or oral depending on severity
- Repeat accuchecks q30–60 minutes depending on severity and likelihood of recurrent hypoglycemia
- Insulin induced hypoglycemia usually can be discharged depending on clinical situation
- Oral hypoglycemic medication induced hypoglycemia usually needs admission or prolonged observation

Serotonin syndrome

Agents

- Meperidine or dextromethorphan + MAOI (monoamine oxidase inhibitors)
- SSRI (selective serotonin reuptake inhibitor) + tricyclic antidepressant
- SSRI + amphetamine
- Tricyclic antidepressant + amphetamine
- MAOI+ amphetamine
- SSRI overdose

Findings

- Altered mental status
- Increased muscle tone
- Hyperreflexia
- Hyperthermia

Treatment

- Remove agent (recent ingestion may give activated charcoal)
- Supportive care (ICU)
  - Oxygen
  - IV fluids
  - Airway support or intubation as needed
  - Continuous cardiac monitoring including QTc and QRS duration

- External cooling measures for hyperthermia, especially > 40C
  - May need neuromuscular paralysis in severe cases
- Serotonin antagonist cyproheptadine
- Severe hypertension can be treated with esmolol or clevidipine
- Acetaminophen and other antipyretics not useful

Cannabinoid Hyperemesis Syndrome

- Intractable vomiting in heavy cannabis users
- Runs hot shower or bath over abdomen for relief history
- THC detectable for up to 72 hours THC for single use and detectable up to 1 month in heavy users
- Illegal synthetic cannabinoids such as "Spice" or "K2" are not detected on urine drug screen for marijuana because chemical structures are different from THC

Treatment

- Haloperidol in doses of 2 – 5 mg IV
  - THC has been shown to increase dopamine synthesis and dopamine cell firing, which may explain clinical improvement with haloperidol
- Topical capsaicin cream
- IV LR or NS for dehydration or acute kidney injury

Evaluation

- Complete history and physical exam
- Contact Poison Control Center
- Cardiac monitoring and EKG with potential toxic ingestions
- Send someone to patient's home to obtain ingestants if necessary
- CMP
- Specific drugs levels if available
- Calculate anion gap: $Na^+ - Cl^- - HCO_3^-$
- CT head for altered mental status not clearly attributable to toxin/overdose/ingestion
- Evaluate for comorbid conditions
- ASA and acetaminophen nomograms as indicated

Anion gap mnemonic — A CAT MUDPILES

A – Alcoholic ketoacidosis
C – Cyanide; carbon monoxide
A – Aspirin; other salicylates
T – Toluene
M – Methanol; metformin
U – Uremia
D – DKA
P – Paraldehyde; phenformin
I – Iron; INH
L – Lactic acidosis
E – Ethylene glycol
S – Starvation

Osmolol gap ≥ 10–20 suspect substance ingestion (Normal < 10)

- Gap = Osmolality measured – Osmolality calculated (calculation equation: $2(Na^+ + K^+)$ + glucose/18 + BUN/2.8; normal 280–300mOsm/L)
- Ethanol measured mg%/4.6 is added to osmolol gap equation if present
- Gap > 50 carries high specificity for toxic alcohol such as methanol, ethylene glycol, or isopropyl alcohol
- Normal gap < 10

Treatment Options

- Nontoxic ingestions: observation and discharge with instructions and follow up
- Suspected toxic ingestions: refer to previous Considerations section and contact Poison Control Center
- IV NS
- Hypotension
  - Adult IV NS 500–1000 cc bolus if hypotensive , may repeat as needed

- Pediatrics 20 cc/kg IV NS bolus, may repeat × 2 prn
- Specific antidotes per poison control center
- Coma cocktail
  - Dextrose
  - Naloxone (Narcan) 0.4–2 mg IV/IM/SQ q2–3 minutes prn (0.01 mg/kg) — NMT 10 mg usually
    - Nasal spray 4 mg (1 spray) alternating nostrils q2–3 minutes prn
  - Thiamine
  - Flumazenil (Is thought to increase seizure in benzodiazepine overdose or chronic users—this is controversial)
    - Recent data suggest low risk of seizure
  - Seizure patients may have keppra or valproic acid treatment with flumazenil

Hemodialysis indications for severe ingestions

- Ethylene glycol or methanol (fomepizole should be given also as treatment)
- Salicylate
  - Level > 90 mg/dL in acute ingestion
  - Level > 80 mg/dL in renal failure
  - Level > 60 mg/dL in chronic ingestion
  - Severe symptoms
  - Unable to alkalinize urine in a less severe ingestion
  - Large ingestion (death may result if not hemodialyzed promptly)
  - Pulmonary edema
  - Seizures
  - Renal failure
  - CNS depression
- Phenobarbital
- Theophylline
- Lithium
- Valproic acid level > 750 or severe symptoms
- Diethylene glycol
- Massive acetaminophen ingestion > 1000 mg/kg if early post-ingestion

Seizures

- Adult: lorazepam 2–6 mg IV; may repeat q10–15 minutes prn
- Pediatric: lorazepam 0.05–0.1 mg/kg IV; may repeat q10–15 minutes prn (NMT 10 mg)
- If no IV available in children, use Diastat (diazepam rectal gel)
  - Age up to 5 years: 0.5 mg/kg
  - Age 6–11 years: 0.3 mg/kg
  - Age > 12 years: 0.2 mg/kg
  - Round up to available dose: 2.5, 5, 7.5, 10, 12.5, 15, 17.5, 20 mg/dose
- Midazolam IV/IM/PR/ET/intranasal 0.1–0.2 mg/kg/dose; not to exceed a cumulative dose of 10 mg)

Antidotes (if clinically indicated)

- **Acetaminophen:** N-acetylcysteine
  - Give if ingestion suspected with elevated ALT
  - Give even if acetaminophen induced hepatic failure present and acetaminophen no longer measurable
- **Anticholinergic**: physostigmine
- **Benzodiazepines:** flumazenil (thought to increase seizure potential — controversial)
  - Recent data suggest low risk of seizure
  - Seizure patients may have keppra or valproic acid treatment with flumazenil
- **Beta**–blockers**:** glucagon
- **Calcium channel blockers:** calcium chloride, insulin
  - Calcium channel blocker severe toxicity
    - CaCl 1–3 gms (10–30 mg/kg) q30 min. prn up to 8 doses
    - High dose insulin therapy
      - Bolus of 0.5–1 Unit/kg, followed by a drip with a rate of 0.5–1 Unit/kg/hr.

        - If blood glucose < 250 give supplemental IV glucose (D10)
        - Accucheck q15 min. to avoid hypoglycemia
    - Levophed IV if hypotensive
- **Carbon monoxide:** 100% FiO_2
    - Consider immediate transfer to hyperbaric facility if
        - Levels above 40%
        - Cardiovascular or neurologic impairment
        - Persistent impairment after 4 hours of oxygen therapy necessitates transfer to a hyperbaric facility
        - Pregnant patients with lower carboxyhemoglobin levels (above 15%)
        - Discuss with physician
- **Coumadin (warfarin):** vitamin K , FFP, Kcentra
    - FFP
        - INR is 1.5
    - Onset of action 13 – 48 hours
    - No clinical benefit in using if INR<1.7
- **Cyanide:** cyanide antidote kit
- **Digoxin (digitalis):** Digibind
    - 20 vials IV over 15–30 minutes in unknown amount ingested
    - Each vial of Digibind or Digifab binds 0.5 mg of digoxin ingested
    - Serum digoxin levels rise after using Digibind—do not use levels afterwards to guide continuing therapy
    - Toxicity during chronic therapy acute distress or for whom a serum digoxin concentration is not available — administer 6 vials
    - Activated charcoal is useful in limiting the absorption of ingested digoxin and is most beneficial if administered within 4 hours of ingestion
    - Phenytoin (Cerebyx PE) 15–20 mg/kg IV at up to 150 mg/minutes can be considered in digoxin toxic dysrhythmias if emergently needed and digibind not available
        - Also can be given for torsades de pointes refractory to magnesium or other medications
    - $MgSO_4$ 1–2 gms IV over 5 minutes and drip 1 gm/hr. can be considered in digoxin toxic dysrhythmias if emergently needed and digibind not available
- **Ethylene glycol and methanol:** fomepizole
    - Osmolol gap ≥ 10 = treatment indicated
    - Large ingestion is indication for stat hemodialysis
    - Serum lactic acid increase may be significant
    - Methanol clinically silent period of 12 - 24 hours
    - Time needed for methanol to be metabolized into formaldehyde and formic acid
- **Iron**: deferoxamine
- **INH:** pyridoxine (vitamin B6)
- **Methemoglobinemia:** methylene blue
- **Organophosphates:** atropine and/or PAM, atrovent aerosol for bronchospasm
- **Tricyclic antidepressants:** $NaHCO_3^-$ drip 0.5 mEq/kg/hour to maintain serum pH between 7.50–7.55
- **Opiates:** narcan (naloxone) for toxic narcotic overdose
    - For adults: Naloxone (Narcan) 0.4–2 mg IV/IM/SQ q2–3 minutes prn (0.01 mg/kg) — NMT 10 mg usually
    - Nasal spray 4 mg (1 spray) alternating nostrils q2–3 minutes prn
    - For pediatrics: narcan (naloxone) 0.1 mg/kg IV or IM (NMT 2 mg)
    - Drip 0.0025 mg/kg/hour if needed or dose used to achieve desired reversal as an hourly rate

Lipid Emulsion Therapy

- Start ACLS
- Mainstream therapy
- Safe
- Used in cardiac arrest due to a single agent
  - Bupivacaine (intra-arterial injection)
  - Verapamil
  - Amitriptyline
  - An unknown agent
- An initial bolus of 20% lipid emulsion at a dose of 1.5 mL/kg
  - Bolus could be repeated 1–2 times for persistent asystole
- Followed by an infusion at a rate of 0.25 ml/kg/min for 30–60 minutes
  - Infusion rate could be increased if the BP declines
- Interferes with some laboratory measurements
  - Serum glucose concentrations when determined by colorimetric testing
  - Serum magnesium
  - Creatinine, lipase, ALT, CPK and bilirubin become unmeasurable

Discharge criteria recommendation

- Psychiatrically cleared
- No toxicity present or is totally detoxified
- Hemodynamically stable
- Good follow up and home situation

Discharge instructions

- Drug or substance ingestion aftercare instructions
- Refer for substance abuse treatment as indicated
- Follow up with PCP within 1 days as needed
- Return if worse

Consult criteria recommendation

- Unstable vital signs
- Metabolic acidosis
- Osmolol gap ≥ 10
- Hypoglycemia secondary to oral hypoglycemic medications
- Altered mental status
- Acetaminophen ingestion
  - Pre-school child of 200 mg/kg or greater
  - Older child and adult > 150 mg/kg or total dose of 7.5 gms
  - Nomogram positive for toxicity
  - Liver function abnormalities
  - Delayed presentation
- Aspirin 150 mg/kg or serum level > 40 mg%
  - Lethal dose 300 mg/kg
  - Stat dialysis for massive ingestions

Notes

____

____

____

REFERENCES:

Lipidrescue.org recommended as reading for those interested in this therapy

Christian MR, et al. *J Med Toxicol* 2013 May 10

Grunbaum AM, et al. *Clin Toxicol (Phila)* 2012;50:812–7

Carbon Monoxide Toxicity Treatment & Management
Author: Guy N Shochat, MD; Chief Editor: Asim Tarabar, MD
emedicine.medscape.com/article/819987

Flumazenil Revisited Williams JS, Lee MA, Schauben J, Nasca L, Kalynynch C/University of Florida, Jacksonville, FL

Beta-Blockers for Cocaine and other Stimulant Toxicity
By John Richards, last update June 19, 2019

Richards JR, et al. *Pharmacotherapy*. 2017 Mar 31

Sorensen Cj, et al. *J Med Toxicol*. 2017 Mar;13(1):71-87

Inayat F, et al. *BMJ Case Rep*. 2017 Jan 4;2017

Witsil JC, et al. *Am J Ther*. 2017 Jan/Feb;24(1):e64-e67

Sorensen CJ, et al. *J Med Toxicol*. 2017 Mar 10

J Med Toxicol, 2017;13:71

J Med Toxicol, epub, 2016 Sep 29

Neuroimaging Clin N Am. 2018;28:435

Neurology

Section Contents

When using any protocol, always follow the Guidelines of Proper Use (page 12).

HEADACHE PROTOCOL

Definition

- Cephalic pain disorder

Differential Diagnosis

- Tension headache
- Migraine headache
- Cluster headache
- Sinusitis
- Otitis media
- Trigeminal neuralgia
- Brain tumor
- Subarachnoid hemorrhage
- Subdural hematoma
- Epidural hematoma
- Temporal arteritis
- Chronic daily headache
- Thunderclap headache
- Analgesic rebound headache
- CVA
- Meningitis
- Encephalitis
- Normal pressure hydrocephalus
- Ventricular peritoneal shunt malfunction
- Temporal mandibular joint disorder

Considerations

- "Functional" or "Primary" headache
  - No detectable cause (common)
  - Migraine
  - Cluster
  - Headache tension type
- "Organic" or "Secondary"
  - From pain sensitive structures; vessels; periosteum
  - Post-concussion headaches
  - Spinal tap headaches
- History is one of the more important tools in headache evaluation
- New headache type in elderly is suggestive of a higher risk process
- Do not use response to therapy to judge seriousness of headache
- Subarachnoid hemorrhage (SAH) up to 1% of all headaches in ED

- Sudden onset and reaching maximal intensity in seconds to minutes
- 1/3 not exertional
- May awake with SAH
- Sentinel leak in SAH headache may improve over time
- CT brain (3rd generation scanner or later) very low miss rate if performed within 6 hours of SAH headache onset
- **ACEP Policy states a negative noncontrast brain CT within first 6 hours in a neurologically intact patient precludes further evaluation for SAH.** If suspicion remains high further workup can be pursued.
  - Criteria for SAH rule-out within 6 hours
    - Hematocrit > 30%
    - Isolated thunderclap headache without seizure, syncope or neck pain
    - 3rd generation or later CT scanner
    - Read by radiologist

Lumbar puncture for possible SAH evaluation

- Xanthochromia is formed by the breakdown of hemoglobin and can take 2-12 hours to develop
- Xanthochromia will be present in up to 20% of patients with SAH who have an LP within 6 hours of headache onset
- Xanthochromia approaches 100% after 12 hours

Red flag headaches

- Sudden onset or onset with exertion
- New, progressive, frequent headaches
- Trauma
- Cancer history
- Immunosuppression/HIV
- Clotting disorders
- First headache
- Worst headache
- Fever

Evaluation

- Complete history and physical exam
- Check gait, motor and sensory exam
- Funduscopic exam

Lab (usually not needed in most headaches)

- CBC
- ESR (age > 50 years: temporal arteritis) — not needed with no changes in chronic headache pattern
- Carbon monoxide level prn
- UCG prn

Benign Headaches — Tension, Migraine, Cluster

General treatment options for all types of benign headaches

- Decadron (dexamethasone) 10 mg IV or IM for adults may be ordered, when not contraindicated, to decrease return visits for same headache
- O_2 therapy can be given for all types of headaches
- Lidocaine 1 cc of a 4% solution placed on a swab in each nostril for 5 minutes is potentially helpful
  - May repeat in 15 minutes

Tension headache

- Pressing or tightening (nonpulsatile quality)
- Frontal-occipital location
- Bilateral: mild/moderate intensity
- Not aggravated by physical activity

Treatment

- NSAID's PO prn
- Tylenol prn
- Fiorinal 1–2 PO q4hr prn not to exceed 6 per 24 hour period
- Midrin 1–2 caps qid PO prn

- Decadron 10 mg IV/IM decreases recurrence of headache at 48–72 hours

Migraine

Associated with:

- Photophobia
- Phonophobia
- Nausea and vomiting
- May be unilateral or bilateral
- Aura occurs 20%
  - Scotoma (blind spots)
  - Fortification (zigzag patterns)
  - Scintilla (flashing lights)
  - Unilateral paresthesia/weakness
  - Hallucinations
  - Hemianopsia
- The unilateral motor weakness associated with a hemiplegic migraine typically lasts from 5 minutes to 72 hours

Migraine risk factors

- Increased levels of C-reactive protein
- Increased body weight
- High blood pressure
- Hypercholesterolemia
- Impaired insulin sensitivity
- High homocysteine levels
- Stroke
- Coronary heart disease

Evaluation

- Don't perform neuroimaging studies in patients with stable headaches that meet criteria for migraine
- Don't perform computed tomography imaging for headache when magnetic resonance imaging is available, except in emergency settings

Indications for neuro imaging

- See related section below

Treatment options

- Compazine (prochlorperazine) 5–10 mg IV or IM (if available)
- Thorazine (chlorpromazine) 75 mg with Benadryl (diphenhydramine) 25 mg IM
  - Thorazine (chlorpromazine) can be given 25–50 mg IV at 1 mg/minute (may cause hypotension)
- Ergots DHE 1 mg IV or IM (caution with hypertension, CAD, kidney or liver disease, pregnancy, sepsis, recent vascular surgery and PAD)
- Reglan (metoclopramide) 10 mg IV or IM, may repeat x 1 in 15 minutes prn
- Sumatriptan 6 mg SQ (do not use with history of coronary artery disease) — read drug information
- Maxalt (rizatriptan) 5–10 mg PO q2h prn for headache not to exceed 30 mg/d. If taking propranolol then NMT 15 mg/day (do not use with history of coronary artery disease) — read drug information
- Nurtec ODT (rimegepant) 75 mg PO qday prn migraine
- Ubrelvy (ubrogepant) 50–100 mg PO x 1, may repeat in ≥ 2 hours if needed (NMT 200 mg per day)
- Ajovy (fremanezumab–vfrm) 225 mg SQ autoinjector qmonth
- Midrin 2 caps PO initially then 1 cap PO q1hr prn not to exceed 5 caps/day (caution with hypertension, tachycardia, MOAI's)
- Toradol (ketorolac) 15–30 mg IM (do not use if creatinine is elevated) —ketorolac therapeutic ceiling is around 10 mg
- Compazine suppository (prochlorperazine) 25 mg PR bid prn
- Don't prescribe opioid or butalbital-containing medications as first-line

treatment for recurrent headache disorders

- Don't recommend prolonged or frequent use of over-the-counter pain medications for headache
- Narcotic prn (not as preferred)
- Decadron 10 mg IV/IM decreases recurrence of headache at 48–72 hours

Intractable migraine (lasting > 72 hours)

- IV valproate up to 1 gm IV
- Dihydroergotamine 1 mg IV/IM/SQ
- May need hospital admission

Cluster

- Grouping of headaches that are lancinating and severe up to 8 times a day
- Sudden onset — peaks in 10–15 minutes
- Unilateral facial
- Duration: 10 minutes to 3 hours per episode
- Character: boring and lancinating to eye
- Distribution: first and second divisions of the trigeminal nerve (approximately 18–20% of patients complain of pain in extratrigeminal regions)
- Frequency: may occur several times a day for 1–4 months (often nocturnal)
- Periodicity: circadian regularity in 47%
- Remission: long symptom-free intervals occur in some patients 2 months to 20 years

Treatment options

- O_2 8 LPM face mask or 100% nonrebreather mask
- Sumatriptan 6 mg SQ (do not use with history of coronary artery disease) — read drug information
- Lidocaine 1 cc of a 10% solution placed on a swab in each nostril for 5 minutes is potentially helpful
- Capsaicin applied intranasally (has a burning sensation side effect)

Trigeminal neuralgia

- Commonly idiopathic
- Shock like severe pains in the distribution of trigeminal nerve
- Onset usually around age 60–70 years of age
- Pains last seconds to less than 2 minutes
- Can be triggered by specific activities such as eating, talking, brushing teeth, etc.
- No associated neurologic deficits
  - A sensory deficit excludes the diagnosis

Glossopharyngeal neuralgia

- Pain is over the distribution of glossopharyngeal nerve triggered by coughing, yawing, swallowing cold liquids

Occipital neuralgia

- Pain is in the posterior scalp region

Treatment options of cranial neuralgias

- Carbamazepine 200 mg PO bid to start (DOC)
  - Titrate increasing dose every 3 days by 200 mg
  - Effective dose is usually 600–1200 mg qday
  - Instruct patient they will need monitoring for aplastic anemia and severe leukopenia
- Dilantin (phenytoin) for carbamazepine failures (lower rate of success in treating neuralgia)
  - Dose of 300–600 mg PO qday (levels need monitoring)
  - Cerebyx (fosphenytoin) 250 mg IV for severe attack
- Lamictal (lamotrigine) 100–400 mg PO qday (NMT 250 mg PO qday in children)

Discharge criteria recommendation

- Uncomplicated cases

Discharge instructions

- Trigeminal neuralgia aftercare instructions
- Follow up with PCP or neurologist in 7–10 days

Consult criteria recommendation

- Complicated cranial neuralgias

Temporal arteritis

- True emergency of the elderly
  - Age of onset 50–70 years of age
  - Six times more common in females than in males
- Headache localized over eye or to scalp
- Fever, malaise and weight loss are associated symptoms
- Jaw claudication is important associated symptom
- Frequently associated with polymyalgia rheumatica (joint and muscles aches)
- ESR 50–100
  - 15% of temporal arteritis patients have normal ESR
- C-reactive protein elevated usually
- Vision loss can occur early in course of disease

Treatment

- Prednisone 40–80 mg PO bid for several months to one year
  - In suspected temporal with normal ESR, treat with steroids

Discharge criteria recommendation

- Minimal symptoms can be treated as outpatient
- Severe symptoms or question of eye involvement should be admitted with IV high dose steroid treatment and ophthalmology consultation obtained

Discharge instructions

- Temporal arteritis aftercare instructions
- Follow up with PCP within 1 day
- Return for visual changes

Consult criteria recommendation

- Discuss all temporal arteritis cases with neurology or ophthalmology

Headaches Prompting CT Brain Scan Consideration

- Worst headache of life — Consider lumbar puncture if CT negative
  - CT in first 6 hours of headache onset with high accuracy of detecting cerebral hemorrhage
- First headache
- New daily or persistent headache
- Change in headache from previous headache symptoms/patterns
- Neurologic complaints
- New onset seizure with headache
- Complaints of altered mental status
- Migraine aura that is sensory or motor
- Change in migraine aura
- Focal deficits
- Headache > 24 hours
- Thunderclap headache
- Headache in elderly
- Posterior headache, especially in children but also in adults
- Red flag Headaches

Indications for lumbar puncture include

- First or worst headache of a patient's life
- Severe, rapid-onset, recurrent headache
- Progressive headache
- Unresponsive or intractable headache

Consider Following "Don't Miss Diagnoses"

(Perform testing for possible diagnoses when suspected)

- Subarachnoid hemorrhage
- Meningitis and encephalitis
- Temporal arteritis
- Acute narrow angle closure glaucoma
- Hypertensive emergencies
- Carbon monoxide poisoning
- Cerebral venous sinus thrombosis (seen for example with OCP use or with women with coagulopathy)
- Trigeminal neuralgia
- Pseudotumor cerebri
- Acute strokes
- Mass lesions

Discharge criteria recommendation

- Benign headache diagnosis and prognosis
- Trigeminal or cranial neuralgias refer to neurologist (website: tna.support.org)

Discharge instructions

- Headache aftercare instructions
- Follow up with PCP or neurologist within 7–10 days as needed
- Return if headache persists > 24 hours

Consult criteria recommendation

- Headache with fever unless consistent with a benign process
- Neck/nuchal rigidity
- Headaches where CT brain scan performed
- Possible High Risk Headache
- Acute neurologic complaints or findings
- Above diagnosis suspected in the "Don't miss diagnosis" section
- Return visit for same headache
- Questionable diagnosis
- Status migrainosus (> 24 hours; dehydration)
- Red flag headaches

Lab consult criteria recommendations

- Adult WBC ≥ 14,000 or < 1,000 neutrophils
- Pediatric WBC ≥ 15,000 or < 1,000 neutrophils
- Bandemia
- Thrombocytopenia — acute
- Metabolic acidosis
- Significant electrolyte abnormality
- Hyperglycemia with metabolic acidosis (decreased serum CO_2 or elevated anion gap)

Notes

REFERENCES:

Brennan KC, Farrell CP, Deough GP, Baggaley S, Pippitt K, Pohl SP, et al. Symptom codes and opioids: disconcerting headache practice patterns in academic primary care. Presented on April 30, 2014 at the Annual Meeting of the American Academy of Neurology, 2014.

Baden EY, et al. Intravenous dexamethasone to prevent the recurrence of benign headache after discharge from the emergency department: a randomized, double-blind, placebo-controlled clinical trial *Can J Emerg Med* 2006;8(6):393–400

Migraine Headache Author: Jasvinder Chawla, MD, MBA; Chief Editor: Helmi L Lutsep, MD emedicine.medscape.com/article/1142556

Loder E, Weizenbaum E, Frishberg B, Silberstein S; the American Headache

Society Choosing Wisely Task Force. Choosing Wisely in Headache Medicine: The American Headache Society's List of Five Things Physicians and Patients Should Question. Headache. Available at onlinelibrary.wiley.com/doi/10.1111/head.12233

Top Magn Reson Imaging, 2015;24:291

J Res Med Sci. 2014 Apr; 19(4): 331–335

Ann of EM, Vol.655:622

JEM, epub, 3/14/19

Ann EM. 2019;74:e41

West J EM. 2019;20:203

Dizziness Protocol

Definitions

- Sensation of being off balance or of movement of body or surrounding environment

Differential Diagnosis

- Vestibular disorder of inner ear
- Cardiac arrhythmia
- Pulmonary embolism
- TIA
- CVA
- Seizures
- Dehydration
- Aortic stenosis
- Hypoglycemia
- Subarachnoid hemorrhage
- Hemorrhage
  - GI bleeding
  - Ectopic pregnancy
- Adrenal insufficiency
- Sepsis
- Hypotension

Considerations

- Vertigo: peripheral ("inner ear") or central
- Disequilibrium: suggests CNS disorder
- Increasingly common in presenting to acute care settings
- Antiemetics and vestibular suppressants should be withdrawn after a few days if possible to hasten vestibular compensation

Can be:

- Near syncope (hypotension)
- Generalized weakness
- Cardiopulmonary (hypotension)
- Neurologic (CVA, TIA)
- Metabolic (acidosis, hyperglycemia, hypoglycemia)
- Emotional disorder

Peripheral Vertigo

- Sensation of movement worsened with head movement or position change
- Horizontal nystagmus; rotary nystagmus
- Nausea and vomiting
- No vital sign abnormalities
- No focal neurologic deficits, neurologic complaints or other significant comorbidities
- No further testing may be needed

Central vertigo

- Gradual onset
- Not worse usually on movement
- Vertical nystagmus
- Tend to be much less intense than those associated with peripheral vertigo
- Infrequent nausea and vomiting
- Central nervous system findings present

Evaluation

- Complete history and physical examination
  - Check for nystagmus, gait abnormalities
  - Hallpike maneuver prn

    - First, the positional change is performed with the patient gazing straight ahead.
    - It is then repeated with the head turned 45° to the right and then 45° to the left.
    - The neck preferably is extended slightly when the patient lies back in the supine position.
    - In contrast to that due to central vertigo, nystagmus due to peripheral disease may not develop immediately after the positional change, and, once it develops, may fatigue quickly and last less than 1 minute
    - If test is negative then central vertigo more likely
- For benign peripheral vertigo no further testing may be needed
- Consider CT brain scan for
    - Ataxia
    - Vertical nystagmus
    - Neurologic deficits or complaints
    - Headache
    - Consult physician
- CBC, BMP, EKG, CXR as indicated for patients that may have a disorder besides peripheral vertigo
- Toxicology screen and medication levels as indicated
- Follow Chest Pain, Dyspnea, TIA, Syncope/Near syncope or other Protocols as indicated

Treatment Options

- Benign Paroxysmal Positional Vertigo: Epley maneuver
- Peripheral benign vertigo: meclizine 25 mg tid prn, or Phenergan (promethazine), or benzodiazepines can be considered
- Consider steroids
- Avoid antihistamines if not peripheral vertigo

Discharge Criteria

- Peripheral vertigo with normal vital signs and O_2 saturation
- Not ataxic
- Acute central nervous system or metabolic disorder not suspected

Discharge instructions

- Provide dizziness aftercare instructions
- Follow up with primary care provider, neurologist or ENT within 10 days as needed

Consult Criteria

- Neurologic abnormalities or complaints
- Visual complaints or findings
- If CT brain scan needed or performed
- Cardiogenic, pulmonary, toxicology cause of dizziness
- Age ≥ 70
- Uncertain or unknown cause of dizziness
- Syncope or near syncope unless vasovagal episode in healthy nonelderly patient
- Refer to General Patient Criteria Protocol (page 15)

Lab and x-ray consult criteria

- New onset renal insufficiency or worsening renal insufficiency
- WBC ≥ 15,000 or < 3,000; Neutrophil count < 1,000
- Bandemia ≥ 15%
- Acute thrombocytopenia
- Increased anion gap
- Metabolic acidosis
- Significant electrolyte abnormally
- Glucose ≥ 400 mg/dL in diabetic patient
- Glucose ≥ 300 mg/dL in non-diabetic patient
- Pleural effusion
- New chest x–ray infiltrate(s) or increased interstitial changes
- New onset renal insufficiency or worsening renal insufficiency

Notes

REFERENCES:

emedicine.medscape.com/article/2149881

Dizziness presentations in U.S. emergency departments, 1995–2004. Acad Emerg Med. 2008; 15(8):744–50

Treatment of vestibular neuritis. Curr Treat Options Neurol. 2009; 11(1):41–5

Transient Global Amnesia Clinical Presentation Updated: Jul 27, 2018
Author: Roy Sucholeiki, MD;

CVA/TIA PROTOCOL

Definition

- TIA — An acute and temporary neurologic dysfunction caused by a focal decrease in blood flow to the central nervous system
- CVA — A neurologic dysfunction caused by a focal decrease in blood flow to the central nervous system that causes neuronal death in the affected area

Differential Diagnosis

- CVA
- Bell's palsy
- Migraine
- Subarachnoid hemorrhage
- Brain tumor
- Multiple sclerosis
- Intracerebral hemorrhage
- Seizure disorder
- Transient global amnesia (TGA)
- Hypoglycemia

Considerations

- TIA always lasts less than 24 hours
  - They usually last 15 minutes to 1 hour in duration
- Up to 40% of patients with TIA have actually had small infarctions by MRI criteria
  - 10.5% of TIA's will have a CVA within 90 days
    - Half of these will occur within 2 days
  - Up to 21 % of CVA's will die or have a major cardiac event
- Up to 16% of TIA patients will have a headache
- Most TIA patients should be hospitalized; especially with a cardiogenic etiology and crescendo TIA's
- Syncope is seldom caused by a TIA
- Acute CVA goal is to complete evaluation and initiate thrombolytics, if indicated, within 60 minutes of patient arrival and within 3–4.5 hours of stroke onset
- Thrombectomy in eligible patients 6 to 24 hours after a stroke

Symptoms and signs

- Acute in onset
- Focal
- Reaching intensity within seconds
- Begin at the same time
- Motor and/or sensory deficit on one side of the body
- Loss of speech or comprehension
- Loss of vision in one eye or one hemifield
- Vertebrobasilar CVA/TIA presenting as syncope is typically associated with other brainstem signs:
  - Diplopia
  - Ataxia

Most common symptoms and signs

- Hemiparesis
- Hemiataxia
- Hemisensory loss
- Speech difficulty

- Visual difficulty — diplopia or visual loss

High risk factors to develop CVA following TIA

- Age > 60
- Diabetes
- TIA lasting > 10 minutes
- Motor weakness
- Speech impairment

TIA mimics

Migraines

- Migraines symptoms usually migrate and grow, without the abrupt symptom onset of TIA

Syncope

- Hypoperfusion usually produces loss of consciousness, but focal deficits can occasionally be seen, especially after an episode of true syncope

Vertigo

- True vertigo without other findings is seldom central. Look especially for other brainstem signs

Epilepsy

- Focal paralysis without motor activity occurs rarely

TGA

- Transient global amnesia without any other neurologic deficit
- Resolves spontaneously
- Imaging to rule out CVA may be performed
- Avoid activities that increase intrathoracic pressure
- Cause uncertain
  - Precipitants of TGA frequently include physical exertion, overwhelming emotional stress, pain, cold-water exposure, sexual intercourse, and Valsalva maneuver. These triggers may have a common physiologic feature: increased venous return to the superior vena cava

Intracerebral hemorrhage

- Symptoms rarely are transient

Multiple sclerosis

- Onset is typically much slower than TIA

Hypoglycemia

- Some alteration in consciousness usually present

Nondescript complaints

- Acute onset of focal symptoms is occasionally a conversion reaction, but be aware of the possibility of embellishment of a real deficit

Evaluation Options

- CBC
- CMP
- EKG
- CT brain scan at time of initial presentation
- Chest x-ray
- C-RP
- ESR
- PT/INR
- Assess for focal neurologic deficits in addition to cardiac and general exam
- Check gait as needed

Assess for other causes

- Migraines
- Seizures
- Vertigo
- TGA
- Medication side effect/toxins
- Multiple sclerosis
- Intracerebral hemorrhage
- Lumbar puncture if subarachnoid hemorrhage is suspected
- Blood cultures if infected emboli are suspected (e.g., SBE)

Acute CVA presentations less than 4.5 hours from onset (notify physician)

- Rapidly perform NIHSS (NIH Stroke Scale) and examine patient

- Order stat CT brain without contrast
- Consult physician and neurologist immediately after ordering CT brain scan
  - If available and appropriate to the specific institution and the patient's clinical situation, order contrast/or perfusion CT brain to be performed after plain CT brain completed per physician (renal patients discuss with physician or radiologist prior to iodinated contrast)
- Determine patient eligibility for t-PA with physician and a course of action if possible
- Repeat NIHSS immediately when patient returns from CT brain scan and discuss with physician
  - To give thrombolysis treatment, blood pressure targets initially are:
    - SBP ≤ 185 mm Hg
    - DBP ≤ 110 mm Hg
- Follow established specific institution's acute stroke policies if present instead of this section
- Oxygen — avoid high flow oxygen
  - Hyperoxia can cause vasoconstriction of the carotid and downstream cerebral arteries
    - Avoid high O_2 saturations caused by supplemental oxygen

Current inclusion guidelines for the administration of t-PA are:

- Diagnosis of ischemic stroke causing measurable neurologic deficit
- Neurologic signs should not be clearing
- Neurologic signs not be minor and isolated
- Symptoms not be suggestive of subarachnoid hemorrhage
- Onset of symptoms < 4.5 hours before beginning treatment
- No history of recent stroke within 3 months (except within 4.5 hours)
- No head trauma or prior stroke in past 3 months
- No MI in prior 3 months
- No GI/GU hemorrhage in previous 21 days
- No arterial puncture in noncompressible site during prior 7 days
- No major surgery in prior 14 days
- No current or history of prior intracranial bleed
- SBP < 185 mm Hg and DBP < 110 mm Hg
- No evidence of acute trauma or bleeding
- Not taking an oral anticoagulant, or if so INR < 1.7
- If taking heparin within 48 hours must have a normal activated partial thromboplastin time (aPTT)
- Platelet count > 100,000 μL
- Blood glucose level greater than 50 mg/dL (2.7 mmol)
- No seizure with residual postictal impairments
- CT scan does not show evidence of multilobar infarction (hypodensity > 1/3 hemisphere) — increased risk of hemorrhagic conversion
- Pregnancy
- The patient and family understand the potential risks and benefits of therapy

Exclusion criteria for t-PA for CVA symptoms 3–4.5 hours of duration (any 1 of the following)

- Patients older than 80 years
- All patients taking oral anticoagulants are excluded regardless of the international normalized ratio (INR)
- Patients with baseline NIHSS score > 25
- Patients with a history of stroke and diabetes
- Patients with imaging evidence of ischemic damage to more than one third of the

middle cerebral artery (MCA) territory

AHA/ASA Guidelines 2018 Update

- Studies showed a clear benefit of "extended window" mechanical thrombectomy for certain patients with large vessel occlusion who could be treated out to 16-24 hours
- The benefits of intravenous (IV) tissue plasminogen activator (tPA) are time-dependent, and treatment for eligible patients should be initiated as quickly as possible (even for patients who may also be candidates for mechanical thrombectomy)
- IV tPA should be administered to all eligible acute stroke patients within 3 hours of last known normal and to a more selective group of eligible acute stroke patients (based on ECASS III exclusion criteria) within 4.5 hours of last known normal
- Centers should attempt to achieve door-to-needle times of <60 minutes in ≥50% of stroke patients treated with IV tPA
- **Prior to initiation of IV tPA in most patients, a noncontrast head computed tomography (CT) and glucose are the only required tests**
  - An INR PTT, and platelet count do not need to have resulted prior to IV tPA initiation if there is no suspicion for underlying coagulopathy
- Centers should attempt to obtain a noncontrast head CT within 20 minutes of arrival in ≥50% of stroke patients who may be candidates for IV tPA or mechanical thrombectomy
- For patients who may be candidates for mechanical thrombectomy, an urgent CT angiogram or magnetic resonance (MR) angiogram (to look for large vessel occlusion) is recommended
  - This study should not delay treatment with IV tPA if indicated
- Patients ≥18 years should undergo mechanical thrombectomy with a stent retriever
  - If they have minimal prestroke disability
  - Have a causative occlusion of the internal carotid artery or proximal middle cerebral artery
  - Have a NIHSS of ≥6
  - Have a reassuring noncontrast head CT
  - Can be treated within 6 hours of last known normal
  - No perfusion imaging (CT-P or MR-P) is required in these patients.
- In selected acute stroke patients within 6-24 hours of last known normal who have evidence of a large vessel occlusion in the anterior circulation, obtaining perfusion imaging (CT-P or MR-P) or an MRI with diffusion-weighted imaging (DWI) sequence is recommended to help determine whether the patient is a candidate for mechanical thrombectomy
- As with IV tPA, treatment with mechanical thrombectomy should be initiated as quickly as possible
- Administration of aspirin is recommended in acute stroke patients within 24-48 hours after stroke onset
  - For patients treated with IV tPA, aspirin administration is generally delayed for 24 hours. Urgent anticoagulation (e.g., heparin drip) for most stroke patients is not indicated

Time targets for t-PA candidates

- Door to Provider: 10 min
- Access to neurologic expertise: 15 min

- Door to CT scan completion: 20 min
- Door to CT scan interpretation: 45 min
- Door to treatment: 60 min
- Admission to monitored bed: 6 hr.
- Preferred thrombolytic treatment window within 3–4.5 hours of stroke onset — may be extended if CT perfusion scan indicates potentially salvageable brain
- From beginning of TPA therapy check BP q15min for 2 hours, then q30min for 6 hours, then q1hr. for 16 hours

TIA Treatment Options

- Aspirin 325 mg per day (if no cerebral hemorrhage)
- Consider Plavix (clopidogrel) for ASA failure or ASA allergy (if no cerebral hemorrhage)
- Aggrenox can be used instead of aspirin or Plavix (clopidogrel)
- Coumadin (warfarin) is more effective than above medications if atrial fibrillation present (or can use newer thrombin inhibitor agents)
    - See Stroke Prevention or atrial fibrillation sections
- Lower head of bed to flat position to improve cerebral circulation (unless intracranial hemorrhage is present)
- Avoid hypotonic IV fluids

Hypertension treatment for TIA and CVA nonthrombolysis candidates

- Consult physician for treatment preferred
    - Treat SBP ≥ 220 mm Hg or MAP ≥ 130 mm Hg carefully (avoid rapid or large decreases in BP > 15%)
    - Avoid treating SBP < 220 mm Hg or MAP < 130 mm Hg
        - Unless AMI, severe CHF, aortic dissection or hypertensive encephalopathy or ICH (intracranial hemorrhage) is present

BP medication options for any CVA or intracerebral hemorrhage patient

- Labetalol 5–20 mg IV over 1–2 minutes — may repeat q10min and double as needed to maximum dose of 150 mg (now controversial) — NMT 300mg/day
    - Infusion is 2mg/minute

<u>OR</u>

- Esmolol 250 mcg/kg bolus and infusion 25–300 mcg/kg/minute

<u>OR</u>

- Nicardipine 5mg/hr. IV and titrate as needed

<u>OR</u>

- Clevidipine 1–2 mg/hr IV, titrate every 2–5 minutes until desired BP is obtained, NMT 21mg/hr.

<u>OR</u>

- Nitroprusside 0.3–10 mcg/kg/min (NMT 10 mcg/kg/min.)—start low

<u>OR</u>

- Hydralazine 5–20 mg q30mn IV prn may be considered

<u>OR</u>

- Enalaprilat 1.25–5 mg IV q6hr prn may be considered

<u>OR</u>

- Nitroglycerin IV 20–400 mcg/minute if heart failure or ACS present

Intracerebral hemorrhage

- Notify physician promptly if present
- Treat SBP > 160–180 mm Hg, DBP > 120 mm Hg or MAP > 130 mm Hg are treated
- Avoid rapids swings in BP
- Do not reduce MAP by > 20% initially
- Reduce BP slowly over 3–6 hours

Admission Criteria

- Acute CVA
- Most TIA's
  - High risk criteria
  - Crescendo/recurrent TIA's
  - Cardiogenic etiology of TIA
  - Recent single TIA's are often offered admission because of the high risk of subsequent stroke and to facilitate rapid work-up
  - Septic emboli diagnosis is a possibility
  - Likelihood that patient would not return for outpatient work-up

Discharge Criteria

- Not surgical or anticoagulation candidate
- Patient declines admission for evaluation
- Fully worked up in recent past
- Neurologically stable

Discharge instructions

- TIA aftercare instructions
- Discharge instructions should include early follow-up along with what signs and symptoms to watch for, and to return immediately for further symptoms

Consult Criteria

- All TIA or CVA patients
- CT brain scan with acute findings
- Unclear diagnosis
- Refer to General Patient Criteria Protocol (page 15)

NIH stroke scale

Do not augment or interpret patient's responses on what you think the patient can do. Only record what the patient exactly does.

1a – Level of consciousness (LOC)

- 0 = **Alert;** keenly responsive
- 1 = **Not alert;** arousable by minor stimulation to obey, answer, or respond
- 2 = **Not alert;** requires repeated stimulation to attend, or is obtunded and requires strong or painful stimulation to make movements (not stereotyped)
- 3 = **Responds only** with reflex motor or autonomic effects or is totally unresponsive, flaccid, and areflexic

1b – LOC questions – asked month and age (must be exact)

- 0 = **Answers** both questions correctly
- 1 = **Answers** one question correctly
- 2 = **Answers** neither question correctly

1c – LOC commands – asked to open and close eyes and then to grip and release non-paretic hand

- 0 = **Performs** both tasks correctly
- 1 = **Performs** one task correctly
- 2 = **Performs** neither task correctly

2 – Best gaze

- 0 = Normal
- 1 = Partial gaze palsy; gaze is abnormal in one or both eyes, but forced deviation or total gaze paresis is not present
- 2 = Forced deviation, or total gaze paresis not overcome by the oculocephalic (doll's eyes) maneuver

3 – Visual

- 0 = No visual loss
- 1 = Partial hemianopsia (quadrantanopsia)
- 2 = Complete hemianopsia
- 3 = Bilateral hemianopsia (blind including cortical blindness)

4 – Facial palsy

- 0 = Normal symmetrical movements
- 1 = Minor paralysis (flattened nasolabial fold, asymmetry on smiling)
- 2 = Partial paralysis (total or near-total paralysis of lower face)
- 3 = Complete paralysis of one or both sides (absence of facial movement in the upper and lower face)

5 – Motor arm (score for each arm)

- 0 = **No drift;** limb holds 90 (or 45) degrees for full 10 seconds
- 1 = **Drift;** limb hold 90 (or 45) degrees, but drifts down before full 10 seconds; does not hit bed or other support
- 2 = **Some effort against gravity;** limb cannot get to or maintain (if cued) 90 (or 45) degrees, drifts down to bed, but has some effort against gravity
- 3 = **No effort against gravity;** limb falls
- 4 = **No movement**
- UN = **Amputation** or joint fusion, explain:

____

6 – Motor leg (score for each leg)

- 0 = **No drift;** leg holds 30–degree position for full 5 seconds
- 1 = **Drift;** leg falls by the end of the 5–second period but does not hit bed
- 2 = **Some effort against gravity;** leg falls to bed by 5 seconds, but has some effort against gravity
- 3 = **No effort against gravity;** leg falls to bed immediately
- 4 = **No movement**
- UN = **Amputation** or joint fusion, explain:

____

7 – Limb ataxia

- 0 = Absent
- 1 = Present in one limb
- 2 = Present in two limbs
- UN = **Amputation** or joint fusion, explain:

____

8 – Sensory

- 0 = **Normal;** no sensory loss
- 1 = **Mild-to-moderate sensory loss;** patient feels pinprick is less sharp or is dull on the affected side; or there is a loss of superficial pain with pinprick, but patient is aware of being touched.
- 2 = **Severe to total sensory loss;** patient is not aware of being touched in the face, arm, and leg

9 – Best Language

- 0 = No aphasia; normal
- 1 = Mild-to-moderate aphasia; some obvious loss of fluency or facility of comprehension, without significant limitation on ideas expressed or form of expression. Reduction of speech and/or comprehension; however, makes conversation about provided materials difficult or impossible. For example, in conversation about provided materials, examiner can identify picture or naming card content from patient's response.
- 2 = Severe aphasia; all communication is through fragmentary expression; great need for inference, questioning, and guessing by the listener. Range of information that can be exchanged is limited; listener carries burden of communication. Examiner cannot identify materials provided from patient response.
- 3 = Mute, global aphasia; no usable speech or auditory comprehension

10 – Dysarthria

- 0 = Normal
- 1 = Mild-to-moderate dysarthria; patient slurs at least some words and, at worst, can

be understood with some difficulty.

- 2 = Severe dysarthria; patient's speech is so slurred as to be unintelligible in the absence of or out of proportion to any dysphasia, or is mute.
- UN = Intubated or other physical barrier, explain:______________________

_

11 – Extinction and Inattention (Neglect)

- 0 = No abnormality
- 1 = Visual, tactile, auditory, spatial, or personal inattention or extinction to bilateral simultaneous stimulation in one of the sensory modalities.
- 2 = Profound hemi-inattention or extinction to more than one modality; does not recognize own hand or orients to only one side of space.

NOTE: If the patient in 1a has a score of 3, then the rest of the exams usually are scored a 3 for each category

Notes

____

____

____

REFERENCES:

www.ninds.nih.gov/doctors/NIH_Stroke_Scale.pdf

Stroke. May 2007;38(5):1655–711

Stroke. 2010;41;2108

Cornet AD, et al. *Crit Care* 2013 Apr 18;17:313

Ischemic Stroke Workup Author: Edward C Jauch, MD, MS, FAHA, FACEP; Chief Editor: Helmi L Lutsep, MD

stroke.ahajournals.org/content/suppl/2013/01/29/STR.0b013e318284056a.DC1/Executive_Summary.pdf

emedicine.medscape.com/article/1160840

Thrombolytic Therapy in Stroke Author: Jeffrey L Saver, MD, FAHA, FAAN; Chief Editor: Helmi L Lutsep, MD

N Engl J Med 2018; 378:11-21 January 4, 2018

N Engl J Med 2018; 378:708-718 February 22, 2018

BELL'S PALSY PROTOCOL

Definition

- Dysfunction or paralysis of the 7th cranial nerve unilaterally of acute onset and usually idiopathic etiology

Differential Diagnosis

- Vascular
  - TIA
  - CVA
  - Aneurysm
- Infectious
  - Lyme disease
  - Herpes zoster
  - Mononucleosis
- Neoplastic
  - Tumor of pons or cerebellopontine angle or acoustic nerve
  - Lymphoma
  - Skull based tumor, cholesteatoma
- Multiple sclerosis

Considerations

- 7th cranial nerve dysfunction
- Affects 1 in 65 persons in a lifetime
- Complete recovery in 65% of patients at 3 months and 85% at 9 months
- Studies have shown the benefit of high-dose corticosteroids for acute cases
- Steroids and Valtrex (valacyclovir) or acyclovir recommended only in the initial 72 hours of symptoms in age 16 years or older, with complete or nearly complete paralysis — not useful otherwise
- Slowly progressive facial paralysis suggestive of cancer
- Recurrent paralysis or bilateral presentation warrants additional workup
- Bilateral 7th nerve weakness excludes Bell's palsy and is suggestive of infectious causes such as Lyme disease or VZV (varicella zoster virus)
- Forehead sparing of motor function usually indicates upper motor neuron lesion (CVA)
- Lyme disease should be considered as a cause in endemic areas
- Bell's palsy can be mimicked by pontine brainstem lesion
- Other associated signs and symptoms:
  - Vestibular signs
  - Diabetes and hypertension higher risk for pontine lesions

Signs and Symptoms

- Typical presentation is subacute weakness of one side of the face
- Often associated with pain near the ear
- No sensory loss although patient may complain of vague sensation disturbance on the face
- Hyperacusis due to paralysis of the stapedius sometimes occurs
- Distortion of taste sometimes occurs although this is seldom a presenting complaint
- Weakness of eye closure is helpful to differentiate Bell's palsy from stroke where eye opening may be impaired
- Asymmetry of mouth movement is most obvious with grimacing and smiling
- Maximal defect is 5 days from onset
- Forehead and lower facial muscles both weak
  - If forehead spared of weakness, suspect central lesion (CVA, tumor)
- Increased tear flow
- Dry eyes
- Rash or vesicles around ear on affected side suggests herpes zoster (Ramsey-Hunt syndrome). Usually significant pain near the ear

Causes

- Idiopathic usually
- Infectious causes
  - Most infectious cases of Bell's palsy are thought to be due to virus infections
    - HSV 1 or 2
    - VZV
  - EBV
  - Lyme disease is a rare cause of Bell's palsy
- Sarcoidosis can present with facial palsy, occasionally can present with bilateral facial weakness.
- Other infections such as osteomyelitis, primary ear infections, and meningitis are less likely
- Neoplasm of local tissues near the ear and skull base or neoplastic meningitis
- Pontine (brainstem) lesion, including cerebellopontine angle lesion
- Aneurysm of the basilar artery or branch with resultant neural compression
- Parotid gland mass lesions

Evaluation Options

- Usually no testing except history and physical exam
- Testing driven by suspected processes or recurrent/bilateral presentations
  - CBC
  - ESR or C-reactive protein
  - Lyme titer
  - HIV test
  - Serum glucose
  - CT brain if suspected central lesion (usually not needed)
  - Lumbar puncture if intracranial or spinal infectious process suspected

Goals of treatment

- Improve facial nerve (seventh cranial nerve) function
- Reduce neuronal damage
- Prevent complications from corneal exposure

Treatment Options

- Artificial tears
- Tape eyelids closed on affected side at night only
- Eye protection if eyelid closure is impaired
- Steroids are commonly used unless specifically contraindicated
  - Prednisone 1 mg/kg/day up to 60 mg/day × 7 days without taper (or may taper to 5 mg/day over 10 days)—use only if symptoms ≤ 3 days
- Antiviral agents (e.g., acyclovir, valacyclovir) may be considered if a herpes viral etiology is suspected, but only in combination with corticosteroids (i.e. herpes zoster rash present, etc.) within the first 72 hours of symptom onset.
  - Valtrex (valacyclovir) 1000 mg PO tid × 5 days
    - Valtrex > age 2 years: 20 mg/kg PO q8hr for 5 days; not to exceed 1 g PO q8hr

      OR
  - Acyclovir 400 mg PO 5 ×/day × 7–10 days

    OR
  - Famciclovir 500 mg tid × 5–10 days
- Physical therapy may be used for patients with moderate to severe deficits

Discharge Criteria

- Isolated 7th nerve palsy

Discharge instructions

- Bell's palsy aftercare instructions
- Follow up with primary care provider or neurologist within 7 to 10 days
- Discharge precautions noted:
  - Return if additional symptoms occur or significant worsening
  - Complete the course of medications prescribed
- Ensure follow-up after discharge

Consult Criteria

- Suspected other causes of nerve palsy
- Central nervous system findings or complaints
- Refer to General Patient Criteria Protocol (page 15) as needed

Notes

____

____

____

REFERENCES:

Baugh RF, Basura GJ, Ishii LE, Schwartz SR, Drumheller CM, Burkholder R, et al. Clinical Practice Guideline: Bell's Palsy Executive Summary. *Otolaryngol Head Neck Surg.* Nov 2013;149(5):656–63.

Sullivan FM, Swan IR, Donnan PT, Morrison JM, Smith BH, McKinstry B, et al. Early treatment with prednisolone or acyclovir in Bell's palsy. *N Engl J Med*. Oct 18 2007;357(16):1598–607.

Engström M, Berg T, Stjernquist-Desatnik A, et al. Prednisolone and valaciclovir in Bell's palsy: a randomised, double-blind, placebo-controlled, multicentre trial. *Lancet Neurol.* Nov 2008;7(11):993–1000

Reconciling the clinical practice guidelines on Bell palsy from the AAO-HNSF and the AAN; Seth R. Schwartz, Stephanie L. Jones, Thomas S.D. Getchius, et. Al. Neurology 2014;1927–1929 May 2, 2014

Adult Seizure Protocol

Definition

- Focal or generalized electrical depolarizations of the brain resulting in focal or generalized neurologic and motor findings with or without loss of consciousness

Differential Diagnosis

- Pseudoseizures
- Migraines
- Encephalitis
- Meningitis
- Transient global amnesia (TGA)
- Psychogenic unresponsiveness
- TIA (rare TIA's can present with focal motor activity or unresponsiveness)
- Syncope
- Hypoglycemia
- Conversion reaction

Considerations

Generalized seizures (most common)

Classic tonic-clonic (grand mal)

- Sustained generalized muscle contractions with loss of consciousness

Absence seizures (petit mal)

- Brief episodes of sudden immobility and blank stares

Partial seizures

Simple

- Brief sensory or motor symptoms without loss of consciousness
  - Focal motor seizures is an example

Complex

- Mental or psychiatric symptoms
- Affect changes
- Confusion
- Automatisms
- Hallucinations
- Impaired consciousness

Status epilepticus (SE)

- Newly defined as seizure > 5 minutes or 2 or more seizures in which patient does not recover consciousness
- Older definition > 30 minutes or 2 or more seizures in which patient does not recover consciousness (controversy exists about definition)
- Mortality 10–12%
- Failure to recognize nonconvulsive SE increases poor outcomes
- Prolonged SE leads to electromechanical dissociation
  - Exhibit minor movements: twitching of eyes, face, hands, feet; coma

Prolactin level

- Helpful if drawn within 10–20 minutes of seizure and elevated 2 times normal
  - Syncope can also elevate prolactin levels
- Normal prolactin level favors pseudoseizure but cannot differentiate seizure from syncope
- Normal prolactin does not rule out seizure however

Pseudoseizures

- Closed eyes during seizure: 96% sensitive; 98% specific in indicating pseudoseizure
- Open eyes during seizure: 98% sensitive; 96% specific in indicating true seizure

First time seizure has 25% recurrence in 2 years

Epilepsy defined as 2 or more seizures not provoked by other illness or causations

Causes

- Idiopathic
- Genetic
- Congenital
- Hypoglycemia or hyperglycemia
- Hypernatremia and hyponatremia
- CVA
- Cerebral mass
- Intracranial hemorrhage — especially subarachnoid or intraparenchymal
- Traumatic brain injury
- Cocaine
- Meningitis
- Encephalitis
- Eclampsia
- Fever
- Prescribed drugs (lowered seizure threshold especially with some antibiotics and analgesics)
- Withdrawal syndromes (drugs and alcohol)

Causes of Seizures Amenable to Treatment

- Hypoglycemia
- Hyponatremia
- Hypocalcemia
- Hypomagnesemia
- Isoniazid ingestion treated with pyridoxine
- Hypertension

Evaluation

- Assess airway and breathing
- Cardiac and O_2 saturation monitoring
- Complete history and physical
  - Lateral tongue bites more specific than distal tongue bites for seizure
- Obtain seizure history and treatment
- Obtain history of associated symptoms
- Drug abuse history

Patients with chronic seizures and no change in typical seizure pattern, without comorbid findings or symptoms

- BMP
- U/A
- Seizure drug levels if acutely measurable

All other seizures with comorbid considerations and new onset seizures

- CMP, Mg^{++}, prolactin level in select patients
- Pregnancy test in childbearing age fertile women
- Consider lumbar puncture (LP) in immunocompromised patient or with meningitis signs
- Consider LP in patients with seizure and fever
- CBC; U/A; chest x-ray as indicated by associated symptoms or findings
- Blood alcohol and drug screen as indicated

- Serum anticonvulsant levels for anticonvulsant therapy that are acutely measurable
- CT brain scan on first seizure if available
- CT brain scan on elderly or patients taking Coumadin or newer anticoagulants
- CT brain scan for head trauma
- Consider stat EEG for suspected nonconvulsive SE

Treatment Options

- Intubation if airway not secure
- IV NS KVO
- Nasal oxygen

Initial treatment

- Lorazepam 2–4 mg (0.1 mg/kg) IV if actively seizing
  - May repeat q3–10 minutes for recurrent seizures prn (NMT 8 mg)
- Diazepam (Valium) 5-10 mg IV/IM q5-10min; not to exceed 30 mg
- Midazolam IV drip 0.05–2 mg/kg/hr. for refractory status epilepticus
  - If no IV available, give midazolam 10 mg IM if patient's weight ≥ 40 kg
    - Nasal 5 mg, may repeat once
    - Buccal route 10 mg once using injectable 5mg/mL
    - Nasal and buccal midazolam are absorbed more rapidly than IM but are not as well studied as IM midazolam in adults

Adjunctive treatments as needed

- Thiamine 100 mg IM/IV for alcoholism history (or if not known)
- Glucose D50W 1 amp if hypoglycemic
- Prophylactic lorazepam can be given in the first 12 hours of alcoholic withdrawal
- Magnesium sulfate 4 gms IV over 5–10 minutes for eclampsia

Status epilepticus (beware of "too slow and too low" treatment)

- Lorazepam 2–4 mg IV — repeat in 3–5 minutes prn (NMT 8 mg total dose)
- Cerebyx (fosphenytoin) 18–20 PE mg/kg IV at 100–150 mg/minute if no response in 3–5 minutes to lorazepam

Drugs that can be used if lorazepam and Cerebyx (fosphenytoin) fail

- Valproic acid 20–30 mg/kg at max rate up to 10mg/kg/minute; (NMT 40 mg/kg) — loading dose
  - 5 mg/kg/hr. drip
- Levetiracetam (Keppra) 30–50 mg/kg at 100 mg/minute (loading dose)
- Phenobarbital 10 mg/kg IV at 100 mg/hr. (seldom used in adults)
- Lidocaine 1 mg/kg up to 100 mg; may be repeated (NMT 3 mg/kg total dose)
- Propofol (intubate patient)
  - 2 mg/kg; may repeat if needed in 3–5 minutes
  - Maintenance 5 mg/kg/hr.
- Ketamine 1–4.5 mg/kg IV over 60 seconds or 4–5 mg/kg IM
- Lorazepam and levetiracetam can be used safely in pregnancy

Management of refractory status epilepticus

- Referral to an intensive care unit
- Anesthetic agents such as midazolam, propofol, barbiturates (thiopental, pentobarbital) or ketamine for generalized convulsive status epilepticus
  - Intermittent ketamine superior to continuous infusion
- Non-anesthetic anticonvulsants such as phenobarbital or

valproic acid for nonconvulsive status epilepticus

ACEP Clinical Policy: Critical Issues in the Evaluation and Management of Adult Patients Presenting to the Emergency Department with seizures (January 2014)

- Intended for emergency departments
- Adult patients ≥ 18 years with generalized convulsive seizure
- Not intended for pediatric patients, complex partial seizures, acute head or multisystem trauma, or brain tumor, immunocompromised or eclamptic patients

Level A recommendations

- Emergency providers should administer an additional antiepileptic medication in emergency department patients with refractory status epilepticus who have failed treatment with benzodiazepines

Level B recommendations

- Emergency providers may administer intravenous phenytoin, fosphenytoin, or valproate in emergency department patients with refractory status epilepticus who have failed treatment with benzodiazepines.

Level C recommendations

- Emergency providers need not initiate antiepileptic medication in the emergency department for patients who have had a first unprovoked seizure
- Precipitating medical conditions should be identified and treated
- Emergency providers need not initiate antiepileptic medication in the emergency department for patients who have had a first unprovoked seizure without evidence of brain disease or injury
- Emergency providers may initiate antiepileptic medication in the emergency department, or defer in coordination with other providers, for patients who experienced a first unprovoked seizure with a remote history of brain disease or injury

Level C recommendations

- Emergency providers need not admit patients with a first unprovoked seizure who have returned to their clinical baseline in the emergency department

Level C recommendations

- Emergency providers may administer intravenous levetiracetam, propofol, or barbiturates in emergency department patients with refractory status epilepticus who have failed treatment with benzodiazepines

Level C recommendations

- When resuming antiseizure medication in the emergency department is advisable, IV or oral route is acceptable at the providers discretion

Discharge criteria recommendation

- Patient with normal neurologic exam and no concerning comorbidities
- No known structural brain disease
- Patients usually do not need to be started on seizure outpatient treatment at that time if patient had single brief seizure without previous seizure history, and has a normal exam, normal imaging and no further seizures
- With treatment, after oral or parenteral load with anticonvulsant
- Without treatment if risk of recurrent seizure is judged to be low

Discharge instructions

- Seizure aftercare instructions
- Advise of seizure precautions/safety issues prior to discharge (for example – no driving, swimming, bathtubs, climbing etc.)
- Referral to neurology

Consult criteria recommendation

- Acute neurologic abnormalities
- Abnormal imaging studies
- Significant abnormal lab tests
- Abnormal vital signs and O_2 saturation < 94% on room air if no history of lung disease (<90% O_2 saturation in COPD patients)

Notes

REFERENCES:

Seizure Assessment in the Emergency Department

Author: M Tyson Pillow, MD, MEd; Chief Editor: Rick Kulkarni, MD

emedicine.medscape.com/article/1609294

American College of Emergency Physicians Clinical Policy: Critical Issues in the Evaluation and Management of Adult Patients Presenting to the Emergency Department With Seizures (January 2014)

American Epilepsy Society (AES) 69th Annual Meeting. Abstracts 3.177 and 1.123

Sathe A, et al. Epilepsia. 2021;62(3):795-806

Gaínza-Lein M, et al. *Seizure*. 2019; 68: 22-30

Uppal P, et al. *Seizure*. 2018; 58: 147-53

Brophy GM, et al. *Neurocrit Care*. 2012;17:3

Hirsch LJ. *N Engl J Med*. 2012;366:659

Neurol Clin. 2021;39:649

PEDIATRIC SEIZURE PROTOCOL

Definition

- Focal or generalized electrical depolarizations of the brain resulting in focal or generalized neurologic and motor findings with or without loss of consciousness

Differential Diagnosis

- Pseudoseizures
- Migraines
- Encephalitis
- Meningitis
- Cat scratch disease
- Amphetamine toxicity
- Cocaine toxicity
- Dystonic reactions
- Heavy metal toxicity
- Syncope
- Brain cancer

Considerations

Generalized seizures (most common)

Classic tonic-clonic (grand mal)

- Sustained generalized muscle contractions followed by loss of consciousness

Absence seizures (petit mal)

- Brief episodes of sudden immobility and blank stares

Partial seizures

Simple

- Brief sensory or motor symptoms without loss of consciousness
  - Focal motor seizures is an example

Complex

- Mental or psychiatric symptoms
- Affect changes
- Confusion
- Automatisms
- Hallucinations
- Impaired consciousness

Status epilepticus (SE)

- Newly defined as seizure > 5 minutes or 2 or more seizures in which patient does not recover consciousness
- Older definition > 30 minutes or 2 or more seizures in which patient does not recover consciousness (controversy exists about definition)
- Most common cause is febrile seizure
- Mortality 10–12%
- Failure to recognize nonconvulsive SE increases poor outcomes
- EEG, CBC, BMP, calcium level, toxicology screen, ABG, anticonvulsant levels, LFT's
- Intubate as needed
- Prolonged SE leads to electromechanical dissociation
  - Exhibit minor movements: twitching of eyes, face, hands, feet; coma

Prolactin level

- Helpful if drawn within 10–20 minutes of seizure and elevated 2 times normal
  - Syncope can also elevate prolactin levels
- Normal prolactin level favors pseudoseizure but cannot differentiate seizure from syncope
- Normal prolactin does not rule out seizure however

Pseudoseizures

- Closed eyes during seizure: 96% sensitive; 98% specific in indicating pseudoseizure
- Open eyes during seizure: 98% sensitive; 96% specific in indicating true seizure

First time seizure has 25% recurrence in 2 years

Epilepsy defined as 2 or more seizures not provoked by other illness or causations

Causes of Seizures Amenable to Treatment

- Hypoglycemia
- Hyponatremia
- Hypocalcemia
- Hypomagnesemia
- Isoniazid ingestion treated with pyridoxine
- Hypertension

Evaluation

- Assess airway and breathing
- Cardiac and O_2 saturation monitoring
- Complete history and physical
  - Lateral tongue bites more specific than distal tongue bites for seizure
- Obtain seizure history and treatment
- Obtain associated symptoms
- Drug abuse history

Patients with chronic seizures and no change in typical seizure pattern, without comorbid findings or symptoms

- BMP
- U/A
- Seizure drug levels if acutely measurable

All other seizures with comorbid considerations and new onset seizures

- CMP, prolactin level in select patients
- Pregnancy test in childbearing age females
- Consider lumbar puncture on the immunocompromised patient or patient that has meningitis signs
- Consider LP in patients with seizure and fever unless it is a benign febrile seizure
- CBC; U/A; chest x-ray as indicated by associated symptoms or findings
- Blood alcohol and drug screen as indicated
- Serum anticonvulsant levels for anticonvulsant therapy that are acutely measurable
- CT brain scan on first time seizures if available
- CT brain scan for head trauma
- Consider stat EEG if no resolution of post-ictal lethargy and for suspected nonconvulsive SE

Treatment Options

- Intubation if airway not secure
- IV NS KVO or INT
- Nasal oxygen

Initial treatment options

- Lorazepam 0.05–0.1 mg/kg IV NMT 4mg per dose; may repeat q3–15 minutes prn (NMT 8 mg)
- Valium (diazepam) 0.2 mg/kg IV/IM q5-10min; not to exceed 30 mg
- Diastat (diazepam rectal gel) if no IV available
  - Age up to 5 years: 0.5 mg/kg
  - Age 6–11 years: 0.3 mg/kg
  - Age > 12 years: 0.2 mg/kg
  - Round up to available dose: 2.5, 5, 7.5, 10, 12.5, 15, 17.5, 20 mg/dose
- Midazolam IV/IM/PR/ET/intranasal 0.1–0.2 mg/kg/dose; not to exceed a cumulative dose of 10 mg
- If no IV available, may give midazolam 10 mg IM if patient's weight ≥ 40 kg and 5 mg IM if 13–39 kg
  - Nasal and buccal midazolam are absorbed more rapidly than IM

Adjunctive treatments as needed

- Dextrose: 0.25–0.5 g/kg/dose (1–2 cc of 25% dextrose) intravenously for hypoglycemia; not to exceed 25 gm/dose
- Naloxone (Narcan): 0.1 mg/kg/dose intravenously preferable (if needed may administer intramuscularly or subcutaneously) for narcotic overdose (do not exceed 2 mg initially)
- Thiamine: 100 mg intramuscularly for possible deficiency
- Pyridoxine (vitamin B6): 50–100 mg IV or IM for possible deficiency
- Rocephin (ceftriaxone) 50–100 mg/kg IV or IM not to exceed 2 grams if meningitis suspected (may use Sanford Guide or databases), initiate treatment with antibiotics prior to cerebrospinal fluid (CSF) analysis or brain imaging
  - Give Decadron (dexamethasone) 15 minutes before antibiotics or with antibiotics

Status epilepticus (beware of "too slow and too low" treatment)

- Lorazepam 0.1 mg/kg IV (NMT 4mg/dose or 8 mg total dose)
- Diazepam 0.2 mg/kg IV
- Cerebyx (fosphenytoin) 15–20 mg/kg PE IV at 100–150 mg/minute if no response in 5 minutes to lorazepam or midazolam (Versed)
  - May repeat in 20 minutes is seizure activity continues at 10 mg/kg PE IV
- Keppra (Levetiracetam) 30-40 mg/kg IV

- 2-5 mg/kg/minute
- NMT 2000 mg

Drugs that can be used if above medications fail

- Pentobarbital 1 mg/kg boluses IV to maximum 5 mg/kg
- Valproic acid 15 mg/kg over 1–5 minutes (NMT 40 mg/kg)
  - 5 mg/kg/hr. drip
- Phenobarbital 20 mg/kg IV at 100 mg/hr.
- Propofol 2 mg/kg IV bolus (patient intubated), may repeat if needed and start 5 mg/kg/hr. infusion if necessary
- Ketamine 1–4.5 mg/kg IV over 60 seconds or 4–5 mg/kg IM
- Lidocaine 1 mg/kg up to 100 mg; may be repeated (NMT 3 mg/kg)

Management of refractory status epilepticus

- Referral to an intensive care unit
- Anesthetic agents such as midazolam, propofol, ketamine or barbiturates (thiopental, pentobarbital) for generalized convulsive status epilepticus
  - Intermittent ketamine superior to continuous infusion
- Non-anesthetic anticonvulsants such as phenobarbital or valproic acid for nonconvulsive status epilepticus

Discharge criteria recommendation

- Patient with normal neurologic exam and no concerning comorbidities
- No known structural brain disease
- Most patients usually do not need to be started on seizure outpatient treatment at time of discharge
- No further seizures
- With treatment, after oral or parenteral load with anticonvulsant
- Without treatment if risk of recurrent seizure is judged to be low

Discharge instructions

- Seizure aftercare instructions
- Advise of seizure precautions/safety issues prior to discharge (for example – no driving)
- Referral to pediatrics or neurology

Consult criteria recommendation

- Acute neurologic abnormalities
- Abnormal imaging studies
- Significant abnormal lab tests
- Abnormal vital signs and O_2 saturation < 94% on room air or respiratory distress

Notes

____

____

____

REFERENCES:

emedicine.medscape.com/article/1179097

Chamberlain JM, Okada P, Holsti M, et al. Lorazepam vs diazepam for pediatric status epilepticus: a randomized clinical trial. *JAMA*. Apr 23–30 2014;311(16):1652–60

emedicine.medscape.com/article/908394

Neurology 2012 Dec 11;79(24):2355-8. doi: 10.1212/WNL.0b013e318278b685. Epub 2012 Nov 28.
Efficacy and safety of ketamine in refractory status epilepticus in children. Rosati A, L'Erario M, Ilvento L, Cecchi C, Pisano T, Mirabile L, Guerrini R

Semin Neurol. 2019;39:73-81

Effectiveness of lidocaine infusion for status epilepticus in childhood: a retrospective multi-institutional study in Japan Brain Dev . 2008 Sep;30(8):504-12

Sathe A, et al. Epilepsia. 2021;62(3):795-806

Gaínza-Lein M, et al. *Seizure*. 2019; 68: 22-30

Uppal P, et al. *Seizure*. 2018; 58: 147-53

Brophy GM, et al. *Neurocrit Care*. 2012;17:3

Hirsch LJ. *N Engl J Med*. 2012;366:659

DELIRIUM (ALTERED MENTAL STATUS) PROTOCOL

Definition

- Acute organic brain syndrome manifested by impaired thinking, confusion, deficits in attention, hallucinations, tremor, fluctuating course, impaired speech and other symptoms and signs of impaired cognition

Causes of delirium

Medications and substances

- Ethanol
- Anticholinergics
- Antihistamines
- Sedatives
- Narcotics
- Antidepressants
- Lithium
- Neuroleptics
- Tagamet (cimetidine)

Withdrawal

- Ethanol
- Benzodiazepines
- Narcotics

Metabolic

- Electrolyte abnormalities (Na^+ and Ca^{++})
- Hypoglycemia and hyperglycemia
- Acid-base disturbance
- Dehydration
- Hypoxia
- End organ insufficiency – liver, kidney and lungs
- Vitamin deficiency – thiamine, folate
- Fever or hypothermia

Infectious

- Urinary tract infection – especially in elderly
- Encephalitis or meningitis
- Pneumonia
- Sepsis
- Influenza

Neurologic

- Brain tumor
- Subdural hematoma
- Intracerebral hemorrhage
- Seizure disorder
- CVA
- Dementia is a risk factor

Endocrine

- Hyperthyroidism
- Hypothyroidism
- Parathyroid – hyper and hypoparathyroidism

Cardiovascular

- Congestive heart failure
- Arrhythmia
- Acute myocardial infarction

Conditions that mimic delirium

- Dementia
- Depression
- Schizophrenia
- Mania
- Wernicke's aphasia

Evaluation of delirium

Mental status examination

OMI HAT (OMI = organic disease; HAT = psychiatric or functional)

- O – Orientation

- M – Memory
- I – Intellect
- H – Hallucinations
- A – Affect disorder
- T – Thought disorder

Functional Disorder

- Age 15–40 years old
- Onset gradual
- Not confused
- Appears depressed

Organic disorder

- Middle age or elderly
- Non-adolescent children
- Labile course
- Confused
- Visual hallucinations
- Vital signs frequently abnormal

Testing Options

- CBC
- CMP
- U/A
- Chest x-ray
- EKG

Tested as indicated

- Drug levels
- Thyroid studies
- Urine drug screen
- Blood alcohol
- Blood cultures
- CT brain
- Lumbar puncture for CSF analysis
- Urine culture

Treatment of delirium

- Treat underlying illness
- Restore any fluid or electrolyte imbalances
- Haloperidol 0.5 mg–5 mg PO, 2–5 mg IM, or 2–10 mg IV depending on severity of symptoms
  - **Do not** use newer atypical antipsychotic medication in **dementia-related psychosis**
- Droperidol 2.5–10 mg IM or IV
- Lorazepam
- Restraints avoided if possible
- Discontinue any unnecessary medication that is contributing to delirium

Consult criteria recommendation for delirium

- Delirium or acute altered mental status patients unless from ethanol or drug abuse

Notes

REFERENCES:

Delirium Author: Kannayiram Alagiakrishnan, MD, MBBS, MHA, MPH; Chief Editor: Iqbal Ahmed, MBBS, FRCPsych (UK)
emedicine.medscape.com/article/288890

American Psychiatric Association. Diagnostic and Statistical Manual of Mental Disorders, Fifth Edition. 5th ed. Washington, DC: American Psychiatric Association; 2013

Back

Section Contents

When using any protocol, always follow the Guidelines of Proper Use (page 12).

Back Pain Protocol

Differential Diagnosis

- Muscular pain
- Aortic aneurysm
- Vertebral infection
- Epidural hematoma
- Epidural abscess
- Herniated nucleus pulposus (HNP)
- Spinal stenosis
- Renal colic
- Pyelonephritis
- Cancer
- Prostatitis
- Perirectal abscess

Considerations

- Most back pain is benign
- Usually is without acute neurologic signs
- Radiculopathy is frequently an associated complaint or finding
- Radicular pain is from inflammation at the nerve compression site
- Fever may be harbinger of spinal or vertebral infection especially with IV drug abuse or recent instrumentation
- Elderly have increased risk of vertebral fractures with or without injury
- Second most common complaint in ambulatory care and third most expensive disorder behind cancer and heart disease

Spinal cord compression signs

- Urinary retention with overflow incontinence or voiding
- Fecal incontinence
- Decreased rectal tone
- Decreased perineal sensation

Cauda equina syndrome

- Urinary retention is most common finding in cauda equina syndrome
- Patients without urinary retention have an approximately 1/10,000 chance of having cauda equina syndrome
- Normal rectal tone usually excludes cauda equina syndrome
- Saddle numbness
- Extreme weakness
- Unilateral sciatica more common than bilateral sciatica

Warning flags in back pain

- Cancer history (Pain not relieved by rest)

- Chronic infections or fever history
- Night pain
- Prolonged pain
- Depression
- HIV history
- Unexplained weight loss
- IV substance abuse
- Disability pursuit
- Urinary retention
- Failure to improve after 6 weeks of conservative therapy

Evaluation

- Complete history and physical examination
- Check reflexes, SLR (straight leg raise), and neurovascular exam
- Check rectal tone; perineal sensation; urinary bladder retention in suspected cauda equina syndrome
- Healthy non-elderly patients without direct blunt trauma usually need no tests
- Elderly frequently need plain spine films (or plain CT) due to higher incidence of vertebral fractures
- Plain back/pelvic films may be needed in falls, MVC's, direct blunt trauma, depending on severity of injury mechanism
- U/A if renal disease suspected or significant injury mechanism
- D-dimer if aortic dissection considered
- CBC, C-RP (or ESR) for fever with vertebral back pain as only other symptom or finding

CT spine

- Acute neurologic complaints or findings
- Compression fracture > 30%
- Burst fracture (goes through entire vertebral body — unstable)
- Posterior vertebral involvement
- Traumatic back pain out of proportion to clinical expectation

MRI for spinal cord findings or symptoms

Treatment Options

- NSAID's more effective long term than opiates
  - Ibuprofen+acetaminophen more effective than hydrocodone 5 mg
  - Dexamethasone 4–6 mg PO qday for 5–10 days prn pain (caution if diabetic)
  - Gabapentin 100 mg qHS, may increase slowly over 2 days up to 300 mg to 600 mg tid as needed and tolerated
    - 1st day start lower dose due to sedation
- Short narcotic course prn for severe pain
- Preferably no prolonged bed rest unless fracture present
- Limit bed rest to no more than 2–3 days if possible (unless compression fracture)
- Return to work with restricted activities or light duty results in better long term outcomes
- Muscle relaxants of questionable usefulness
- Salmon calcitonin for compression fractures that can be discharged

Discharge criteria recommendation

- Uncomplicated presentation and findings
- Ability to control pain and ambulate

Referral

- Orthopedic referral for fractures
- Interventional radiology may treat compression fractures with vertebroplasty
- Pain management (Anesthesiologist) for possible epidural steroid injections if indicated for facet joint pain and radicular pain
- If HNP suspected refer to neurosurgeon, orthopedic spine surgeon or pain management specialist (Anesthesiologist)

- Chiropractor referral may be considered for back pain without fracture
- Physical therapy

Discharge instructions

- Follow up within 10 days as needed
- Back pain aftercare instructions

Consult criteria recommendation

- Severe pain with inability to ambulate
- Neurologic deficits
- Signs of cauda equina syndrome
- Signs of spinal cord compression or injury
- Evidence of infectious, vascular, or neoplastic etiologies
- Nontraumatic pediatric back pain
- Fracture
- Suspected aortic disease as cause of pain
- Refer to General Patient Criteria Protocol as needed

Notes

REFERENCES:

emedicine.medscape.com/article/822462

Chaparro LE, Furlan AD, Deshpande A, Mailis-Gagnon A, Atlas S, Turk DC. Opioids compared to placebo or other treatments for chronic low-back pain. *Cochrane Database Syst Rev.* Aug 27 2013;8:CD004959

Kinkade S. Evaluation and treatment of acute low back pain. Am Fam Physician. Apr 15, 2007;74(8):1181–8

Am J EM. 2020;38:143

FLANK PAIN PROTOCOL

Differential Diagnosis

- Renal colic
- Renal infarction
- Biliary colic
- Aortic aneurysm
- Mechanical back pain
- Herpes zoster
- Pyelonephritis
- Renal vein thrombosis
- Retroperitoneal bleeding
- Appendicitis
- Splenic infarction or injury

Considerations

- Renal colic is most common misdiagnosis of ruptured abdominal aortic aneurysm
- Aortic disease cause more frequent in elderly
- No hematuria on U/A with 10–15% of kidney stones
- Flank ecchymosis indicative of intra-abdominal bleeding

Evaluation

- Detailed abdomen, back, flank, and neurovascular exam

Musculoskeletal suspected as cause

- No tests unless blunt injury occurred
- Blunt trauma consider imaging
- CBC and U/A as indicated

Kidney stone suspected

- KUB
- UA
- Noncontrast CT abdominal/pelvis may be considered

CT abdominal/pelvis scan considered

- In elderly
- Unclear diagnosis

- Aortic cause suspected
- Inadequate response to pain medications

D-dimer

- Can be used as screening test to rule out aortic disease if negative (98% specific)
- Coumadin (warfarin) can cause false negative D-dimer
- Elderly have a positive D-dimer > 50% of the time without acute process
  - D-dimer increases 10 mcg/L for every year over 50 years of age if the upper cutoff is 500 mcg/L (for example an 80 year old with d-dimer 700 mcg/L would be in the normal range)
  - If another assay used, then 2% increase/year over age 50 may be used to adjust upper limit for age

U/A

- UTI symptoms
- Obtain urine C&S if pyelonephritis suspected or a diabetic with UTI

Treatment Options

- Toradol (ketorolac) 10–15 mg IV with or without
  - Ketorolac therapeutic ceiling is around 10 mg
  - Do not use Toradol (ketorolac) if creatinine is elevated
- Dilaudid (hydromorphone) 0.5–1 mg IV (or other equipotent narcotic) and Phenergan (promethazine) 6.25 mg or Zofran (ondansetron) 4 mg IV for suspected renal colic
- Ketorolac 10 mg PO qid prn not to exceed 5 days
- Musculoskeletal pain can be treated with Tylenol, OTC medication, NSAID or short narcotic course
- Narcotic short course prn on discharge for renal colic pain, with or without Toradol (ketorolac)
- Phenergan (promethazine) prn
- Flomax (tamsulosin) 0.4 mg PO every day for 2–4 weeks for ureteral calculus

Simple UTI

- Septra DS bid PO for 3 days
- Amoxicillin-clavulanate (Augmentin) 875 mg/125 mg PO BID for 7 days
- Cefdinir 300 mg PO BID for 7 days
- Ciprofloxacin 250 mg bid PO for 3 days
- Levofloxacin (Levaquin) 250 mg PO qday for 3 days
- Nitrofurantoin (Macrobid) 100 mg PO BID for 5 days
- Fosfomycin (Monurol) 3 g PO with 3-4 oz. of water X 1 dose
- Pyridium: 100–200 mg TID prn urinary symptoms — do not dispense more than 6 for acute cystitis (avoid in renal insufficiency)

Pyelonephritis (mild to moderate)

- Septra DS bid PO for 14 days
- Amoxicillin-clavulanate (Augmentin) 875 mg/125 mg PO BID for 14 days
- Cefdinir 300 mg PO BID for 7 days
- Cephalexin 500mg PO qid for 14 days
- Ciprofloxacin 500 mg bid PO for 7 days (mild infection)
- Ciprofloxacin 500 mg bid PO for 10–14 days (moderate infection)
- Levofloxacin (Levaquin) 500 mg PO qday for 5 days (mild infection)
- Levofloxacin (Levaquin) 500 mg PO qday for 10–14 days (moderate infection)
- IV Rocephin (ceftriaxone) 1–2 gms IV or IM × 1 can be given initially
- Invanz (ertapenem) × 1 can be given initially

Pyelonephritis (severe)

- Needs hospitalization

  - Invanz (ertapenem) 1 gm IV qday for 14 days or IM qday for 7 days
  - IV Rocephin (ceftriaxone) 1 gm q12hr. or 2 gms q24hr. IV or IM for 14 days
  - Ciprofloxacin (Cipro) 400 mg IV q12h for 10-14d
  - Levofloxacin (Levaquin) 250 mg IV q24h for 10d
  - Levofloxacin (Levaquin) 750 mg IV q24h for 5d
  - Tobramycin 3-6 mg/kg/day IV/IM divided q8hr (with normal renal function)
- Herpes zoster Rx as indicated

Discharge Criteria

- Renal colic controlled
- Simple cystitis
- Pyelonephritis in nontoxic patient and able to hold down medication at home
- Benign musculoskeletal disorder

Discharge instructions

- Flank pain aftercare instructions
- Refer to primary care provider or urologist as indicated within 1–7 days

Consult Criteria

- Unknown cause of moderate to severe flank pain
- Unable to hold oral fluids down at home
- Heart rate ≥ 110, hypotension or relative hypotension (SBP < 105 with history of hypertension)
- Suspected vascular cause of flank pain
- Toxic UTI patient
- Unable to hold down medications at home
- WBC ≥ 15,000
- New onset anemia
- Inadequate renal colic relief
- Age ≥ 60 without firm diagnosis
- New onset renal insufficiency or worsening renal insufficiency
- Solitary kidney with ureteral calculus
- Pyelonephritis with ureteral calculus

Notes

REFERENCES:

emedicine.medscape.com/article/1958746–overview

Causes of Flank Pain Author: J Stuart Wolf Jr, MD, FACS; Chief Editor: Bradley Fields Schwartz, DO, FACS

Age-Adjusted D-Dimer Cutoff Levels to Rule Out Pulmonary Embolism: The ADJUST-PE Study *JAMA.* 2014;311(11):1117-1124. doi:10.1001/jama.2014.2135

Gastrointestinal

Section Contents

When using any protocol, always follow the Guidelines of Proper Use (page 12).

Abdominal Pain Protocol

Differential Diagnosis

- See below locations of pain

Considerations

- Appendicitis may have normal WBC
  - WBC ≥ 10,000 with left shift in 80–90% of patients
- WBC is a poor predictor of surgical disease
- Consider EKG in epigastric pain with CAD risk factors and a benign exam
- Constitutional history important

Diagnostic pitfall

- Diagnosing UTI with mildly elevated urinary WBC's in the general range of 7–15 WBC's (or so) on U/A as the cause of moderate to severe abdominal pain and/or tenderness, especially in females and those without infectious urinary complaints, frequently is erroneous

Locations of pain

RUQ

- Gallbladder disease
- Liver disease
- Peptic ulcer disease

Epigastric

- Peptic ulcer
- Cardiac ischemia
- Gallbladder disease
- Pancreatitis
- Aortic aneurysm
- Mesenteric ischemia
- Small bowel disorder
- Gastroparesis

LUQ

- Colon disorder
- Spleen disorder
- Liver disease
- Constipation

Right and left flanks

- Renal colic
- Pyelonephritis
- Aortic aneurysm

Periumbilical

- Pancreatitis
- Peptic ulcer
- Mesenteric ischemia
- Aortic aneurysm
- Intussusception

RLQ

- Appendicitis
- Mesenteric adenitis
- Diverticulitis
- Renal colic
- Ectopic pregnancy
- Ovarian cyst rupture
- Colitis
- Constipation
- Intussusception

LLQ

- Diverticulitis (most common area)
- Renal colic
- Ectopic pregnancy
- Ovarian cyst rupture
- Colitis
- Intussusception
- Constipation

Suprapubic

- Cystitis
- Prostatitis
- Proctitis
- Perirectal abscess
- Constipation/fecal impaction

Groin

- Inguinal hernia
- Femoral hernia
- Inguinal ligament strain
- Femoral pseudoaneursym post cardiac catheterization

Appendicitis

- See Appendicitis Protocol

Diverticulitis

- Prevalence increases with age
- Usually pain and tenderness in LLQ of abdomen
- Fever may occur
- WBC may not be elevated in 60% of patients
- CT abdominal/pelvis imaging study of choice
  - With children start with abdominal ultrasound for radiation considerations
    - Ultrasound used to rule in appendicitis; do not use to rule out appendicitis (if negative and appendicitis a consideration, then CT abdomen/pelvis)
- Patients with mild to moderate diverticulitis without systemic signs of infection or peritoneal signs may be discharged home on antibiotics and a clear liquid diet for 2–3 days and advanced as tolerated
  - Flagyl (metronidazole) 500 mg PO qid for 10 days
  - Cipro (ciprofloxacin) 500 mg PO bid or Levaquin (levofloxacin) 500–750 mg PO qday with Flagyl (metronidazole) for 10 days
  - Septra DS PO bid can be used instead of Cipro (ciprofloxacin) or Levofloxacin if needed
  - Augmentin (amoxicillin/clavulanate) 875 mg PO bid for 10 days may be

used instead of other antibiotics
  - May use Sanford guide or antibiotic database also

Biliary colic and cholecystitis

- See Gallbladder Disease Protocol

Pancreatitis

- Major causes are gallstones lodged in common bile duct and ethanol consumption
- 2 of the 3 following criteria
  - Characteristic abdominal pain
  - Serum amylase or lipase > 4 times the upper limit of normal
  - Imaging findings suggestive of acute pancreatitis
- Severe pain usually in central abdomen and vomiting very common
- Chronic pancreatitis may develop (alcoholics)
  - Lipase may remain elevated with a normal amylase
- Lipase may remain elevated up to 12 days whereas amylase will return to normal after acute pancreatitis has resolved
- Level of lipase and amylase do not indicate severity of disease
- Fever may occur
- Obtain CBC, amylase, lipase, LFT's, LDH and U/A
  - Amylase may be normal early
  - Lipase and amylase elevated more than 4 times normal is diagnostic of acute pancreatitis
- Ultrasound if cholecystitis or choledocholithiasis suspected
- Treatment options
  - IV NS or LR 250–400 cc/hour for adults
    - Lactated ringers (LR) may be preferred over NS
    - Caution in heart failure and renal failure patients, etc.
  - If patient hypotensive then more aggressive fluid resuscitation needed
  - Phenergan (promethazine) 6.25 mg IV or 25–50 mg IM

OR

  - Zofran (ondansetron) 4–8 mg IM or IV
  - Stadol (butorphanol) 0.25–1 mg IV or 2 mg IM (avoid in opiate addiction)

OR

  - Dilaudid (hydromorphone) 0.25–2 mg IV or 1–2 mg IM
  - Small narcotic doses for very elderly

Mesenteric ischemia

- Mortality high – 70–90%, especially with low flow circulatory states such as CHF
- Causes are arterial embolism, arterial thrombosis, non-occlusive mesenteric ischemia and venous thrombosis which all lead to ischemia/reperfusion syndrome of the bowel
- Order CBC, BMP, lactate level, amylase, lipase and CT abdomen/pelvis
- Severe pain with less than expected tenderness on exam (may only have mild tenderness)
- Vomiting and diarrhea frequently present
- Risk factors are CHF, atrial fibrillation, and atherosclerotic disease
- May have metabolic acidosis secondary to bowel infarction (elevated lactic acid and/or elevated anion gap)
- Intestinal angina may occur after a meal

Small bowel obstruction (SBO)

- Usually from postsurgical adhesions
- Pain is usually severe if obstruction is complete
- Vomiting is very common
- Hyperactive bowels sounds seen early in process
- Abdominal distension common
- Check for hernias
- Order CBC, amylase, lipase and CMP
- Obtain flat and upright plain abdominal films — may be negative in 30%

- Consider CT abdomen/pelvis if SBO suspected and plain films nondiagnostic
- May need N-G tube to low suction though can be managed frequently without suction.
  - Latest data suggest suction may not be as effective as was thought in the past

Large bowel obstruction

- 60% from malignancy, 20% from diverticulitis and 5% from cecal volvulus
- Abdominal distension is significant
- Abdomen is hyperresonant on percussion
- Fever, rebound tenderness and rigidity suggest perforation
- Order CBC, CMP, lactate level if acidotic, and flat and upright abdominal films
- Ogilvie syndrome is colonic pseudoobstruction
  - Needs to be decompressed to avoid perforation

Hernia

Differential diagnosis

- Epididymitis
- Hydrocele
- Lymphogranuloma Venereum
- Testicular torsion
- Pseudoaneurym of femoral artery
- Varicocele
- Groin abscess

Considerations

- Reducible hernia can have contents returned to abdominal cavity
- Incarcerated hernia cannot be reduced
  - Not strangulated
  - Bowel obstruction not uncommon
  - Painful
- Strangulated hernia
  - Blood flow compromised with possible necrosis of bowel
  - Significant pain and tenderness
  - If reduced, pain and tenderness persists

Types of hernia

- Umbilical
  - Through umbilical ring
  - Common in childhood
  - Usually resolves by age 2 years
- Inguinal
  - Indirect inguinal hernia
    - Through inguinal ring into the inguinal canal following spermatic cord to scrotum
  - Direct inguinal hernia
    - Through Hasselbach's triangle (above inguinal ligament
- Femoral
  - Through femoral canal
  - Frequently become incarcerated or strangulated
- Ventral or incisional hernia
  - Post-surgical complication
  - Usually without pain or incarceration

Gastroenteritis

- See Gastroenteritis Protocols for adults and pediatrics

Flank pain or kidney stone pain (renal colic) see respective Protocols

Elderly abdominal pain

- Pain perception and abdominal exam altered in elderly
- Admissions and surgery rates are higher
- Consider mesenteric and cardiac ischemia
- Elderly may have normal WBC with serious disease
- Appendicitis missed 50% of the time
- CT abdominal/pelvis commonly ordered as serious organic disease is more prevalent
- Diverticulitis: WBC is normal 50% of the time
- Consider ruptured aortic aneurysm especially with flank pain thought to be renal colic

- Polypharmacy and medication side effects can be a cause of abdominal complaints

Pediatric abdominal pain

- Peritonitis patient is immobile
- Colic patient is writhing
- Absence of fever does not rule out serious illness
- In children start with abdominal ultrasound for radiation exposure considerations
  - Ultrasound used to rule-in appendicitis; do not use to rule-out appendicitis (if negative and appendicitis a consideration, then CT abdomen/pelvis)

Pediatric appendicitis

- Frequently missed in age < 2 years
- With abdominal pain, fever is most useful sign in appendicitis
- CBC may be normal
- Absolute neutrophil count < 6750 significantly decreases the likelihood of appendicitis
- Less than 50% have classic presentation
- Missed appendicitis is second most common reason for pediatric malpractice suits in the emergency department
- Perforation occurs in majority of patients < 4 years of age with appendicitis
- Treatment delayed > 36 hours increases rate of perforations up to 65% in appendicitis cases
- C-reactive protein is nonspecific and not helpful if positive in determining cause of inflammation or abdominal pain
- U/A can have pyuria, bacteriuria or hematuria in 20–40% of patients
- MRI has a high accuracy for the diagnosis of acute appendicitis, with a sensitivity and specificity of 96% and 96% in children
- CT abdomen/pelvis if needed

Gastroparesis

- Frequently seen in diabetes, but occurs in other conditions
- Abdominal pain more so in upper abdomen

Treatment

- IV hydration as needed
- Metoclopramide 10 mg IV/IM/PO q6hr 30 minutes before meals and at bedtime
  - Use injectable dosing only if severe symptoms are present
- Erythromycin 250-500 mg PO three times daily before meals (very expensive)

General Evaluation

History

- Pain onset and duration
- Location and migration
- Appetite
- Exacerbating factors
- Prior surgical, medical and medication history
- Vomiting and fever history
- Bowel and urinary history
- Constitutional history
- Melena or bleeding
- Last normal menstrual cycle
- Menstrual abnormalities

Physical examination

- Observe for distension
- Auscultation for bowel sounds and arterial bruits
- Gently palpate entire abdomen
- Percuss for liver size; and for ascites if present
- Perform rectal exam for masses; tenderness; prostate disease; gross blood; occult blood when indicated
- Palpation of entire abdomen and document any findings of:
  - Tenderness location and severity
  - Rebound tenderness
  - Voluntary and involuntary guarding
  - Pulsatile masses
  - Abdominal masses

Objective testing

Benign findings and complaints in nonelderly healthy patient

- Consider no tests

Moderate complaints and findings, or if diabetic

- CBC and CMP

Urine or renal disease

- U/A
- CBC and BMP if pyelonephritis suspected
- Urine culture as indicated

Pancreatitis

- Amylase and lipase
- CBC and CMP

Gallbladder disease

- Gallbladder ultrasound as needed
- CBC and BMP
- Amylase, lipase and LFT's

Hepatic or metastatic malignant disease

- Liver function tests
- CBC and BMP

Fertile female

- UCG

Constipation or obstruction

- KUB or flat/upright films

Consider CT scan in adults for

- Suspected appendicitis or diverticulitis
- Flank pain of unknown etiology
- Rebound tenderness in adults
- Suspected bowel obstruction not seen on plain flat and upright abdominal films
- Elderly with moderate to severe pain

Caution in ordering pediatric CT scans – ultrasound can be used for appendicitis evaluation instead to rule-in appendicitis (not rule-out), depending on the institution

Outpatient Treatment Considerations

- OTC medications
- Hydrocodone or synthetic codeine derivatives short course (≤3 days) as needed
- Avoid Demerol (meperidine)
- Phenergan (promethazine) or Zofran (ondansetron) prn nausea or vomiting

Parenteral Treatment Considerations

- IV NS for adults as clinically indicated
- IV NS 1–2 times maintenance in children if stable if indicated
- Nausea or vomiting (adjust for children)
  - Phenergan (promethazine) 6.25 mg IV (adult or pediatrics) or 25–50 mg IM adult or 0.5 mg/kg IM for children

    OR

  - Zofran (ondansetron) 4 mg ODT, IM or IV (adults and pediatrics)
- Pain control (adjust for children)
  - Stadol (butorphanol) 0.25–1 mg IV or 1–2 mg IM for adults (avoid in opiate addiction)

    OR

  - Dilaudid (hydromorphone) 0.25–1 mg IV or 1–2 mg IM for adult or 0.015 mg/Kg IV or IM for pediatrics
  - Reduced narcotic and Phenergan (promethazine) doses for the very elderly

Discharge criteria recommendation

- Mild pain and tenderness in nonelderly healthy patient with normal vital signs consider symptomatic treatment if benign disease process suspected

- Biliary colic with normal vital signs and exam that resolves with treatment may not require labs, or has normal CBC and LFT's, may be discharged frequently
- Acute and self-limited process suspected such as gastroenteritis in stable nontoxic patient
- Reducible hernia with resolution of pain and no strangulation initially present

Discharge instructions

- To primary care provider or surgeon for follow-up in 1 day if pain is moderate to severe, otherwise in 5–7 days
- To primary care provider for abnormal lab within 1 week unless chronic in nature
- Abdominal pain aftercare instructions

Consult criteria recommendation

- Abdominal pain that develops hypotension or relative hypotension (SBP < 105 with history of hypertension)
- Toxic appearance
- Dehydration
- Significant GI blood loss or melena
- Acute surgical abdomen or rebound tenderness
- Severe pain of uncertain cause
- Severe pain with any diagnosis
- Intractable vomiting
- Return ED or clinic visit within 14 days for same acute abdominal pain complaint

Discuss with surgeon or physician if following suspected or diagnosed

- Appendicitis
- Cholecystitis
- Pancreatitis
- Diverticulitis
- Aortic aneurysm
- Bowel obstruction
- Ectopic pregnancy
- Intra-abdominal abscess
- Mesenteric ischemia
- Incarcerated or strangulated hernia

Lab consult criteria recommendation (if checked)

- Hemoglobin decrease > 1 gm or creatinine increase> 0.5 from baseline
- Significant acute hemoglobin decrease
- Elevated LFT's
- Elevated amylase or lipase
- WBC ≥ 14,000
- Bandemia
- Increased anion gap
- Metabolic acidosis
- Elevated lactic acid
- Significant electrolyte abnormally
- Hyperglycemia with metabolic acidosis (decreased serum CO_2 or elevated anion gap)
- Acute thrombocytopenia

Notes

____

____

____

REFERENCES:

Tenner S, Baillie J, Dewitt J, et al. American College of Gastroenterology Guidelines: Management of Acute Pancreatitis. *Am J Gastroenterol.* Jul 30 201

Wu BU , et al. Â C*lin Gastroenterol Hepatol* 2011; 9:710

emedicine.medscape.com/article/181364

JICS;15(3):226-230

Diabetic Neuropathy Updated: Jul 23, 2019

Author: Dianna Quan, MD; Chief Editor: Romesh Khardori, MD, PhD, FACP

Mayo Clin Proc. 2021;96:1052

CT Abdominal Scan Issues

Cancer Risk from One CT Depending on Type

- Adults: 1/500–2000
- Children under 1 year of age: 1/500
- Decreasing risk with increasing age

Oral contrast considerations

- Adds little if anything to interpretation
  - Oral contrast located immediately adjacent to the bowel wall can make assessment of the degree of IV contrast enhancement difficult
  - IV contrast extravasating into bowel lumen can be masked by dense positive oral contrast
- Some radiologists uncomfortable without it
- Appendicitis diagnosed without vs. with contrast
  - Sensitivity 95% vs. 92%
  - Specificity 97% vs. 94%
  - Accuracy 97% vs. 89%
- Message: Non-oral contrast CT is better in diagnosing appendicitis

IV contrast considerations

- Does not improve accuracy of noncontrast studies
- In very thin patients without much body fat IV contrast is needed

There is no connection between seafood and/or shellfish allergy and IV contrast allergy

Treatment of Allergy to IV Contrast

- Benadryl (diphenhydramine) 50 mg in adult or weight based in children
- Decadron (dexamethasone) 10 mg IV in adult or 0.6 mg/kg IV in children (not to exceed 10 mg)
- May not be effective since steroid dosing should be done 12 hours before IV contrast

Prior History of Asthma

- 1/1000 chance of severe reaction to IV contrast
- No reason to withhold contrast study

Creatinine Considerations

- Majority of patients do not need a creatinine measurement
- Needed with history of **risk** factors
  - Renal insufficiency
  - Elderly
  - Diabetes
  - Multiple myeloma
  - Volume depletion
  - Diuretic therapy
  - NSAID's use
  - ACE inhibitor use
  - CHF
  - Anemia

Prevention of Contrast-induced Nephropathy (CIN)

- There is a lack of good data
- Defined as creatinine increase of 0.5mg/dL or 1.0 mg/dL over baseline depending on literature source or 25% increase 1–5 days after contrast
- Risk with creatinine levels
  - Creatinine < 1.5 mg/dL = 0.6% risk
  - Creatinine 1.5–4.5 mg/dL = 9.2% risk

  - Creatinine >4.5 mg/dL = 39% risk
- Dialysis is required in less than 1% of contrast usage
- IV hydration NS 1–1.5 ml/kg/hr. 3 hours before contrast and continued 6–24 hours after reduces nephropathy
- Considerations for 0 or 1 risk factor above
  - Before procedure: 1 liter of D5W mixed with 3 amps of $NaHCO_3^-$ IV at 3 cc/kg for 1 hour
  - During procedure: low volume iso-osmolar contrast
  - After procedure: 1 liter of D5W mixed with 3 amps $NaHCO_3^-$ IV at 1 cc/kg for 6 hours
- Considerations for 2 or more risk factors — do above

  PLUS
  - N-acetylcysteine 150 mg/kg IV 30 minutes before procedure

    and 600–1200 mg PO bid × 2 doses after procedure

  OR
  - Vitamin C 3 gms PO 2 hours before procedure and bid PO after procedure for 1 day

Metformin and IV contrast

- No increase in lactic acidosis if creatinine normal

Notes

REFERENCES:

xrayrisk.com/calculator/calculator.php

Ionizing Radiation Exposure with Medical Imaging Author: Edward B Holmes, MD, MPH, MSc; Chief Editor: Caroline R Taylor, MD emedicine.medscape.com/article/1464228

Friedewald VE, Goldfarb S, Laskey WK, et al. The editor's roundtable: contrast-induced nephropathy. *Am J Cardiol.* Aug 1 2007;100(3):544–51

Emerg Radiol, epub 5/11/16

ADULT GASTROENTERITIS PROTOCOL

Definition

- Acute inflammatory or infectious process of the stomach and intestines

Differential Diagnosis

- Appendicitis
- Cholecystitis
- Pancreatitis
- Mesenteric ischemia
- Aortic aneurysm
- Peptic ulcer disease
- GERD
- Biliary colic
- Renal colic
- Bowel obstruction
- Inflammatory bowel disease
- Excessive cannabis use
- Rheumatoid Colitis

Definitions

- Diarrhea > 3 loose bowel movements (BM's) per day
- Acute diarrhea is < 14 days
- Dysentery
  - Disorders with intestinal inflammation (usually colon)
  - Abdominal pain
  - Tenesmus
  - Frequent BM's with blood and mucus in stool
- Enteritis — small bowel inflammation
- Gastritis — stomach inflammation

- Gastroenteritis symptoms
  - Abdominal pain
  - Weakness
  - Nausea
  - Diarrhea
  - Anorexia
  - Fever

Considerations

- Diarrhea most common manifestation (virus most common cause — norovirus)
- Enteritis — often with bloating, periumbilical pain, nausea/vomiting (viral most common cause)
- Colitis — can have localized left sided pain, rectal bleeding
- Antibiotics can cause diarrhea — C. difficile (antibiotic-associated or "pseudomembranous" colitis)
- Association between antibiotic use, enterohemorrhagic Escherichia coli and hemolytic-uremic syndrome has various study conclusions
  - Shiga toxin-producing E.coli. (STEC) is the most common infectious bloody diarrhea in the United States.
  - Antibiotics are not recommended for toxin-producing bacteria, especially STEC, due to risk of hemolytic uremic syndrome and bacterial lysis leading to worsening illness or symptom prolongation
- Probiotics and prebiotics not recommended for acute diarrhea or mild travelers–associated diarrhea except for postantibiotic–diarrhea

Diarrhea Red Flags

- Bloody stools or pus in stool
- Infant refuses to drink anything for more than 3 to 4 hours
- Signs of dehydration and/or acute weight loss
- Abdominal pain that comes and goes over extended period of time, or is severe
- Any fever >102°F (39°C) or a fever >101°F (38.4°C) that persists for more than 3 days
- Decreased responsiveness or lethargy
- Chronic diarrhea
- Recent antibiotic use
- Weight loss over past 1–2 months

Invasive bacteria — frequently with occult or gross blood

- Campylobacter
- Salmonella
- Shigella
- Vibrio
- Yersinia

Food-borne disease

- Staph aureus most common: 1–6 hours post food ingestion
- Bacillus cereus: 1–36 hours post food ingestion
- Cholera: profuse rice water stools
  - Ciprofloxacin 1 gm PO once or doxycycline 300 mg PO once or Septra DS (TMP160 mg/SMX 800 mg) bid PO for 5–7 days
- Ciguatera: Fish — 5 minutes–30 hours post food ingestion
- Traveler's diarrhea: E. coli usually
- Camping: Giardia, water ingestion, beavers
  - Tinidazole 2 gm PO once or Nitazoxanide 500 mg PO q12hr for 3 days or metronidazole 250 mg tid PO for 5–7 days

Evaluation

- Travel, food and antibiotic history
- Healthy patient without toxicity and with acute onset of symptoms and mild to no tenderness and normal vital signs may not require further testing
- Consider CBC, CMP if vital signs abnormal or with significant tenderness
- Consider stool WBC, RBC, cultures for fever; blood in stool
- Consider rectal exam
- Imaging usually not necessary unless

- Obstruction suspected
  - Abdominal flat and upright films
  - Consider CT abdomen/pelvis if bowel obstruction suspected and plain films negative
- Consider CT abdomen/pelvis with significant abnormal vital signs and/or significant tenderness or pain

Treatment Options

Dehydration

Oral Rehydration Therapy (ORT) for mild to moderate dehydration

- Oral rehydration formula (WHO, Rehydralyte or Pedialyte) for mild to moderate dehydration or serum CO_2 13–18 mEq/L or Na^+ 146–152 mEq/L — if able to take PO fluids
- Zofran (ondansetron) 8 mg chewable tablet if vomiting or 4–8 mg IM
- 15–30 cc every 1–2 minutes for 1–4 hours for age > 12 — start 20 minutes after Zofran (ondansetron) given
- Hold ORT 10 minutes if vomiting occurs then resume
- Re-assess for urine production, improved heart rate, and absence of severe vomiting
- Recheck serum CO2 if initially < 17 mEq/L or anion gap > 21
- Mild dehydration give 20 cc/kg in < 4 hours
- Moderate dehydration give 20–40 cc/kg in 1–4 hours
- Severe dehydration give IV NS 200–500 cc/hour over 2–4 hours or 1000 cc/hour for 1 hour
- Hypotension or signs of poor organ perfusion (lactic acid > 2) give NS at 500–1,000 cc/hour up to 2 liters (can start with IV 500–1,000 cc bolus)

Diarrhea

- Nontoxic, non-dehydrated healthy patients with mild abdominal tenderness, benign vital signs and diarrhea may be discharged without further testing
- Treat with oral rehydration if tolerated, or IV rehydration if needed
- **Empirical antibiotic treatment not recommended for routine acute diarrhea or mild traveler–associated diarrhea**
- Persistent diarrhea 15–30 days evaluated with culture and non–independent microbiologic testing
- Community acquired acute diarrhea usually is viral and does not need antibiotic treatment

Traveler–associated diarrhea

- **Mild diarrhea does not usually need antibiotics**
- Pepto-Bismol — good for traveler's diarrhea
- Loperamide recommended if antibiotic therapy is started to decrease duration of diarrhea
- Prophylactic antibiotics only for travelers going outside of U.S. or Europe who are at high risk for traveler's diarrhea, especially if the illness may pose a threat for serious health morbidities or affect the purpose of travel
- Fluoroquinolone such as ciprofloxacin 500 mg PO bid
  - 1, 3 or 5 day course, especially with traveler's diarrhea
  - Fluoroquinolones significantly increase incidence of C. difficile colitis
- Azithromycin 500 mg once or qday for 3 days as effective as quinolone and is recommended if fever present
- Septra DS 1 PO bid for 5 days (DOC for age < 18 years or for **shigella)**

- Septra (TMP/SMZ) 8-12 mg TMP/kg/dose or 0.5 cc/LB BID PO for PO q12hr for 5-10 days for children
- Contraindicated in ages < 2 months
- Rifaximin – Xifaxan 200 mg PO q8hr. for 3 days
  - Better safety profile than fluoroquinolones (ciprofloxacin etc.) with C. difficile and extended β–lactamase producing Enterobacteriaceae (ESBL–PE)
  - ESBL–PE 12–69% of travelers become colonized with antibiotic treatment and may last 6–9 months
- If C. difficile colitis suspected from recent antibiotic use:
  - See Antibiotic–associated Colitis Protocol
  - Mild to moderate symptoms
    - Flagyl (metronidazole) 500 mg PO tid × 10 days
    - Florastor PO bid × 10 days (OTC)

Antibiotic therapy

- World Health Organization currently recommends empiric antimicrobial therapy in the setting of febrile acute bloody diarrhea in young **children**
  - Infections by enteropathogenic *E coli*, when having a prolonged course — septra or ceftriaxone
  - Enteroinvasive E coli, based on the serologic, genetic, and pathogenic similarities with *Shigella* — septra or ceftriaxone
  - Yersinia infections in subjects with sickle cell disease — septra or cipro or ceftriaxone or doxycycline (avoid doxycycline in age <8 years)
  - *Salmonella* infections in very young infants, if febrile or with positive blood culture findings — ceftriaxone
  - Most salmonella infections do not require antibiotics and they may prolong the illness
- Clostridium difficile proven or clinically suspected — metronidazole (30 mg/kg/d divided qid for 7 d) can be used as a first-line agent, with oral vancomycin reserved for resistant infections
  - Stop offending antibiotic
  - See primary care provider within 1–2 days for follow-up

Antimotility agents

- Loperamide (most preferred due to safety profile)
- Diphenoxylate (heme negative stools only)

Vomiting in gastroenteritis

- Phenergan (promethazine) PO/PR/IM (if IV give no more than 6.25 mg/dose as single dose)
- Zofran (ondansetron) 4–8 mg PO/IM/IV

Cannabinoid Hyperemesis Syndrome

- Intractable vomiting in heavy cannabis users
- Runs hot shower or bath over abdomen for relief
- THC in single use detectable for up to 72 hours and up to 1 month in heavy users
- Illegal synthetic cannabinoids such as "Spice" or "K2" are not detected on urine drug screen for marijuana because chemical structures are different from THC

Treatment

- Haloperidol in doses of 2 – 5 mg IV/IM
  - THC has been shown to increase dopamine synthesis and dopamine cell firing, which may explain clinical improvement with haloperidol
- Topical capsaicin cream
- IV LR or NS for dehydration or acute kidney injury

Abdominal pain treatment outpatient considerations

- OTC medications
- Hydrocodone or synthetic codeine derivatives as needed
- Avoid Demerol (meperidine)

Abdominal pain parenteral treatment considerations

- Stadol (butorphanol), Nubain (nalbuphine) or Dilaudid (hydromorphone): IV or IM
  - Stadol and Nubain may cause acute opiate withdrawal in opiate addicted patients
- Give Phenergan (promethazine) 6.25 mg (if IV) or Zofran (ondansetron) as needed for nausea
- Adjust doses for weight in pediatrics

Discharge criteria recommendation

- Healthy nontoxic patient with stable vital signs

Discharge instructions

- Gastroenteritis aftercare instructions
- Resume regular diet as soon as possible
- Follow-up in 1–2 days if symptoms are moderate to severe if discharged, otherwise within 5–7 days if symptoms persist
- Follow up for abnormal lab within 1 week unless chronic in nature
- Return within 3 days if symptoms not improving

Consult criteria recommendation

- Toxic appearance
- Dehydration > 5%
- Significant blood loss or melena
- Suspected or diagnosed appendicitis, cholecystitis, pancreatitis, diverticulitis, aortic aneurysm, bowel obstruction or admittable diagnosis
- Acute surgical abdomen
- Moderate pain of uncertain cause
- Severe pain
- Intractable vomiting
- Return visit within 14 days for same acute abdominal pain complaint

Lab consult criteria recommendation (if checked)

- Metabolic acidosis (increased anion gap)
- Elevated lactic acid
- Hemoglobin decrease > 1 gm or creatinine increase> 0.5 from baseline
- Elevated LFT's
- Elevated amylase or lipase
- WBC ≥ 15,000
- Bandemia
- Significant electrolyte abnormally
- Hyperglycemia with metabolic acidosis (decreased serum CO_2 or elevated anion gap)
- Acute thrombocytopenia

Vital sign consult criteria recommendation

- Adult heart rate > 110 post-treatment
- Hypotension or relative hypotension (SBP < 105 with history of hypertension)
- Orthostatic vital signs

Notes

___

___

___

REFERENCES:

Payne DC, Vinjé J, Szilagyi PG, Edwards KM, Staat MA, Weinberg GA. Norovirus and medically attended gastroenteritis in U.S. children. *N Engl J Med.* Mar 21 2013;368(12):1121–30

Author: Arthur Diskin, MD; Chief Editor: Steven C Dronen, MD, FAAEM emedicine.medscape.com/article/775277

Richards JR, et al. *Pharmacotherapy*. 2017 Mar 31

Sorensen Cj, et al. *J Med Toxicol*. 2017 Mar;13(1):71-87

Inayat F, et al. *BMJ Case Rep*. 2017 Jan 4;2017

Witsil JC, et al. *Am J Ther*. 2017 Jan/Feb;24(1):e64-e67

Sorensen CJ, et al. *J Med Toxicol*. 2017 Mar 10

J Med Toxicol, 2017;13:71

Mayo Clin Proc.2021;96:E1

Irritable Bowel Syndrome Protocol

Definition

- A functional bowel disorder without specific pathology of abdominal pain and altered bowel habits

Differential Diagnosis

- Anxiety disorder
- Biliary colic
- Inflammatory bowel disease
- Ischemic colitis
- Antibiotic-associated colitis
- Endometriosis
- Gastroenteritis
- Food allergies
- Malabsorption
- Porphyria
- Colon carcinoma
- Thyroid disease

Considerations

- Is a disorder of exclusion of other disease processes
- Hypersensitivity to pain and symptoms
- Association with psychopathology is common
- Is a chronic relapsing disorder
- Females 2–3 times more likely to have the disorder than males

Common Symptoms and Findings

- Abdominal pain
- Diarrhea
- Constipation
- Mucus in stool
- Abdominal distension
- Stress related commonly
- Fibromyalgia is frequently present
- Postprandial bowel movement urgency

Symptoms not consistent with IBS

- Middle age or later onset
- New symptom presentations
- Fever
- Weight loss
- Nocturnal symptoms
- Progressive symptoms
- Rectal bleeding
- Painless diarrhea

Patterns of IBS

- IBS-D (diarrhea predominant)
- IBS-C (constipation predominant)
- IBS-M (mixed diarrhea and constipation)
- IBS-A (alternating diarrhea and constipation)

Evaluation

- History and physical examination
- Rectal examination for occult blood as indicated
- Testing not recommended in age < 50 years with typical IBS symptoms and no weight loss, or family history of serious bowel

diseases (colon cancer, inflammatory bowel disease, etc.)

Lab test options

- CBC
- BMP
- LFT's
- Thyroid panel as indicated
- Plain flat and upright x-rays as indicated
- Amylase and lipase as indicated
- CT abdominal and pelvis scan as indicated (usually not needed)

Treatment Options

- Add fiber to diet
- Reassurance regarding symptoms and diagnosis
- Stress management suggestions
- Consider psychiatric referral

Antispasmodic agents

- Bentyl (dicyclomine) 10–40 mg PO qid ac (before meals) or with pain onset
- Levsin (hyoscyamine) 0.125–0.25 mg q4hr and or prn (NMT 1.5 pills/day) for adults
- Levsin (hyoscyamine) 1/2–1 pill qid PO q4hr or prn (NMT 6 tabs/day) for age 2–12 years

Antidiarrheal agents

Lomotil (diphenoxylate/atropine)

- Age > 12 years: 1–2 tabs PO qid ac prn
- Age 8–12 years: 2 mg PO 5 times qday prn
- Age 5–7 years: 2 mg PO qid prn
- Age 2–4 years: 2 mg PO tid prn

Imodium (loperamide)

- Adult: 4 mg PO after 1st loose stool, then 2 mg PO after each following loose stool prn (NMT 16 mg/day)
- Pediatric: 0.1 mg/kg PO after each loose stool not to exceed adult total daily dose

Other agents

- SSRI's
- Elavil (amitriptyline) 10–100 mg PO qday prn (start with low dose)
- Rifaximin – Xifaxan 550 mg PO q8hr for 14 days (nonabsorbed antibiotic) — read drug information
- Lubiprostone – Amitiza 8 mcg PO q12hr in women ≥ 18 years with IBS–C (constipation type) — read drug information
- Linaclotide – Linzess 290 mcg PO qday at least 30 minutes before first meal of the day for adults for the treatment of irritable bowel syndrome with constipation
- Eluxadoline – Viberzi 100 mg bid PO with food for diarrhea-predominant irritable bowel syndrome (IBS-D) in adult men and women
  - Stop if constipation > 4 days
  - 75 mg bid for cholecystectomy patients or hepatic impairment

Discharge criteria recommendation

- No other concerning disease process diagnosed

Discharge instructions

- Irritable bowel syndrome aftercare instructions
- Follow up within 10 days or as needed

Consult criteria recommendation

- Elevated WBC
- Severe pain
- Heart rate > 110
- Dehydration
- Patient appears toxic
- Fever
- Weight loss
- Progressive symptoms
- Rectal bleeding

Notes

REFERENCES:

Brandt LJ, Chey WD, Foxx-Orenstein AE, Schiller LR, Schoenfeld PS, Spiegel BM, et al. An evidence-based position statement on the management of irritable bowel syndrome. *Am J Gastroenterol*. Jan 2009;104 Suppl 1:S1–35

Irritable Bowel Syndrome Author: Jenifer K Lehrer, MD; Chief Editor: Julian Katz, MD
emedicine.medscape.com/article/180389–overview

APPENDICITIS PROTOCOL

Definition

- Inflammation of the appendix secondary to luminal obstruction

Differential Diagnosis

- Pelvic inflammatory disease
- Ruptured ovarian cyst
- Endometriosis
- Mesenteric adenitis
- Inflammatory bowel disease
- Colon carcinoma
- Mesenteric ischemia
- Ureteral colic
- Pyelonephritis
- Biliary colic
- Abdominal abscess
- Diverticulitis
- Ectopic pregnancy
- Ovarian torsion
- Constipation

Considerations

- Appendicitis is missed 50% of the time in elderly
- In patients with suspected acute appendicitis, use clinical findings (signs and symptoms) to risk-stratify patients and guide decisions about further testing and management
- In adult patients undergoing a CT scan for suspected appendicitis, perform abdominal and pelvic CT scan with or without contrast IV
  - Patients with little body fat may need IV contrast
  - In children, use ultrasound to confirm acute appendicitis but not to definitively exclude acute appendicitis
    - In children, use an abdominal and pelvic CT to confirm or exclude acute appendicitis if ultrasound does not rule-in appendicitis
- The duration of symptoms is less than 48 hours in approximately 80% of adults
  - Frequently longer in elderly persons and in those with perforation
- Approximately 2% of patients report duration of pain in excess of 2 weeks
- A history of similar pain is reported in as many as 23% of cases, and this history of similar pain should not be used to rule out the possibility of appendicitis
- If mesenteric adenitis is diagnosed, it can be treated with supportive care or in more severe cases antibiotics
  - Metronidazole, clindamycin, or Unasyn

Presentations

- Abdominal pain is most common symptom
- Migration of pain from periumbilical area to RLQ has sensitivity and specificity of 80%
- Nausea present in 61–92% of patients

- Vomiting that precedes pain suggests intestinal obstruction instead
- Anorexia present in 74–78% of patients
- Diarrhea or constipation noted in around 18% of patients
- Common to have either low-grade fever or no fever
- High fever develops with abscess formation secondary to appendiceal rupture
- Fecaliths and lymphoid hyperplasia most common causes of luminal obstruction

Physical findings

- 96% of patients with RLQ tenderness — most specific sign
- The most specific exam findings are guarding, percussion tenderness, rebound tenderness and rigidity
- Rosving, Obturator, Psoas signs present in minority of patients and their absence should not be used to rule out appendicitis

Lab findings

- Normal C-reactive protein after abdominal pain for 24 hours has a high negative predictive value ruling out appendicitis
- Urinary complaints and U/A showing WBC's not uncommon in appendicitis

Pregnancy and appendicitis

- First trimester pain in RLQ
- Second trimester pain at level of umbilicus
- Third trimester pain in RUQ
- Anorexia in one-third to two-thirds of patients
- Nausea usually present
- MRI has a high accuracy for the diagnosis of acute appendicitis, with a sensitivity and specificity of 94% and 97%, respectively, in pregnant patients

Pediatric appendicitis

- Frequently missed in age < 2 years
- With abdominal pain, fever is most useful sign in appendicitis
- CBC may be normal
  - WBC >10,500 in 80–85% of adults with appendicitis
  - Less than 4% of patients with appendicitis have a WBC count less than 10,500 and neutrophilia less than 75% of WBC's
- Absolute neutrophil count < 6750 significantly decreases the likelihood of appendicitis
- Less than 50% have classic presentation
- Missed appendicitis is second most common reason for pediatric malpractice suits in the emergency department
- Perforation occurs in majority of patients < 4 years of age with appendicitis
- Treatment delayed > 36 hours increases rate of perforations up to 65% of appendicitis cases
- C-reactive protein is nonspecific and not helpful if positive in determining cause of inflammation or abdominal pain
  - Very high levels of CRP in patients with appendicitis indicate gangrenous appendix, especially if it is associated with elevated WBC and neutrophils
- Appendicitis: U/A can have pyuria, bacteriuria or hematuria in 20–40%
- MRI has a high accuracy for the diagnosis of acute appendicitis, with a sensitivity and specificity of 96% and 96% in children

Evaluation

- History and physical examination
  - Specific attention to onset and progression of symptoms

Testing

- No testing if signs and symptoms not consistent with possible appendicitis
- CBC
- BMP
- U/A

- UCG in fertile females (includes those with history of bilateral tubal ligation)
- LFT's as indicated
- Amylase and lipase as indicated
- Plain flat and upright if obstruction suspected
- CT abdominal and pelvic scan in adults as needed
- CT abdominal and pelvic scans in pediatrics need serious consideration of the risk potential for later cancer development — discuss with physician before ordering
    - Ultrasound has usefulness in pediatric appendicitis depending on radiologist experience

Discharge Criteria

- None

Consult Criteria

- All appendicitis or suspected appendicitis patients

Notes

REFERENCES:

Howell JM, Eddy OL, Lukens TW, Thiessen ME, Weingart SD, Decker WW, American College of Emergency Physicians. Clinical policy: critical issues in the evaluation and management of emergency department patients with suspected appendicitis. Ann Emerg Med. 2010 Jan;55(1):71–116

Appendicitis Clinical Presentation
Author: Sandy Craig, MD; Chief Editor: Barry E Brenner, MD, PhD, FACEP
emedicine.medscape.com/article/773895

AJR,2016;206:508

Antibiotic-Associated Colitis Protocol

Definition

- Inflammation of the bowel secondary to Clostridium difficile and usually recent antibiotic use or hospitalization

Differential Diagnosis

- Crohn's disease
- Ulcerative colitis
- Irritable bowel syndrome
- Gastroenteritis
- Toxic megacolon
- Diverticulitis

Considerations

- 20% of hospitalized patients acquire the infection
    - Diarrhea develop in 30% of these
- Colitis is caused by a toxin produced by C. difficile
- Should be considered with antibiotic use past 2 months or hospitalization in past 3 days
- Asymptomatic colonization occurs in 1–3% of the healthy population
- Do not routinely test for Clostridium difficile in age < 12 months where rates can exceed 40% in asymptomatic patients
    - By age 2–3 years carrier rate of Clostridium difficile are 1–3%
    - Test in symptomatic patients with evidence of pseudomembranous colitis, toxic megacolon or clinically significant diarrhea
- A brief exposure to an antibiotic can cause C. difficile colitis
    - Symptoms usually start 3–9 days after antibiotic initiation
- Age ≥ 60 years is a risk factor
- Relapse after treatment is common

- Recurs in 15 – 35% of patients with one previous episode and 33 – 65% of patients with more than two episodes
- Elevated WBC is found in 50–60% of patients

Symptoms and Findings

- Mild to moderate watery diarrhea
  - Usually not bloody
- Crampy abdominal pain
- Loss of appetite
- Fever usually in severe cases
- Lower abdominal tenderness
  - Rebound tenderness suggests bowel perforation

Evaluation

- History and physical examination
- Lab test options
  - CBC
  - CMP
  - U/A
  - Stool cultures for C. difficile and other pathogens
  - PCR testing
  - Enzyme immunoassay for C. difficile A and B toxins
    - Available in 2.5 hours
    - Sensitivity 75–80%
- Imaging options
  - Plain upright and flat x-rays if toxic megacolon suspected
  - CT abdominal and pelvis scan may be needed

Treatment Options

- Stop antibiotics (consult physician if antibiotic treatment crucial in treating another condition)
  - May be all that is needed in mild cases without fever, abdominal pain and elevated WBC
- No treatment of asymptomatic carriers of C. difficile
- Mild to moderate diarrhea or colitis
  - First episode of non–severe clostridium difficile diarrhea may be treated with vancomycin 125 mg PO qid for 10 days
  - Flagyl (metronidazole) 500 mg PO tid for 10–14 days — IV can be used if needed but not as effective as PO
  - Florastor PO bid for 10–14 days (over the counter)
- More severe cases
  - Vancomycin 125 mg PO qid for 10 days
  - Florastor PO bid for 10–14 days (over the counter)
- Recurrent infection
  - Vancomycin 125 mg PO qid for 10 days

    OR
  - Vancomycin 125 mg PO qid for 10–14 days, then 125 mg PO bid for 7 days, then 125 mg PO qday for 7 days
- Antidiarrheal antimotility agents should be avoided, though if used, should have antibiotics already started
- Analgesics
- Symptoms improve usually in 3 days on above antibiotics
- Recurrent and/or intractable symptomatic C difficile infection can be treated with fecal-microbiota transplant

Discharge Criteria

- Mild to moderate C. difficile or antibiotic-associated colitis
- See General Patient Criteria Protocol (page 15)

Discharge instructions

- Antibiotic-associated colitis aftercare instructions
- Stop current antibiotics
- Follow up with primary care provider within 3–5 days
- Return if symptoms worsen or do not improve
- Wash hands frequently with soap and water

Consult Criteria

- Fever
- WBC ≥ 13,000
- Severe pain
- Rebound tenderness
- CT scan shows colitis
- Dehydration

Notes

REFERENCES:

Clostridium Difficile Colitis
Author: Faten N Aberra, MD, MSCE; Chief Editor: Julian Katz, emedicine.medscape.com/article/186458–overview

Sloan LM, Duresko BJ, Gustafson DR, Rosenblatt JE. Comparison of real-time PCR for detection of the tcdC gene with four toxin immunoassays and culture in diagnosis of Clostridium difficile infection. *J Clin Microbiol.* Jun 2008;46(6):1996–2001

Debast SB, Bauer MP, Kuijper EJ. European Society of Clinical Microbiology and Infectious Diseases (ESCMID): update of the treatment guidance document for Clostridium difficile infection (CDI). *Clin Microbiol Infect.* Oct 5 2013

AHQR Comparative Effectiveness Review, 172, March 2016

McDonald LC, et al. *Clin Infect Dis.* 2018 Feb 15

Fecal-Microbiota Transplant Beats Antibiotics for Recurrent C Diff - Medscape - Jan 15, 2019

Inflammatory Bowel Disease Protocol

Definition

- Inflammatory disorder of unknown cause — ulcerative colitis or Crohn's disease

Differential Diagnosis

- Appendicitis
- Diverticulitis
- Endometriosis
- Pelvic inflammatory disease
- Colon carcinoma
- Antibiotic-associated colitis
- Irritable bowel syndrome
- Ischemic colitis

Considerations

- Ulcerative colitis is limited to the large intestine
- Crohn's disease can be anywhere in the gastrointestinal tract
- Kidney stone incidence is increased in Crohn's disease
- Smoking increases the risk Crohn's flares and severity of disease

Ulcerative colitis presentations and findings

- Bloody diarrhea
- Abdominal pain and cramping
- Fever in more severe cases
- Rectal tenesmus or urgency
- Nausea and vomiting
- Dehydration
- Anemia
- Total colectomy is curative
- Test for C. difficile infection

Crohn's disease

- Insidious onset
- Usually nonbloody diarrhea
- Half of cases have perianal fistulas or abscesses
- Weight loss

- Skip regions of intestinal involvement
- Fever
- Arthritis
- Uveitis
- Hepatitis
- Anemia

Evaluation

- History and physical examination
- Lab test options
  - CBC
  - BMP
  - LFT's
  - Amylase and lipase
  - U/A
- Imaging options
  - Plain upright and flat x-rays if toxic megacolon suspected or obstruction suspected
  - CT abdominal and pelvis scan
    - Also perform if obstruction suspected
    - No CT scan if ESR+5 x CRP ≤ 10 in crohn's disease
      - Negative predictive value of 98.1% for missing serious complications

Treatment

Step therapy

- Step 1 –aminosalicylates
- Step 2 – corticosteroids
- Step 2 – immunomodulators

Crohn's disease

Mild disease

- Sulfasalazine 0.5–1.5 gms PO 2–4 times a day for mild to moderate disease in colon
  - Caution with sulfasalazine hypersensitivity, renal insufficiency, coagulation abnormalities, pyloric stenosis, PUD, and liver disease
  - Read drug information in database
- Mesalamine (Asacol HD) 1.6 g three times daily for small bowel for remission induction of active mild to moderate – read PDR or databases
- Antidiarrheal medications qid for diarrhea without active colitis (avoid if possible)
  - Imodium (loperamide) 2 mg PO qid prn
  - Lomotil (diphenoxylate/atropine) 5 mg PO qid prn

Moderate disease

- Prednisone 30–60 mg PO qday 7–10 days
- Flagyl (metronidazole) 250–500 mg PO qid for fistula complications for 1 month

Disease not responsive to usual treatment

- Vedolizumab (Entyvio) at 0, 2 and 6 weeks, then 300 mg IV q8weeks — read drug information
- Biologics (TNF inhibitors) read drug information and discuss with physician
  - Infliximab (Remicade)
  - Adalimumab – Humira

Ulcerative colitis

Mild disease

- Sulfasalazine 0.5–1.5 gms PO 2–4 times a day for mild to moderate disease in colon
  - Contraindications
    - Hypersensitivity to mesalamine or salicylates
    - Breastfeeding
    - Rectal suspension: Patients with history of sulfite hypersensitivity
    - Children with chickenpox or flulike symptoms
  - Caution with sulfasalazine hypersensitivity, renal insufficiency, coagulation abnormalities, pyloric stenosis, PUD, and liver disease
- Disease confined to the rectum, topical mesalamine (Asacol) given by suppository is the preferred therapy

- Antidiarrheal medications qid for diarrhea without active colitis (avoid if possible)
  - Imodium (loperamide) 2 mg PO qid prn
  - Lomotil (diphenoxylate/atropine) 5 mg PO qid prn
- Mesalamine (Asacol HD) for mild to moderate disease with differing doses depending on disease activity – read PDR or databases

Moderate disease

- Prednisone 30–60 mg PO for 7–14 days followed by taper of 5 mg/week (should see PCP within 1–3 days after discharge)

Disease not responsive to usual treatment

- Vedolizumab (Entyvio) 300 mg IV at 0, 2 and 6 weeks, then 300 mg IV q8weeks — read drug information
- Biologics (TNF inhibitors) read drug information and discuss with physician
  - Infliximab (Remicade)
  - Adalimumab – Humira

Discharge Criteria

- Mild to moderate disease
- Prior history of Crohn's disease or ulcerative colitis
- Heart rate ≤ 110 for age ≥ 14 years

Discharge instructions

- Crohn's disease or ulcerative colitis aftercare instructions
- Smoking cessation for Crohn's disease patients
- Follow up within 1–3 days as needed
- Refer perianal disease to surgeon within 7–10 days

Consult Criteria

- Severe pain
- Fever
- Heart rate > 110/minute for age ≥ 14 years
- WBC ≥ 13,000
- Dehydration
- Hypotension
- Appears toxic
- Toxic megacolon
- Unable to self–hydrate
- Vomiting
- Progressive anemia
- Hemoglobin < 10 gms

Notes

____

____

____

REFERENCES:

Mayo Clin Proc, June 2011, pg. 557

Inflammatory Bowel Disease
Author: William A Rowe, MD; Chief Editor: Julian Katz, MD
emedicine.medscape.com/article/179037–overview

Ford AC, Bernstein CN, Khan KJ, et al. Glucocorticosteroid therapy in inflammatory bowel disease: systematic review and meta-analysis. *Am J Gastroenterol.* Apr 2011;106(4):590–9

Ulcerative Colitis Treatment & Management
Author: Marc D Basson, MD, PhD, MBA, FACS; Chief Editor: Julian Katz, MD
emedicine.medscape.com/article/183084

Govani SM, Guentner AS, Waljee AK, Higgins PD. Risk stratification of emergency department patients with Crohn's disease could reduce computed tomography use by nearly half. Clin Gastroenterol Hepatol. 2014 Oct. 12(10):1702-1707.e3

ACG Clinical Guideline: Ulcerative Colitis in Adults
David T. Rubin, MD, FACG1, Ashwin N. Ananthakrishnan, MD, MPH2, Corey A.

Siegel, MD, MS3, Bryan G. Sauer, MD, MSc (Clin Res), FACG (GRADE Methodologist)4 and Millie D. Long, MD, MPH, FACG

Gastroesophageal Reflux Disease (GERD) Protocol

Definition

- When the amount of gastric juice that refluxes into the esophagus exceeds the normal limit, causing symptoms with or without associated esophageal mucosal injury

Differential Diagnosis

- Acute coronary syndrome
- Biliary colic
- Peptic ulcer disease
- Esophagitis
- Esophageal spasm
- Achalasia
- Irritable bowel syndrome
- Asthma from aspiration

Considerations

- 40% of the population experience GERD monthly
- Most patients with hiatal hernias do not experience clinically significant reflux
- Acid secretion is the same with or without GERD

Causes and effects

- Obesity
- Smoking
- Decrease in lower esophageal sphincter (LES) tone or function (most common cause)
- Erosive gastritis
- Esophageal stricture
- UGI bleeding
- Recurrent pneumonia
- Asthma

Medications that can cause GERD:

- Calcium channel blockers
- Nitrates
- Beta–blockers
- Theophylline

Foods and beverages that can cause GERD:

- Coffee
- Chocolate
- Tea
- Alcohol
- Tomato products
- Citrus products

Signs and Symptoms

- Heartburn (burning from epigastrium up into chest and throat at times)
- Dysphagia
- Odynophagia
- Regurgitation
- Belching
- Worse bending over or lying down
- Usually transiently relieved with antacids

Evaluation

- Consider high risk differential diagnoses and test as indicated

Treatment Options

- Weight loss if obese
- Antacids
- Analgesics (excluding NSAID's or aspirin)
- Avoid late night or heavy meals
- Eat last meal ≥ 3 hours before laying down
- Stop smoking and alcohol intake
- Avoid drugs and foods/beverages that decrease LES
- Reglan (metoclopramide) — caution with long term usage — tardive dyskinesia)
- H2 blockers prn
- Proton pump inhibitors prn
- Elevate head of bed 6–8 inches
- Fundoplication (refer to surgery as outpatient)

Discharge Criteria

- Uncomplicated GERD
- Follow up with primary care provider or gastroenterologist within 1–3 weeks as needed

Discharge instructions

- GERD aftercare instructions

Consult Criteria

- UGI bleeding
- Esophageal obstruction
- Dehydration
- Toxic appearing patients
- Uncertain diagnosis as cause of patient complaints
- Refer to General Patient Criteria Protocol (page 15) as needed

Notes

REFERENCES:

Gastroesophageal Reflux Disease

Author: Marco G Patti, MD; Chief Editor: Julian Katz, MD

emedicine.medscape.com/article/17659 5

DeVault KR, Castell DO. Updated guidelines for the diagnosis and treatment of gastroesophageal reflux disease.*Am J Gastroenterol.* Jan 2005;100(1):190–200

Agency for Healthcare Research and Quality. Comparative Effectiveness of Management Strategies for Gastroesophageal Reflux Disease - Executive Summary. AHRQ pub. no. 06–EHC003–1. December 2005

PEPTIC ULCER DISEASE AND GASTRITIS PROTOCOL

Definition

- Inflammatory changes in the gastric mucosa or a discrete mucosal defect in the stomach or duodenum

Differential Diagnosis

- GERD
- Gastroenteritis
- Acute coronary syndrome
- Biliary colic
- Peptic ulcer disease
- Esophagitis
- Esophageal spasm
- Irritable bowel syndrome
- Abdominal aortic aneurysm
- Mesenteric ischemia
- Hepatitis
- Inflammatory bowel disease
- Pancreatitis
- Pulmonary embolism

Considerations

- Consider high risk differential diagnoses and test as indicated

Causes

- H. pylori responsible for 90–95% of duodenal ulcers and 80% of gastric ulcers with NSAID use
- NSAID's interfere with prostaglandin synthesis and lead to breakdown in mucosa
- Smoking
- Alcohol intake
- Aspirin
- Steroids
- Long term PPI therapy associated with chronic kidney disease (CKD)

Signs and Symptoms

- Epigastric pain and burning 80–90%
- Epigastric tenderness
- Gastric ulcer pain worsened by food
- Duodenal ulcer pain improved by food
- Nausea
- Vomiting
- UGI bleeding
- Hematemesis
- Melena
- Peritonitis with perforation
- Anemia

Evaluation Options

- Mild symptoms and findings with normal vital signs treat symptomatically
- H. pylori testing if available
- Moderate or severe symptoms or tenderness
  - CBC
  - BMP
  - Amylase
  - Lipase
  - Consider LFT's
- Peritonitis findings
  - Upright chest x-ray and abdominal films to evaluate for free air
  - CT abdominal and pelvis if diagnosis is uncertain or age ≥ 65 years
- EKG
  - Age ≥ 45 years with unimpressive abdominal exam and no cardiac risk factors
  - Any adult with cardiac risk factors for coronary artery disease with unimpressive abdominal exam
  - Consider CT abdominal/pelvis scan with age ≥ 70 if diagnosis not reasonably certain

Treatment Options

- Unstable patient notify physician immediately
- Stable nonacute patient
- Antacids prn
- H2 blockers
- Proton pump inhibitors (PPI) × 1–2 months
  - Omeprazole
    - Duodenal ulcer 20 mg PO 30-60 minutes before meal q day for 4 weeks
    - Gastric ulcer 40 mg PO bid 30-60 minutes before meal for 4–8 weeks
    - GERD 20 mg PO before meal qday for NMT 4 weeks
  - Other PPIs are pantoprazole, dexlansoprazole, esomeprazole, lansoprazole etc.

Antibiotics with PPI only if H. pylori documented with testing

- Biaxin (clarithromycin) 500 mg PO × 14 days
- Flagyl (metronidazole) 500 mg PO × 14 days

OR

- Biaxin (clarithromycin) 500 mg PO bid × 14 days
- Amoxicillin 1,000 mg bid × 14 days

2017 American College of Gastroenterology (ACG) guidelines for the treatment of H. pylori infection

- 10-14 days of bismuth quadruple therapy (bismuth, proton pump inhibitor [PPI], tetracycline, and metronidazole), particularly in those with previous macrolide exposure or are penicillin allergic
- Recommended option — 10-14 days of concomitant PPI, clarithromycin, amoxicillin, and metronidazole
- 14 days of clarithromycin triple therapy (clarithromycin, a PPI, and amoxicillin or metronidazole) should be reserved for patients with no

previous history of macrolide exposure who live in regions where clarithromycin resistance among *H pylori* isolates is known to be low (< 15%)

- Suggested option — 5-7 days of sequential therapy with a PPI and amoxicillin, followed by 5-7 days with clarithromycin, a PPI, and metronidazole
- Suggested option — 7 days of a hybrid therapy with a PPI and amoxicillin, followed by 7 days with a PPI, amoxicillin, clarithromycin, and metronidazole
- Suggested option — 10-14 days of levofloxacin triple therapy (levofloxacin, a PPI, and amoxicillin)
- Suggested option — 5-7 days of fluoroquinolone sequential therapy (a PPI and amoxicillin), followed by 5-7 days of a PPI, fluoroquinolone, and nitroimidazole (metronidazole or others of this class)

Discharge Criteria

- Uncomplicated exam and findings consistent with gastritis or peptic ulcer disease

Discharge instructions

- Peptic ulcer or gastritis aftercare instructions
- Follow up with primary care provider in 1 day if pain is moderate to severe, otherwise in 5–7 days
- Follow up with primary care provider for abnormal lab within 1 week unless chronic in nature
- Return within 3 days if not improving

Consult Criteria

- GI bleeding
- Moderate pain with age ≥ 70 years
- Abdominal pain that develops hypotension or relative hypotension (SBP < 105 with history of hypertension)
- Toxic appearance
- Dehydration
- Significant blood loss or melena
  - Melena can occur with as little as 50 ml of upper GI blood loss
- Suspected or diagnosed appendicitis, cholecystitis, pancreatitis, diverticulitis, aortic aneurysm, bowel obstruction
- Acute surgical abdomen or rebound tenderness
- Moderate to severe pain of uncertain cause
- Severe pain with any diagnosis
- Intractable vomiting
- Return visit within 14 days for same acute abdominal pain complaint

Lab consult criteria (if checked)

- Hemoglobin decrease > 1 gm or creatinine increase> 0.5 from baseline
- Elevated LFT's
- Elevated amylase or lipase
- WBC ≥ 15,000
- Bandemia
- Increased anion gap
- Significant electrolyte abnormally
- Glucose ≥ 450 mg/dL in diabetic patient
- Glucose ≥ 300 mg/dL in non-diabetic patient
- Hyperglycemia with metabolic acidosis (decreased serum CO_2 or elevated anion gap)
- Acute thrombocytopenia

Notes

REFERENCES:

Peptic Ulcer Disease

Author: BS Anand, MD; Chief Editor: Julian Katz, MD

emedicine.medscape.com/article/181753

Chey WD, Wong BC. American College of Gastroenterology guideline on the management of Helicobacter pylori infection. *Am J Gastroenterol.* Aug 2007;102(8):1808–25

Chey WD, Leontiadis GI, Howden CW, Moss SF. ACG Clinical Guideline: Treatment of Helicobacter pylori infection. *Am J Gastroenterol.* 2017 Feb. 112(2):212-39

Gallbladder Disease Protocol

Definition

- Disease of gallbladder from gallstone obstruction of cystic duct or infection and inflammation of the gallbladder without gallstones

Differential Diagnosis

- Peptic ulcer disease
- Acute myocardial infarction
- Angina
- Right-sided pulmonary embolism
- Right-sided pneumonia
- Right renal colic
- Hepatitis
- Mesenteric ischemia
- Cholangitis
- Right pyelonephritis
- Gastroenteritis
- Abdominal aortic aneurysm
- Pancreatitis

Considerations

- Common in females age ≥ 40 years
- 90% of cholecystitis is from gallstones
- Moderate to severe pain and tenderness RUQ of abdomen
- Nausea and vomiting very common
- Charcot's triad: (1) Jaundice, (2) Fever, (3) RUQ abdominal pain
- Fever occurs with advanced disease
- Increased morbidity and mortality in **diabetes**
- Ascending cholangitis is a life threatening infection of common bile duct
- May increase LFT's, amylase, lipase and bilirubin with common duct gallstones
- Acalculus cholecystitis has a higher mortality than cholecystitis with gallstones
  - Seen more in elderly and diabetic patients
- Elderly may present with vague and diminished symptoms
- Emphysematous cholecystitis more common with diabetes

Evaluation

- History for
  - Onset
  - Severity
  - Duration
  - Associated symptoms
  - Previous episodes
- Abdominal exam for
  - Tenderness
  - Guarding
  - Rebound tenderness
  - Distension

Testing options

- CBC
- U/A
- UCG if fertile female
- LFT's
- Amylase
- Lipase
- Gallbladder ultrasound may be needed, especially with elevated WBC, and if amylase or lipase elevated
- If pain, tenderness and vomiting resolve with treatment, testing may not be needed

Treatment Options

- IV NS or LR 1 liter bolus if hypotensive (notify physician promptly)

- Pain and vomiting treatment
  - Dilaudid (hydromorphone) 0.5–2 mg IV/IM prn
  - Stadol (butorphanol) 0.5–2 mg IV or 1–4 mg IM prn (Stadol and Nubain may cause acute opiate withdrawal in opiate addicted patients)
  - Nubain (nalbuphine) 10–20 mg IV/IM/SQ prn (may give ¼ dose in opioid dependent patients to see if withdrawal is precipitated
  - Phenergan (promethazine) or Zofran (ondansetron) prn

Discharge Criteria

- Resolution of pain, tenderness, vomiting
- Gallbladder ultrasound without findings of cholecystitis or choledocholithiasis (if performed)
- No fever or chills
- Diagnosis reasonable certain for biliary colic

Discharge instructions

- Gallbladder disease aftercare instructions
- Return within 1 day if pain persists or worsens
- Refer to general surgeon or primary care provider within 7 days

Consult Criteria

- WBC ≥ 13,000
- Bandemia ≥ 15%
- Rebound tenderness
- Intractable nausea or vomiting
- Pain not resolved with treatment
- Cholecystitis
- Choledocholithiasis
- Cholangitis
- Gallstone pancreatitis

Lab consult criteria

- Hemoglobin decrease > 1 gm or creatinine increase> 0.5 from baseline
- Elevated LFT's
- Elevated amylase or lipase
- Increased anion gap
- Acute thrombocytopenia
- Significant electrolyte abnormally
- Glucose ≥ 300 mg/dL in diabetic patient
- Glucose ≥ 200 mg/dL in non-diabetic patient
- Hyperglycemia with metabolic acidosis (decreased serum CO_2 or elevated anion gap)
- Lactic acidosis

Vital sign and age consult criteria

- Adult HR ≥ 110 post treatment
- Hypotension or orthostatic vital signs

Notes

REFERENCES:

Cholecystitis Author: Alan A Bloom, MD; Chief Editor: Julian Katz, MD emedicine.medscape.com/article/171886

Huffman JL, Schenker S. Acute acalculous cholecystitis - a review. *Clin Gastroenterol Hepatol*. Sep 9 2009

ACUTE HEPATITIS PROTOCOL

Definition

- Inflammation of the liver

Differential Diagnosis

- Biliary colic
- Cholecystitis
- Cholangitis
- Peptic ulcer disease
- Gastritis
- Gastroenteritis

- Aortic aneurysm
- Pancreatitis

Considerations

- Frequently asymptomatic
- Ranges from asymptomatic to fulminate hepatitis and liver failure
- Misdiagnosed frequently as nonspecific viral syndrome
- Viral causes are most frequent: hepatitis A – 40%, hepatitis B – 30%, hepatitis C – 20%
  - Hepatitis A: fecal-oral transmission most common cause
  - Hepatitis B: exposure to infected blood or body fluids most common cause
  - Hepatitis C: percutaneous exposures most common cause
- Screening for hepatitis B and HCV recommended in high risk patients
- Chronic hepatitis develops in 75% of acute hepatitis C patients
  - Contacted largely from IV drug abuse or contaminated needles. Less often from tattoos, sharing razors, acupuncture or blood transfusions
- Autoimmune disorders can cause hepatitis
- Toxic causes
- Acetaminophen is a frequent worldwide cause (can cause liver failure)
- Ethanol (causes 50% of end-stage liver disease in U.S.)
- Isoniazid
- Ecstasy (MDMA)
- Industrial solvents and cleaning solutions
- Iron

Viral hepatitis

Risk factors

- Male homosexuality
- Hemodialysis
- IV drug abuse
- Raw seafood
- Blood product transfusion
- Tattoos or body piercing
- Foreign travel
- Sexual exposure to hepatitis B carrier

Preicteric phase

- Flu-like illness with fever, chills and malaise
- Nausea, vomiting, anorexia

Icteric phase

- Dark urine
- Light stools
- Pruritus
- Right upper quadrant tenderness
- Tender hepatomegaly

Nonalcoholic fatty liver most common cause of elevated LFT's in U.S. (ALT > AST frequently)

- Associated with obesity, Type-II DM, and/or hyperlipidemia
- Most patients asymptomatic
- Bilirubin rarely elevated
- Can lead to hepatic cirrhosis
- Treatment is weight loss
- Usually a benign course though common cause of hepatic cirrhosis

Evaluation

- Complete history and physical exam
- Alcohol and drug history
- Special attention to acetaminophen or acetaminophen containing medicines
- Check acetaminophen level if ALT elevated with possible history of acetaminophen containing medication usage
- CBC
- BMP
- LFT's (SGOT/AST is commonly 2 times > SGPT/ALT in alcoholic hepatitis)
  - ALT > AST in fatty liver usually
- PT/PTT/INR
- Ammonia level if encephalopathic
  - Ammonia may not correlate with severity of encephalopathy

- Rectal exam if encephalopathic for stool blood or if BUN elevated out of proportion to creatinine level
- U/A
- Consider viral serology
- Monospot if pharyngitis present
- Acetaminophen level if suspected usage

Treatment Options

- IV D50W 1 amp if hypoglycemic
- Hypotension give 250–500 cc NS bolus and notify physician
- Treat ongoing hypoglycemia with D5 1/2NS drip of 100–150 cc/hour
- Usually supportive
- Acetadote for acetaminophen toxicity as indicated
  - May need treatment if ALT elevated with history of recent acetaminophen containing medication usage, even if acetaminophen level is 0
- Cessation of ethanol use
- No acetaminophen

Discharge Criteria

- Stable patient
- PT < 3 seconds elevation
- INR < 1.5
- See General Patient Criteria Protocol (page 15)

Discharge instructions

- Hepatitis aftercare instructions
- Primary care provider within 1–2 days
- Gastroenterology within 1–2 days unless chronic liver disease without acute exacerbation

Consult Criteria

- Toxic acetaminophen level on nomogram or elevated ALT regardless of level if acetaminophen containing medication usage is suspected
- Hypoglycemia
- Altered mental status
- PT prolonged > 3 seconds
- INR > 1.5
- Bilirubin > 5
- Intractable vomiting
- Significant comorbid conditions
- Significant electrolyte or fluid disturbances
- Age ≥ 70
- Ascites
- GI bleeding
- Immunosuppression
- Fever
- LFT's > 5 times normal

Notes

____

____

____

REFERENCES:

Hepatitis B Author: Nikolaos T Pyrsopoulos, MD, PhD, MBA, FACP, AGAF; Chief Editor: Julian Katz, MD emedicine.medscape.com/article/177632

Centers for Disease Control and Prevention. Hepatitis B information for health professionals: hepatitis B FAQs for health professionals cdc.gov/hepatitis/HBV/index.htm

[Guideline] Ghany MG, Strader DB, Thomas DL, Seeff LB. Diagnosis, management, and treatment of hepatitis C: an update. *Hepatology.* Apr 2009;49(4):1335–74

GASTROINTESTINAL BLEEDING PROTOCOL

Differential Diagnosis

- Peptic ulcer disease
- Esophagitis
- Mallory-Weiss tear
- Esophageal varices

- Diverticular disease
- Colon cancer
- Colon polyps
- Arteriovenous malformation
- Aortoenteric fistula
- Hemorrhoids

Considerations

- Upper gastrointestinal (UGI) bleeding as little as 50 ml can cause melena
  - Melena may be produced from proximal large intestine also
- UGI bleeding
  - Rapid transit can cause gross blood per rectum
  - Elevates BUN out of proportion to creatinine
    - BUN/creatinine ratio of >30:1 suggests UGI bleeding
  - Can lead to hepatic encephalopathy in hepatic cirrhosis patients
  - FFP should not be used in esophageal variceal bleeding with hepatic cirrhosis patients that have a high INR
    - Actually cirrhotic patients can be hypercoagulable due to imbalance of thrombotic and antithrombotic factors
- Lower gastrointestinal (LGI) bleeding
  - Bright or dark red gross blood
  - Frequently painless
  - Frequently from a colon diverticular source in elderly (30–65% of all GI bleeding)
- Hemorrhoidal bleeding usually bright red and not mixed with stools
- Can present with dyspnea, chest pain; syncope, altered mental status

Lower GI Bleeding and Risk of Severe Bleeding

- Heart rate 100 beats per minute or more (1 point)
- SBP ≤ 115 mmHg (1 point)
- Patient had associated syncope (1 point)
- Blood per rectum during first 4 hours of evaluation (1 point)
- Patient on aspirin (1 point)
- 3 or more comorbid conditions present (1 point)

0 points = 9% risk

1–3 points = 43% risk

4–6 points = 84% risk

Evaluation

- Complete history and physical exam (including rectal exam for hemoccult testing or gross bleeding)
- Medication history
- Prior GI history
- CBC
- BMP
- PT/INR
- PTT if on heparin
- Ammonia and LFT's if mental status altered
- Type and screen for history of significant bleeding
- Type and cross if
  - Hypotensive
  - Adult heart rate ≥ 120
  - Orthostatic vital signs
- Multidetector CT scan accurate to determine bleeding site if active bleeding at time of scan
- EGD and/or colonoscopy may be indicated depending on degree of bleeding
  - Timing up to GI doctor
- Hemorrhoidal bleeding with benign bleeding history and normal vital signs may not need lab tests
- Angiography for treatment

Treatment Options

- IV NS 500cc bolus if hypotensive adult (notify physician promptly) — see Bleeding Protocol
- Avoid > 1 liter of isotonic fluids for acute blood loss before blood products transfusion started if possible
- Avoid hypertension

- Target systolic blood pressure of 80-90 mm Hg until major bleeding has been stopped
- Target Hgb of 7-9 g/dl after termination of major bleeding
  - Maintain HGB > 7 g/dL in most patients. Consider transfusion threshold of 9 g/dL in patients with significant coexisting disease (such as ischemic CAD)
- Pediatric: 20 cc/kg IV NS bolus, start blood and plasma for continued hypotension and bleeding (notify physician promptly)
- Protonix (pantoprazole) IV for upper GI bleeding or peptic ulcer disease/gastritis/esophagitis
- Transfusion with PRBC's/FFP/platelets 1:1:1 ratio if hypotension persists or significant acute anemia
  - Recommendations range from 4:1:1 to 1:1:1 (consult physician promptly first)
- Consider N-G tube for UGI bleeding (consult physician)
- Somatostatin IV for UGI bleeding as needed
- 45 - 66% cirrhotic patients with upper GI bleeding develop bacterial infection within the first 5-7 days of the bleeding episode
  - Ceftriaxone IV or other broad spectrum antibiotics decrease infection, improves bleeding, prevents rebleeding and improves survival
- Angiography for embolization in unstable or potentially unstable patients
- Surgery if bleeding not able to be successfully treatment with above methods

Hemorrhoids

External hemorrhoids

Medical treatment for mild to moderate painful thrombosed hemorrhoids

- Warm soaks (sitz baths) or hot towel applied in lateral decubitus position
- Stool softeners
- Anusol, Anusol HC or Protofoam HC topical preparations
- Tuck's pads prn (witch hazel)
- Analgesics
- Nupercainal (dibucaine) ointment 1% tid–qid prn
- Avoid exacerbating activities

Excisional treatment for severe painful acute thrombosed hemorrhoids (usually within 72 hours of symptoms)

- Prep area with betadine
- Spread buttocks with assistant's help or use tape
- Infiltrate base of hemorrhoid with 2–5 cc of 1% lidocaine with epinephrine (use plain lidocaine in coronary artery disease patients)
- Infiltrate into the hemorrhoid with 1–2 cc of lidocaine with epinephrine (use plain lidocaine in coronary artery disease patients)
- Elliptical incision (preferred) in roof/top of hemorrhoid 2–3 mm wide radially in line from anus
  - Avoid deeper anal verge and sphincter
- Remove clots(s) by expressing or with forceps
- May be packed with 0.25 gauze (removed in 6 hours) or have gelfoam applied as needed
- Analgesics

Internal hemorrhoids

Medical treatment similar to external hemorrhoid treatment

Discharge Criteria

- Healthy patient
- Normal vital signs
- Stable CBC if checked

- Normal coagulation studies if checked
- Good follow up
- Negative or insignificant blood on rectal exam

Discharge instructions

- GI bleeding or hemorrhoid aftercare instructions
- Refer to primary care provider or GI physician within 5–7 days

Consult Criteria

- Significant blood loss or melena present
- Hematemesis
- Suspected or diagnosed aortic aneurysm
- Acute surgical abdomen
- Moderate to severe pain of uncertain cause
- Severe pain with any diagnosis
- Return ED visit within 14 days for same complaint

Vital signs and age consult criteria

- Age ≥ 70
- SBP < 90 or relative hypotension (SBP < 110 with history of hypertension)
- Adult heart rate > 100
- Orthostatic vital signs
- Pediatric heart
  - 0–4 months ≥ 180
  - 5–7 months ≥ 175
  - 6–12 months ≥ 170

Lab consult criteria

- Hemoglobin < 12 gms unless chronic
- Hemoglobin decrease > 1 gm
- Bandemia ≥ 15%
- Metabolic acidosis
- Significant electrolyte abnormally
- Glucose ≥ 400 mg/dL in diabetic patient or > 300 mg/dL in non-diabetic patient
- Hyperglycemia with metabolic acidosis (decreased serum CO_2 or elevated anion gap)
- Acute thrombocytopenia (common in alcoholics)
- Elevated coagulation studies
- Creatinine increase > 0.5 from baseline
- Elevated LFT's

Notes

____

____

____

REFERENCES:

JAMA, Vol.307:1072–1079

Strate LL, Orav EJ, Syngal S. Early predictors of severity in acute lower intestinal tract bleeding. *Arch Intern Med.* 2003; 163: 838–43

Scottish Intercollegiate Guidelines Network (SIGN). *Management of acute upper and lower gastrointestinal bleeding. A national clinical guideline.* (SIGN publication; no. 105). Edinburgh (Scotland): Scottish Intercollegiate Guidelines Network (SIGN); Sep 2008

Hemorrhoids Treatment & Management
Author: Scott C Thornton, MD; Chief Editor: John Geibel, MD, DSc, MA
emedicine.medscape.com/article/775407

Imperiale TF, Birgisson S. Somatostatin or octreotide compared with H2 antagonists and placebo in the management of acute nonvariceal upper gastrointestinal hemorrhage: a meta-analysis
Ann Intern Med 1997 Dec 15;127(12):1062–1071

Tripodi A, et al. *N Engl J Med* 2011;365:147-156

Nadim. Management of the critically ill patient with cirrhosis: A multidisciplinary perspective. *Journal of Hepatology* 2016;64(3):717-735

Jalan R, et al. *J Hepatol* 2014;60(6):1310-24

Chavez-Tapia, N.C., et al. *Cochrane Database Syst Rev* 2010; 9: CD002907

Rossaint R, Bouillon B, Cerny V, Coats TJ, Duranteau J, Fernández-Mondéjar E, et al. The European guideline on management of major bleeding and coagulopathy following trauma: fourth edition. *Crit Care*. 2016 Apr 12. 20 (1):100

Gastrointestinal Foreign Body Protocol

Definition

- Ingestion of a foreign body that may or may not be impacted

Considerations

- Most pass without assistance or danger once past the pylorus
- Sharp objects > 5 cm or multiple in number may need endoscopic removal
- Plastic clips (e.g. bread bag fasteners) mandate immediate endoscopic or surgical removal regardless of location
  - High risk of bowel perforation, hemorrhage and obstruction

Esophageal foreign body

Symptoms

- Foreign body sensation
- Dysphagia

Areas of narrowing

- Cricopharyngeus muscle (most common)
  - C6
- Aortic arch and tracheal carina
  - T4
  - T6
- Lower esophageal sphincter (GE junction)
  - T11

Evaluation options

Chest x-ray findings

- Coins
  - Tracheal foreign body
    - Oriented anterior–posterior
  - Esophageal foreign body
    - Oriented transversely
- Bones may be seen on chest x-ray

Gastrograffin or barium swallow

- For nonopaque foreign bodies

CT scan

- For nonopaque foreign bodies
- Superior to gastrograffin or barium swallow

Button battery

- Must be removed immediately if lodged in esophagus
  - If passed esophagus does not need immediate removal
  - If passed pylorus in 48 hours does not need removal
- Rapid burns occur within 6 hours if impacted
- Lithium batteries have worse outcomes
- Consult GI physician immediately for retained esophageal button battery
  - **Intranasal button batteries need immediate removal**

Esophageal food impaction

- Esophageal disease present usually
  - Esophageal stricture from GERD common
- Complete obstruction patient cannot hold saliva down

Treatment options

- Endoscopic removal

- Glucagon (not too successful)
  - Adult 1–2 mg IV may repeat in 10–20 minutes if needed
  - Pediatric 0.02–0.03 mg/kg IV (NMT 0.5 mg)
- Foley catheter removal
  - Do not use
    - If esophageal disease present
    - Foreign body present more than 72 hours

Discharge criteria recommendation

- Resolved foreign body impaction
- Benign foreign body that will likely pass
- Button battery
  - If passed esophagus
  - If passed pylorus in 48 hours

Discharge instructions

- Esophageal or gastrointestinal foreign body aftercare instructions
- Refer to GI or PCP within 48 hours to assess foreign body evacuation

Consult criteria recommendation

- Retained esophageal foreign bodies
- Sharp foreign bodies
- Button battery in esophagus
- Unresolved esophageal food impaction
- Continued symptoms of foreign body
- Continued dysphagia
- Foreign bodies unlikely to spontaneously pass

Notes

REFERENCES:

Gastrointestinal Foreign Bodies Workup

Author: David W Munter, MD, MBA; Chief Editor: Steven C Dronen, MD, FAAEM

Emedicine.medscape.com/article/776566

Disk Battery Ingestion Follow-up

Author: Daniel J Dire, MD, FACEP, FAAP, FAAEM; Chief Editor: Asim Tarabar, MD

emedicine.medscape.com/article/774838

Anorectal Disorder Protocol

Conditions

- Hemorrhoids
- Anal Fissure
- Perianal/perirectal abscess
- Rectal prolapse
- Pruritus ani
- Pilonidal cyst/abscess

Hemorrhoids

Definition

- Disease caused by pathologic swelling and inflammation of veins in the anorectum

Differential diagnosis

- Rectal prolapse
- Proctitis
- Crohn's disease and ulcerative colitis
- Condyloma acuminata
- Pregnancy related vein engorgement

Considerations

- Symptoms range from none to severe pain
- External hemorrhoids develop distal to the dentate line
  - Are bluish-purplish in color

- Internal hemorrhoids are above the dentate line
  - No sensory innervation and usually painless
  - Usually cannot be felt when not prolapsed
- Bright blood that drips into toilet or as streaks on stool is commonly from internal hemorrhoids
- Commonly thought to be from constipation or straining, but this is controversial
- Blood is not mixed inside stool

Internal hemorrhoid grading

- 1st degree = projects into canal
- 2nd degree = protrudes with defection then retracts
- 3rd degree = protrudes with straining but only retracts by manual manipulation
- 4th degree = prolapsed and cannot be reduced

Evaluation options

- Usually history and physical examination with rectal exam is all that is needed
- CBC for tachycardia or history of moderate to severe bleeding
- PT/INR if on Coumadin (warfarin)

Treatment options

External hemorrhoids

Medical treatment for mild to moderately painful thrombosed hemorrhoids

- Warm soaks (sitz baths) or hot towel applied in lateral decubitus position
- Stool softeners
- Anusol, Anusol HC or Proctofoam HC topical preparations
- Tuck's pads prn (witch hazel)
- Analgesics
- Avoid exacerbating activities

Excisional treatment for severe painful acute thrombosed hemorrhoids (usually within 72 hours of symptoms)

- Prep area with betadine
- Spread buttocks with assistant's help or use tape
- Infiltrate base of hemorrhoid with 2–5 cc of 1% lidocaine with epinephrine
- Infiltrate into the hemorrhoid with 1–2 cc of lidocaine with epinephrine
- Elliptical incision (preferred) in roof/top of hemorrhoid 2–3 mm wide radially in line from anus
  - Avoid the deeper anal verge and sphincter
- Remove clots(s) by expressing or with forceps
- May be packed with 0.25 inch gauze (removed in 6 hours) or have gelfoam applied as needed
- Analgesics

Internal hemorrhoids

Medical treatment similar to external hemorrhoid treatment

Surgical referral and treatment

- Failure of conservative treatment
- Excessive and/or prolonged bleeding
- Gangrenous 4th degree hemorrhoid (emergency)
- Concurrent anal fistula or fissure
- 3rd and 4th degree internal hemorrhoids with severe symptoms
- Patient requests referral

Discharge criteria recommendation

- Uncomplicated internal and external hemorrhoids

Discharge instructions

- Warm soaks (sitz baths) or hot towel applied in lateral decubitus position
- Stool softeners and bulk laxatives (psyllium fiber)
- Anusol, Anusol HC or Proctofoam HC topical preparations
- Hemorrhoid aftercare instructions

Consult criteria recommendation

- See surgical referral above

Anal fissure

Definition

- Superficial linear tear of the anus

Differential diagnosis

- Crohn's disease
- Ulcerative colitis
- Carcinoma
- Syphilis, gonorrhea and other STD
- HIV and AIDS
- Herpes simplex
- Rectal foreign bodies (as a cause)
- Pilonidal cyst or sinus
- Proctitis

Considerations

- Most common cause of painful rectal bleeding
- Distal to the dentate line
- Usually occur in posterior anal midline (90%) or anterior anal midline (10%)
    - If not in midline consider other diseases
- Most resolve in 2–4 weeks (may last several months)
- Refractory cases may require surgery
- Causes increased anal sphincter pressures

Evaluation

- Usually only need history and rectal exam

Treatment options

- WASH regimen
    - Warm water, shower or sitz bath after bowel movement
    - Analgesics
    - Stool softener
    - High-fiber diet
- Topical 0.5% nitroglycerin ointment bid topically applied for up to 6–8 weeks if failure of WASH regimen
- Botulinum toxin injection locally
- Topical application of clove oil cream for chronic anal fissure

Discharge criteria recommendation

- Uncomplicated anal fissure

Discharge instructions

- Anal fissure aftercare instructions
- WASH regimen

Consult criteria recommendation

- Refractory anal fissure
- Other disease process suspected
- Anal fistula

Perianal abscess

Definition

- Infection and collection of pus just outside the anus

Differential diagnosis

- Perirectal abscess
- Squamous cell carcinoma
- Crohn's disease

Considerations

- May be associated with a fistula tract into rectum
- Peak incidence is third to fourth decade of life
- Males affected more than females
- Common in infants
- Arises from obstruction of the anal crypts
- Usually patient is afebrile

Evaluation

- Usually history and physical exam is all that is needed

Treatment

- Incision and drainage of abscess avoiding anal verge
  - Pack abscess for 1–2 days (patient removes pack or return visit for removal)
- Antibiotics usually are not necessary
- Analgesics prn

Discharge criteria recommendation

- Uncomplicated perianal abscess

Discharge instructions

- Sitz baths 3 times a day and after bowel movements for 3–4 days
- Stool softeners
- Perianal abscess aftercare instructions

Consult criteria recommendation

- Perirectal abscess suspected
- Anal fistula
- Other disease process suspected
- Fever
- Immunocompromised patient

Perirectal abscess

Definition

- Abscess in the deeper perirectal spaces

Differential diagnosis

- Perianal abscess
- Crohn's disease
- Inflammatory bowel disease
- Rectal carcinoma
- Foreign body
- Sexually transmitted disease
- Proctitis
- Hemorrhoids
- Necrotizing fasciitis

Considerations

- Caused by obstruction of the anal crypts
- Fever and leukocytosis common (WBC can be normal)
- Severe pain present
- Sepsis can occur
- Increased pain with sitting, coughing or bowel movement
- Rectal or perirectal drainage in ¼ of patients
- Severe tenderness in rectum on digital examination
- May or may not be palpable
- Results in fistula in 25–50% of patients
- Urinary retention in 5% of patients

Evaluation options

- History and physical examination including rectal exam
- CBC
- BMP if diabetic
- Blood cultures if toxic appearing or immunocompromised
- CT abdomen/pelvis scan if diagnosis is in doubt on history and physical examination
- If in doubt and CT not performed, an 18 or 20 gauge needle aspiration of the most tender and/or swollen area after sterile skin prep can be used to help diagnose abscess (not to be used for definitive treatment

Treatment

- Per surgeon
- Analgesics parentally prn

Discharge criteria recommendation

- Do not discharge unless directed by surgeon

Consult criteria recommendation

- All perirectal abscess patients

Rectal prolapse

Definition

- Mucosal or full thickness prolapse of rectal tissue through anus

Differential diagnosis

- Hemorrhoids
- Proctitis
- Intussusception

Considerations

- Fecal incontinence and constipation commonly develop after prolapse
- Ulceration of rectal tissue may occur
- May be caused by staining and constipation
- 90% of children with rectal prolapse will spontaneously resolve
- Peak incidence is the 4th and 7th decades of life
- Much more common in females (80–90% of total)
- Children peak incidence less 1 year of age
  - Cystitis fibrosis associated with prolapse

Findings

- Protruding rectal mucosa
- Thick concentric mucosal ring
- Gap noted between anal canal and rectum
- Decreased anal sphincter tone

Evaluation

- History and physical examination including rectal exam
- Barium enema (preferred) or colonoscopy
- Tests for any associated conditions as needed

Treatment

- Adults are treated surgically
- Children usually treated nonsurgically and underlying condition is treated
- Attempt gentle digital reduction of rectum
  - Granulated table sugar applied to the rectal tissue causes an osmotic shift of fluid out of the mucosa decreasing the swelling in a few minutes that facilitates reduction of the prolapse
- Stool softeners

Discharge criteria recommendation

- Reducible mucosal or rectal prolapse

Discharge instructions

- Rectal prolapse aftercare instructions if available
- Stool softeners

Consult criteria recommendation

- All patients should be referred to surgeon
- Emergency consultation if incarcerated, ischemic or perforated rectal tissue

Pruritus ani

Definition

- Chronic anal itching

Differential diagnosis

- Eczema
- Psoriasis
- Pinworm infestation
- Scabies
- Urticaria
- Contact dermatitis
- Hemorrhoids

Considerations

- Worse at night usually
- Can be caused by increased moisture around anus or fecal leakage
- May be from certain foods, clothing, poor rectal hygiene, or medications

Evaluation options

- Cellophane tape when waking up in morning for pinworms if suspected
- 10% KOH skin scraping for fungus

Treatment options

- Diphenhydramine or hydroxyzine prn for itching
- Hydrocortisone cream 1% course bid prn for 5–10 days
- Avoid offending foods, clothing or agents
- Treat underlying condition if known
- Clean anus completely post-defecation
- Corn starch powder to dry skin

Discharge criteria recommendation

- Uncomplicated cases

Discharge instructions

- Pruritus ani aftercare instructions

Consult criteria recommendation

- Refractory cases refer to gastroenterologist

Pilonidal cyst/abscess

Definition

- A cyst that develops from hair penetration in the skin of the sacrococcygeal region 4–5 cm posterior to the anus

Differential diagnosis

- Anal fistula
- Perirectal abscess
- Hidradenitis suppurativa

Considerations

- Thought to be an acquired condition for folliculitis from hair that gets impacted into the skin
- More common in males
- Affects 26 out of 100,000 persons in the U.S.
- Occurs most commonly in late teens and early twenties
- Painful when acutely infected

Evaluation

- History and physical examination is usually all that is needed

Treatment

- For abscess perform I&D off midline, angulating into abscess cavity
  - See Soft Tissue Abscess section in book
- Remove any hair and granulation tissue
- Pack with gauze (medicated ribbon gauze has no added benefit)
  - Remove packing in 1–2 days
- No I&D for asymptomatic patients
- Phenol injection into cyst by experience Providers

Hidradenitis suppurativa

Definition

- Hidradenitis suppurativa is a disorder of the terminal follicular epithelium in the apocrine gland–bearing skin (intertriginous areas usually)

Considerations

- Involves 1 or more areas — axilla, genitofemoral area, perineum, gluteal area and in women inframammary area
  - May occur on shoulders, scalp, areola or umbilicus
- Recurrent painful or suppurating lesions occurring > 2 times in 6 months
- Usually staph infection
- Classic lesion double comedone "black head" with 2 surface openings, tender with or without purulent discharge

Treatment options

- Warm compresses
- Burrow solution
- Weight loss if indicated
- Doxycycline 100 mg PO qday or bid, or tetracycline 500 mg PO bid, or minocycline 100 mg qday or bid PO if cellulitis present (usually needed for several months)
  - Clindamycin and rifampin PO for suppurative disease not responsive to tetracyclines
- Topical clindamycin 2%, topical corticosteroids, or topical antiseptic
- Benzoyl peroxide 5 or 10% or chlorhexidine wash daily
- Biologics SQ or IV respectfully for moderate to severe disease
  - Humira (adalimumab) SQ
  - Remicade (infliximab) IV
- Oral contraceptives for women
- Dexamethasone 6 mg qday x 10–14 days, may taper last 7

days for acute inflammation if needed
- Incision and drainage as needed
- Loose fitting clothes
- Good personal hygiene

Admission criteria

- Severe disease
- Requires surgery acutely

Referral

- Dermatology or general surgery as indicated

Discharge criteria recommendation

- Uncomplicated pilonidal cyst, abscess or hidradenitis suppurativa
- Asymptomatic patients

Discharge instructions

- Pilonidal cyst aftercare instructions
- Return if pain returns or fever develops
- Refer to surgeon for definitive treatment

Consult criteria recommendation

- Pilonidal abscess near anus
- Patient toxicity
- Fever ≥ 101°F (38.3°C)

Notes

____

____

____

REFERENCES:

Hemorrhoids Treatment & Management
Author: Scott C Thornton, MD; Chief Editor: John Geibel, MD, DSc, MA
emedicine.medscape.com/article/775407

Pilonidal Disease Treatment & Management
Author: James de Caestecker, DO; Chief Editor: John Geibel, MD, DSc, MA
emedicine.medscape.com/article/192668

Anal Fissure Treatment & Management
emedicine.medscape.com/article/196297

Schiano di Visconte M, Munegato G. Glyceryl trinitrate ointment (0.25%) and anal cryothermal dilators in the treatment of chronic anal fissures. *J Gastrointest Surg*. Jul 2009;13(7):1283–91

Rectal Prolapse Author: Jan Rakinic, MD; Chief Editor: John Geibel, MD, DSc, MA
emedicine.medscape.com/article/2026460

CONSTIPATION PROTOCOL

Definition

- A gastrointestinal motility disorder resulting in 2 of the following
  - Less than 3 bowels movements per week
  - Hard lumpy stools
  - Straining
  - Incomplete defecation sensation
  - Anorectal obstruction sensation
  - Manually assisted defecation

Differential diagnosis

- Large bowel obstruction
- Abdominal hernia
- Hypothyroidism
- Irritable bowel syndrome
- Anxiety disorders
- Toxic megacolon
- Colon cancer
- Diverticulitis

Considerations

- Most common digestive complaint
- Affects 15% of the U.S. population

- Usually treated medically with improvement in symptoms
- 30% higher incidence in nonwhite population
- May be asymptomatic or have pain with above definition symptoms

Red flag symptoms

- Unexplained weight loss
- Vomiting
- Inability to pass flatus
- Abdominal pain
- Rectal bleeding

Types

Primary or idiopathic constipation

- Normal transit constipation
- Slow transit constipation
    - Infrequent stools and decreased urgency
    - Impaired phasic colon activity
- Pelvic floor dysfunction
    - Dysfunction of pelvic floor or anal sphincter

Secondary constipation

- Caused by
    - Low fiber diet
    - Decreased fluid intake
    - Lack of exercise
    - Anal fissures
    - Diabetes mellitus, hypothyroidism
    - Stroke, spinal cord injuries, multiple sclerosis
    - Parkinson's disease
    - Antidepressants
    - Anticholinergics
    - Narcotics
    - Calcium channel blockers
    - Antacids
    - NSAID's
    - Depression

Evaluation options

- Usually history and examination is all that is needed
- CBC for weight loss, fever or bleeding
- CMP for diabetes mellitus or vomiting or weight loss
- Abdominal flat and upright films for vomiting
- CT abdominal/pelvic scan for vomiting, weight loss or unusually severe pain

Treatment options

Prevention

- Good fluid intake
- Exercise
- High fiber diet
- Avoid constipating medications
- Fiber supplements

Acute ED or office treatment

- Fleets mineral oil enema
    - Adult 1 bottle
    - Pediatric 30–60 ml (Age 2–11 years)
- Fleet bisacodyl enema
    - Adult 30 ml (1 bottle)
    - Pediatric (2–12 years) 15 ml
- Fleet enema
    - Adult 118 ml (1 bottle)
    - Pediatric 5–12 years Pedia-Lax 1 bottle 59 ml
    - Pediatric 2–5 years Pedia-Lax ½ bottle
    - Do not use in megacolon, CHF, ascites, renal failure or intestinal obstruction
- Glycerin suppository
    - Age > 6 years 1 suppository
    - Age 2–6 years Fleet's Babylax applicator (4 ml)
- Digital disimpaction
- Milk and molasses enema in children not allergic to milk

Acute home treatment

- Dulcolax suppository or tablet
- Colace
- Fleet's enema
- Prune juice
- Glycerin suppository

Chronic home treatment

- High fiber diet
- Psyllium (Metamucil)

- < 6 years 1 gm PO qday-tid in water or juice
- Age 6–11 years 1.7 gm (powder) in water or juice PO qday-tid or 1 oral wafer, increase slowly as needed
- > 12 years 2–6 caps qday-tid or 2 wafers PO qday increasing as needed

- Magnesium hydroxide (Milk of magnesia)
  - Age 6–11 years 15–30 ml PO qday prn
  - Age > 12 years 30–60 ml PO qday prn
- Polyethylene glycol (MiraLax)
  - Age < 17 years – 0.8 gm/kg in 8 oz. of liquid PO qday prn up to 4 days
  - Age ≥ 17 years – 1 capful in 8 oz. liquid PO qday prn up to 4 days
- Lubiprostone (Amitiza 24 mcg PO q12hr for chronic constipation; IBS-C 8 mcg PO q12hr
- Lactulose 15–30 mL (10–20 g) PO once daily; may be increased to 60 mL (40 g) once daily
  - Children 0.7–2 g/kg/day (1–3 mL/kg/day) PO in divided doses; not to exceed 40 g/day (60 mL/day)

Constipation induced by opioids with advanced illness

- Methylnaltrexone (Relistor) weight-base dosing

Discharge criteria

- Uncomplicated findings
- Normal vital signs

Discharge instructions

- Constipation aftercare instructions
- See Gastroenterologist referral criteria

Consult criteria

- Red flag symptoms
- Fever
- Vomiting
- Tachycardia
- Metabolic acidosis
- Significant gross rectal bleeding
- Melena
- Rebound abdominal tenderness
- Moderate to severe tenderness

Referral to gastroenterologist criteria

- Recent onset
- Rectal bleeding
- Weight loss
- Recent bowel habit changes

Notes

____

____

____

REFERENCES:

Constipation Author: Marc D Basson, MD, PhD, MBA, FACS; Chief Editor: Julian Katz, MD emedicine.medscape.com/article/184704

Noguera A, Centeno C, Librada S, Nabal M. Screening for Constipation in Palliative Care Patients. *J Palliat Med.* Sep 11 2009

[Guideline] North American Society for Pediatric Gastroenterology, Hepatology and Nutrition. Evaluation and treatment of constipation in children: summary of updated recommendations of the North American Society for Pediatric Gastroenterology, Hepatology and Nutrition. *J Pediatr Gastroenterol Nutr.* Sep 2006;43(3):405–7

Pediatric Constipation Medication Author: Stephen Borowitz, MD; Chief Editor: Carmen Cuffari, MD emedicine.medscape.com/article/928185

Urinary and Male Genitourinary

Section Contents

When using any protocol, always follow the Guidelines of Proper Use (page 12).

KIDNEY STONE PROTOCOL

Definition

- Ureteral colic produced by passage of renal calculus from kidney into the ureter

Differential Diagnosis

- Biliary colic
- Aortic aneurysm
- Mechanical back pain
- Herpes zoster
- Pyelonephritis
- Renal vein thrombosis
- Renal infarction
- Retroperitoneal bleeding
- Appendicitis
- Pulmonary embolism
- Testicular and ovarian torsion
- Ectopic pregnancy

Considerations

- Calcium stones account for 75% of kidney stones
- Sudden pain onset located in the lateral mid to lower back or lower quadrant with occasional radiation to the groin
- Nausea or vomiting usually occurs
- Fever usually absent
- Groin pain felt when kidney stone at ureterovesicular junction (UVJ)
  - Most common location of impaction
- Aortic aneurysm can mimic ureteral colic
  - Renal colic is most common misdiagnosis of ruptured abdominal aortic aneurysm
- Retained kidney stones in the renal calyces asymptomatic and rarely cause pain
- Hematuria on U/A absent 10–15% of the time
- KUB reveals approximately 30–60% of the kidney stones (calcium stones)

- Pelvic calcifications commonly are phleboliths (benign)
- Abdominal exam frequently benign
- Abdominal tenderness can occur with high grade ureteral obstruction
- Flomax (tamsulosin) 0.4 mg qday Rx outpatient allows larger kidney stones to pass frequently — up to 1 cm
  - Flomax (tamsulosin) may be given for 2–4 weeks to pass ureteral calculus
- Most kidney stones pass given time
- Stones up to 1 cm can be managed conservatively in the absence of fever, infection and renal failure if pain is controlled
  - Most large stones will need removal by urology
- CT abdomen/pelvis 97% accurate
- Thrombocytosis can occur with ureteral obstruction with pyelonephritis

Evaluation Options

U/A and KUB

- More useful in patients with known kidney stone disease
- May be all that is needed on healthy patients with typical presentation

Ultrasound in children and pregnant patients

- Sensitivity of 98.3% and specificity of 100% in study of 318 patients
- Failed to find stones in 40% of children

UCG in sexually active fertile females

BMP and CBC for any below

- Diabetic patient
- Fever present
- Tachycardia present
- Hypotension present
- SBP < 105 with history of hypertension

Consider CT abdomen and pelvis without contrast

- Uncertain diagnosis
- Age ≥ 60
- Abdominal pulsatile mass
- Possibility of aortic aneurysm considered
- CT has a sensitivity of 94% to 100% and specificity of 92% to 100% in evaluating urinary and non-urinary flank pain

Urine culture if fever or pyuria present

Treatment Options

Acute treatment

- Toradol (ketorolac) 10–15 mg IV with or without Dilaudid (hydromorphone) 0.5– 1 mg (or equipotent narcotic IV) and Phenergan (promethazine) 6.25 mg IV or Zofran (ondansetron) 4 mg IV; may repeat narcotics × 2 prn if stable vital signs and no significant altered mental status or any respiratory depression
- Toradol (ketorolac) 15–30 mg IM with or without Dilaudid (hydromorphone) 1–2 mg IM (or equipotent narcotic) and Phenergan (promethazine) 25 mg IM or Zofran (ondansetron) 4 mg IM if IV access not readily available
  - Do not use Toradol (ketorolac) if creatinine is elevated
  - Ketorolac therapeutic ceiling is around 10 mg
- Do not give increased IV fluids except as needed for dehydration or hypotension

Discharge treatments

- Flomax (tamsulosin 0.4 mg PO each day for 2–4 weeks if discharged home (can cause passage of larger stones)
- UTI antibiotics if lower urinary tract infection present without pyelonephritis or fever

Discharge symptom treatment options

- Toradol (ketorolac) 10 mg PO QID prn up to 5 days
  - Do not use Toradol (ketorolac) if creatinine is elevated
- Hydrocodone or oxycodone 5–10 mg PO QID prn up to 3 days
- Phenergan (promethazine) 12.5–25 mg QID PO/PR prn nausea or vomiting

Discharge Criteria

- Pain resolved or tolerable by patient and the patient is agreeable to go home
- No upper tract urinary infection
- No solitary kidney
- No acute renal dysfunction

Discharge instructions

- Kidney stone aftercare instructions
- Increase or additional oral hydration 1–2 liters per day
- Low salt, low protein diet if type of stone not known
- Follow up within 7–10 days with urologist
- Urine strainer and turn in any stone for analysis

Consult Criteria

- Ureteral stone ≥ 6 mm
- Pain and/or vomiting not controlled to clinician or patient's satisfaction
- Uncertain diagnosis
- Concurrent upper tract urinary infection (pyelonephritis)
- Solitary functioning kidney with ureteral calculus
- Pyelonephritis
- Fever

Vital sign and age consult criteria

- Age ≥ 75
- Fever
- Adult heart rate ≥ 110
- Developing hypotension or relative hypotension (SBP < 105 with history of hypertension)

Lab consult criteria

- WBC ≥ 14,000
- Bandemia
- Metabolic acidosis
- Significant electrolyte abnormality
- Glucose ≥ 400 mg/dL in diabetic patient
- Glucose ≥ 300 mg/dL in non-diabetic patient
- Hyperglycemia with metabolic acidosis (decreased serum CO_2 or elevated anion gap)
- Hemoglobin decrease > 1 gm
- Creatinine increase > 0.5 from baseline
- Renal insufficiency
- Acute thrombocytosis
- Acute thrombocytopenia

Notes

REFERENCES:

Medical therapy for calculus disease BJU INTERNATIONAL Volume 107, Issue 3, February 2011, Pages: 356–368, Shrawan K. Singh, Mayank Mohan Agarwal and Sumit Sharma

Talner L, Vaughn M. Nonobstructive renal causes of flank pain: findings on noncontrast helical CT (CT KUB). Abdom Imaging. 2003; 28:210–216

Tamm EP, Silverman PM, Shuman WP. Evaluation of the patient with flank pain and possible ureteral calculus. Radiology. 2003;228(2): 319–329 (Clinical radiologic review)

Park SJ, Yi BH, Lee HK, et al. Evaluation of patients with suspected ureteral calculi using sonography as an initial diagnostic tool: how can we improve diagnostic accuracy? Ultrasound Med. 2008; 27:1441–1450 (Prospective study; 318 patients

(Am J Emerg Med, epub, 7/18/20)

URINARY TRACT INFECTION PROTOCOL

Definition

- Bacteriuria with the presence of symptoms

Differential Diagnosis

- Cystitis
- PID
- Ovarian cyst pain
- Gonococcal urethritis
- Nonspecific urethritis (chlamydia or ureaplasma)
- Renal colic
- Bladder outlet obstruction
- Neurogenic bladder
- Pelvic pain disorder
- Endometriosis
- Vaginitis
- Orchitis
- Epididymitis

Considerations

- Female > male incidence until age 50
- 0–3 months of age associated with 30% incidence of sepsis (80% of time the U/A may be normal in neonates with UTI)
- E. coli most common cause
- Sexually active males frequently have prostatitis or urethritis as cause of urinary symptoms (frequently gonorrhea or chlamydia)
- Asymptomatic bacteriuria present in 20% women > 65 years of age
  - Borderline WBC counts of 6-10 cells/mL may reflect the state of hydration such as in patients with oliguria or anuria (dialysis) will usually have some degree of pyuria
    - WBCs may also be seen with moderate hematuria
- Elderly often have atypical presentation
  - Altered mental status
  - Confusion
  - Acute incontinence
  - GI symptoms
  - Urinary retention
- Fever and/or vomiting suggest upper tract urinary infection
- Gross hematuria usually present in lower tract infection
- Acute thrombocytosis with upper tract infection (pyelonephritis) may indicate obstruction from ureteral calculus

UTI facts

- Visual inspection of urine clarity is not useful in diagnosing UTI in women
- Foul-smelling urine is an unreliable indicator of infection in catheterized patients
- Asymptomatic bacteriuria is common in all ages and frequently over-treated
- Virtually 100% of patients with an indwelling Foley catheter are colonized within 2 weeks of placement with 2–5 organisms
- Younger women with true recurrent UTI, bacteriuria may be "protective" for future UTI from more pathogenic organisms
- Leukopenia patients may have artificially low urine WBC
- Noninfectious conditions may result in pyuria — for example acute renal failure, STD, or noninfectious cystitis from a catheter
- Pyuria is a nonspecific, frequent finding in older patients with or without bacteriuria and is not diagnostic of UTI or indicate a need for antibiotics
  - The absence of pyuria has a negative predictive value of > 95% to rule out UTI

- Urine nitrates should not be used alone to start antibiotics
  - Bacteriuria, as noted above, does not define a clinically significant UTI
- Occurrence of candiduria in the catheterized patient is common, and most often reflects colonization or asymptomatic infection
  - Treatment of candida in the urine should occur only in rare situations, such as clear signs and symptoms of infection and no alternative source of infection
- Attributing altered mental status to bacteriuria can result in failure to identify the true cause
  - Without clinical instability or other signs or symptoms of UTI, AMS in elderly can reasonably be observed for resolution of confusion for 24-48 hrs. without antibiotics, while searching for other causes of confusion

Children with UTI admission criteria recommendation

- Patients who are toxic or septic
- Patients with signs of urinary obstruction or significant underlying disease
- Patients who are unable to tolerate adequate oral fluids or medications
- Infants younger than 2 months with febrile UTI (presumed pyelonephritis)
- All infants younger than 1 month with suspected UTI, even if not febrile

High risk

- Diabetes
- **Pregnancy**
  - Higher incidence of premature rupture of membranes and fetal demise with UTI (even if asymptomatic)
- Renal failure
- Sickle cell anemia
- Immunocompromised

Complicated UTI

- High risk criteria listed above
- Structural abnormalities
- Mechanical (catheter, stones, stents, instrumentation)
- Functional (reflux or neurogenic bladder)
- Males
- Resistant pathogens

Acute urethral syndrome

- Dysuria without pyuria
- Empiric treatment for STD

Differential of acute urethral syndrome

- Chlamydia
- Gonorrhea
- Herpes
- Vaginitis

Evaluation

- Complete history and physical exam
- Abdominal and costovertebral exam
- Pelvic exam in females and genital exam in males if STD suspected
- U/A – clean catch; catheter specimen if contamination suspected
  - Positive nitrite highly specific (low false positives)
- CBC if vomiting, fever or tachycardia present
- BMP if diabetic or for dehydration/tachycardia if present
- Prostate and urethral meatus exam in males at risk for STI

Urine culture

- For high risk patient or complicated UTI
- Symptoms after > 2 days of treatment or relapse
- Pyelonephritis

Treatment Options

Asymptomatic bacteriuria do not treat unless

- Pregnant (obtain culture)
- Neutropenic
- Abnormal renal functions
- Transplant patient
- Undergoing urologic procedure
- Children (treat 5–7 days)

Uncomplicated UTI options (Simple UTI)

- Septra DS bid PO for 3 days (trimethoprim/sulfamethoxazole)
  - Pediatric age > 2 months 0.5 ml/kg bid (max dose 20 ml) or 8 mg TMP/kg/day PO divided q12hr for 7-10 days
- Amoxicillin-clavulanate (Augmentin) 875 mg/125 mg PO BID for 7 days
- Ciprofloxacin 250 mg bid PO for 3 days
  - Children treat 5–7 days (not first line antibiotic due to arthropathy)
- Levofloxacin (Levaquin) 250 mg PO qday for 3 days
- Macrobid (nitrofurantoin) × 5 days — do not use in renal impairment or in upper tract infections
- Cephalexin age >15 years give 250 mg PO q6hr for 7 days
  - Cephalexin 20–50 mg/kg/day for 7 days pediatrics not to exceed adult dose
- Cefdinir 300 mg PO BID for 7 days
  - Pediatric cefdinir 7mg/kg up to 43 kg for 7 days
- Fosfomycin (Monurol) 3 gm PO with 3-4 oz. of water X 1 dose
- Avoid quinolones if locally high resistance > 10%
- May use Sanford Guide or antibiotic database

Urinary analgesia

- Pyridium: 100–200 mg TID prn urinary symptoms — do not dispense more than 6 tablets for acute cystitis (avoid in renal insufficiency)

Complicated UTI

- Cystitis same as uncomplicated UTI but for 5–7 days of antibiotics (excluding Fosfomycin and nitrofurantoin)
- Ertapenem (Invanz) 1 gm IV
- Ciprofloxacin or levofloxacin may be used if known resistance is < 10%
  - Not first line antibiotic in children due to potential complications of arthropathy
- Obtain culture

Pyelonephritis (mild to moderate)

- Obtain culture
- Septra DS bid PO for 14 days
- Amoxicillin-clavulanate (Augmentin) 875 mg/125 mg PO BID for 14 days
- Cefdinir 300 mg PO BID for 7 days
- Cephalexin 500mg PO qid for 14 days
- Ciprofloxacin 500 mg bid PO for 7 days (mild infection)
  - Pediatric cefdinir 7mg/kg up to 43 kg for 7 days
- Ciprofloxacin 500 mg bid PO for 10–14 days (moderate infection)
  - Ciprofloxacin ≥ 1 year of age (PO) 10-20 mg/kg q12hr; individual dose not to exceed 750 mg q12hr for 10-21 days (not first line antibiotic due to arthropathy)
- Levofloxacin (Levaquin) 500 mg PO qday for 5 days (mild infection)
- Levofloxacin (Levaquin) 500 mg PO qday for 10–14 days (moderate infection)
- IV Rocephin (ceftriaxone) 1–2 gms IV or IM × 1 can be given initially
- Invanz (ertapenem) 1 gm IV × 1 can be given initially
- Do not use fosfomycin or nitrofurantoin

Pyelonephritis (severe) antibiotic choices

- Needs hospitalization
- Invanz (ertapenem) 1 gm IV qday for 14 days or IM qday for 7 days — adjust for renal dosing
- Rocephin (ceftriaxone) 1 gm q12hr. or 2 Gms q24hr. IV or IM for 14 days in adults
  - 50 mg/kg in children – not to exceed adult dose)

- Ciprofloxacin (Cipro) 400 mg IV q12h for 10-14 days
- Levofloxacin (Levaquin) 250 mg IV q24h for 10 days
- Levofloxacin (Levaquin) 750 mg IV q24h for 5 days
- Tobramycin 3 mg/kg/day IV/IM divided q8hr (with normal renal function)
- Ciprofloxacin or levofloxacin may be used if known resistance is < 10%
  - Not first line antibiotic in children due to potential complications of arthropathy
- Do not use fosfomycin or nitrofurantoin
- Obtain culture

Sexually transmitted diseases

- See Sexually Transmitted Disease Protocol

Pain and nausea medication prn

- Narcotics short course
- OTC medications
- Pyridium (phenazopyridium) 100–200 mg TID (NMT 6 pills)
  - Avoid in renal insufficiency—can cause renal failure
- Phenergan (promethazine) — may need suppository if actively vomiting)
- Zofran (ondansetron)

Discharge criteria recommendation

- Uncomplicated UTI without toxicity
- Able to hold PO intake and medications down
- Healthy patients with uncomplicated pyelonephritis

Discharge instructions

- UTI aftercare instructions
- Follow up primary care provider or urologist within 7 days as needed

Consult criteria recommendation

- Complicated UTI
- Toxic appearance or septic
- Failed outpatient treatment
- Immunocompromised
- Persistent vomiting
- Unable to hold PO meds down
- Unable to self-hydrate
- Pregnancy
- Progressive renal insufficiency
- Poor follow-up
- Male children with first UTI

Vital signs and age consult recommendations

- Age < 3 months
- Adult heart rate ≥ 110
- Hypotension (or relative hypotension: SBP < 105 in patient with hypertension history)

Lab consult criteria recommendations

- WBC ≥ 20,000 or < 3,000; neutropenia < 1,000
- Bandemia ≥ 15%
- Acute thrombocytopenia
- Acute thrombocytosis
- Creatinine increase > 0.5 from baseline
- Renal insufficiency
- Increased anion gap
- Significant electrolyte abnormality
- Glucose ≥ 300 mg/dL in diabetic patient
- Glucose ≥ 200 mg/dL in non-diabetic patient
- Hyperglycemia with metabolic acidosis (decreased serum CO_2 or elevated anion gap)
- Lactic acidosis

Notes

____

____

____

REFERENCES:

International Clinical Practice Guidelines For The Treatment Of Acute Uncomplicated Cystitis And Pyelonephritis In Women: A 2010

Update By The Infectious Diseases Society Of America And The European Society For Microbiology And Infectious Diseases. Clinical Infectious Diseases. 2011;52(5):e103–e120

Management Of Suspected Bacterial Urinary Tract

Infection In Adults. A National Clinical Guideline.1

Scottish Intercollegiate Guidelines Network. 2012.

Sign.ac.uk/pdf/sign88 pdf

Cystitis in Females

Author: John L Brusch, MD, FACP; Chief Editor: Michael Stuart Bronze, MD

emedicine.medscape.com/article/233101

American College of Obstetricians and Gynecologists (ACOG). 2008. Treatment of urinary tract infections in nonpregnant women

Gupta K, Hooton TM, Naber KG, et al. International clinical practice guidelines for the treatment of acute uncomplicated cystitis and pyelonephritis in women: A 2010 update by the Infectious Diseases Society of America and the European Society for Microbiology and Infectious Diseases. Clin Infect Dis. Mar 2011;52(5):e103–20

Urinary Tract Infection in Males Medication

Author: John L Brusch, MD, FACP; Chief Editor: Michael Stuart Bronze, MD

emedicine.medscape.com/article/231574

Pediatric Urinary Tract Infection

Author: Donna J Fisher, MD; Chief Editor: Russell W Steele, MD emedicine.medscape.com/article/969643

Schulz L, et al. *Journal of Emerg Med,* April 7 2016. [Epub]

Nicolle LE, et al. *Clin Infect Dis.* 2005; 40: 643–654

Emedhome.com Clinical Pearls: 6 UTI Myths

Published April 13, 2016

JEM, 7/16:25

NEJM,2016;374:562

CHRONIC RENAL FAILURE PROTOCOL

Definition

- Decreased kidney glomerular filtration rate (GFR) of less than 60 mL/min

Differential Diagnosis

- Acute renal failure
- Acute on chronic renal failure

Considerations

- Normal glomerular filtration rate (GFR) in healthy adult is 120 cc/minute
- Uremia occurs when GFR is 10–20 cc/minute

Chronic kidney disease classification (CKD)

- Stage 1: Kidney damage with normal or increased GFR (>90 mL/min/1.73 m ^{2})
- Stage 2: Mild reduction in GFR (60-89 mL/min/1.73 m ^{2})
- Stage 3a: Moderate reduction in GFR (45-59 mL/min/1.73 m ^{2})
- Stage 3b: Moderate reduction in GFR (30-44 mL/min/1.73 m ^{2})
- Stage 4: Severe reduction in GFR (15-29 mL/min/1.73 m ^{2})
- Stage 5: Kidney failure (GFR < 15 mL/min/1.73 m ^{2} or dialysis)

Main causes

- Diabetes
- Hypertension
- Obstruction (usually in men)
- Polycystic kidney disease (inherited)

- NSAIDs are among the most common causes of drug-induced renal injury
  - Prostaglandin-induced renal vasodilation is critical for maintaining renal perfusion
    - Prostaglandin inhibition by NSAIDs impairs this vasodilation — magnified in hypovolemic patients or those taking ACE inhibitors

Signs, Symptoms and Associated Disorders

- Malaise; weakness; fatigue
- Anorexia; nausea; vomiting
- Gastritis and peptic ulcer disease
- Peripheral neuropathy
- Anemia
- Pruritus
- Volume overload
- CHF
- Hypocalcemia
- Increased infections
- Dialysis catheter infections
- Pericarditis
- Peritonitis in peritoneal dialysis (CAPD) patients

Dialysis disequilibrium syndrome

- Overdialysis
- Weakness
- Dizziness
- Headache
- Mental status changes in severe cases

Hyperkalemia

- EKG cannot reliably predict K^+ level
- Caused frequently by medications (ACEI/ARB/spironolactone/eplerenone)
- May be caused by potassium supplements

K^+ level

- 5.5–6.5 mEq/L — T wave peaking; shortening QTc interval
- 6.5–8.0 mEq/L — PR interval prolongation; loss of P waves; QRS widening
- Greater than 8.0 mEq/L — IVCD; bundle branch blocks; sine wave complex

Evaluation

- Complete history and physical exam
- Last dialysis noted if currently being treated
- BMP

Testing options

- CBC
- BMP
- Troponin (frequently elevated due to volume overload and CHF only)
- BNP or NT–ProBNP (commonly very elevated and of questionable utility)
- U/A if producing urine and UTI suspected (cath urine sample for fever or lower abdominal pain)
- Chest x-ray if volume overload suspected
- EKG if K^+ elevated
- DO NOT ORDER IV CONTRAST unless approved by physician
- Digoxin level if taking it

Treatment Options

Emergent hypertension (consult physician promptly)

- Treat with nitroglycerin SL (NTG) up to 3 doses prn
- NTG paste 1–2 inches prn
- Nitroprusside drip IV
- Dialysis if due to volume overload and patient is on dialysis. Usually an urgent treatment and other steps need to be taken first

Asymptomatic hypertension

- Per Hypertension Protocol (usually no treatment needed)

Hyperkalemia > 5.5 mEq/L (consult physician)

- EKG with peaked T waves or widened QRS complex may or may not be seen
- EKG may not reflect degree of hyperkalemia
- Emergent treatment is indicated if the ECG is abnormal even before the lab test returns
  - Emergent treatment is otherwise not indicated without the lab results
  - Frequently no treatment acutely needed with $K^+ <$ 6.0–6.5 mEq/L unless EKG changes or cardiotoxicity present or symptomatic

Calcium gluconate (safer peripheral IV than CaCl) or calcium chloride up to 1 amp IV over 2–3 minutes with patient on monitor

- Calcium chloride 3 three times more potent than calcium gluconate
  - Give 10 ml of calcium gluconate or 5 ml of calcium chloride initially — may repeat as needed per physician
- Duration of action 30–60 minutes
- May be repeated in 5–10 minutes if EKG not improved
- Does not lower serum potassium levels
- Stabilizes cardiac membranes from effects of high potassium
- Controversial whether dangerous or not in Digoxin (digitalis) toxic patients — give Digibind as indicated

D50W 1 amp (if patient not hyperglycemic) followed by regular insulin 5–10 units IV

- **In chronic kidney disease patients use regular insulin 5 units IV to avoid hypoglycemia**
- Starts to lower K^+ by 0.5–1.5 mEq/L in 15 minutes
- Peak effect in 60 minutes
- Effect lasts 4–6 hours
- Recheck blood glucose in 60–75 minutes for hypoglycemia
- If initial blood glucose is ≥ 250, then D50W is not given
- Check K^+ and glucose every 2 hours

Albuterol aerosol inhalation

- 10–20 mg of Albuterol in chamber with a few cc's of NS
- Onset of action within 20–30 minutes
- Peak effect in 90 minutes and lasts 2 hours
- May cause tachycardia

Sodium bicarbonate not acutely effective in treating hyperkalemia in renal failure patients

Kayexalate

- 30–60 gms in 20% sorbitol or water PO
  - Onset of action 1–3 hours
- 60 gms without sorbitol PR
  - Longer onset of action than PO
- Recent controversy on effectiveness
- May cause colonic necrosis

Patiromer (*Veltassa*, Relypsa)

- New agent approved in 2015
- Binds medications so need at least 6 hour delay from taking other medications
- Not for emergency treatment of hyperkalemia due to delay in action

Dialysis

CHF and volume overload (consult physician prior to treatment)

- BNP or NT–ProBNP usually elevated even in asymptomatic patients

Hypertension treatment options

- NTG SL
- NTG paste 1–2 inches
- NTG drip IV
- Dialysis best treatment

Hypotension

- Rule out sepsis
- IV NS 200 bolus if not in clinical fluid overload
- Notify physician promptly

Bleeding

- Direct pressure
- DDAVP (more for oozing than brisk bleeding)

CAPD peritonitis

- Consult physician

Discharge Criteria

- Chronic renal failure patient who is stable and at baseline without acute significant electrolyte abnormalities

Discharge instructions

- Chronic renal failure aftercare instructions
- Avoid potassium supplements
- See Hyperkalemia Protocol

Consult Criteria (with supervising physician)

- Hyperkalemia
- Volume overload
- Heart failure
- Significant electrolyte abnormalities or active comorbidities
- Abnormal vital signs or O_2 desaturation

Notes

REFERENCES:

Weisberg LS. Management of severe hyperkalemia. *Crit Care Med* 2008;36:3246–3251

Sood MM, et al. Emergency Management and Commonly Encountered Outpatient Scenarios in Patients With Hyperkalemia *Mayo Clin Proc* 2007;82:1553–1561

Annals Int Med 110(6):426, March 15, 1989

Levine M, et al. The Effects of Intravenous Calcium in Patients with Digoxin Toxicity *J Emerg Med* 2011 Jan;40(1):41–6

Dialysis Complications of Chronic Renal Failure

Author: Richard S Krause, MD; Chief Editor: Erik D Schraga, MD emedicine.medscape.com/article/1918879

Int J Nephr Renovas Dis,7:459

LaRue H, et al. *Pharmacotherapy*. 2017 Oct 4

Li T, et al. *Clin Kidney J*. 2014 Jun;7(3):239-41

Allon M, et al. *Kidney Int* 1990; 38(5): 869-872

Hyperkalemia Treatment & Management Updated: Jun 20, 2018 Author: Eleanor Lederer, MD, FASN; Chief Editor: Vecihi Batuman, MD, FASN

MALE GENITOURINARY PROTOCOL

Urethritis and Epididymoorchitis

Definition

- Infection or inflammation of the urethra, epididymis or testicle

Differential diagnosis for epididymoorchitis

- Testicular torsion
- Mumps
- Trauma
- Hernia
- Tumor — usually painless

Considerations

- Gonorrhea and chlamydia are the main causes and coexist 25–50% of the time
- Urethral discharge
- Tender and swollen epididymis and/or testicle

Gonorrhea

- Dysuria
- Thick purulent discharge from urethra
- Gram negative intracellular diplococci

Chlamydia

- Thinner discharge from urethra
- Little to no discomfort

Evaluation

- Sexual history
- Genital exam
- Smear with intracellular gram negative diplococci can be performed
- Culture
- RPR prn

Treatment options

- Follow CDC guidelines
- Analgesics prn
- Rocephin (ceftriaxone) 500 mg
  - Ceftriaxone 1 gm IM if weight > 150 kg
- IM route not available may use 800 mg cefixime PO once
- Cephalosporin allergy may use gentamicin 240 mg IM plus azithromycin single 2 g PO
- Add doxycycline 100 mg PO bid × 7 days if chlamydia not excluded for urethral, cervical, rectal and pharyngeal uncomplicated infections
- If concerned about syphilis coinfection then doxycycline 100 mg bid PO for 15 days
- A test-of-cure is unnecessary for persons with uncomplicated urogenital or rectal gonorrhea who are treated with any of the recommended or alternative regimens; however, for persons with pharyngeal gonorrhea, a test-of-cure is recommended, using culture or nucleic acid amplification tests 7–14 days after initial treatment

Discharge criteria

- Nontoxic patient

Discharge instructions

- Epididymoorchitis aftercare instructions
- Return if worse
- Follow up with PCP or urologist in 3–7 days
- If STD present, sexual partners in the previous 60 days should be tested and treated. Patients should have no sexual contact until treatment is completed, or 7 days after single-dose treatment.

Consult criteria

- Systemic toxicity
- Refer to General Patient Criteria Protocol prn (page 15)

Testicular Torsion

Definition

- Torsion of the testicle and spermatic cord with subsequent loss of blood flow to the testicle causing loss of testicular function and eventual testicular death and necrosis

Differential diagnosis

- Torsion of testicular or epididymal appendage (blue dot sign in light skinned patients may be present) — can be discharged home if diagnosed
- Epididymitis
- Epididymoorchitis
- Orchitis
- Hydrocele
- Testicular tumor or carcinoma
- Scrotal edema
- Inguinal hernia
- Fournier gangrene
- Testicular trauma
- Henoch-Schonlein Purpura
- Varicocele
- Appendicitis

Considerations

- True urologic emergency
- Complete torsion occurs with ≥ 360° rotation
- Partial torsion occurs with < 360° rotation
- Testicular salvage rate 90–100% with detorsion within 6 hours of pain onset
- Testicular viability 20–50% after 12 hours
- Peak age is 14 years of age, with second peak in first year of life
- Most torsions rotate inward and toward midline

Signs and symptoms

- Usually rapid onset of unilateral severe testicular pain
- Can occur from activity or trauma
- Can occur during sleep
- High-riding testicle occurs on affected side
- Scrotal swelling
- Nausea and/or vomiting
- Abdominal pain around 20–30%
- Fever not very common
- Cremasteric reflex absent on affected side

Evaluation

- Clinical diagnosis if classic history and findings
- Ultrasound color flow Doppler if unsure of diagnosis
  - 94% sensitive
  - 96% specific

Lab tests not usually very useful (used to evaluate for inflammatory processes with low suspicion of torsion)

- CBC – can be normal or elevated in torsion
- U/A – can have WBC's in 30% of torsions
- C-reactive protein – not too helpful

Treatment

- Pain control
- Manual rotation of testicles outward like opening a book
  - May need to be repeated 2–3 times to obtain relief
- Emergent surgery if unable to detorse testicle
- Urgent surgery if testicle detorsed
- All testicular torsion patients should have surgery and not be discharged

Consult criteria

- Discuss suspected testicular torsion with physician or urologist immediately

Prostatitis

Definition

- Infection or inflammation of the prostate gland

Differential diagnosis

- Prostate cancer
- Urethritis
- Mechanical back pain

- UTI

Considerations

- Gonorrhea and chlamydia are the main causes in men age < 35 years and coexist 25–50% of the time
- Prostate tender (caution with vigorous palpation if fever or toxicity present)
- Age > 35 years the usual cause is bacterial
- Nonbacterial prostatitis is an inflammatory condition without infection
- Chronic prostatitis
  - Increases risk of UTI and BPH

Acute bacterial prostatitis age > 35 years

- Fever
- Chills
- Perineal prostatic pain
- Dysuria
- Obstructive bladder symptoms
- Low back pain
- Low abdominal pain
- Spontaneous urethral discharge

Evaluation options

- U/A
- CBC

Treatment options

General supportive treatment

- Sitz baths, stool softeners, NSAIDs, Flomax or similar alpha blockers to assist in urine flow and decrease recurrence, and hydration

Age < 35 years

- Follow CDC guidelines
- Analgesics prn
- Rocephin (ceftriaxone) 500 mg IM

+

- Doxycycline 100 mg PO bid × 14–28 days
- Treatment for sexual partners or refer for treatment for STD

Age > 35 years

- May use Sanford Guide or other drug databases
- Septra DS 1 PO bid × 14–28 days (chronic bacterial prostatitis 4–6 weeks)

OR

- Ciprofloxacin 500 mg PO bid for 14–28 days
- Doxycycline 100 mg PO bid for 14-28 days for chronic bacterial prostatitis if cultures show susceptible organisms

  Metronidazole 2 gm orally in a single dose for men if trichomonas in the urine or on prep
- NSAID's and/or narcotics prn
- May give Pyridium for discomfort prn

Discharge criteria

- Nontoxic patient
- Refer to General Patient Criteria Protocol prn (page 15)

Discharge instructions

- Prostatitis aftercare instructions
- Return if worse
- Follow up with PCP or urologist in 3–7 days
- If STD present, sexual partners in the previous 60 days should be tested and treated. Patients should have no sexual contact until treatment is completed, or 7 days after single-dose treatment. Testing is repeated 3 months after treatment

Consult criteria

- Systemic toxicity
- Urinary retention

Priapism

Definition

- Persistent erection unrelated to sexual desire that is usually painful

Differential considerations

- Penile implant

- Urethral foreign body
- Peyronie's disease
- Erection from sexual arousal

Causes

- Idiopathic 35–50% of the time
- Sickle cell anemia
- Leukemia
- Trauma
- Spinal cord injury
- Vasoactive drugs

Low-flow priapism

- Painful
- Ischemia and impotence can occur
- From venous obstruction

High-flow priapism

- From arterial high flow state in penis
- Not usually painful
- Less common than low-flow priapism
- Trauma most frequent cause

Evaluation of priapism

- CBC
- Sickle prep or screen if suspected as a cause
- Color flow ultrasound if not sure if high or low-flow priapism

Treatment options

Low-flow priapism

- Analgesia
- Sickle cell patients may need exchange transfusion
- Terbutaline 0.25 mg SQ may help
- Pseudoephedrine 30–60 mg PO may help
- 1–2 ml of 1% lidocaine with epinephrine 1/100,000 premix injected into proximal corpora cavernosa on lateral penile shaft (one side only) post betadine and alcohol prep — use 27 gauge needle or smaller if possible
    - Aspirate some blood to ensure corpora cavernosa has been entered before injection
    - Caution with coronary artery disease history
    - Hold pressure 30–60 seconds post injection
- Phenylephrine 250–500 mcg can be used instead of 1% lidocaine with epinephrine
- Corpora cavernosa injections usually resolve priapism in 5–15 minutes

High-flow priapism

- Analgesia prn
- Ice packs

Discuss with physician and consult urology immediately

Paraphimosis

Definition

- Entrapment and inability of foreskin to be pulled back (forward) over the glans penis from the shaft in uncircumcised or partially uncircumcised males

Differential diagnosis

- Anasarca
- Balanitis
- Cellulitis
- Insect bite
- Carcinoma
- Penile fracture
- Penile hematoma
- Contact dermatitis
- Hair tourniquet

Considerations

- True emergency
- Can result in penile necrosis

Treatment

- Manual reduction after 5 minutes of ice in exam glove — pushing glans penis under foreskin while holding foreskin in place successful up to 90% of the time
- Dorsal slit of foreskin (consult physician)

Discharge criteria

- Successful reduction of paraphimosis
- No ischemic tissue damage

Discharge instructions

- Referral to urology for circumcision within 7–14 days

Consult criteria

- Inability to reduce the paraphimosis
- Penile tissue ischemic injury

Phimosis

Definition

- Inability to retract foreskin over glans penis

Considerations

- Can lead to venous congestion and eventually tissue damage
- Can lead to paraphimosis

Treatment

- Small hemostat can be passed into foreskin orifice to dilate it and deliver glans penis

Discharge criteria

- Usually can be discharged

Discharge instructions

- Refer to urology

Consult criteria

- Tissue ischemia
- Cellulitis

Hydrocele

Definition

- Collection of serous fluid in scrotum in up to 1% of males

Differential diagnosis

- Orchitis
- Testicular torsion
- Indirect inguinal hernia
- Epididymitis
- Trauma

Considerations

- Usually asymptomatic or subclinical
- Located anterior and superior to testicles
- A light shines through the hydrocele
- Most pediatric cases are congenital
- Can be from trauma, orchitis, or epididymitis

Evaluation options

- History and physical examination only may be all that is needed (transillumination)
- CBC
- U/A
- Ultrasound can be used if diagnosis uncertain

Treatment

- Usually no acute treatment needed

Discharge criteria

- Nonpainful, non-inflamed scrotal hydrocele

Discharge instructions

- Hydrocele aftercare instructions
- Refer to urology

Consult criteria

- Painful scrotum
- Scrotal cellulitis
- Fever

Notes

REFERENCES:

Lewis AG, Bukoswki TP, Jarvis PD et al. Evaluation of the acute scrotum in the emergency department. J Pediatr Surg 1995;30:2:277–82

Orchitis; Author: Nataisia Terry, MD; Chief Editor: Erik D Schraga, MD; emedicine.medscape.com/article/777456

Paraphimosis Treatment & Management Author: Jeffrey M Donohoe, MD, FAAP; Chief Editor: Bradley Fields Schwartz, DO, FACS emedicine.medscape.com/article/442883

Roberts JR, Price C, Mazzeo T. Intracavernous epinephrine: a minimally invasive treatment for priapism in the emergency department. *J Emerg Med.* Apr 2009;36(3):285–9

Chronic Bacterial Prostatitis Medication Author: Sunil K Ahuja, MD; Chief Editor: Edward David Kim, MD, FACS emedicine.medscape.com/article/458391

Prostatitis Author: Paul J Turek, MD; Chief Editor: Jeter (Jay) Pritchard Taylor, III, MD emedicine.medscape.com/article/785418

Update to CDC's Treatment Guidelines for Gonococcal Infection, 2020 *Weekly* / December 18, 2020 / 69(50);1911–1916

CCJM. Vol.86:733

Sexually Transmitted Infections Treatment Guidelines, 2021 Recommendations and Reports / July 23, 2021 / 70(4);1–187

Acute Urinary Retention Protocol

Definition

- Acute or subacute inability to voluntarily void sufficiently causing significant retention in the urinary bladder often requiring immediate attention and intervention

Considerations

Causes (some)

- Benign prostatic hypertrophy (BPH) most common cause in men of acute urinary retention (AUR) — most common cause overall
- Bladder masses, gynecologic surgery, and pelvic prolapse most common cause in women (relatively uncommon cause of AUR)
- AUR rarely secondary to spinal cord compression
- Diabetic neuropathy may cause AUR
- Urethral stricture
- Herpes genitalis

Medications causing AUR

- Anticholinergics or antihistamines that inhibit detrusor muscle activity
- Sympathomimetic drugs that increase alpha-adrenergic tone in the prostate
- NSAIDs that may inhibit prostaglandin-mediated detrusor muscle contraction
- Chronic opioid therapy causing a reduced bladder-fullness sensation

Symptoms

- Abdominal pain and/or distension
- Back pain may be confused with renal pathology or spinal tumors
- Urinary complaints (e.g., frequency, dribbling)
- Genital pain

Evaluation

- History of medications
- Voiding history
- Associated symptoms such as fever, chills, dysuria, new onset constipation, low back pain
- Rectal and genital exam as indicated
- U/A
- CBC, BMP as needed to assess renal function and for SIRS
- Bladder scan and possibly renal ultrasound (if needed)
- CT abdomen/pelvis without contrast if ureteral calculi or other significant disease process suspected

Treatment

- Double lumen foley catheter
- Coude catheter for significant BPH and difficulty passing standard foley
- Triple lumen foley catheter if irrigation needed (16F-20F)
- Tamsulosin (Flomax) 0.4 mg PO qday with catheter
  - Improves spontaneous voiding when catheter removed
- Antibiotics not needed unless existing UTI is present
- No evidence for the need to clamp foley with rapid bladder emptying
- 70% of men had a recurrent episode of AUR within 1 week if the bladder was drained only temporarily and initially on presentation
- BPH and AUR catheterized for ≤ 3 days had greater success with spontaneous voiding than those catheterized for > 3 days

Discharge criteria

- Resolution of AUR with foley
- No significant comorbidities

Discharge instructions

- Follow up with urologist ≤ 3 days
- Foley instructions
- Leg bag
- Return if fever, increased pain, vomiting or other concerning symptoms occur

Consult criteria

- Inability to pass foley
- Fever
- Pyelonephritis
- SIRS
- Significant comorbid disease processes or causes of AUR

Notes

REFERENCES:

Vilke GM, Ufberg JW, Harrigan RA, et al. Evaluation and treatment of acute urinary retention. J Emerg Med. 2008;35(2):193–198. (Review)

Afonso AS, Verhamme KM, Stricker BH, et al. Inhaled anticholinergic drugs and risk of acute urinary retention. BJU Int. 2011;107(8):1265–1272

Kaplan SA. AUA guidelines and their impact on the management of BPH: an update. Rev Urol. 2004;6 Suppl 9:S46–S52

Nyman MA, Schwenk NM, Silverstein MD. Management of urinary retention: rapid versus gradual decompression and risk of complications. Mayo Clin Proc. 1997;72(10):951–956

Breum L, Klarskov P, Munck LK, et al. Significance of acute urinary retention due to intravesical obstruction. Scand J Urol Nephrol. 1982;16(1):21–24

An Evidence-Based Approach To The Emergency Department Management of Acute Urinary Retention in Men and Women January 2014 review article; EB Medicine

Electrolyte and Acid/Base Disturbances

Section Contents

When using any protocol, always follow the Guidelines of Proper Use (page 12).

Hyperkalemia Protocol

Definition

- Elevated serum potassium levels

Differential Diagnosis

- Hypocalcemia
- Acute tubular necrosis
- Acute renal failure
- Chronic renal failure
- Metabolic acidosis
- Digoxin toxicity
- Burns
- Rhabdomyolysis
- Tumor lysis syndrome
- Head trauma

Considerations

- EKG cannot reliably predict K^+ level
  - K^+ level
    - 5.5–6.5 mEq/L — T wave peaking; shortening QTc interval
    - 6.5–8.0 mEq/L — PR interval prolongation; loss of P waves; QRS widening
    - Greater than 8.0 mEq/L — IVCD; bundle branch blocks; sine wave complex

Causes

- Renal failure
- K^+ supplementation
- Medications (ACEI/ARB/spironolactone/eplerenone)
- High potassium foods
- Hemolysis from blood draw

- Hemolysis
- DIC
- Tissue injury or ischemia

Evaluation

- Complete history and physical exam
- Last dialysis noted if being currently treated
- BMP
- Chest x-ray if volume overload suspected
- EKG

Testing options

- CBC
- Troponin questionable value (frequently elevated due to volume overload and CHF only)
- BNP questionable value (commonly very elevated)
- U/A if producing urine (cath urine sample for fever or lower abdominal pain)
- DO NOT ORDER IV CONTRAST STUDIES UNLESS APPROVED BY PHYSICIAN

Treatment Options

Hyperkalemia > 5.5 mEq/L (consult physician)

- EKG with peaked T waves or widened QRS complex may or may not be seen
- EKG may not reflect degree of hyperkalemia
- Emergent treatment is indicated if the ECG is abnormal even before the lab test returns
  - Emergent treatment is otherwise not indicated without the lab results
  - Frequently no treatment acutely needed with K^+ < 6.0–6.5 mEq/L unless EKG changes or cardiotoxicity present

Calcium gluconate (safer peripheral IV than CaCl) or calcium chloride up to 1 amp IV over 2–3 minutes with patient on monitor

- Calcium chloride 3 three times more potent than calcium gluconate
  - Give 10 ml of calcium gluconate or 5 ml of calcium chloride initially — may repeat as needed per physician
- Duration of action 30–60 minutes
- May be repeated in 5–10 minutes if EKG not improved
- Does not lower serum potassium levels
- Stabilizes cardiac membranes from effects of high potassium
- Controversial whether dangerous or not in Digoxin (digitalis) toxic patients — give Digibind

D50W 1 amp (if patient not hyperglycemic) followed by regular insulin 5–10 units IV

- **In chronic kidney disease patients use regular insulin 5 units IV to avoid hypoglycemia**
- Starts to lower K^+ by 0.5–1.5 mEq/L in 15 minutes
- Peak effect in 60 minutes
- Effect lasts 4–6 hours
- Recheck blood glucose in 60–75 minutes for hypoglycemia
- If initial blood glucose is ≥ 250, then D50W is not given
- Check K^+ and glucose every 2 hours

Albuterol aerosol inhalation

- 10–20 mg of Albuterol in chamber with a few cc's of NS
- Onset of action within 20–30 minutes
- Peak effect in 90 minutes and lasts 2 hours.
- May cause tachycardia

Sodium bicarbonate not acutely effective in treating hyperkalemia in renal failure patients

Kayexalate

- 30–60 gms in 20% sorbitol or water PO
  - Onset of action 1–3 hours
- 60 gms without sorbitol PR
  - Longer onset of action than PO
- May cause colonic necrosis
- Some controversy about effectiveness and has FDA warning about combining with sorbitol

Patiromer (*Veltassa*, Relypsa)

- New agent approved in 2015
- Binds medications so need at least 6 hour delay from taking other medications
- Not for emergency treatment of hyperkalemia due to delay in action

Dialysis

Discharge Criteria

- Mild hyperkalemia < 6.0 mEq/L
- Acceptable treatment response
- Further potassium rises not anticipated

Discharge instructions

- Close follow up
- Hyperkalemia aftercare instructions
- Chronic renal failure aftercare instructions if indicated

Consult Criteria

- Discuss with supervising physician if potassium > 5.5 mEq/L
- End-stage renal disease with abnormal vital signs or O_2 desaturation
- Significant comorbidities

Notes

REFERENCES:

Weisberg LS. Management of severe hyperkalemia. *Crit Care Med* 2008;36:3246–3251

Sood MM, et al. Emergency Management and Commonly Encountered Outpatient Scenarios in Patients With Hyperkalemia *Mayo Clin Proc* 2007;82:1553–1561

Annals Int Med 110(6):426, March 15, 1989

Levine M, et al. The Effects of Intravenous Calcium in Patients with Digoxin Toxicity *J Emerg Med* 2011 Jan;40(1):41–6

Dialysis Complications of Chronic Renal Failure

Author: Richard S Krause, MD; Chief Editor: Erik D Schraga, MD; emedicine.medscape.com/article/1918879

FDA Asks for Drug Interaction Studies on Kayexalate

medscape.com/viewarticle/853117

LaRue H, et al. *Pharmacotherapy*. 2017 Oct 4

Li T, et al. *Clin Kidney J*. 2014 Jun;7(3):239-41

Allon M, et al. *Kidney Int* 1990; 38(5): 869-872

Hyperkalemia Treatment & Management Updated: Jun 20, 2018 Author: Eleanor Lederer, MD, FASN; Chief Editor: Vecihi Batuman, MD, FASN

Hypokalemia Protocol

Definition

- Serum potassium level < 3.5 mEq/L

Differential Diagnosis

- Cushing syndrome
- Hypocalcemia
- Hypomagnesemia

Considerations

- Very common
- Increases dysrhythmias
- Increases Digoxin (digitalis) toxicity effects
- Mild 3.0–3.4 mEq/L
- Moderate 2.5–2.9 mEq/L
- Severe < 2.5 mEq/L
- Serum potassium decreases by 0.3 mEq/L for each 100 mEq of potassium reduction in total-body stores, but the response is extremely variable

Causes

- Diuretics
- Hyperventilation
- Hypomagnesemia
- Poor nutrition
- Diarrhea
- Metabolic alkalosis
- Renal tubular acidosis
- Adrenal conditions
- Hyperaldosteronism
- Gastrointestinal losses (vomiting, diarrhea, NG suction)
- Familial Periodic Hypokalemia Paralysis

Signs and Symptoms

- Severe weakness — $K^+ < 2.5$ mEq/L
- Paralysis can occur with rapid development of $K^+ < 2.0$ mEq/L
- Paresthesias
- Muscle weakness
- Muscle cramps
- Constipation
- Cardiac dysrhythmias
- EKG changes
  - Low voltage T waves
  - ST segment depression
  - U waves
  - Small P waves
  - PAC's
  - PVC's

Evaluation

- BMP
- EKG if potassium < 2.5 mEq/L
- Magnesium level not needed usually

Treatment Options

- Oral replacement preferred when indicated
- Oral potassium 40–60 mEq can raise serum potassium 1–1.5 mEq/L; 135–160 mEq PO raises serum potassium 2.5–3.5 mEq/L (transient elevation since potassium taken up in cells)
- Potassium level < 2.5 mEq/L can give IV replacement no faster than 10 mEq per hour
- $MgSO_4$ (magnesium sulfate) replacement can improve potassium replacement
  - 2–4 gms IV over 30 minutes if needed
  - Mg gluconate 200–400 mg PO TID prn if hypokalemia is asymptomatic (adults)

Discharge Criteria

- Asymptomatic patient
- Able to replenish potassium orally
- Potassium level > 2.5 mEq/L

Discharge instructions

- Hypokalemia aftercare instructions
- Follow up with primary care provider within 2–3 days

Consult Criteria

- Potassium ≤ 2.5 mEq/L
- Symptomatic patient
- EKG changes

Notes

REFERENCES:

Hypokalemia in Emergency Medicine
Author: David Garth, MD; Chief Editor: Erik D Schraga, MD
emedicine.medscape.com/article/767448

Agarwal A, Wingo CS. Treatment of hypokalemia *N Engl J Med* 1999;340: 154-5

Gennari FJ. Hypokalemia *N Engl J Med* 1998;339:451-458

Nicolis, GL, et al. Glucose-induced hyperkalemia in diabetic subjects *Arch Intern Med* 1981;141:49

HYPERNATREMIA PROTOCOL

Definition

- Serum Na^+ level > 145 mEq/L

Differential Diagnosis

- Hyperglycemic hyperosmolar state
- Diabetes insipidus
- Salt ingestion
- Hypertonic dehydration

Considerations

Dehydration

- Secondary to volume depletion
- Poor oral intake of fluids
- Commonly seen in nursing home patients
- PEG tube feeding patients
- Bedridden patients
- Stroke patients
- Patients unable to care for themselves
- Medication induced diuresis
- Accompanied by metabolic acidosis frequently
- High risk condition for mortality in elderly
- Usually in patients with significant comorbidities
- Na^+ 150–170 mEq/L usually indicates dehydration
- Na^+ > 170 mEq/L usually indicates diabetes insipidus
- Na^+ > 190 mEq/L usually indicates long term salt ingestion

Diabetes insipidus

Decreased ability of kidneys to concentrate urine

- Lithium
- Sickle cell anemia
- Post obstructive diuresis after treatment of bladder outlet obstruction
- Na^+ > 170 mEq/L usually indicates diabetes insipidus

Decreased secretion of ADH (antidiuretic hormone)

- Brain tumors
- Brain injury
- Cerebral infectious processes

Signs and symptoms

- Altered mental status
- Decreased responsiveness
- Tachycardia
- Hypotension may occur
- Tachypnea
- Poor skin turgor
- Decreased capillary refill
- Dry mucous membranes
- Decreased urine output
- Hard stools

Evaluation Options

- BMP
- CBC
- U/A

- Chest x-ray usually performed to rule out concurrent disease process
- CT brain scan if central process suspected
- Urine specific gravity < 1.005 and osmolarity <200 mOsm/kg if serum sodium > 170 mEq/L (usually indicates diabetes insipidus)

Treatment Options

- Restore plasma volume first
- Oral rehydration therapy (ORT) preferred over IV in mild to moderate dehydration if appropriate to patient's condition and ability to self-hydrate

Serum Na^+ correction no more than 1 mEq/L per hour

- Too rapid correction may cause cerebral edema

Adult dehydration

Oral Rehydration Therapy (ORT) for mild to moderate dehydration if able to self-hydrate

- Oral rehydration formula (WHO formula, Rehydralyte or Pedialyte) for mild to moderate dehydration or serum CO_2 is 14–18 mEq/L or NA^+ 146–152 mEq/L
  - Zofran (ondansetron) 8 mg chewable tablet or 4–8 mg IM if vomiting
  - 15–30 cc every 1–2 minutes for adults (age > 12) for 1–4 hours — start 20 minutes after Zofran (ondansetron) given
  - Hold ORT 10 minutes if vomiting occurs then resume
  - Reassess for urine production, improved heart rate, and absence of severe vomiting
  - Recheck serum CO_2 if initially < 17 mEq/L
  - Mild dehydration give 50 cc/kg in < 4 hours
  - Moderate dehydration give 50–100 cc/kg in 1–4 hours

IV rehydration

- Moderate to severe dehydration (Na^+ > 152 mEq/L), give IV NS or LR 150–300 cc/hour over 2–4 hours
  - Normal saline has 154 mEq/L of sodium
  - Lactated ringers has 130 mEq/L of sodium
- Hypotension or signs of poor organ perfusion, give NS or LR at 500–1000 cc/hour up to 2 liters (consult physician promptly) — caution if CHF history

Pediatric dehydration

Dehydration assessment

Mild ≤ 5%

- Alert
- Mucous membranes variable dry
- Skin turgor normal
- Fontanel flat
- Blood pressure normal
- Heart rate normal
- Capillary refill < 2 seconds
- Urine output decreased

Moderate 6–9%

- Irritable
- Mucous membranes dry
- Skin turgor variably reduced
- Fontanel depressed
- Blood pressure variably orthostatic
- Heart rate tachycardic
- Capillary refill 2–3 seconds
- Urine output decreased — oliguria

Severe ≥ 10%

- Lethargic
- Mucous membranes dry
- Skin turgor reduced
- Fontanel depressed
- Blood pressure orthostatic or hypotensive
- Heart rate markedly tachycardic

- Capillary refill ≥ 4 seconds
- Urine output decreased – oliguria/anuria

Oral Rehydration Therapy (ORT) for mild to moderate dehydration

- Zofran (ondansetron) oral chewable tablet in ED for frequent vomiting
  - 2 mg for 8–15 kg; 4 mg for 15–30 kg; 8 mg for > 30 kg
  - Zofran (ondansetron) 2–4 doses can be prescribed for home if indicated

Oral rehydration formula for mild to moderate dehydration; serum CO_2 14–18 mEq/L or serum Na^+ 146–155 mEq/L

- 5 cc every 1–2 minutes for small children by caretaker for < 4 hours — start 20 minutes after Zofran (ondansetron) given
- 5–10 cc every 1–2 minutes for larger children by caretaker for 1–4 hours
- Hold ORT 10 minutes if vomiting occurs then resume
- Reassess for urine production, weight gain, improved HR and alertness, and absence of severe vomiting
- Recheck serum CO_2 if initially < 17
- Mild dehydration give 50 cc/kg in < 4 hours
- Moderate dehydration give 50–100 cc/kg over 1–4 hours

Severe dehydration give IV NS bolus 20 cc/kg; may repeat × 2

Exclusion Criteria for Oral Rehydration Therapy

- Age < 6 months of age
- Hematemesis
- Bilious vomiting
- Bloody diarrhea
- VP shunt
- Head trauma
- Focal RLQ tenderness (possible appendicitis)
- Severe dehydration
- Patient vomits 3 or more times after starting ORT

IV therapy criteria and treatment for moderate to severe dehydration

- IV NS hydration for CO_2 < 14 mEq/L or Na^+ > 155 mEq/L
- ORT failure
- IV NS 20 cc/kg bolus, may repeat × 2
- Consult physician
- Maintenance IV with D5NS (dextrose decreases return visits)

Discharge Criteria

- Patient responds to rehydration
- Healthy without significant comorbid conditions
- Good social support systems
- Unlikely to acutely become hypernatremic post discharge

Discharge instructions

- Dehydration or hypernatremia aftercare instructions
- Follow up with primary care providers within 1–3 days

Consult Criteria

Discuss with physician

- Patients with significant comorbid conditions or findings
- Serum Na^+ > 150 mEq/L
- Age > 60
- Age < 6 months
- Diabetes insipidus

Vital signs consult criteria

- Adult heart rate > 100 post treatment
- Hypotension or relative hypotension (SBP < 105 with history of hypertension)
- Orthostatic vital signs
- Pediatric heart rate
  - 0–4 months ≥ 180
  - 5–7 months ≥ 175

- 8–12 months ≥ 170
- 1–3 years ≥ 160

Notes

____

____

____

REFERENCES:

Hypernatremia in Emergency Medicine Author: Zina Semenovskaya, MD; Chief Editor: Romesh Khardori, MD, PhD, FACP

emedicine.medscape.com /article/76668

HYPONATREMIA PROTOCOL

Definition

- Serum sodium level < 135 mEq/L

Differential Diagnosis

- SIADH
- Hepatitis cirrhosis
- Adrenal insufficiency
- Adrenal crisis
- CHF
- Water intoxication
- Gastroenteritis
- Renal failure
- Hypothyroidism
- Nephrotic syndrome

Considerations

- Acute hyponatremia is more symptomatic
- Chronic hyponatremia can be asymptomatic
- Central pontine myelinolysis can occur from too rapid correction of hyponatremia
  - Dysarthria
  - Dysphagia
  - Seizures
  - Altered mental status
  - Quadriplegia
  - Hypotension
- Correction of severe symptomatic hyponatremia should not raise serum sodium level more than 4 mEq/L acutely
- Chronic hyponatremia usually does not need rapid correction (can be dangerous to do so)
- Chronic hyponatremia is much more common than acute hyponatremia
- Serum Na^+ is lowered 1.6 mEq/L for every blood glucose level increase of 100 mg% over normal
  - Will correct with correction of hyperglycemia alone
- Children more prone to iatrogenic water intoxication by parents giving excessive water to replace GI fluid losses

Signs and symptoms

- Mild or none in some chronic hyponatremic patients with Na^+ > 120 mEq/L

Acute hyponatremia

- Serum sodium > 120 mEq/L
  - Headache
  - Nausea; vomiting
  - Muscle cramps
  - Weakness
  - Anorexia
  - Rhabdomyolysis
- Serum sodium 110–120 mEq/L
  - Hyperventilation
  - Decreased responsiveness
  - Hallucinations
  - Behavior disturbances
  - Incontinence
  - Ataxia
- Serum sodium < 110 mEq/L
  - Posturing
  - Hypertension
  - Bradycardia
  - Impaired temperature regulation
  - Seizures
  - Coma

- Respiratory arrest

Causes

Hypovolemic

- Excess fluid losses replaced with hypotonic solutions by patient
  - Vomiting
  - Diarrhea
  - Third spacing of fluids
  - Burns
  - Excessive sweating
  - Diuretics

Hypervolemic

- Excessive water intake (water intoxication)
- Hepatic cirrhosis
- CHF
- Nephrotic syndrome
- Renal insufficiency

Euvolemic

- Hypothyroidism
- Adrenal insufficiency
- SIADH
- Psychogenic polydipsia

Medications

- Diuretics
- NSAID's
- Oral hypoglycemic agents
- ACE inhibitors
- ARB's
- PPI's

Sodium Requirement (mEq/L)

- Na^+ deficit is total body water (Kg × 0.6) times (desired Na^+ – Serum Na^+)

Hypertonic saline

- 513 mEq/L of NaCl

Normal saline

- 154 mEq/L of NaCl

Lactated ringers

- 130 mEq/L of Na^+

Evaluation

- BMP
- Urine spot Na^+ level (consider if SIADH suspected)
- Urine osmolarity (if SIADH suspected, which has inappropriately concentrated urine)
- Serum cortisol level if adrenal insufficiency suspected
- TSH and thyroid function tests if hypothyroidism suspected

Treatment Options

Chronic hyponatremia with mild to moderately severe symptoms

(Do not increase serum Na^+ by more than 10–12 mEq/L in first 24 hours)

- Hypovolemia: IV NS
- Hypervolemia: restrict free water and sodium
- Euvolemia: restrict free water — may add Lasix (furosemide) short term

Acute hyponatremia — Na^+ < 120 mEq/L with severe symptoms (or chronic hyponatremia with severe symptoms such as seizures, coma, severe altered mental status) consult physician

- 3% saline at 100 cc/hr. × 2 hours and recheck serum sodium for adults
- Pediatric calculation of TBW (kg × 0.6) × 4 mEq/L = acute Na^+ deficit to be replenished over 2 hours
- Do not raise Na^+ acutely more than 4 mEq/L

Discharge Criteria

- Asymptomatic serum sodium > 125 mEq/L without comorbid conditions

Discharge instructions

- Follow up within 1–3 days for serum sodium < 130 mEq/L with primary care provider

- Hyponatremia aftercare instructions

Consult Criteria

- Serum sodium ≤ 125 mEq/L
- Comorbid conditions or symptoms
- Refer to General Patient Criteria Protocol prn (page 15)

Notes

REFERENCES:

Hyponatremia in Emergency Medicine Clinical Presentation

Author: Sandy Craig, MD; Chief Editor: Romesh Khardori, MD, PhD, FACP

emedicine.medscape.com/article/767624

Verbalis JG, Goldsmith SR, Greenberg A, Schrier RW, Sterns RH. Hyponatremia treatment guidelines 2007: expert panel recommendations. *Am J Med.* Nov 2007;120(11 Suppl 1):S1–21

Metabolic Acidosis Protocol

Definition

- Disease process with an increase in plasma acidity

Differential Diagnosis

- See A CAT MUDPILES below

Considerations

- Normal pH is 7.39–7.41 (~7.35–7.45 depending on lab)
- Kidneys excrete H^+ and reabsorb HCO_3^- normally

Metabolic acidosis

- pH lower than normal unless over-compensated by a primary metabolic or respiratory alkalosis (unusual) — can occur with aspirin overdose initially
- Elevated H^+ concentration in guise of various acids
- Low HCO_3^-
- Goal of therapy is to raise pH to 7.2 usually by treating the process causing the acidosis
  - HCO_3^- not used unless pH < 7.0 (check with physician)
- K^+ may be elevated and will decrease sometimes significantly when acidosis is treated whether initially elevated or not

Nonanion gap acidosis

- Diarrhea
- Renal tubular acidosis
- Carbonic anhydrase inhibitors — Diamox (acetazolamide)
- Hypoaldosteronism

Anion gap calculation

- Na^+ minus (HCO_3^- – Chloride)
- Normal range 5–12 ± 3 mEq/L

Respiratory compensation

- Expected pCO_2 is $1.5[HCO_3^-]+8$
- If higher, then primary respiratory acidosis exists and there is inadequate respiratory compensation
- Death can result from intubation and ventilation that does not adequately compensates enough for severe metabolic acidosis (or maintains sufficient respiratory compensation with hyperventilation if intubated)

Respiratory acidosis

- Acute: HCO_3^- increased by 1 mEq/L for each 10 mm Hg increase in pCO_2
- Chronic: HCO_3^- increased by 4 mEq/L for each mm Hg increase in pCO_2

Anion gap mnemonic — A CAT MUDPILES

A – Alcoholic ketoacidosis
C – Cyanide; carbon monoxide
A – Aspirin; other salicylates
T – Toluene
M – Methanol; metformin
U – Uremia
D – DKA
P – Paraldehyde; phenformin
I – Iron; INH
L – Lactic acidosis (dehydration or tissue ischemia commonly)
E – Ethylene glycol
S – Starvation

Osmolol gap > 10–20 suspect substance ingestion (Normal < 10)

- Gap = Osmolality measured – Osmolality calculated (calculation equation: $2(Na^{+}+K^{+})$ + glucose/18 + BUN/2.8; normal 280–300 mOsm/L)
- Ethanol mg%/4.6 is added to osmolol gap equation if present
- Gap > 50 carries high specificity for toxic alcohol such as methanol, ethylene glycol, or isopropyl alcohol
- Normal gap < 10
- Refer to Toxicology Protocol

Signs and Symptoms

- Tachypnea or Kussmaul respirations
- Tachycardia
- Confusion
- Depends on the degree and type of acidosis

Evaluation

- Complete history and physical examination
- CBC
- BMP
- Serum ketones if diabetic
- Lactic acid level
- ABG for
  - Severe acidosis
  - Altered mental status
  - Significant tachycardia
- Chest x-ray if indicated
- EKG if indicated
- Toxicology tests as indicated

Treatment Options

- Treat underlying process
- pH < 7.0 can consider IV HCO_3^- (some controversy over degree of acidosis needing this treatment) — consult physician immediately
- See Adult and Pediatric Gastroenteritis Protocols

Discharge Criteria

- Resolving metabolic acidosis with treatable outpatient process
- HCO_3^- > 17
- Anion gap ≤ 19
- No significant comorbidities
- Nontoxic

Discharge instructions

- Aftercare instructions relevant to cause of acidosis
- Follow up with primary care provider within 1 day

Consult Criteria

- HCO_3^- < 18
- Anion gap ≥ 20
- Age ≥ 60
- Condition not likely to improve as outpatient
- Respiratory acidosis
- Hypotension or relative hypotension (SBP < 105 with history of hypertension)
- Toxic appearance
- Adult heart rate ≥ 110
- Pediatric heart rate
  - 0–4 months ≥ 180
  - 5–7 months ≥ 175
  - 8–12 months ≥ 170
  - 1–3 years ≥ 160
  - 4–5 years ≥ 145
  - 6–8 years ≥ 130
  - 9–11 years ≥ 125
  - 12–15 years ≥ 115
  - 16 years or older ≥ 110

Notes

REFERENCES:

Metabolic Acidosis Author: Christie P Thomas, MBBS, FRCP, FASN, FAHA; Chief Editor: Vecihi Batuman, MD, FACP, FASN
emedicine.medscape.com/article/242975

Metabolic Acidosis in Emergency Medicine
Author: Antonia Quinn, DO; Chief Editor: Romesh Khardori, MD, PhD, FACP
emedicine.medscape.com/article/768268

Head Trauma and Neck Pain

Section Contents

When using any protocol, always follow the Guidelines of Proper Use (page 12).

Adult Minor Head Trauma Protocol

Definition

- Head trauma with Glasgow coma scale ≥ 14 and no focal neurologic deficits or complaints

Differential Diagnosis

- Subarachnoid hemorrhage
- Subdural hematoma
- Epidural hematoma
- Cerebral contusion
- Skull fracture

Considerations

- Loss of consciousness (LOC), amnesia, headache, vomiting and seizures have low sensitivity and specificity for detecting intracranial injury
- Cervical spine exam and evaluation important
- Skull films mainly replaced by CT evaluation of adult head trauma — may consider skull films for laceration > 5 cm or that extends deep to the skull
  - Violent mechanism of injury
- Significant maxillofacial injuries can coexist

Concussion Definitions

Grade 1 concussion

- Transient confusion
- No LOC
- Duration of mental status abnormalities < 15 minutes

Grade 2 concussion

- Transient confusion
- No LOC
- Duration of mental status abnormalities > 15 minutes

Grade 3 concussion

- Loss of consciousness

Postconcussion Syndrome

- Symptoms of headache, dizziness, trouble concentrating days to weeks following a concussion and can persist for months
- Can occur in up to 30% of concussions
- Anxiety and depression reported by patients

- Issues of compensation and litigation associated at times with persistent symptoms
- Disequilibrium and vertigo from vestibular concussion
- Reassurance decreases incidence and duration of symptoms
- Avoid narcotics
- Can use mild analgesics
- Can use meclizine or Phenergan (promethazine) for vestibular symptoms
- Rarely seen in young children
- Countries with low litigation have low postconcussion syndrome disability

Evaluation

- **CT brain scan**
  - For concussion with loss of consciousness
  - Patients on Coumadin (warfarin), DOAC agents (dabigatran, apixaban, or rivaroxaban) or Plavix (clopidogrel) with more than trivial injury
  - Suspected intracranial injury
  - Glasgow coma scale < 15
  - Retinal exam: hemorrhages present in 65–90% with abuse inflicted head injury
- Evaluate for other injuries, especially C-spine
- Detailed neurologic exam
- INR if on Coumadin (warfarin)
- Evaluate for other injuries, especially C-spine
- Detailed neurologic exam
- INR if on Coumadin (warfarin)

ENT exam

- Check for hemotympanum
- CSF rhinorrhea
- Battle's sign
- Cranial nerve palsy

CT Head Rules (your choice)

New Orleans CT brain criteria (for ordering noncontrast CT brain)

- Normal neurologic exam and one of the following
  - Abnormal GCS
  - Headache
  - Vomiting
  - Age > 60
  - Persistent anterograde amnesia
  - Drug or alcohol intoxication
  - Visible trauma above the clavicle
  - Seizure

Canadian CT Head Rule

- Any positive below then perform head CT
  - GCS < 15 at 2 hours after injury
  - Suspected or open skull fracture
  - Signs of basilar skull fracture
  - Vomiting ≥ 2 episodes
  - Age ≥ 65 years
  - Pre–impact amnesia ≥ 30 minutes
  - Dangerous mechanism

Noncontrast CT brain scan for acute brain injury

(From ACEP/CDC Clinical Policy)

Order noncontrast CT brain scan

- Loss of consciousness
- No loss of consciousness with one of the following:
  - Headache
  - Vomiting
  - Age > 60 years
  - Persistent anterograde amnesia
  - Focal neurologic deficit
  - Coagulopathy
  - Drug or alcohol intoxication
  - Visible trauma above the clavicle
  - Posttraumatic seizure
  - GCS < 15

Consider noncontrast CT brain scan with no LOC and one of following

- Signs of basilar skull fracture
- Age > 65 years

- Dangerous mechanism of injury (includes)
  - Motor vehicle ejection
  - Pedestrian struck by motor vehicle
  - Fall from > 3 feet or 5 stairs
- Patients on warfarin
  - Minor head trauma patients on warfarin or DOAC type anticoagulation with a normal initial CT brain, it is recommended that 24 hours observation and repeat CT brain scan be performed
  - Higher risk with INR > 3.0 for delayed intracranial bleeding

Treatment Options

- Tylenol (no ASA or NSAID's for 36 hours)
- Avoid more potent analgesics so progression of symptoms can be detected
- Head injury instruction sheet
- Return for any neurologic changes
- Follow up with primary care provider or neurologist/neurosurgeon
- Aerobic exercise protocols and visio-vestibular rehabilitation within the first week helps recovery in concussion and decreases post–concussion symptoms

Discharge Criteria

- Stable condition
- Normal neurologic exam
- No other significant trauma
- No radiologic abnormalities

Discharge instructions

- Head injury aftercare instructions

Consult Criteria

- Age > 65
- Bleeding potential from medications or preexisting disease processes
- Patients on warfarin therapy or DOAC's
- Concussions with loss of consciousness should be discussed with physician
- Dementia
- Persistent vomiting
- Severe persistent headache
- Focal neurologic deficits
- Inadequate home observation

Notes

____

____

____

REFERENCES:

Ann of Emergency Medicine, June 2012 (Vol. 59 | No. 6 | Pages 451–455)

ACEP Clinical Policy: Neuroimaging and Decision making in Adult Mild Traumatic Brain Injury in the Acute Setting

Head Trauma Treatment & Management
Author: David W Crippen, MD, FCCM; Chief Editor: John Geibel, MD, DSc, M
emedicine.medscape.com/article/433855

Closed Head Trauma
Author: Leonardo Rangel-Castilla, MD; Chief Editor: Allen R Wyler, MD
emedicine.medscape.com/article/251834

PEDIATRIC MINOR HEAD TRAUMA PROTOCOL

Definition

- Head trauma with Glasgow coma scale ≥ 14 and no focal neurologic deficits or complaints

Differential Diagnosis

- Subarachnoid hemorrhage
- Subdural hematoma
- Epidural hematoma
- Cerebral contusion
- Skull fracture
- Child abuse and neglect

Considerations

- Loss of consciousness (LOC), amnesia, headache, vomiting and seizures have low sensitivity and specificity for detecting intracranial injury
- Children < 2 years have a higher risk of skull fracture and intracranial injury after minor mechanisms of injury
  - Skull fracture associated with a 20–fold increase in intracranial injury
  - Most skull fractures are associated with scalp hematomas
- Scalp hematomas indicative of skull fractures is the most sensitive predictor of intracranial injury of the clinical signs of brain injury
- Infant's clinical signs of brain injury less reliable

Postconcussion Syndrome

- Symptoms of headache, dizziness, trouble concentrating days to weeks following a concussion and can persist for months
- Anxiety and depression reported by patients
- Issues of compensation and litigation associated at times with persistent symptoms
- Disequilibrium and vertigo from vestibular concussion
- Reassurance decreases incidence and duration of symptoms
- Avoid narcotics
- Can use mild analgesics
- Can use meclizine or Phenergan (promethazine) for vestibular symptoms
- Rarely seen in young children
- Countries with low litigation have low postconcussion syndrome disability

Evaluation

- Evaluate for other injuries besides head
- Retinal exam: hemorrhages present in 65–90% with abuse inflicted head injury
- ENT exam for:
  - Hemotympanum
  - CSF rhinorrhea
  - Battle's sign
  - Cranial nerve palsy
- Awake, alert and asymptomatic children without LOC usually do not require imaging

CT scan rules

Pecarn Algorithm Age < 2 years

- Order CT head if any positive
  - Abnormal GCS
  - Palpable skull fracture
  - Signs of altered mental status
  - Occipital, parietal or temporal scalp hematoma
  - History of loss of consciousness ≥ 5 seconds
  - Severe mechanism
  - Not acting normally

Pecarn Algorithm Age ≥ 2 years for pediatric head trauma

- Order CT head if any positive
  - Abnormal GCS
  - Palpable skull fracture
  - Signs of altered mental status
  - History of loss of consciousness
  - History of vomiting
  - Severe mechanism
  - Severe headache

CT brain scan other considerations

- Anticoagulation therapy

- Preexisting CNS disease such AVM or ventriculoperitoneal shunt
- Retinal exam: hemorrhages present in 65–90% with abuse inflicted head injury
- Hemotympanum
- CSF rhinorrhea
- Battle's sign
- Cranial nerve palsy or neurologic abnormalities

Treatment Options

- Tylenol (no ASA or NSAID's for 36 hours)
- Avoid more potent analgesics so progression of symptoms can be detected
- Quiet play or activities can be resumed if no significant symptoms
- Head injury instruction sheet
- Return for any neurologic changes
- Follow up with primary care provider or neurologist
- Aerobic exercise protocols and visio-vestibular rehabilitation within the first week helps recovery in concussion and decreases post–concussion symptoms

Discharge Criteria

- Stable condition
- Normal neurologic exam
- No other significant trauma
- No radiologic abnormalities

Discharge instructions

- Head injury aftercare instructions
- Refer or arrange for follow-up with primary care physician or provider for concussion

Consult Criteria

- Concussion
- Skull fracture
- CT findings of intracranial injury
- Acute neurologic abnormalities
- Intracranial bleeding potential
- Persistent vomiting
- Severe persistent headache
- Focal neurologic deficits
- Inadequate home observation
- Serial visits for head injury symptoms needed
- Patients on warfarin or other anticoagulation therapy

Concussion Definitions and Return-to-sports Recommendations

Grade 1 concussion

- Transient confusion
- No loss of consciousness (LOC)
- Duration of mental status abnormalities < 15 minutes

Grade 2 concussion

- Transient confusion
- No LOC
- Duration of mental status abnormalities > 15 minutes

Grade 3 concussion

- Loss of consciousness

Return to Sports Stages (CISG 2017)

For all concussions

- Rest no more than 24–48 hours
- Symptom limited activities that do not provoke symptoms ≥ 24 hours followed by
- Light aerobic activities ≥ 24 hours (no resistance training) followed by
- Sport–specific exercise ≥ 24 hours (i.e. running, skating but no head impact activity) followed by
- Non–contact exercises ≥ 24 hours (i.e. passing drills, resistance training) followed by
- Full contact exercises after medical clearance

If symptoms recur in any stage then go back to prior stage and try to progress again after 24 hours

Notes

REFERENCES:

Kuppermann N, Holmes JF, Dayan PS, et al. Identification of children at very low risk of clinically-important brain injuries after head trauma: a prospective cohort study. *Lancet*. Oct 3 2009;374(9696):1160–70

Pediatric Head Trauma
Author: Michael J Verive, MD, FAAP; Chief Editor: Timothy E Corden, MD emedicine.medscape.com/article/907273

AMERICAN ACADEMY OF PEDIATRICS
The Management of Minor Closed Head Injury in Children Committee on Quality Improvement, American Academy of Pediatrics Commission on Clinical Policies and Research, American Academy of Family Physicians

The Use of Computed Tomography in Pediatric Patients with Minor Head Injury - Micelle J. Haydel, MD Assistant Residency Director, Section of Emergency Medicine Clinical Assistant Professor of Medicine Louisiana State University Health Science Center at New Orleans

Consensus statement on concussion in sport—the 5th international conference on concussion in sport held in Berlin, October 2016

JAMA,306(1):79-86

Pediatr Neurol. 2015 Apr 11

NEJM, Vol. 356, pg. 166

NECK PAIN PROTOCOL

Definition

- Various disorders causing neck pain

Differential Diagnosis

- Muscle strain
- "Whiplash" injury
- Cervical fracture
- HNP
- Soft tissue infection
- Retropharyngeal abscess
- Cervical lymphadenitis
- Spinal stenosis
- Rheumatoid arthritis
- Endocarditis
- Thoracic outlet syndrome

Considerations

- Common neck pain causes
  - Torticollis ("wry neck") from muscle spasm
  - Cervical disc disease
  - Soft tissue disorder
  - Cervical spine injury
  - Muscular and ligament strain
  - Ankylosing spondylitis
    - Can have cranial–cervical disassociation
    - Put in Philadelphia or rigid cervical collar
    - Exercise caution with patient's neck

Torticollis

- Discomfort caused by cervical spine motion frequently related to muscular etiology
- May be secondary to:
  - C-spine injury
  - Muscle injury
  - Ligamentous injury

- Usually acute in children and of muscular etiology
- Infectious causes
  - URI
  - Cervical adenitis
  - Pharyngitis
  - Retropharyngeal abscess
    - Measurements of retropharyngeal space:
      - At C2: < 7 mm
      - At C6: < 22 mm in adults; < 14 mm in children
  - Epiglottitis
  - Upper lobe pneumonia
  - Meningitis
  - Dystonic reaction to medication (treat with Benadryl)

Evaluation

- Neurologic and neck exam
- If fever present order
  - CBC
  - Soft tissue neck films
  - C-reactive protein if diagnosis not evident
  - CT neck for severe pain and possible deep space infection
- No fever
  - C-spine plain films if injured
  - CT C-spine scan if
    - Significant pain and mechanism of injury
    - Neurologic deficit or complaint

Treatment options

- Benign infectious processes treat per Protocols
- Benign muscular etiology treat with NSAID's and heat or ice
- May try muscle relaxants such as Skelaxin (metaxalone) 800 mg PO tid (age ≥ 12 years) or Norflex (orphenadrine) 100 mg PO bid (adults)

Discharge criteria

- Benign process
- Chronic stable condition
- Cervical radiculopathy controlled with analgesics

Consult criteria

- Fever
- Meningitis concerns
- Airway concerns
- Severe pain
- Epiglottitis
- Retropharyngeal abscess
- Neurologic deficit

Neck Trauma

Cervical strain

- Neck pain increases at 12–72 hours
- Perform neurologic exam
- Plain films if trauma is minor
- CT cervical scan for significant mechanism of injury, concern for fracture or dislocation

Quebec Taskforce on Whiplash-Associated Disorders classification

- Grades 0–2 no special imaging recommended
- 0: No neck pain complaints, no physical signs
- 1: Neck pain complaints, only stiffness or tenderness, no other physical signs
- 2: Neck complaints and musculoskeletal signs (decreased range of motion [ROM] and point tenderness)
- 3: Neck complaints and neurologic signs (weakness, sensory and reflex changes) — CT C–spine
- 4: Neck complaints with suspected fracture and/or dislocation — CT C–spine

Treatment options

- NSAID's +/– acetaminophen
- Ice packs first 72 hours
  - May alternate with heat if helpful after 72 hours
- Muscle relaxants
- Physical therapy
- Soft cervical collar

Penetrating neck trauma

- Consult physician unless very superficial laceration
- Do not explore Zone 2 penetrating deep neck injuries

- Angle of mandible to cricoid cartilage
- Consult physician/surgeon
- Stop any bleeding with pressure

Cervical spine trauma

- Leave cervical collar on until patient examined and cleared of cervical vertebra/spine injury
- Plain C-spine x-ray 3 views

Exclusionary criteria for C-spine films

- No neurologic deficit
- No distracting injuries
- No evidence of intoxication
- Normal mentation
- No posterior midline tenderness

CT C-spine indications

- Moderate to high risk of cervical fracture
- Significant mechanism of injury
- Fracture on plain C-spine films
- Neurologic deficit or complaint
- Inadequate plain C-spine films
- Whiplash-Associated Disorders classification
  - 3: Neck complaints and neurologic signs (weakness, sensory and reflex changes)
  - 4: Neck complaints with suspected fracture and/or dislocation
- Severe neck pain with normal plain C-spine films
- Patient will not move neck actively (on their own) without external support of patient's hands ("head in hand sign")
- Obtunded patients

Flexion-extension plain films

- Significant pain with negative plain and CT imaging after the acute trauma has subsided for subacute presentations
- Evaluates for ligamentous instability

MRI C-spine if spinal cord findings or symptoms present and CT scan unremarkable (consult physician)

Treatment options

- If C-spine cleared: analgesics and ice packs prn

Discharge criteria

- Benign neck injury
- No fracture

Discharge instructions

- Neck pain or injury aftercare instructions
- Refer to primary care provider or neurosurgeon within 3 days if not improving
- Avoid discharging with cervical collar if possible

Consult criteria

- Cervical fracture or dislocation/subluxation
- Neurologic deficit or complaint
- Significant pain
- Significant mechanism of injury

Notes

REFERENCES:

Torticollis Author: Michael C Kruer, MD; Chief Editor: Selim R Benbadis, MD emedicine.medscape.com/article/1152543

Spitzer WO, Skovron ML, Salmi LR, et al. Scientific monograph of the Quebec Task Force on Whiplash-Associated Disorders: redefining "whiplash" and its management. *Spine*. Apr 15 1995;20(8 Suppl):1S-73S

Cervical Sprain and Strain Workup Author: Oregon K Hunter Jr, MD; Chief Editor: Consuelo T Lorenzo, MD

emedicine.medscape.com/article/30617
6

Cervical Spine Sprain/Strain Injuries
Author: Gerard A Malanga, MD; Chief
Editor: Sherwin SW Ho, MD;
emedicine.medscape.com/article/94387

HEENT

Section Contents

When using any protocol, always follow the Guidelines of Proper Use (page 12).

Sore Throat Protocol

Definition

- Pain located or perceived in the throat or anterior neck region

Differential Diagnosis

- GABHS (Group A beta–hemolytic streptococcus)
- Mononucleosis
- Gonococcal pharyngitis
- Peritonsillar abscess
- Epiglottitis
- Retropharyngeal abscess
- Diphtheria (rare)
- Cervical lymphadenitis
- Thyrotoxicosis
- Gastroesophageal reflux

Considerations

- Viral 40%
- Bacterial 30%
- Strep throat – Group A beta–hemolytic Strep (GABHS)
  - 15–30% childhood pharyngitis
  - 5–10% of adult pharyngitis
  - Peak ages 4–11 years
  - Peak months January – May
  - Associated symptoms and findings
    - Sudden onset
    - Odynophagia
    - Fever
    - Headache
    - Abdominal pain
    - Nausea and vomiting
- Viral pharyngitis
  - Cough
  - Rhinorrhea
  - Lack of cervical adenopathy
- Lemierre's syndrome — spread of pharyngitis infection (usually Fusobacterium necrophorum) to cause septic thrombophlebitis of internal jugular vein
  - Up to 50% mortality
  - Septic emboli can occur if unrecognized

Viral Pharyngitis

URI

- Treat symptomatically

Mononucleosis

Findings

- Exudative tonsillitis
- Fever
- Posterior cervical chain lymphadenopathy considered diagnostic
- Monospot
  - 90% sensitive age > 5 years
  - 75% sensitive age 2–4 years
  - Less than 30% sensitive age < 2 years
- Consider CMV and EBV IgM/IgG serology for age < 10 years
- CBC: 50% lymphocytes, 10% atypical lymphocytes
- Liver function tests elevated in 80–85% of patients up to 3 times normal
- Splenomegaly
- Hepatomegaly
- Encephalitis
- Meningitis

Treatment options

- Treat symptomatically
- No contact sports or gym for 4 weeks after onset of illness
  - Follow up with primary care provider before resuming sports or gym
- Ampicillin or amoxicillin rash can occur if prescribed
- Steroids may decrease symptoms and swelling but may also delay recovery and there is a concern for association with development chronic EBV syndrome
- Steroid dosing if used:
  - Adult or patients heavier than 40 kg: prednisone 40 mg PO or dexamethasone 6 mg PO daily for 4 days
  - May increase risk of secondary bacterial infection
  - Pediatrics: prednisone 1 mg/kg PO daily for 4 days (NMT 40 mg)

Strep throat — GABHS

- Rheumatic fever can be prevented if antibiotic treatment started within 9 days of onset—very rare now
- Number needed to treat to prevent one case of acute rheumatic fever would be 1,430,000 on 2003 review
- Glomerulonephritis cannot be prevented with antibiotic treatment
- Reason for antibiotic treatment is the prevention of rheumatic fever and complications such as abscess
- Without antibiotic therapy, symptoms typically resolve in 3 -5 days for most patients
- Antibiotics have been found to reduce symptoms by 12-16 hrs. when compared to placebo

Evaluation

Modified Centor criteria

- Tonsillar exudates
  +1 point
- Tender anterior cervical lymphadenopathy
  +1 point
- Fever by history
  +1 point
- Absence of cough
  +1 point
- Age < 15 years
  +1 point
- Age ≥ 45 years
  – point
- **Centor score (excludes age)**
  - If 3 present: 40–60% have GABHS—antibiotic
  - If 3 or 4 absent: 80% negative predictive value—no antibiotic
  - None or one criterion present: No testing or treatment needed for GABHS

Modified Centor Score (includes age)

- 0 = Do not test or treat
- 1 = Do not test or treat
- 2 = Treat if rapid strip test positive
- 3 = option 1: treat if rapid test result is positive or option 2 treat empirically
- 4 = Treat empirically

Considerations of Rapid Strep Tests

- Sensitivity 85–95%
- Specificity 96–99%
- May be positive with carriage state and another cause of acute pharyngitis besides GABHS may exist

Treatment options

- Per Sanford Guide or drug database
- Antibiotic treatment without rapid strep testing permissible if 3 or 4 Centor criteria score present
- Treatment of symptomatic household contacts if patient has positive GABHS testing for 10 days is recommended
- Pen VK or cephalexin or Augmentin or cefdinir
  - Third generation cephalosporin with improved cure rates and significantly less recurrence
- Clindamycin if penicillin allergic is usually safe
- Zithromax and erythromycin less effective due to resistance
- Steroids one dose (controversial)
  - Prednisone 40–60 mg PO > 40 kg
  - Prednisone or prednisolone 1 mg/kg PO (NMT 60 mg)
  - Decadron (dexamethasone) 10 mg IM if unable to take PO
  - Decadron (dexamethasone) 0.06 mg/kg IM (NMT 10 mg) if unable to take PO

Epiglottitis or suspected epiglottitis

- Now more common in adults than children
- Adults may not be in distress
- Constitutes an airway emergency — consult anesthesia and ENT
- Do not agitate or aggressively exam
- If patient is in distress
- Drooling present
- Tripod position or sniff position present
- Pain on moving thyroid cartilage
- Lateral neck films findings — only obtain in stable patient
- Thumb sign
- Vallecula sign — loss of vallecula
- False positives may occur with x-ray being rotated slightly
- Consider CT neck if needed (may do prone if supine position not tolerated)
- Review or listen to radiology report
- Extreme caution if epiglottitis suspected or patient in distress

Peritonsillar abscess

- Sore throat 100%
- Fever 26–97%
- Voice change (hot potato)
- Dysphagia
- Drooling
- Headache
- Trismus
- Uvular deviation and peritonsillar bulge
- Asymmetric lymphadenopathy
- Peritonsillar phlegmon
- Neck CT scan may be required to delineate abscess from necrotic lymph node
- **Needs drainage**
- Antibiotic choices
  - Clindamycin or augmentin or cefdinir
- Dexamethasone dose may be considered

Retropharyngeal abscess

- Usually age 3–5 years

Complications

- Airway compromise
- Aspiration pneumonia
- Internal jugular vein thrombosis
- Carotid artery erosion
- Cranial nerve palsies

History and findings

- Fever
- Dysphagia
- Decreased oral intake
- Stridor or dyspnea
- Neck swelling
- Neck motion pain
- Ill appearing
- Duck-like voice

X-ray findings

- Neck CT scan much more sensitive than lateral neck plain films
- Lateral soft-tissue neck films (neck flexion may cause false positive reading)
- Retropharyngeal space anterior to C2 > 7 mm or > half the width of vertebral body
- Space anterior to C6 > 14 mm in preschool children or > 22 mm in adults

Treatment

- Supplemental oxygen (avoid patient agitation)
- Keep child calm
- ENT stat consult

Discharge Criteria for Sore throat

- Nontoxic
- No airway obstruction concerns
- Can tolerate oral intake
- Benign diagnosis

Discharge instructions

- Sore throat or pharyngitis aftercare instructions
- Follow up with primary care provider or ENT surgeon within 5 days as needed

Consult Criteria for Sore throat

- Airway compromise
- Toxic
- Respiratory distress
- Dehydration > 5%
- Suspected epiglottitis
- Peritonsillar or retropharyngeal abscess consult ENT immediately
- Unable to tolerate oral intake
- Immunosuppression

Vital signs consult recommendations

- Hypotension
- O_2 saturation < 95% on room air in nonCOPD patient

Lab consult criteria recommendation

- Acute thrombocytopenia
- Metabolic acidosis

Notes

REFERENCES:

Practice Guidelines for the diagnosis and management of group A streptococcal pharyngitis

Clin Infect Dis. 2002;35(2):113–125 Guideline statement

[Guideline] Gerber MA, Baltimore RS, Eaton CB, et al. Prevention of rheumatic fever and diagnosis and treatment of acute Streptococcal pharyngitis: a scientific statement from the American Heart Association Rheumatic Fever, Endocarditis, and Kawasaki Disease Committee of the Council on Cardiovascular Disease in the Young, the Interdisciplinary Council on Functional Genomics and Translational Biology, and the Interdisciplinary Council on Quality of Care and Outcomes Research: endorsed by the American Academy of

Pediatrics. *Circulation*. Mar 24 2009;119(11):1541–51

Pharyngitis Treatment & Management Author: John R Acerra, MD; Chief Editor: Pamela L Dyne, MD; emedicine.medscape.com/article/764304

Del Mar CB, Glasziou PP, Spinks AB. Antibiotics for sore throat (Review). *The Cochrane Collaboration*. 2007;(1):1–41

Retropharyngeal Abscess Author: Joseph H Kahn, MD; Chief Editor: Robert E O'Connor, MD, MPH medicine.medscape.com/article/764421

Epiglottitis Clinical Presentation Author: Sandra G Gompf, MD, FACP, FIDSA; Chief Editor: Pamela L Dyne, MD emedicine.medscape.com/article/763612

Ducic Y, Hébert PC, MacLachlan L, Neufeld K, Lamothe A. Description and evaluation of the vallecula sign: a new radiologic sign in the diagnosis of adult epiglottitis. *Ann Emerg Med*. Jul 1997;30(1):1–6

Gottlieb M, et al. *J Emerg Med*. 2018 Mar 6. [Epub ahead of print]

Pelucchi, C, et al. Clin Microbiol Infect. 2012;18: 1-28

Del Mar, CB, et al. *Cochrane Database Syst Rev*. 2006; CD000023

Otitis Externa Protocol

Definition

- Inflammation of the external auditory canal

Differential Diagnosis

- Auditory canal foreign body
- Otitis media with perforation
- Cholesteatoma
- Chondroma
- Herpes zoster

Considerations

- Caused by breakdown in protective barrier of ear canal
  - Pseudomonas; staph; strep species; fungi
- Pain increased with movement of external ear or touching external ear canal
- Discharge common
- Fever uncommon

Malignant Otitis Externa

- Elderly
- Diabetes
- Immunocompromised — pseudomonas frequent concern
- Marked swelling
- Headache
- Possible cranial nerve deficit

Clinical Practice Guideline: acute otitis externa executive summary

- Distinguish diffuse acute otitis externa (AOE) from other causes of otalgia, otorrhea, and inflammation of the external ear canal
- Assess the patient with diffuse AOE for factors that modify management (non-intact tympanic membrane, tympanostomy tube, diabetes, immunocompromised state, prior radiotherapy)

- Assess patients with AOE for pain and recommend analgesic treatment based on the severity of pain
- Do not prescribe systemic antimicrobials as initial therapy for diffuse, uncomplicated AOE unless there is extension outside the ear canal or the presence of specific host factors that would indicate a need for systemic therapy
- Use topical preparations for initial therapy of diffuse, uncomplicated AOE
- Inform patients how to administer topical drops and should enhance delivery of topical drops when the ear canal is obstructed by performing aural toilet, placing a wick, or both
- Non-intact tympanic membrane when the patient has a known or suspected perforation of the tympanic membrane, including a tympanostomy tube, the clinician should recommend a non-ototoxic topical preparation (fluoroquinolone suspension drops)
- If the patient fails to respond to the initial therapeutic option within 48–72 hours the clinician should reassess the patient to confirm the diagnosis of diffuse AOE and to exclude other causes of illness
- Avoid water in ear

Evaluation

- Usually none except otoscope and external ear exam
- Serum glucose if diabetic
- Suspected malignant otitis externa
  - CBC
  - C-reactive protein
  - Cultures

CT scan indications

- Neurologic abnormalities
- Toxic appearing patient
- Malignant otitis externa
- Fever

Treatment Options

- Clean ear canal (most important aspect of treatment)
- Irrigate or ear loop curettage (may be difficult due to pain)
  - Use ½ peroxide and ½ water (or water only) — if TM (tympanic membrane) visible and intact (keep liquid near body temperature)
- Can use ear wick if canal markedly swollen — remove in 3 days; replace if canal still very swollen
- NSAID's or narcotics prn

Antibiotic choices

- Acetic acid 2% (Domeboro otic) 4–6 drops q4–6h for 7–10 days or until ear canal normal for 2 days
- Otic suspension or solution of hydrocortisone/polymyxin b /neomycin (neomycin can cause allergy) 4 drops qid for 7–10 days or until ear canal normal for 2 days
- Ofloxin 5 drops bid for 7–10 days or until ear canal normal for 2 days (drug of choice for TM perforation)
- Dexamethasone/ciprofloxacin (Ciprodex) age > 6 months: 4 drops in affected ear q12hr for 7 days
  - For acute otitis media with tympanostomy tube
  - Not for use < 6 months of age
- Oral antibiotics for facial or neck cellulitis, significant edema of ear canal, or when TM (tympanic membrane) cannot be visualized
- Diabetics may be treated also with ciprofloxacin PO for 10–14 days
- May use Sanford Guide or drug database

Discharge Criteria

- Benign otitis externa

Discharge instructions

- Otitis externa aftercare instructions
- Keep ear dry for 3 weeks (no swimming) — cotton with Vaseline in ears during showers
- Prophylaxis for future OE after swimming with rubbing alcohol or acetic acid 2% if no TM (tympanic membrane) perforation
- Follow up with primary care provider or ENT surgeon within 7–10 days if needed

Consult Criteria

- Malignant external otitis (needs ENT consultation and IV antibiotics)
- Fever
- Return visit for same episode
- Glucose ≥ 400 mg/dL in diabetic patient
- Hyperglycemia with metabolic acidosis (decreased serum CO_2 or elevated anion gap)

Notes

____

____

____

REFERENCES:

Rosenfeld RM, Schwartz SR, Cannon CR, Roland PS, Simon GR, Kumar KA, et al. Clinical practice guideline: acute otitis externa executive summary. *Otolaryngol Head Neck Surg.* Feb 2014;150(2):161–8

Wall GM, Stroman DW, Roland PS, Dohar J. Ciprofloxacin 0.3%/dexamethasone 0.1% sterile otic suspension for the topical treatment of ear infections: a review of the literature. *Pediatr Infect Dis J.* Feb 2009;28(2):141–4

Otitis Externa Medication

Author: Ariel A Waitzman, MD, FRCS(C); Chief Editor: Arlen D Meyers, MD, MBA emedicine.medscape.com/article/994550

Eye Protocols

Considerations

- Most conjunctival infections are viral
- Allergic manifestations common
- Contact lens keratitis can be bacterial or from oxygen deficit of cornea

Evaluation

- Visual acuity if complaints of decreased vision
- Examination of
  - Conjunctiva
  - Cornea
  - Pupils
  - Extraocular motion
  - Any discharge
  - For consensual photophobia (light shined in unaffected eye causes pain in affected eye — have affected eye closed during exam)
  - Periorbital tissues
  - Anterior and posterior chambers
  - Visual fields examination as indicated
- See specific conditions below

Conjunctivitis

Allergic

- Itching and redness; watery
- Papillary hypertrophy

Treatment options

- Systemic antihistamine
- Remove offending agent if known
- Choices:
  - Naphcon-A ophthalmic 1–2 drops qid prn
  - Ketorolac ophthalmic 1 drop qid prn

- Low dose steroid eye drops prn — short course
  - Dexamethasone ophthalmic 1–2 drops tid-qid prn or similar ophthalmic steroid
  - Contraindications:
    - Herpes simplex infection (corneal dendrite)
    - Glaucoma
    - Fungal infection

Discharge criteria

- Benign presentation and findings

Consult criteria

- Photophobia
- Visual changes

Viral

- Adenovirus most common
  - Viral conjunctivitis due to adenoviruses (65% - 90% of VC cases) is highly contagious
  - Spreads through direct contact via contaminated fingers, swimming pool water, medical instruments, or personal items
- Watery mucus discharge
- Gritty or foreign body sensation
- HSV: vesicles eyelid margins or periorbital skin; corneal dendrites

Treatment options

- Usually no specific therapy
- Artificial tears prn
- HSV
  - Viroptic ophthalmic drops 1 gtt q2h not to exceed 9 gtts qday
  - Consult physician if herpes infection present
  - Ophthalmology referral within 1 day for HSV infection

Bacterial

- Purulent discharge
- Staph most common
- Gonorrhea: profuse purulent discharge
- Chlamydial: mucopurulent discharge; photophobia occasionally
- Contact lens: pseudomonas possible

Treatment options

Common drugs

- Erythromycin eye ointment
- Sulfa eye drops
- Gentamicin eye drops 1–2 drops q4h for 7–10 days (ointment ½ inch) bid–tid
- All medications given for 7 days

Contact lens complications

- Remove lens until eye normal for 2 days
- Ciloxan 1–2 drops QID × 7–12 days
- Consult physician

Chlamydia

- Doxycycline 100 BID × 3 weeks

OR

- Erythromycin 500 mg QID PO × 3 weeks (erythromycin pediatric dose 50 mg/kg PO divided into 4 doses × 14 days — NMT 500 mg per dose)
- May give azithromycin 1 gm PO once instead of doxycycline or erythromycin
- Azithromycin ophthalmic solution: Instill 1 drop BID for 2 days, then 1 drop for 5 days in addition to PO medications
- Mother of children and other close contacts at risk — treat with doxycycline 100 mg BID × 7 days in age > 8 years, otherwise erythromycin treatment

Gonococcal

- Doxycycline 100 BID × 3 weeks or erythromycin 500 mg QID PO × 3 weeks
- Rocephin (ceftriaxone) 1000 mg IM (can be given daily for 3 days)

- Neonates: Rocephin (ceftriaxone) 50 mg/kg IV daily for 7 days; erythromycin eye ointment QID × 14 days
- May use Sanford Guide or other drug databases

Discharge criteria

- Benign, non-herpetic conjunctivitis

Discharge instructions

- Conjunctivitis aftercare instructions
- Warm moist compresses as needed for discomfort or swelling
- Follow up with primary care provider or ophthalmology within 1 day for contact lens complications, gonococcal or chlamydial infections

Consult criteria

- Visual change
- Photophobia
- Suspected gonococcal or chlamydial infection
- Significant pain
- Contact lens complications

Infectious Keratitis

Causes

- HSV
- Staph
- Herpes zoster

Evaluation

- Direct visualization
- Fluorescein staining and wood's lamp
- Look for dendritic lesions

Treatment options

HSV

- Viroptic 1 drop q2hr while awake (NMT 9 drops qday)
- Follow up with ophthalmologist within 24 hours

Bacterial

- Ciloxan 1–2 gtts q15 minutes x 6 hr, then 2 gtts q30 minutes rest of the day, then 1gtt q2hr. 2nd day, then q4hr. days 3–14 (may use other quinolone ophthalmic solutions)
- Homatropine 2% or 5% solution 1–2 gtts bid–tid or q3–4hr. for 1–4 days

Discharge instructions

- Appropriate keratitis aftercare instructions if discharged

Consult criteria

- All infectious keratitis with ophthalmology before discharge

Episcleritis

- Episcleritis is an inflammatory condition affecting the episcleral tissue that lies between the conjunctiva and the sclera
- Mild and self-limiting but may be recurrent
- Usually idiopathic
  - 1/3 have an underlying systemic condition
  - May be caused by exogenous inflammatory stimuli
- Mainly based on clinical findings
- Edema of the episcleral tissue and injection of superficial episcleral vessels
- Nontender
- Mild to moderate discomfort
- Normal visual acuity

Examination

- Redness and injected vessels
- Radial orientation of blood vessels (scleritis is violet tinged redness of sclera and loss of radial oriented vessels)
- Episcleritis blanches with instillation of 10% phenylephrine ophthalmic drops, but not in scleritis (scleritis much more serious disorder requiring ophthalmology consult)
- Nodular episcleritis well demarcated and slightly raised border of erythema
- Lab tests may be performed for rheumatoid disorders if

suspected with ANA, rheumatoid factor, ESR, CBC, U/A etc.

Treatment

- May not need treatment
- Treat underlying disease if present
- Ophthalmic ketorolac 0.5% 1 gtt qid prn
- Prednisolone acetate 1% 1-2 gtt bid to qid (controversial due to rebound after completed) — second line
- NSAID's PO (third line)
- Oral steroids (fourth line)

Disposition

- Usually discharged and follow-up with ophthalmology as outpatient in a few days
- Consult ophthalmology is not sure if scleritis is present (painful, destructive, inflammatory disorder)
  - Scleritis needs admission usually

Blepharitis, Hordeolum (Stye) and Chalazion

Stye

- Painful, swollen, tender and red eyelid
- Staph 90–95% of the time
- Usually will drain spontaneously

Treatment options

- Warm soaks 3–4 days a day until resolved
- Erythromycin eye ointment or sulfa eye drops or gentamicin eye drops (all for 7–10 days)
- Clean eyelid margins with baby shampoo
- Oral cephalexin or staph medications for 7–10 days if infection spread beyond hordeolum or lymph nodes are swollen
- Refer to ophthalmologist in 10–14 days if not resolved

Chalazion

- Treatment similar to Stye

Blepharitis

- Treatment similar to Stye

Discharge instructions

- Appropriate aftercare instructions

Periorbital (Preseptal) Cellulitis

- Usually from S. aureus
- More common in children
- Age < 3 years can progress to bacteremia
- Is anterior to orbital septum

Signs

- Red swollen eyelid
- No vision changes
- Ocular mobility normal
- Conjunctival discharge may be present
- May have minimal pain
  - More severe with orbital cellulitis and helps to differentiate between the two
- Chemosis (conjunctival swelling)
- Fever

Evaluation

- Detailed ocular exam
  - Anterior and posterior chambers
  - Extraocular motion
  - Pupillary examination
  - CT scan may be needed if unable to differentiate from orbital cellulitis
- CBC and blood culture if age < 5 years
- Culture of eye discharge if present

Treatment options

- Most children need IV antibiotics
- Augmentin (amoxicillin/clavulanate) 45 mg/kg/day divided bid PO for 10–14 days
- Vancomycin IV
- Rocephin (ceftriaxone)
- Clindamycin 150–300 mg PO qid for 7–10 days

- May use Sanford Guide or other drug databases

Discharge instructions

- Periorbital or preseptal cellulitis aftercare instructions
- Follow up in 24 hours with PCP or ophthalmologist

Orbital Cellulitis

- Most commonly from ethmoid sinusitis spread

Findings and symptoms

- May have toxic appearance
- Proptosis
- Limited extraocular motion
- Diplopia
- Significant pain
- Dark red eyelids
- Decreased vision
- Increased intraocular pressure

Complications

- Meningitis
- Cavernous sinus thrombosis
- Vision loss

Evaluation

- Detailed ocular exam
  - Anterior and posterior chambers
  - Extraocular motion
  - Pupillary examination
  - CT scan may be needed if unable to differentiate from orbital cellulitis
- CBC and blood culture if age < 5 years
- Culture of eye discharge if present

Treatment

- Ceftin (cefuroxime) IV and/or per Sanford Guide or other drug databases
- Admission to hospital

Consult criteria

- All suspected or diagnosed orbital cellulitis patients

Corneal Ulcer or Lesions

- Consult physician
- Ciloxan 2 gtts q15min,for 6 hours, then q30min. for 18 hours, then q1hr for 1 days, the q4hr for 12 days for bacterial ulcer
- No patching

Discharge instructions

- Corneal ulcer aftercare instructions

Iritis

- Photophobia — is consensual (light shined into opened normal eye causes pain in closed affected eye due to pupillary reflex)
- Ciliary flush (red injection at edge of cornea circumferentially)
- Cells and flare in anterior chamber; hypopyon more rare
- Miosis
- 50% associated with systemic disease
- Slit lamp exam helpful

Treatment

- Homatropine eye drops 2–5% 1 drop TID for 7–10 days
- Steroid eye drops per ophthalmologist (controversy whether beneficial)
- Biologics have off-label recommendation recently
- Consult physician

Discharge instructions

- Iritis aftercare instructions
- Close ophthalmology follow-up

Corneal Abrasion

- Can detect with direct ophthalmoscopy or fluorescein staining
- No consensual photophobia unless iritis present
- Heals in 24–48 hours
- If corneal pain recurs in 2–3 days, it may indicate sloughing of corneal epithelium

Treatment

- No patching (may need patching for > 50% or cornea or pediatric patient who rub eyes)
  - No patching in contact lens patients

- Can use local anesthetic eye drops at time of exam only (do not prescribe for home pain control since it is mildly cytotoxic and will prevent healing)
- Narcotics PO prn × 2–3 days
- Antibiotic drops for contact lens patient — ofloxacin ophthalmic
    - Days 1-2: 1-2 gtt q30min while awake, awaken 4-6 hours after retiring
    - Days 3-7: 1-2 gtt q1hr while awake
    - Days 7-9: 1-2 gtt four times daily until clinical cure
    - No contact lens until lesion resolved

Extensive corneal abrasion

- Homatropine 2% sol 1–2 gtt to achieve cycloplegia (pupil dilation) — may repeat q15 min. × 2 prn
    - Can prescribe 1–2 gtt QID up to 3 days

Discharge instructions

- Corneal abrasion aftercare instructions
- Follow up in 2–3 days for recheck with primary care provider or ophthalmologist

Ultraviolet Keratitis (Band Keratitis)

- Usually from welding or tanning beds
- Acular (ketorolac) or Voltaren (diclofenic) eye drops 1 gtt QID for several days until eye corneal pain resolved (not longer than 2 weeks)
- Homatropine 2% or 5% solution 1–2 gtts bid–tid or q3–4hr. may be used for photophobia prn
- Similar evaluation and treatment as corneal abrasion

Discharge instructions

- Ultraviolet (flash burn) keratitis aftercare instructions

Eye Foreign Body

- Usually a foreign body sensation is the chief complaint
- Anesthetic eye drops with proparacaine or tetracaine immediately relieves symptoms for 15 minutes or so
- Patient may or may not be able to localize the foreign body

Examination

- Evert eyelids as needed to locate the foreign body
- If foreign body is not identified, flush under eyelids with eye irrigation fluids to see if symptoms can be resolved
- If foreign body persists after eye flush, use moistened sterile cotton swab to gently swab under eyelids to see if any foreign bodies are found or the patient's symptoms of foreign body sensation resolve
- Check lacrimal duct opening for retained eyelash

Discharge criteria

- Foreign body removed
- No visual changes or significant residual discomfort

Discharge instructions

- Eye foreign body aftercare instructions

Consult criteria

- Retained intraocular foreign body, discuss with physician
- Significant residual pain post foreign body removal
- Acute visual changes or complaints

Corneal Foreign Body

- If an iron containing metallic foreign body is present, a rust ring may develop in a few hours
- Examine anterior and posterior ocular chambers — if abnormal discuss with physician or ophthalmologist
- Fluorescein staining can be used as needed to locate foreign bodies and abrasions
- The Provider may opt to not remove small residual rust rings outside of visual axis, and refer to an ophthalmologist for further treatment in 1–3 days

Removal instructions

- After 3–4 drops of eye anesthetic over 1 minute are instilled into the affected eye and the patient has no further complaints of a foreign body sensation or pain, a sterile moistened cotton swab is used to swab across the foreign body to effect removal
- If the cotton swab does not remove the corneal foreign body, an experienced Provider may use a blunt eye spud or eye burr to remove the foreign body
- Consult a physician if not experienced with using a blunt eye spud or eye burr
- If a metallic foreign body has rusted, a residual rust ring will be left after the majority of the central rust area has been removed with the cotton swab
  - A blunt eye spud or eye burr can be used to remove some of the residual rust left, although it is not unusual to not be able to remove it all
- Fresh rust rings are more difficult to remove and after sterile cotton swabbing the residual rust ring can be left to mature in 1–3 days and the patient can then be referred to an ophthalmologist for follow-up

Discharge instructions

- Corneal foreign body aftercare instructions
- Refer to ophthalmology within 3 days
- Return if pain worsens, or photophobia or visual changes develops

Consult criteria

- Discuss with the physician if the residual rust ring is in the visual axis

Corneal Laceration

- Protective rigid eye shield
- Consult physician and ophthalmologist immediately
- Analgesia and vomiting control IM or IV prn to decrease valsalva

Eyelid Lacerations

Findings to discuss with physician (usually needs referral treatment)

- Tarsal plate involvement
- Eyelid margin
- Tear duct injury
- Orbital septum injury
  - Fat can protrude
- Tissue loss

Globe Injury

- History is important of what patient was doing at time of injury
- Globe injury can be obvious with uveal tissue prolapsing from a wound or pupil, or the eye or papillary shape can be grossly abnormal, or the injury may be subtle
- Small eyelid lacerations can cover or mask perforations of globe
  - Do not close laceration until globe injury is ruled out
- Assess eye motion and visual acuity
  - Visual acuity can be counting fingers at 18 inches or light perception if necessary
  - Critical to avoid pressure on the eye
  - Palpate orbital rims for deformity and crepitus
  - Do not remove any foreign bodies that have penetrated the globe
  - Conjunctival hemorrhage covering 360 degrees of the bulbar conjunctiva can indicate globe rupture
  - Assess pupils for size, shape, afferent defect, direct and indirect pupillary light reflex and the red reflex
  - Examine anterior chamber
  - CT orbital scans are the preferred imaging to evaluate for occult globe injury

Treatment

- Place protective rigid eye shield immediately after assessment with no touching the eyelids

Disposition

- Consult physician and ophthalmologist immediately
- Analgesia and vomiting control IM or IV prn to decrease valsalva and minimize intraocular pressure increases

Chemical Eye Injuries

Alkali burns most serious

- Causes immediate liquefaction necrosis if the pH is very high
- Penetrates the tissue deeply
- Immediate eye lavage with NS for one hour (Morgan lens)
- Exam after lavage
- Notify physician promptly

Acid burns

- Cause coagulation of proteins which can limit depth of injury
- Can use fluorescein to evaluate cornea (exam after lavage if needed)
- Weak acids burns usually managed as outpatient

Evaluation

- Inspection
- After lavage if strong alkali: fluorescein or slit lamp
- Check visual acuity

Treatment

- Significant burns flush with NS using Morgan lens for 30–60 minutes
- Check pH at 5 and 30 minutes of eye lavage to achieve pH 7.3–7.5
- Mild burns with weak acids can be lavaged less (with or without Morgan lens) depending on symptoms
- Use topical eye anesthetic for pain of examination and treatment as needed
- Gentamicin plus erythromycin or bacitracin ophthalmic ointment tid × 5–10 days or until healed for significant chemical burns
- Mild burns without significant damage can be managed with one topical eye antibiotic ointment
- Narcotics or NSAID's PO prn pain

Discharge criteria

- Mild conjunctivitis and keratitis from weak acid chemical burns
- Discuss with physician all chemical eye injuries

Discharge instructions

- Chemical eye injury aftercare instructions
- Refer to ophthalmologist within 1 day if indicated

Consult criteria

- Alkali burns
- Acid burns of moderate or worse severity
- Visual acuity changes

Glaucoma

- Severe pain, ipsilateral visual defects and may see halos around objects
- Nausea and vomiting common with acute closed angle glaucoma
- Steamy and cloudy cornea
- Increase IOP (normal IOP 10–22 mm Hg)
- Mid-dilated pupil and firm globe
- Consult physician promptly

Orbital Blowout Isolated Fracture

- Orbital wall composed of 7 bones
- Occurs usually with larger object than the orbit (baseball; fist)
- Can result in diplopia

Evaluation

- Neurologic exam
- Extraocular motor exam
- Evaluate for associated ocular injuries (present 20–40% of the time)
- CT head, facial and orbital films (CT scan gold standard) if CT

not available then plain facial (water's view best)
- Ocular anterior and posterior chamber exam
- TM's (tympanic membrane) exam for hemotympanum
- Grasp upper teeth and palate and pull to assess for Lefort fractures (movement noted)
- Dental exam
- C-spine films prn (see Neck Pain Practice Guide)

Treatment
- Most patients can be followed as outpatient with plastic surgeon or ophthalmologist in a timeframe determined by the surgeon
- Discuss with physician
- No nose blowing
- Amoxicillin/clavulanate 500 mg TID PO × 10 days or Levaquin (levofloxacin) 750 mg qday PO × 10 days
- Pediatric amoxicillin/clavulanate dose — 12.5 mg/kg PO bid × 10 days
- Analgesics PO prn
- Ice prn for swelling
- Tetanus if not up to date (see Tetanus Protocol)

Discharge criteria
- Uncomplicated inferior blowout fracture without extraocular muscle entrapment or other facial fractures or associated conditions

Discharge instructions
- Head injury aftercare instructions
- Orbital blowout fracture aftercare instructions
- Referral to Ophthalmology or plastic surgeon within 7 days

Consult criteria
- Discuss all facial fractures except simple nasal fracture with physician

Subconjunctival Hemorrhage
- No treatment
- Check PT/INR if on Coumadin (warfarin)
- CBC if constitutional symptoms present

Retinal Detachment

Causes
- Tear in retina

Risk factors
- Near sighted
- Advanced age
- Diabetes
- Sickle cell anemia
- Prior retinal detachment history

Findings and symptoms
- Painless
- Light flashes
- Decreased peripheral vision
- Floaters
- Lowering of curtain over vision in affected eye

Examination includes
- Direct ophthalmoscopy (may need pupils dilated)
- Bedside ultrasound with vascular probe can detect retinal detachment (see Acute Care Ultrasound chapter)

Treatment
- Elevate head of bed for inferior detachment
- Lay flat for superior detachment

Consult criteria
- Consult physician and ophthalmologist promptly

Central Retinal Artery Occlusion
- True emergency
- Usually from emboli
- 90 minutes to restore vision before irreversible damage
- Evaluate for sickle cell anemia and temporal arteritis

Findings

- Sudden loss of vision in one eye
- Pupil reacts consensually
- Afferent defect to light in affected eye (pupil does not constrict)
- Increased intraocular pressure
- Pale fundus
- Dilated pupil
- Retinal artery may have "box cars" appearance
- Macula has enhanced cherry red appearance (different blood supply)

Treatment

- Gentle massage on globe to attempt dislodging emboli
  - Apply direct pressure for 5-15 seconds, then release. Repeat several times
  - Ocular massage can move the embolus further down the arterial circulation and improve perfusion
- Rebreathing bag or mask to increase CO_2
- Hyperbaric oxygen if < 2 hours of symptoms, but can be used for vision loss if < 12 hours

IOP treatment

- Timoptic (timolol)
- Diamox (acetazolamide)
- Ophthalmology paracentesis of anterior chamber

Consult criteria

- Notify physician immediately
- Ophthalmologist consult immediately

Central Retinal Vein Occlusion

- Rapid and painless vision loss of one eye
  - Slower onset than retinal artery occlusion
  - From thrombosis of central retinal vein

Findings

- Retinal hemorrhages
- Impressive appearance of fundus with bloody engorgement
  - Optic disc edema

Treatment

- Aspirin

Consult criteria

- All central retinal vein occlusion patients
- All patients with acute vision loss

Hyphema and Hypopyon (Blood or Pus in Anterior Chamber)

- Consult physician

Hyphema

- Eye shield
- Elevate head of bed 30–45 degrees
- Avoid NSAID's
- Tranexamic acid (caution in CKD)
- Cycloplegics (1% cyclopentolate or 1% atropine eye drops 1–3 times a day for 5 days)

Notes

REFERENCES:

Acute Conjunctivitis: Author: Michael A Silverman; Chief Editor: Barry E Brenner, MD, PhD, FACEP

emedicine.medscape.com/article/797874-overview

Iritis and Uveitis Author: Keith Tsang, MD; Chief Editor: Rick Kulkarni, MD

emedicine.medscape.com/article/798323

[Best Evidence] Islam N, Pavesio C. Uveitis (acute anterior). *Clin Evid (Online)*. November 2009;04:705

Ophthalmology Volume 121, Issue 3, Pages 785-796.e3, March 2014

Levy-Clarke G, Jabs DA, Read RW, Rosenbaum JT, Vitale A, Van Gelder RN. Expert Panel Recommendations for the Use of Anti-Tumor Necrosis Factor Biologic Agents in Patients with Ocular Inflammatory Disorders. *Ophthalmology*. Dec 17 2013

Orbital Fracture in Emergency Medicine Medication

Author: Thomas Widell, MD; Chief Editor: Rick Kulkarni, MD

emedicine.medscape.com/article/825772

Orbital Floor Fractures (Blowout)

Author: Adam J Cohen, MD; Chief Editor: Deepak Narayan, MD, FRCS emedicine.medscape.com/article/1284026

[Best Evidence] Turner A, Rabiu M. Patching for corneal abrasion. *Cochrane Database Syst Rev*. Apr 19 2006;(2):CD004764

Corneal Abrasion Author: Arun Verma, MD; Chief Editor: Hampton Roy Sr, MD emedicine.medscape.com/article/1195402

Preseptal Cellulitis

Author: Geoffrey M Kwitko, MD, FACS, FICS; Chief Editor: Hampton Roy Sr, MD
emedicine.medscape.com/article/1218009

Fraser SG, Adams W. Interventions for acute non-arteritic central retinal artery occlusion. Cochrane Database of Systematic Reviews 2009, Issue 1. Art. No.: CD001989. DOI: 10.1002/14651858.CD001989.pub2

Hyperbaric oxygenation combined with nifedipine treatment for recent-onset retinal artery occlusion. Eur J Ophthalmol. 1993; 3(2):89-94 (ISSN: 1120-6721)

Duma SM, Jernigan MV. The effects of airbags on orbital fracture patterns in frontal automobile crashes. Ophth Plast Reconst Surg. 2003;19(2):107-111

Francis DO, Kaufman R, Yueh B, et al. Air bag-induced orbital blow-out fractures. Laryngoscope. 2006;116:1966-1972. (Case series of 150 orbital fractures derived from 2739 crashes in CIREN database)

Hackl W, Fink C, Hausberger K, et al. The incidence of combined facial and cervical spine injuries. J Trauma. 2001;50:41-45

JAMA,310(16):1721-1730

Hordeolum and Stye in Emergency Medicine Treatment & Management Updated: Jul 24, 2018 Author: Michael J Bessette, MD, FACEP; Chief Editor: Gil Z Shlamovitz, MD, FACEP

Episcleritis Updated: Jul 15, 2019
Author: Ellen N Yu-Keh, MD; Chief Editor: Andrew A Dahl, MD, FACS
emedicine.medscape.com/article/1228246

NOSEBLEED PROTOCOL

Definition

- Bleeding from nostril, nasal cavity or nasopharynx

Differential Diagnosis

- Nasal foreign body
- Sinusitis
- Barotrauma
- Thrombocytopenia
- Leukemia
- Anticoagulation therapy

- Cocaine abuse
- NSAID use
- ASA use
- Hemophilia
- Von Willebrand's disease
- Trauma

Considerations

- 90% of nosebleeds are anterior
- Most common cause is nose picking
- Hypertension common
- Anticoagulant or antiplatelet agents contribute to bleeding
- Look for foreign body in young children (suspect if foul smell or unilateral discharge present)
- Posterior Epistaxis
  - Less common than anterior Epistaxis
  - Associated with
    - Elderly
    - Hypertension
    - Atherosclerosis

Evaluation

- Attempt visualization of bleeding
- Use nosebleed tray equipment or otoscope
- Have patient clear blood by forcefully blowing nose
- Use suction prn
- Cocaine intranasally can be used for hemostasis and pain control
  - May use afrin spray with or without pledget
- If bleeding has stopped and site unknown, take moistened cotton swab and gently stroke suspected area to elicit bleeding
- CBC if suspected significant blood loss or patient is tachycardic or orthostatic
- PT/INR if on Coumadin (warfarin). PTT if on heparin or has Von Willebrand's disease or hemophilia

Treatment options

- Control anterior nosebleed by pinching all of nose below nasal bone or use nasal clamp, up to at least 3–5 minutes
  - May apply ice to dorsal nose or pressure under upper lip
- Patients with significant hemorrhage should receive an IV NS 250–500 ml bolus and transfusion as indicated
  - See Bleeding Protocol
  - Continuous cardiac monitoring and pulse oximetry for significant bleeding
- Patients frequently present with an elevated blood pressure
  - Significant reduction can usually be obtained with analgesia and mild sedation alone
  - May treat hypertension if > SBP 180 or DBP > 110 and not decreasing
    - Repeat BP 10–15 minutes initially, before treatment, to see if BP decreases sufficiently without medication
- IV NS if vital signs or CBC reflect significant bleeding

Silver nitrate

- Silver nitrate stick cautery directly on bleeding site for 5–7 seconds, and then in a circle around bleeding site, holding 5–7 seconds each spot, to form a solid eschar
  - Then hold 2 dry cotton swabs side by side for 60 seconds over cauterized area with enough pressure to stop any bleeding (usually mild pressure is all that is needed)
  - May repeat in places that continue bleeding with more cautery and cotton swab pressure until bleeding stops
  - Complication is septal perforation with too vigorous cautery

Additional treatments

Use Rapid Rhino anterior or posterior balloons (or similar balloons) if silver nitrate cautery not used or ineffective

- Anterior epistaxis balloons are available in different lengths
- Carboxycellulose outer layer promotes platelet aggregation
- As efficacious as nasal tampons, easier to insert and remove, and more comfortable for the patient
- Soak outer layer with water, insert it along the floor of the nasal cavity aiming down to the level of the ear lobe, and inflate it slowly with air until the bleeding stops.

Merocel packing

- Trim the compressed sponge to fit snugly through the naris
- Moisten the tip with surgical lubricant or topical antibiotic ointment
- Firmly grasp the length of the sponge with a bayonet forceps, spread the naris vertically with a nasal speculum, and advance the sponge along the floor of the nasal cavity
- Once wet with blood or a small amount of saline, the sponge expands to fill the nasal cavity and tamponade the bleeding

Afrin type nasal spray or cocaine pledgets can be used for hemostasis (caution in CAD)

Epistaxis thrombin kit for intranasal application

- Consider Floseal in thrombocytopenic or coagulopathic patients

Tranexamic acid

- Put tranexamic acid that is used for injection on a pledget and allow to be in contact with bleeding site for 20-30 minutes before removal
- May use as an aerosolized spray
- May give 1000 mg or 10 mg/IV for uncontrollable bleeding over 20 minutes (no faster than 100 mg/minute)

- Septra DS or sinusitis medication Rx per Sanford Guide or database for 5–7 days if packing or balloon used

Discharge criteria recommendation

- Successful treatment of anterior bleeding
- Hemodynamically stable
- No respiratory distress

Discharge instructions

- Nosebleed or epistaxis aftercare instructions
- Packing removal in 2–3 days
- Refer to ENT or primary care provider in 2–3 days
- Antibiotic ointment on bleeding site twice a day for 7–10 days for cautery only or after packing removed — very gently applied

Consult criteria recommendation

- Unable to stop bleeding
- Posterior nasal bleeding or packing
- Significant blood loss per CBC or vital signs abnormalities
  - Tachycardia, hypotension or orthostatic vital signs
- Coagulopathy secondary to Coumadin (warfarin) or DOACs
- Bleeding site not identified or not known whether anterior or posterior (if packing not effective then likely is a posterior nosebleed)
- Admit patients with large posterior packing or bilateral deep packing for observation and oxygen saturation monitoring

- Posterior nasal packing is particularly uncomfortable for the patient and promotes hypoxia and hypoventilation
- Failure to admit and appropriately monitor all patients who require large posterior packing (e.g. nasostat or large gauze packing) may result in mortality

Vital sign recommendations

- Significant sinus tachycardia
- SBP < 90 or relative hypotension (SBP < 105 with history of hypertension)

Lab consult criteria recommendations

- Acute hemoglobin decrease of > 1 gm
- Thrombocytopenia
- INR > 1.2
- PTT > 1.2 times normal

Notes

REFERENCES:

Acute Epistaxis Author: Ola Bamimore, MD; Chief Editor: Steven C Dronen, MD, FAAEM
emedicine.medscape.com/article/764719

Brinjikji W, Kallmes DF, Cloft HJ. Trends in Epistaxis Embolization in the United States: A Study of the Nationwide Inpatient Sample 2003–2010. *J Vasc Interv Radiol.* May 3 2013

ENT EMERGENCY PROTOCOL

Ludwig's Angina

Definition

- Cellulitis (occasionally abscess) involving submandibular and sublingual spaces

Considerations

- Mortality has declined to < 10% since penicillin was introduced
- Can result in elevation of tongue to obstruct airway
- Increased association with diabetes; SLE; neutropenia; alcoholism
- Polymicrobial infection is usual
- Infection of 2nd and 3rd molars most common cause — 80% of cases
- Is a clinical diagnosis
- Assess airway status — may need anesthesia or ENT if difficult intubation likely
- Ability of tongue to be protruded beyond vermillion border excludes sublingual space infection usually

Signs

- Bilateral submandibular swelling – All (firm floor of mouth)
- Elevated or protruding tongue – 19/20
- Fever – 9/10
- Increased WBC – 17/20
- Recent dental extraction or toothache – 8/10
- Neck swelling – 7/10
- Dysphagia – 5/10
- Trismus – 5/10
- Neck pain – 1/3
- Respiratory (stridor; dyspnea; tachypnea) – 7/20
- Dysphonia and dysarthria – 1/5

Evaluation

- Is a clinical diagnosis

- Airway management takes precedence over testing
- CT scanning best modality if needed
- Soft tissue neck and panorex useful when CT not available
- CBC
- BMP

Treatment options

- Antibiotics effective
  - Penicillin + Flagyl (metronidazole)
  - Unasyn
  - Clindamycin
- Surgery
  - Needed 20–65% of time
  - If abscess identified
- Airway management if needed
  - Endotracheal intubation
  - Cricothyroidotomy by physician
  - Notify physician immediately for suspected airway compromise

Complications

- Aspiration
- Mediastinitis
- Pneumonia
- Empyema
- Bacteremia
- Septic emboli
- Pericarditis
- Cavernous sinus thrombosis
- Cerebral abscess

Consult criteria

- All Ludwig's angina cases
- If imminent airway concern, notify physician immediately

Angioedema of Oropharyngeal Area

Considerations

- Affects deeper tissues
- Localized non-pitting edema
- 25% of population experiences urticaria or angioedema during lifetime
- Localized swelling resolves in several days
- Typically involves face and upper lip
- GI tract involvement causes
  - Nausea
  - Vomiting
  - Diarrhea
  - Abdominal pain
  - Esophageal involvement can cause chest pain
- Neurologic involvement rare
- Upper respiratory involvement responsible for mortality

Types of angioedema

- Histamine mediated
  - Allergic/immunogenic
- Bradykinin mediated
  - ACE inhibitors
  - Hereditary
    - Decreased C1 esterase inhibitor (or poorly functioning C1 esterase inhibitor) allowing overproduction of bradykinin
      - Cryoprecipitate may help (contain C1 esterase inhibitor)
  - Acquired
  - Bradykinin metabolized mainly by angiotensin converting enzyme
- Physically induced
- Idiopathic

Predictors of need for airway intervention

- Increased age
- Tongue swelling
- Oropharynx swelling
- Odynophagia
- Hoarseness/voice change

Signs

- Respiratory distress
- Stridor
- Voice changes
- Dysphagia

Causes

- Hereditary angioedema (HAE)

- Angiotensin converting enzyme inhibitors (ACE) around 70% of patients
  - Increased incidence in African-Americans and women
  - Most occur in first week of therapy, but can occur anytime

Treatment options

- Medical management usually suffices
- Stop offending agent if known — ACE inhibitor most common
- Examining the airway aggressively may precipitate airway obstruction in advanced oropharyngeal angioedema
  - Double set–up with ET tube and cricothyrotomy equipment if patient in distress

Histamine mediated angioedema (allergic)

- **Epinephrine**
  - Caution if history of coronary artery disease
  - Adult: 0.3–0.5 mg SQ; (if respiratory distress notify physician promptly)
  - Pediatrics: 0.01 mg/kg SQ not to exceed adult dose; give IV or IM (anterior thigh) if respiratory distress present (notify physician promptly)
- **Antihistamines** (diphenhydramine 50 mg IV/IM) helpful in IgE/histamine mediated (may have pruritus)
  - Benadryl (diphenhydramine) 50 mg PO or IM adult; continue for 5–7 days PO
  - Benadryl (diphenhydramine) 0.625–1.25 mg/kg PO or IM pediatrics; continue for 5–7 days PO qid prn (NMT 50 mg/dose)
  - Pepcid (famotidine) 20 mg IV/PO – 40 mg PO for adult
  - Pepcid (famotidine) 0.25 mg/kg IV/PO for pediatric (NMT 20mg IV or 40 mg PO)
- Consider steroids
  - Prednisone 40–60 mg PO qday for 5–7 days (> 40 kg)
  - Prednisone/prednisolone 1 mg/kg PO qday (children < 40 kg) for 5–7 days
  - Dexamethasone 10 mg IV
    - Onset of action IV is 1 hour. PO onset of action is 1–2 hours
    - Duration of action is 36–54 hours
    - Dexamethasone 6mg =prednisone 40 mg

Bradykinin mediated (ACE inhibitor induced most common)

- May respond to fresh frozen plasma (jumbo unit) or C1 esterase inhibitor concentrate
- Tranexamic acid1 gm IV over 10 minutes may be effective (no faster than 100 mg/minute)
- Less responsive to treatment than histamine mediated angioedema with below agents
  - Attempt treatment with
    - Diphenhydramine 50 mg PO or IM adult; continue for 5–7 days PO
    - Diphenhydramine 0.625–1.25 mg/kg PO or IM pediatrics; continue for 5–7 days PO qid prn (NMT 50 mg/dose)
  - Additional treatments if needed
  - Pepcid (famotidine) 20 mg IV/PO – 40 mg PO for adult
  - Pepcid (famotidine) 0.25 mg/kg IV/PO for pediatric (NMT 20mg IV or 40 mg PO)
- Consider steroids
  - Prednisone 40–60 mg PO qday for 5–7 days (> 40 kg)
  - Prednisone/prednisolone 1 mg/kg PO qday (children < 40 kg) for 5–7 days
  - Dexamethasone 10 mg IV for adults and pediatric 0.6

mg/kg IV or IM (NMT 10 mg)

- Airway compromise or significant oropharyngeal swelling (notify physician immediately)
  - Epinephrine
    - Caution if coronary artery disease history present
    - Adult: 0.3 mg SQ; (notify physician promptly)
    - Pediatrics: 0.01 mg/kg SQ – do not exceed adult dose (notify physician promptly)
    - Oxygen prn
- **Stop ACE inhibitors if currently taking**

Consult physician promptly for posterior oropharyngeal angioedema, respiratory distress or hoarseness (may need anesthesiologist for intubation standby)

Discharge criteria

- Observation for 4–6 hours
- Discharge mild lip or non-oropharyngeal angioedema with normal vital signs and no distress

Discharge instructions

- Angioedema aftercare instructions
- Refer to primary care provider within 1 day if not improving, otherwise 3–4 days if improving

Consult criteria

- Discuss all patients with physician

Barotitis Media and Barosinusitis

- Caused by relative negative pressures from descent during flying usually with a coexistent URI or positive pressures from ascent during diving
- Findings that may be seen
  - Loss of TM (tympanic membrane) landmarks, congestion around umbo, hemorrhage into middle ear

Valsalva maneuver

- On airplane descent can be used to prevent occurrence (nostrils pinched and patient blows against a closed mouth forcing air into Eustachian tubes with tympanic membranes feeling the pressure and subsequently moving – do not perform if vertigo present

Treatment options

- For tympanic membrane congestion only
  - Nasal and oral decongestants
- For hemorrhage into middle ear
  - Adult: prednisone 60 mg PO qday for 6 days then taper over 7–10 days (may use dexamethasone)
  - Children: prednisone 1 mg/kg PO for 6 days then taper over 7–10 days (do not exceed adult dose) — may use dexamethasone
- Otitis media antibiotics are prescribed if tympanic membrane perforation or discharge noted
  - Keep ear dry
- Narcotics and/or NSAID's prn for pain

Discharge instructions

- Barotitis or barosinusitis aftercare instructions
- Refer to ENT surgeon if perforation or vertigo present – refer to PCP otherwise
- No altitude traveling or scuba diving till symptoms and findings resolve

Consult criteria

- Discuss with physician immediately any patient with joint pain or swelling, chest pain or dyspnea (order chest x-ray), dizziness, headache, altered mental status or hypotension after diving

Notes

REFERENCES:

Seidmann MD. Christopher AL. Sarpa JR. Potesta E. Angioedema related to angiotensin converting enzyme inhibitors. Otolaryngology – Head & Neck Surgery. 102:727–31, 1990.

Brown NJ. Ray WA. Snowden M. Griffin MR. Black Americans have an increased rate of angiotensin converting enzyme inhibitor-associated angioedema. Clinical Pharmacology & Therapeutics. 60(1):8–13, 1996 Jul

World Allergy Organization Guidelines for the Assessment and Management of Anaphylaxis

World Allergy Organ J. Feb 2011; 4(2): 13–37.

Acute Epistaxis Author: Ola Bamimore, MD; Chief Editor: Steven C Dronen, MD, FAAEM

emedicine.medscape.com/article/764719

Brinjikji W, Kallmes DF, Cloft HJ. Trends in Epistaxis Embolization in the United States: A Study of the Nationwide Inpatient Sample 2003–2010. *J Vasc Interv Radiol*. May 3 2013

Wang K, et al. *Am J Emerg Med*. 2020 Oct 21. Online ahead of print.

Beauchene J, et al. *Rev Med Interne*. 2018;39(10): 772-776.

Long BJ, et al. *West J Emerg Med*. 2019;20(4): 587-600.

NASAL AND FACIAL FRACTURES PROTOCOL

Considerations

- The incidence of concomitant major injuries is reported to be as high as 50% in high-impact facial fracture, compared to 21% for lower impact fractures.
- Fractures are more commonly associated with motor vehicle collisions, rather than other blunt trauma
- Airbag deployment considerably decreases the incidence and severity of orbital fractures for front-seat occupants in frontal automobile crashes
- Bleeding control imperative
- Up to 10% of patients with significant blunt facial injuries will also have cervical spine injury
- Blood or edema resulting from the injury can cause upper airway obstruction
- The tongue may obstruct the airway in a patient with a mandibular fracture
- A fractured free-floating maxilla can fall back, obstructing the airway
- Tooth fragments may migrate to the airway

Nasal Fractures

- Most common fracture
- X-rays may miss around 50%

Complications

- Septal hematoma
- Associated orbital wall blowout fractures
- Facial fractures with CSF (cerebrospinal fluid) leak — cribriform plate fracture
- Hyphema
- Retinal detachment
- Subconjunctival hemorrhage

CSF rhinorrhea

- Cribriform plate fracture
- Increased by leaning forward
- Increased with jugular compression
- Ring sign (2 rings formed when CSF placed on filter paper) — blood is inner circle and CSF is clearer ring outer
- Dipstick findings — CSF glucose > 30mg%

Evaluation options

- Physical examination
- Clear nares of blood
- Evaluate for septal hematoma
- CT facial bones if suspected facial fractures
- CT head injury protocols
- C-spine films prn (see Neck Pain Protocol)
- Plain nasal films not usually needed but can be ordered
- CBC if significant blood loss suspected or tachycardia/hypotension
- Tympanic membranes for hemotympanum
- Eye exam of anterior and posterior chambers if suspected eye injury or complaints
- Excessive tearing may indicate nasolacrimal duct injury — if suspected instill fluorescein in eye and examine posterior pharynx (with Wood's light if needed) to see if dye flows into pharynx through intact duct

Treatment options

- Epistaxis controlled with pinching nares together for 2–5 minutes
- Septal hematoma needs immediate drainage
  - Can be drained with 18 gauge needle after cocaine topical anesthesia
  - Rolled cotton swab can help decompress hematoma
  - Packing after drainage for 3–5 days
  - Antibiotics to prevent sinusitis (same as otitis media antibiotics)
- Analgesics prn
- Tetanus if not up to date (see Tetanus Protocol)

Discharge criteria

- Simple nasal fractures

Discharge instructions

- Nasal fracture aftercare instructions
- Refer to ENT within 7–10 days
- Head injury instructions
- No nose blowing with facial fractures for 1 week

Consult criteria

- Septal hematoma
- Associated facial fractures
- Other associated injuries
- Significant blood loss

Orbital Blowout Fractures

- Orbital wall composed of 7 bones
- Occurs usually with larger object than the orbit (baseball; fist)
- Can result in diplopia

Evaluation

- Neurologic exam
- Extraocular motor exam
- CT head, facial and orbital films (CT scan gold standard) if CT not available then plain facial (water's view best)
- CT head injury guidelines
- Ocular anterior and posterior chamber exam
- TM's (tympanic membrane) for hemotympanum
- Grasp upper teeth and palate and pull to assess for Lefort fractures (movement noted)
- Check orbital rim for step off and for malar flattening
- Dental exam
- C-spine films or CT cervical spine (see Neck Pain Protocol)
  - In any fall induced facial fracture (especially elderly)

Treatment

- Antibiotics (same as sinusitis treatment)
- Analgesics prn
- Tetanus if not up to date (see Tetanus Protocol)

Discharge criteria

- Uncomplicated inferior blowout fracture without extraocular muscle entrapment or other facial fractures or associated conditions
- Head injury instructions should be given to competent alert patient or family member or personal significant person

Discharge instructions

- Head injury aftercare instructions
- Orbital blowout fracture aftercare instructions
- Referral to Ophthalmology or plastic surgeon within 7 days
- No nose blowing

Consult criteria

- Discuss all facial fractures except uncomplicated nasal fracture with physician
- Vision changes
- EOM entrapment
- Referral to Ophthalmology within 7 days

Mandible dislocation

- May be traumatic or spontaneous
- Unilateral dislocation the mandible is tilted
- Bilateral dislocation patient appears to have an underbite
- Teeth cannot be closed or occluded
- Mandible films or panorex

Treatment

- Prep skin and inject 2% lidocaine if desired for masseter spasm and pain

Facing patient technique

- Back of head supported by wall if possible
- Pad thumbs gauze taped on
- Place thumbs on lower posterior molars
- Lock elbows and push down on lower molars with bending knees and using your weight

Behind patient technique

- May need conscious sedation
- Place heavily padded thumbs **behind** last molar
- Grab mandible anteriorly and push caudally

Syringe technique

- 5 or 10cc syringe placed across posterior molars and patient instructed to bite down and roll syringe back and forth
  - 30 of 31 patients had success with this method

Mandible Fracture

- Third most common facial fracture
- 20–40% of mandibular fracture patients have associated injuries
- Children age 4–11 years at risk for facial growth disturbance if fracture missed
- The tongue may obstruct the airway in a patient with a mandibular fracture
- Tooth fragments can become may migrate to the airway

Findings

- Facial asymmetry
- Malocclusion of teeth
- Paresthesia to lower lip or gums indicate inferior alveolar nerve damage
- Blood in mouth suggests open fracture
- Jaw may deviate to side of fracture

Evaluation

- Airway exam — notify physician immediately if any airway concerns
- Dental exam
- Neurologic exam
- Plain mandible films or panorex
- CT mandible if the plain films not helpful in suspected fracture

- CT head and facial bones per head injury protocols or abnormal neurologic exam
- Chest x-ray if missing teeth cannot be located
- C-spine films or CT cervical spine (see Neck Pain Protocol)
  - In any fall facial fracture (especially elderly)

Treatment

- Dental antibiotics choices
  - Pen VK 500 mg PO qid × 7–10 days
  - Amoxicillin 875 mg PO bid × 7–10 days
  - Cleocin (clindamycin) 300 mg PO qid × 7–10 days
  - Cephalexin 500 mg PO qid × 7–10 days
  - Erythromycin 250 mg PO qid × 7–10 days (very expensive)
- Tetanus if not up to date (see Tetanus Protocol)
- See Dental Injury Protocol

Discharge criteria

- Simple nondisplaced mandible fractures
- Soft diet
- Analgesics prn

Discharge instructions

- Mandible fracture aftercare instructions
- Referral to oral surgeon within 1–4 days
- Head injury instructions

Consult criteria

- Discuss all mandible fractures with physician or oral surgeon

Notes

REFERENCES:

Orbital Fracture in Emergency Medicine Medication
Author: Thomas Widell, MD; Chief Editor: Rick Kulkarni, MD
emedicine.medscape.com/article/825772

Orbital Floor Fractures (Blowout)
Author: Adam J Cohen, MD; Chief Editor: Deepak Narayan, MD, FRCS emedicine.medscape.com/article/1284026

Bartkiw TP, Pynn BR, Brown DH. Diagnosis and managment of nasal fractures. Int J Trauma Nurs. 1995;1:11–18. (Review article)

Duma SM, Jernigan MV. The effects of airbags on orbital fracture patterns in frontal automobile crashes. Ophth Plast Reconst Surg. 2003;19(2):107–111

Francis DO, Kaufman R, Yueh B, et al. Air bag-induced orbital blow-out fractures. Laryngoscope. 2006;116:1966–1972. (Case series of 150 orbital fractures derived from 2739 crashes in CIREN database)

Hackl W, Fink C, Hausberger K, et al. The incidence of combined facial and cervical spine injuries. J Trauma. 2001;50:41–45

Gorchynski J, Karabidian E, Sanchez M. The "syringe" technique: a hands-free approach for the reduction of acute nontraumatic temporomandibular dislocations in the emergency department. J Emerg Med. 2014;47(6):676-681. (Prospective convenience sample, multicenter study

DENTAL INJURY PROTOCOLS

Considerations

- Injury to primary teeth common in toddlers

- Older children dental injuries commonly from sports
- Assess for other injuries
- Primary tooth eruption from 7 months to 2–3 years of age
- Malocclusion of teeth is a mandible or maxilla fracture until proven otherwise

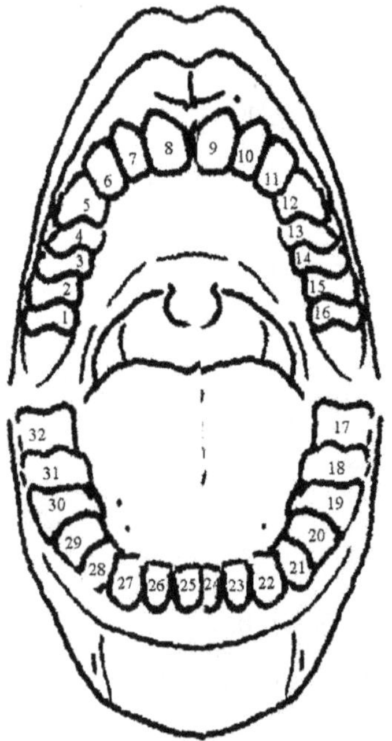

Tooth Fractures

- Ellis class 1: enamel injured only
- Ellis class 2: dentin involved
- Ellis class 3: pulp involved (bloody dental tissue seen)

Dental Avulsions of Permanent Teeth

- 1% loss of successful reimplantation of avulsed tooth per minute that tooth is not replaced in socket
- More than 15 minutes out of socket has poor salvage rate
- After 60 minutes of being out of socket there usually is no salvage rate
- Avulsed teeth should be handled by crown only
- Put in either Hank's solution, milk, or normal saline as a temporizing measure
    - Tooth can be held in buccal mucosa side of mouth if no other means to keep it stored, making sure not to swallow it
- Leave the socket alone as much as possible.
- If extraoral time is 20–60 minutes, soak in Hanks solution for 30 minutes before attempting reimplantation
- Put tooth back immediately after aspirating any clot and irrigating the socket
- If the tooth can be replaced in the prehospital setting, the root should be gently rinsed off first to remove any debris (preferably with saline)
    - The root should not be wiped off as this removes the periodontal ligament
- Apply a mouth guard (sports mouth guard acceptable)
    - Coe Pak splinting
- Antibiotics: Pen VK 500 mg PO qid for 10 days or other oral antibiotics such as amoxicillin, clindamycin or cephalexin, and see dentist or oral surgeon within one day for further treatment
- It is preferable to discuss with dentist at time of injury

Dental Avulsions of Primary Teeth

- Leave out of mouth

Gingival Lacerations

- Heal well
- Reapproximate with chromic or Vicryl sutures
- Antibiotics are not indicated

Lip and Intraoral Lacerations

- Repair from inside out then close skin
- Use absorbable sutures intraorally
- Line up vermillion border if involved
- Antibiotics are not indicated

- Refer to Laceration Protocol

Evaluation

- Dental history important to know to determine if teeth worth saving
- Time of injury important
- Palpate and lightly percuss teeth (should be a ping sound normally)
- Remove blood clots
- Check for intraoral lacerations and any through and through involvement
- Check facial bones for looseness (Lefort fractures) by pulling forward on palate or upper maxillary rim
- Plain x-rays for
  - Bony abnormalities
  - Aspirated teeth
  - Foreign bodies (tooth fragments) in lacerations
- Panorex films if available
- CT of facial bones may be needed for more extensive injury
- Check posterior molar's occlusion are normal
- Refer to Head Injury Protocols

Treatment

- Enamel fractures do not require immediate treatment
- Class 2 fractures
  - Cover with Dycal (calcium hydroxide paste)
- Class 3 fractures
  - Anesthetize tooth
  - Immediate covering with Dycal
  - Antibiotics choices
    - Adult
      - Pen VK 500 mg PO qid × 10 days
      - Clindamycin 300 mg PO tid × 10 days
      - Amoxicillin 875 mg PO bid × 10 days
    - Weight adjustment of above antibiotics for pediatrics
- Analgesics prn
- Loose teeth are referred to dentist and prescribe a soft diet
  - Chlorhexidine rinses
- Can use mouth guard to splint very loose teeth
  - Coe Pak splinting
- Move displaced teeth into position post local anesthesia
- Tetanus prophylaxis: (High risk = every 5 years; Low risk = every 10 years)
  - Tetanus IG 250–500 units IM if high risk and less than 3 tetanus or unknown history of immunizations previously in life — usually with the elderly
- Refer to health department or primary care provider to complete tetanus primary vaccination series if < 2 vaccinations given in past
  - See Tetanus Protocol

Discharge Criteria

- Ellis class 1 and 2 fractures
- Primary tooth avulsions
- Mildly loose teeth
- Refer to dentist or oral surgeon
  - Ellis class 2 fractures within 24 hours for primary dental avulsions and loose teeth
  - Ellis class 3 fractures need dental referral ASAP, no more than next day if possible
- Give avulsed teeth that are not reimplanted to patient to take to dentist

Consult Criteria

- Displaced teeth
- Avulsed permanent teeth
- It is preferable to discuss with dentist at time of injury
- Discuss with physician or dentist Ellis class 2 and 3 fractures

Notes

REFERENCES:

Barrett EJ, Kenny DJ. Avulsed permanent teeth: a review of the literature and treatment guidelines. *Endod Dent Traumatol* 1997Aug;13(4):153–163

Krasner P. Modern treatment of avulsed teeth by emergency physicians. *Am J Emerg Med* 1994 Mar;12(2):241–246

ebmedicine.net/topics.php?paction=showTopic&topic_id=543

DENTAL PAIN PROTOCOL

Differential diagnosis

- Periapical abscess
- Trigeminal neuralgia
- Masticator space infection
- Ludwig's angina
- Retropharyngeal space infection
- Infection after a root canal
- Dental caries

Considerations

- Dental abscess is rare in children
- Abscess can spread more deeply to
  - Bone (osteomyelitis)
  - Cavernous sinus (thrombosis)
  - Maxillary sinus
  - Floor of mouth (Ludwig's angina)
  - Adjacent facial spaces and planes
- Advanced dental disease in children could indicate diabetes mellitus or HIV infection
- Lower third molar most common abscess site followed by other lower posterior teeth
  - Upper teeth uncommon source of dental abscess

Evaluation options

- Usually history and physical exam only
- Percussion tenderness present
- CBC when patient is toxic appearing or cellulitis present
- BMP for tachycardia or history of diabetes or suspicion of undiagnosed diabetes
- Panorex
- CT face and/or neck for suspected deeper infections
- Needle aspiration (remove 1–2 drops of pus for diagnosis of abscess being present, if further drainage is to be attempted, to leave I&D area large as possible)

Periapical abscess

- Most common dental infection
- Very painful

Treatment options

- I&D with needle if abscess seen
  - Tap water as effective as normal saline for irrigation
- Antibiotics (choose one below)
  - Pen VK 250 mg PO qid for 7–10 days
  - Amoxicillin 875 mg PO bid 7–10 days
  - Clindamycin 150–450 mg PO qid for 7–10 days
  - Metronidazole 500 mg PO bid for 7–10 days
  - Azithromycin 5 day dose pak
- NSAID's prn
- Hydrocodone or oxycodone prn up to 3 days

Discharge criteria

- Nontoxic patient
- Most dental pain patients

Discharge instructions

- Warm salt water rinses very frequently for 1–5 days. Hold in mouth for several minutes as tolerated
- Warm compresses to painful area several times a day
- May use Orajel (benzocaine) for toothache
- Follow up with dentist within 48 hours

Consult criteria

- Deep space infection diagnosed or suspected
- Fever
- Potential for airway compromise
- Immunocompromised
- Systemic involvement

Notes

REFERENCES:

Dental Abscess Empiric Therapy
Author: Jane M Gould, MD, FAAP; Chief Editor: Thomas E Herchline, MD
emedicine.medscape.com/article/2060395

HealthPartners Dental Group guideline for diagnosing and treating endodontic emergencies. Minneapolis (MN): HealthPartners; 2009 Sep 1. 11

Trauma

Section Contents

When using any protocol, always follow the Guidelines of Proper Use (page 12).

Motor Vehicle Accident Protocol

Considerations

- Leading cause of death ages 1–37 years
- Complete exam important even when single isolated injury suspected
- Initial assessment critical in determining life threatening processes
- Comorbidities should be addressed
- Liver and spleen most common intra-abdominal injuries followed by small and large intestine in blunt abdominal trauma
- Cervical and lumbar strains common in minor MVA
- Seatbelt marks may indicate deeper injuries
- Early coagulopathy in trauma from shock and tissue damage
  - Activated protein C and t-PA released

Evaluation

- Patients seen only by the practitioner should have minor injuries preferably
- Patients on spine boards can be moved carefully if no evident spinal cord injury
  - Log roll patient off spine board within 60 minutes of arrival with team of 4 persons with 1 person maintaining inline cervical immobilization to prevent pressure tissue damage from board
- Notify physician immediately for Glasgow scale < 15

Primary survey

- Airway
- Breathing
- Circulation/bleeding
- Disability (neurologic exam)
- Exposure/environment (expose patient and hypothermia evaluation)

- Contact physician immediately if any serious findings found on primary survey
- Significant hemorrhagic vital sign findings, contact physician immediately

- See Permissive hypotension section below (consult physician immediately)

Secondary survey

- Complete physical exam
- Palpate and inspect all body areas
- Complete neurovascular exam

AMPLE mnemonic for historical key elements

A – Allergies
M – Medications
P – Past history
L – Last meal
E – Events leading to presentation

Estimated Blood and Fluid losses (adults)

	Class I	Class II	Class III	Class IV
Blood loss (cc)	Up to 750	750–1000	1500–2000	> 2000
Blood loss %	Up to 15%	15–30%	30–40%	> 40%
Pulse rate	< 100	> 100	> 120	> 140
Blood pressure	Normal	Normal	SBP < 90	SBP < 70
Capillary refill	Normal	Normal	Delayed	Absent
Pulse pressure	Normal/incr	Decreased	Decreased	Decreased
Respiratory rate	14–20	20–30	30–40	> 35
Urine output (cc/hr.)	> 30	20–30	5–15	Negligible
Mental status	Anxious	Anxious	Confused	Lethargic

(Derived from Advanced Trauma Life Support)

Lethal triad for bleeding (each contributes to the others)

- Hypothermia
- Acidosis
- Coagulopathy (frequently too much crystalloid without blood product replacement)

Imaging and Lab Tests (As indicated by exam, history, and mechanism of injury)

- C-spine
- Extremities
- Chest x-ray
  - Deep sulcus sign may indicate pneumothorax when one is not seen in periphery
    - Costophrenic angle deeper than normal
- CT head and CT C-spine
- CT abdomen/pelvis; chest if indicated (physician should be involved)
- See Acute Care Ultrasound chapter

Lab if indicated

- CBC
- BMP
- LFT's
- U/A
- Type and screen or cross

Treatment Options

- Analgesics prn
  - Dilaudid (hydromorphone) 0.5–1 mg IV or 1–2 mg IM (may repeat prn, monitor respiratory drive)
    - Stadol (butorphanol) 0.5–1 mg IV or 1–2 mg IM (avoid in opiate addiction)
  - Toradol (ketorolac) 10–15 mg IV or 15–30 mg IM (if no bleeding possibility present)
    - Do not use Toradol (ketorolac) if creatinine is elevated
    - Ketorolac therapeutic ceiling is around 10 mg
- NSAID's or PO narcotics prn (outpatient treatment)

- Tetanus prophylaxis: (High risk = every 5 years; Low risk = every 10 years) Tetanus IG 250–500 units at different site if high risk and less than 3 tetanus or unknown history of immunizations previously in life — usually with the elderly
- Refer to health department or primary care provider to complete tetanus primary vaccination series if < 2 vaccines given in past
  - See Tetanus Protocol

Blood/fluid replacement for hemorrhage

- PRBC's/FFP/platelets 1:1:1 ratio

Permissive hypotension

- Administering 2 liters of crystalloid in hypotensive trauma patients worsens coagulopathy and should be replaced by permissive hypotension
- Normotensive patients receive no fluid resuscitation
- Hypotensive patients have fluid withheld until SBP approaches 80 mm Hg, at which point 250 – 500 ml boluses of blood or plasma are given to maintain SBP between 80 – 90 mmHg
- Avoid > 500 ml of NS for acute blood loss and shock before blood products transfusion started if possible
  - NS used if blood products not readily available
  - Avoid hypertension
  - Use blood warmer
  - Uncrossed match blood for hemorrhagic shock if needed emergently
  - Tranexamic acid 1 gm/10 minutes IV then 1 gm over 8 hours given within first 3 hours of trauma (no faster than 100 mg/minute)

    OR
  - 10 mg/kg IV followed by infusion of 1mg/kg/h
  - Use lab to guide ongoing resuscitation after initial resuscitation if available

Head Trauma

Considerations

- Loss of consciousness (LOC), amnesia, headache, vomiting and seizures have low sensitivity and specificity for detecting intracranial injury
- Cervical spine exam and evaluation important
- Skull films mainly replaced by CT evaluation of head trauma
- Evaluate for significant maxillofacial injuries

Concussion definitions

Grade 1 concussion

- Transient confusion
- No LOC
- Duration of mental status abnormalities < 15 minutes

Grade 2 concussion

- Transient confusion
- No LOC
- Duration of mental status abnormalities > 15 minutes

Grade 3 concussion

- Loss of consciousness

Evaluation

- CT per head injury protocols
- Evaluate for other injuries, especially C-spine
- Retinal exam: for hemorrhages
- Detailed neurologic exam

ENT exam

- Check for hemotympanum
- CSF rhinorrhea
- Battle's sign
- Cranial nerve palsy

CT head scanning rules (choose)

Nexus 2 CT Head Rule (age 1 or greater)

- Any positive below then perform head CT
- Age ≥ 65 years
- Coagulopathy

- Evidence of significant skull fracture
- Scalp hematoma
- Neurologic deficit
- Abnormal behavior
- Altered level of alertness
- Persistent vomiting

New Orleans CT head criteria

- Normal neurologic exam and one of the following
  - Decreased GCS
  - Headache
  - Vomiting
  - Age > 60
  - Persistent anterograde amnesia
  - Drug-alcohol intoxication
  - Visible trauma above the clavicle
  - Seizure

Canadian CT Head Rule

- Any positive below then perform head CT
- GCS < 15 at 2 hours after injury
  - Suspected or open skull fracture
  - Signs of basilar skull fracture
  - Vomiting ≥ 2 episodes
  - Age ≥ 65 years
  - Pre–impact amnesia ≥ 30 minutes
  - Dangerous mechanism

Pecarn Algorithm Age < 2 years

- Order CT head if any positive
  - Abnormal GCS
  - Palpable skull fracture
  - Signs of altered mental status
  - Occipital, parietal or temporal scalp hematoma
  - History of loss of consciousness ≥ 5 seconds
  - Severe mechanism
  - Not acting normally

Pecarn Algorithm Age ≥ 2 years for pediatric head trauma

- Order CT head if any positive
  - Abnormal GCS
  - Palpable skull fracture
  - Signs of altered mental status
  - History of loss of consciousness
  - History of vomiting
  - Severe mechanism
  - Severe headache

Discharge criteria

- Stable condition
- Normal neurologic exam
- No other significant trauma
- No radiologic abnormalities

Discharge instructions

- Head injury aftercare instructions
- Tylenol (no ASA or NSAID's for 36 hours)
- Avoid more potent analgesics so progression of symptoms can be detected
- Return for any neurologic changes
- Follow up with primary care provider or neurologist

Consult criteria

- Age ≥ 70 or < 2 years of age
- Bleeding potential
- Concussions
- Dementia
- Persistent vomiting
- Severe persistent headache
- Focal neurologic deficits
- Inadequate home observation

Neck Trauma

Penetrating neck trauma

- Consult physician unless very superficial laceration
- Do not explore Zone 2 penetrating deep injuries
  - Angle of mandible to cricoid cartilage
  - Consult physician

- Surgical treatment may be needed

Cervical spine trauma

- Leave cervical collar on until patient examined and cleared
- Plain C-spine x-ray 3 views

Exclusionary criteria for C-spine films

- No neurologic deficit
- No distracting injuries
- No evidence of intoxication
- Normal mentation
- No posterior midline tenderness

CT C-spine indications

- Moderate to high risk of cervical fracture
- Significant mechanism of injury
- Fracture on plain C-spine films
- Neurologic deficit or complaint
- Inadequate plain C-spine films
- Severe neck pain with normal plain C-spine films
- Patient will not move neck actively (on their own) without external support of patient's hands ("head in hand sign")
- Obtunded patients
- Facial fractures

Flexion-extension plain films

- Significant pain with negative plain and CT imaging in subacute patients only
- Evaluation for ligamentous instability

Treatment

- C-spine cleared: analgesics and ice packs

Discharge criteria

- Benign cause of neck pain

Discharge instructions

- Neck injury aftercare instructions
- Refer to primary care provider or neurosurgeon within 3 days if not improving
- Avoid discharging with cervical collar if possible

Consult criteria

- Cervical fracture or dislocation/subluxation
- Neurologic deficit or complaint
- Significant pain
- Significant mechanism of injury

Extremity Trauma

- Refer to specific protocols

Lacerations and Cutaneous Wounds

- Refer to Laceration and Cutaneous Wound Protocol

Discharge Criteria for MVA

- No significant injury that needs admission or acute consultation

Discharge Instructions for MVA

- MVA aftercare instructions
- Refer to appropriate physician specialty within 7–10 days as needed

Consult Criteria for MVA

- As in above sections
- Notify physician immediately for suspected severe trauma or bleeding
- Significant injuries or mechanism of injury should be seen by physician initially and throughout length of stay
- Severe pain
- Moderate abdominal pain
- Refer to General Patient Criteria Protocol (page 15)
- Hemorrhage from more than minor simple laceration
- Fractures
- Dislocations
- Neurovascular injuries
- Tendon injuries

Notes

REFERENCES:

Advanced Trauma Life Support

Hemorrhagic Shock Author: John Udeani, MD, FAAEM; Chief Editor: John Geibel, MD, DSc, MA emedicine.medscape.com/article/432650

ACEP Clinical Policy: Neuroimaging and Decisionmaking in Adult Mild Traumatic Brain Injury in the Acute Setting

Head Trauma Treatment & Management
Author: David W Crippen, MD, FCCM; Chief Editor: John Geibel, MD, DSc,
emedicine.medscape.com/article/433855

Closed Head Trauma
Author: Leonardo Rangel-Castilla, MD; Chief Editor: Allen R Wyler, MD emedicine.medscape.com/article/251834

NEJM. 2019;380:763

LACERATION AND CUTANEOUS WOUND PROTOCOL

Considerations

- Scalp lacerations with arterial bleeding can cause shock
  - Suture initially instead of pressure dressings if significant arterial bleeding present
- Tap water (potable) is a safe and cost effective means of wound flushing
- Tissue adhesives, adhesive strips, staples, and hair apposition are cost-effective techniques for wound closure
- Wounds closed with absorbable sutures do not have worse cosmetic outcomes
- Most traumatic wounds do not require antibiotic prophylaxis
- Patients with high-risk bite wounds should receive prophylactic antibiotics

Anesthetics

- There are two major types of local anesthetics: amides and esters — little cross reactivity
- Maximum safe doses of local anesthetics
  - Lidocaine plain — 4.5 mg/kg
    - Lidocaine with epinephrine — 7 mg/kg
  - Marcaine plain — 2 mg/kg
    - Marcaine (bupivacaine) with epinephrine — 3 mg/kg

Duration of anesthesia

- Lidocaine without epinephrine lasts 15 minutes locally
  - Regional block lasts longer
- Lidocaine with epinephrine lasts 2–3
- Marcaine (bupivacaine) lasts 90 minutes to 12 hours

Digital block

- Prep site with betadine alcohol or chlorhexidine
- Volar aspect of hand
- Just proximal to MCP flexion crease (distal palmar flexion crease may be used instead)
- 3-5 ml of lidocaine 1% or 2% with or without epinephrine (half bupivacaine may be used with lidocaine if desired) injected SQ (usually suffices for complete block)
  - Lidocaine with epinephrine is safe in digital blocks as long as no underlying arterial disease

- May take 5–10 minutes to take effect
  - If desired, 3–4 ml SQ may be further injected a distance of 2 cm either side of initial site injection
  - Dorsal SQ injection corresponding opposite volar side may be also performed if needed

Local anesthetic tips

- If lidocaine mixed with $NaHCO_3^-$ in 9:1 ratio (90% lidocaine and 10% $NaHCO_3^-$) it will yield a pH closer to body pH that will not burn with injection
- Warming local anesthetic to body temperature decreases pain of injection
- Topical tetracaine in wound for 20–30 minutes decreases pain of injection and may by itself be superior to local anesthetic injection
- Lidocaine with epinephrine can be used in fingers and toes

Increased infection risk with

- Foreign body
- Crush injury
- Human or animal bite

Lacerations

Sutures

Nonabsorbable (nylon; polypropylene)

- Retains strength > 60 days; low tissue reactivity
- Use 6'0 on face
- Use 4'0 on rest of body
- May use 3'0 on very high tension areas except on face

Absorbable

- Synthetic is less reactive
- Synthetic has increased strength vs. cat gut
- Wound retains 50% of strength in < 1 week to 2 months
- Plain 5'0–6'0 gut sutures can be used to close the skin margins on children's facial lacerations
  - Avoid using plain gut in high tension areas
  - Vicryl retains strength to 21 days which is too long for external facial lacerations
- Vicryl rapide may be used for oral lacerations
- Plain gut retains strength for 4–5 days

Deep sutures

- Helps relieve skin tension
- Decreases dead space and hematoma formation
- May improve cosmetic outcomes
- Recommend liberal use of deep sutures to approximate skin edges before closure with either skin sutures or tissue adhesives

Staples

- Considered for scalp; trunk; extremity lacerations
- When saving time is essential

Tissue adhesives (Dermabond)

- Reduces the need of suturing in up to 1/3 of lacerations
- Sloughs in 7–10 days
- Not to use if skin margins cannot be manually approximated or held together without a lot of tension
- Use 3–4 coats
- Keep out of laceration
- Caution: excessive amount applied can cause too much heat to be released from the exothermic reaction
- Can be removed with bathing, petroleum or antibiotic gel, or acetone if rapid removal necessary
- May take shower after 24 hours, but avoid bathing or swimming until the adhesive

sloughs — usually within 7 days

Evaluation

- Assess for other injuries
- X-ray for foreign bodies or fractures as indicated by history and exam
- Ultrasound may be used to detect foreign bodies depending on level of experience
- Record neurovascular exam prior to anesthesia
- Examine and document any deeper structures involvement
- Tendon involvement or injuries, consult physician
- High pressure injection injuries, consult physician promptly **(do not discharge)**

Treatment Options

Wound preparation

- All foreign material needs to be removed as much as possible
- Flush lacerations deeply with 0.1% betadine sol. (diluted betadine), NS or municipal tap water
  - PSI 5–8 flush is sufficient and superior to high pressure flush, as long as foreign material is removed
  - Flush with at least 50–100 ml/cm of laceration
- Municipal potable tap water is safe and effective to flush wounds (if doubt of water quality then use sterile flush)
  - May have lower infection rate than other methods of flush
- Hemostasis by direct pressure
  - Elevation of extremity helpful with point pressure to stop persistent extremity bleeding

Closure techniques

- Keep wound margins flat or everted with the closure (corner suture may be used for V or X shaped laceration)
- Avoid wound margin inversion
- Partial muscle injury can be closed by using fascia of muscle
- Lacerations with high risk of infection may need to be left partially or fully open
- Steri–strips or tissue adhesive can be used as indicated

Simple Suture

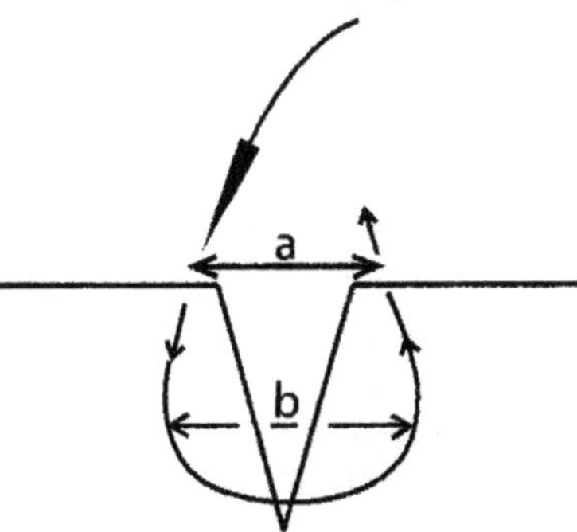

The distance of line (a), the skin entry and exit points, is less than line (b) at the base of the laceration.

- This creates wound eversion which is cosmetically desirable.
- Wound inversion creates a shadow in the laceration site after healing.

Vertical Mattress Suture

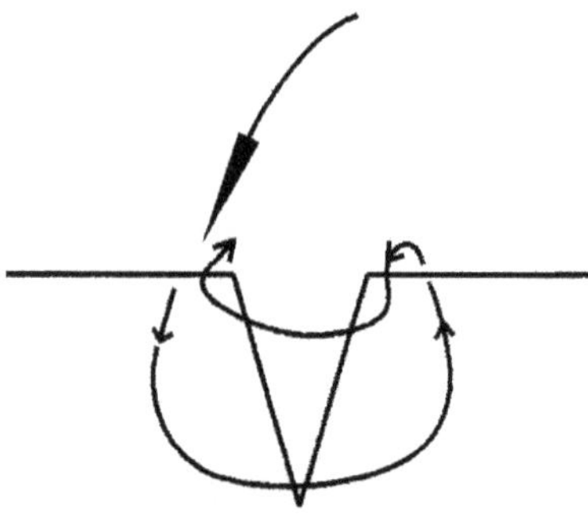

Vertical mattress is used for high tension wounds and when laceration margin eversion is needed.

Antibiotics for

- Tendon or bone involvement
- Septic contamination
- Animal/human bites

Aftercare

- Laceration aftercare instructions
- Sutured or stapled lacerations keep clean and gently cleansed after 24–48 hours
- Sutured or stapled lacerations should be protected with nonadherent dressing for 48 hours
- Air dry lacerations after 48 hours of dressing (cover dressing when in contaminated environment)
- Sutured or stapled laceration infection incidence may be reduced with topical antibiotic ointments
- Splint if there is a fracture or tendon injury and prn otherwise
- No antibiotics for clean, simple lacerations that are not animal or human bites or from a contaminated source

Suture and Staple Removal

- Face 3–5 days
- Neck 4–6 days
- Scalp and trunk 7–10 days
- Upper extremity 10–14 days
- Lower extremity 14–21 days
- Joints 10–21 days

Consult criteria

- Wounds beyond the practitioner's ability to treat
- See General Consult Criteria below

Skin tears

- Common among elderly and long term steroid therapy
- Skin tears can be closed with tissue adhesive if within 8 hours

Class 1 skin tear

- No tissue loss
- Close with surgical tape
- Cover with nonadherent dressing

Class 2 skin tear

- Partial tissue loss
- Manage with absorbent dressings (petroleum based, hydrogels, foams, or hydrocolloids, etc.) for 5–7 days
  - Change daily if needed
  - Use elastic tubular nets to hold in place

Class 3 skin tear

- Complete tissue loss
- Manage same as Class 2 skin tear

Discharge instructions

- Skin tear aftercare instructions
- Follow up with primary care provider or surgeon within 2–5 days as needed

Consult criteria

- Large amount of tissue loss

Plantar puncture wounds

- Rate of cellulitis 2–10%
  - Usually staph or strep
  - Use dicloxicillin or Sanford Guide or other drug databases
- Cleaning alone may be effective
- If foreign body suspected, use plain x-rays if radiopaque, or CT

or ultrasound scan otherwise if needed

- Punctures through sweaty moist tennis shoes carries risk of pseudomonas osteomyelitis
  - May prescribe antipseudomonal antibiotic such as Cipro (ciprofloxacin)
- Frequent cleansing and topical antibiotic as treatment at home
- Do not core out puncture wound

Discharge instructions

- Puncture wound aftercare instructions
- Close follow-up within 2–3 days for suspected deep punctures

Consult criteria

- Neurovascular or bone injury
- Unable to remove foreign body

Subungual hematomas

- Treat with nail trephination (burr hole)
- Nail may be removed for disruption of nail or surrounding nail folds

Discharge instructions

- Subungual hematoma aftercare instructions

General Consult Criteria

- Open fracture
- Neurovascular or tendon injuries or deficits
- Muscle bundle totally severed
- Practitioner is uncomfortable repairing laceration
- Human or animal bites
- Degloving injury

Vital signs and age consult criteria

- Adult heart rate > 110
- SBP < 90 or relative hypotension (SBP < 105 with history of hypertension)

Lab consult criteria

- Acute hemoglobin decrease of > 1 gm or significant blood loss
- Hemoglobin < 10 gm unless chronic and stable
- Thrombocytopenia
- INR > 1.5 if checked

Notes

REFERENCES:

Emergency management of skin and soft tissue wounds : an illustrated guide Ernest N Kaplan; Vincent R Hentz

Weiss EA, Oldham G, Lin M, et al. Water is a safe and effective alternative to sterile normal saline for wound irrigation prior to suturing: a prospective, double-blind, randomised, controlled clinical trial. BMJ Open. 2013;3(1):1-6. (Randomized controlled trial; 663 patients)

Liu JX, Werner JA, Buza JA 3rd, et al. Povidone-iodine solutions inhibit cell migration and survival of osteoblasts, fibroblasts, and myoblasts. Spine (Phila Pa 1976). 2017. (In vitro study

ebmedicine.net/topics.php?paction=showTopic&topic_id=558

Epinephrine in digital nerve block
Emerg Med J. 2007 Nov; 24(11): 789–790.

Bleeding Protocol

Considerations

- Active hemorrhage may be apparent or unsuspected
- Scalp lacerations with arterial bleeding can cause shock

- Suture initially instead of pressure dressings with significant arterial bleeding
- Medical therapy can precipitate or worsen bleeding
- Early coagulopathy in trauma from shock and tissue damage
    - Activated protein C and t-PA released

Estimated Blood and Fluid losses (adults)

	Class I	Class II	Class III	Class IV
Blood loss (cc)	Up to 750	750–1000	1500–2000	> 2000
Blood loss %	Up to 15%	15–30%	30–40%	> 40%
Pulse rate	< 100	> 100	> 120	> 140
Blood pressure	Normal	Normal	SBP < 90	SBP < 70
Capillary refill	Normal	Normal	Delayed	Absent
Pulse pressure	Normal/incr	Decreased	Decreased	Decreased
Respiratory rate	14–20	20–30	30–40	> 35
Urine output (cc/hr.)	> 30	20–30	5–15	Negligible
Mental status	Anxious	Anxious	Confused	Lethargic

(Derived from Advanced Trauma Life Support)

Lethal triad for bleeding (each contributes to the others)

- Hypothermia
- Acidosis
- Coagulopathy

Evaluation

- CBC
- PT/INR/PTT if on anticoagulant or have comorbid conditions contributing to bleeding
- Type and screen or cross depending on level of hemorrhage

Treatment

- Direct pressure of bleeding site for 2–5 minutes if actively bleeding when possible
- Tourniquet for exsanguination from extremities where direct pressure ineffective

Blood/fluid replacement for hemorrhage

- May use uncrossed matched blood if transfusion needed immediately (O neg)
- PRBC's/FFP/platelets 1:1:1 ratio (recommendations range from 4:1:1 to 1:1:1)
    - 1:1:1 ratio yields estimated hematocrit of 29%, platelet count of 90,000 and coagulation factors 62% of whole blood
- Avoid > 1 liter of isotonic fluids for acute blood loss before blood products transfusion started if possible
- Avoid hypertension
- Target systolic blood pressure of 80-90 mm Hg until major bleeding stopped
- Target Hgb of 7-9 g/dl after termination of major bleeding
- Pediatric: 20 cc/kg IV NS bolus, start blood and plasma for continued hypotension and bleeding
- Use blood warmer
- Uncrossed match blood for hemorrhagic shock if needed emergently
- Tranexamic acid 1 gm/10 minutes IV then 1 gm every 8 hours (no faster than 100 mg/minute)
    - Give within first 3 hours of trauma

OR

- 10 mg/kg followed by infusion of 1 mg/kg/hour
- Use lab to guide ongoing resuscitation after initial resuscitation

Reversal of anticoagulation

Elevated INR for patient on warfarin (vitamin K antagonists)

- INR 4.5–10 without bleeding — no vitamin K treatment
  - Hold warfarin until in therapeutic range
- INR > 10 without bleeding give oral vitamin K 5–10 mg
  - Hold warfarin until in therapeutic range
- INR 2–3 will be normal after holding warfarin for 4–5 days
  - Warfarin half-life is 1.5–2 days
- For major bleeding — see below

Warfarin reversal

- Major bleeding give 4 factor prothrombin complex concentrate (Kcentra) if available over FFP
- Vitamin K 10 mg IV over 10 minutes (not faster than 1 mg/minute) or IM/SQ/PO prn — time of onset for vitamin K 1–2 hours parenterally and 6–12 hours PO with normal clotting factor synthesis
- **FFP** 10–15mL/kg — FFP unit usually is 250 mL
  - FFP INR is 1.5
  - Onset of action 13 – 48 hours
  - No clinical benefit in using if INR<1.7
- FEIBA 500 units (Factor VIII inhibitor bypassing activity) when INR was < 5 or 1,000 units of FEIBA when INR was ≥ 5

Heparin reversal

- Protamine 1 mg IV for each 100 units of heparin given to reverse anticoagulation prn
  - Do not exceed 50 mg in a single dose

Timing for dosage

- Heparin given
  - < 30 minutes ago — protamine 1U/100U heparin
  - 30–60 minutes — protamine 0.75U/100U heparin
  - 60–120 minutes — protamine 0.5U/100U heparin
  - > 120 minutes give protamine 0.25U/100U heparin

Low Molecular Weight Heparin

- Last dose < 4 hours give protamine 1 mg for each 1 mg of enoxaparin
  - If bleeding continues give ½ the dose in 4 hours
- Last dose 4–8 hours ago give 0.5 mg for each 1 mg of enoxaparin

t-PA reversal

- No universal accepted guideline (empirical)
- Cryoprecipitate 0.15 U/kg if fibrinogen < 150 mg/dL
- Tranexamic acid 1000 mg IV/10minutes (inhibits plasminogen activation) — no faster than 100 mg/minute
- Platelet transfusion for platelet count < 100,000 or platelet dysfunction suspected

Dabigatran (thrombin inhibitor)

- Half-life 14–16 hours
- Praxbind (idarucizumab) is reversal agent (for life threatening bleeding or uncontrolled bleeding)
- Supportive care
- Activated charcoal if dabigatran taken within past 2 hours
- Hemodialysis

Other direct Xa inhibitors (DOAC'S) rivaroxaban or apixaban reversal

Andexxa low dose

- Initial IV bolus: 400 mg IV; target infusion rate of 30 mg/min
- Follow-on IV infusion: 4 mg/min IV for up to 120 min

Andexxa high dose

- Initial IV bolus: 800 mg IV; target infusion rate of 30 mg/min
- Follow-on IV infusion: 8 mg/min IV for up to 120 min

Andexxa dose based on rivaroxaban or apixaban dosing

- Use low dose described above
  - Rivaroxaban dose ≤10 mg (any timing from last dose)
  - Apixaban dose ≤5 mg (any timing from last dose)
  - Rivaroxaban >10 mg or dose unknown (≥8 hr from last dose)
  - Apixaban >5 mg or dose unknown (≥8 hr from last dose)
- Use high dose described above
  - Rivaroxaban >10 mg or dose unknown (<8 hr from last dose or unknown)
  - Apixaban >5 mg or dose unknown (<8 hr from last dose or unknown)

Treatment considerations

- Rivaroxaban half-life ~ 5 - 13 hours
  - Andexxa — Coagulation factor Xa recombinant, inactivated-zhzo (for life threatening bleeding or uncontrolled bleeding)
    - Very expensive — hospital pharmacies may not stock
    - Half-life of Andexxa is far shorter than the FXa inhibitors (onset of action within 2 minutes)
    - Anti-FXa activity starts to resume to baseline after the 2-hour infusion and goes back to the baseline by 4 hours after drug initiation, so further bleeding may resume
    - Prothrombotic
      - Arterial and venous thromboembolic events
      - Ischemic events, including AMI and stroke
      - Cardiac arrest
      - Sudden death
- Apixaban half-life ~ 8 - 15 hours
  - Andexxa — Coagulation factor Xa recombinant, inactivated-zhzo (for life threatening bleeding or uncontrolled bleeding)
    - Very expensive — hospital pharmacies may not stock
    - Half-life of Andexxa is far shorter than the FXa inhibitors (onset of action within 2 minutes)
    - Anti-FXa activity starts to resume to baseline after the 2-hour infusion and goes back to the baseline by 4 hours after drug initiation, so further bleeding may resume
    - Prothrombotic
      - Arterial and venous thromboembolic events
      - Ischemic events, including AMI and stroke
      - Cardiac arrest
      - Sudden death
- Consider PCC (Kcentra prothrombin complex concentrate or recombinant activated factor VII) if Andexxa not available for life threatening bleeding (not a specific antidote)
- Normal PT rules out significant clinical effect

Admission criteria recommendation

- Massive ingestion of anticoagulant
- Long acting anticoagulant
  - Hydroxycoumadin > 0.05 mg
  - Indandione > 5 mg
  - Warfarin > 0.5 mg/kg
- Rapid or severe increase in PT
- Any significant bleeding
- Risk of falls

Discharge criteria recommendation

- Bleeding without effect on vital signs or hemoglobin level
- Further significant bleeding unlikely
- No coagulopathy

Consult criteria recommendation

- Significant bleeding
- SBP < 90 or relative hypotension (SBP < 110 with history of hypertension)
- Significant tachycardia

Notes

REFERENCES:

Advanced Trauma Life Support

Saver JL. Stroke 2007;38(8):2279–2283

French KF, et al. Neurocrit Care 2012;17(1):107–111

Fugate JE, et al. Mayo Clin Proc, epub, April 28 2014

Hirsh J, Warkentin TE, Shaughnessy SG, et al. Chest 2001;119:64S-94S

Borgman J Trauma 2007: 63; 805
Chest 2012;141(2_suppl):e152S-e184S
JEM, Vol. 45, pg. 467

https://reference.medscape.com/drug/eliquis-apixaban-999805#5

https://reference.medscape.com/drug/xarelto-rivaroxaban-999670#5

https://reference.medscape.com/drug/pradaxa-dabigatran-342135#5

Hemorrhagic Shock in Emergency Medicine Guidelines
Updated: May 06, 2016 Author: William P Bozeman, MD; Chief Editor: Trevor John Mills, MD, MPH

Rossaint R, Bouillon B, Cerny V, Coats TJ, Duranteau J, Fernández-Mondéjar E, et al. The European guideline on management of major bleeding and coagulopathy following trauma: fourth edition. *Crit Care*. 2016 Apr 12. 20 (1):100

JEM, epub, 3/20319

Key Points to Consider When Evaluating Andexxa for Formulary Addition
Harry Peled, Nhu Quyen Dau and Helen Lau

BURN PROTOCOL

Considerations

- In children consider child abuse
- Electrical burns may be much worse than suspected
- Evaluate airway and pulmonary system with enclosed building fire or with facial burns
- Consider possible carbon monoxide and cyanide poisoning in enclosed areas
- Difficult to tell difference between deep second degree burn and third degree burn
- Second degree deep partial thickness burn can become a third degree burn
- Body surface area (BSA) of burn use rule of 9's or the palmer surface of patient is approximately 1% BSA
- Rule of nines for BSA burned is for patients ≥10 years of age
- Depth of burn frequently underestimated
- Size of burn frequently overestimated

- Carbon monoxide (CO) has affinity for hemoglobin 230 times that of oxygen
  - Pulse oximetry not accurate in CO poisoning
  - Treat with 100% oxygen

Burn depth

First degree

- Epidermis only; no blisters
- Sensation — painful
- Bleeding on pinprick — brisk
- Appearance — light red and dry
- Blanching to pressure — brisk

Second degree superficial partial thickness

- Dermis involved with blisters
- Sensation — painful
- Bleeding on pinprick — brisk
- Appearance — moist and pink
- Blanching to pressure — slow return

Second degree deep partial thickness

- Dermis involved with blisters
- Sensation — dull
- Bleeding on pinprick — delayed
- Appearance — mottled pink or red; waxy white
- Blanching to pressure — none

Third degree full thickness

- Sensation — none
- No bleeding on pinprick
- Appearance — white, charred and dry
- Blanching to pressure — none

Fourth degree

- Involves muscle, fascia or bone

Thermal Burns

Evaluation

Enclosed space fire with smoke

- Airway evaluation
- O_2 saturation
- CO (carbon monoxide) level
- CBC
- BMP
- Lactic acid
- Chest x-ray
- Notify physician promptly

BSA burn < 10%

- Physical exam usually all that is needed if no smoke inhalation history or findings

Treatment options

- Clean with soap and water
- Cool burn with cold tap water
  - Decreases pain
  - Decreases depth and extent of injury
  - Do not use ice or ice water

Blister management

- Leave blisters intact ≤ 3 cm in size
  - Heals faster
- Totally debride any ruptured blisters
- May sterilely aspirate blisters > 3 cm

First degree burns

- Aloe vera and NSAIDs can be used for 1st burns

Superficial 2nd degree burns

- Topical antibiotic or absorptive occlusive dressing
  - Absorptive occlusive dressing is less painful and results in faster healing than antibiotic ointment

Deep 2nd and 3rd degree burns

- Topical antibiotic and refer to surgeon
- Silvadene (silver sulfadiazine) ointment qday for 5–7 days (not on face)
- Aquacel dressing superior to plain Silvadene in healing burns and reducing pain and may be used instead (releases silver sulfadiazine slowly)

Parkland formula for IV fluid resuscitation

- 4 ml NS x kg x % BSA burned in 24 hours
  - Give ½ IVF in first 8 hours
  - Give rest of NS in following 16 hours
  - If patient presents, for example, 2 hours after burn, then give first ½ of IVF in 6 hours (8 hours-2 hours)

Tetanus prophylaxis

- Tetanus toxoid (ADT) or Tdap 0.5 cc IM if last dose > 5 years
- Tetanus immune globulin 250–500 units IM at different site if < 3 or unknown previous tetanus immunizations
- Refer to health department or primary care provider to complete tetanus primary vaccination series if < 2 vaccines given in past
  - See Tetanus Protocol

Discharge criteria

- First degree burns
- Second degree superficial burns < 15% in adults and < 10% in children age 10 or less

Discharge instructions for burns

- Burn aftercare instructions
- Wash burn with soap and water qday and change dressing qday for 5–7 days
- Facial burns use triple antibiotic ointment or polysporin ointment 5–7 days
- Antibiotic PO or IM not usually needed
- Pain treatment with NSAID's and/or narcotics prn (hydrocodone, oxycodone)

Consult criteria

- Second degree superficial burns ≥ 10% in adults and 5% or greater in children
- Deep second degree and third degree burns unless extremely small (<2 cm)
- Burns involving hand; joints; perineum; genitalia; face; eyes; ears
- Comorbid conditions such diabetes, immunosuppression
- Circumferential burns
- Age < 12 months
- All inhalation injuries
- Carbon monoxide poisoning

Electrical Burns

Considerations

- Household electrical injury can be lethal
- Difficult to estimate degree of injury
- Causes tetany of muscles
- Traumatic injuries common (falls)

Compartment syndrome

- From increased pressure in a muscle or other internal compartment
- Not all signs and symptoms are needed to make diagnosis
- High pressures > 8 hours leads to tissue damage
- Normal tissue pressure is < 10 mm Hg
- Capillary blood flow is compromised at > 20 mm Hg
- Intracompartmental pressures > 30 mm Hg or within 10–30 mm Hg of DBP

Signs and symptoms (not diagnostic)

- Pain
  - Out of proportion to injury
  - On passive stretch of muscles
- Pallor
- Paresthesias
- Paralysis
  - Sensory and motor findings are late signs
- Poikilothermia — decreased temperature
- Pulselessness
  - Usually not lost until muscle necrosis has occurred

  - Last sign to develop
- Tense muscle compartment on palpation

Treatment

- Consult physician if suspected
- Keep extremity at level of heart
- Do not use ice if suspected
- Remove cast and padding
- Surgery fasciotomy is usually necessary

Evaluation

- Complete history and physical exam
- Degree of burn and voltage
- Length of time of electrical injury
- Neurologic exam
- EKG and monitor
- CBC
- BMP
- CPK
- U/A for myoglobin if hemoglobin dipstick positive
- Serum myoglobin if U/A positive for hemoglobin

Treatment options

- Treat skin burns same as thermal injuries
- IV NS 200 cc/hr. if significant burn injury or suspicion for significant injury for adults and 2 times maintenance rate for pediatrics
- Tetanus toxoid (ADT) 0.5 cc IM if last dose > 5 years
- Tetanus immune globulin 250–500 units IM different site if < 3 or unknown history of previous tetanus immunizations
- Refer to health department or primary care provider to complete tetanus primary vaccination series if < 2 vaccines given in past
  - See Tetanus Protocol
- Pain treatment with NSAID's and/or narcotics prn

Discharge criteria

- Low voltage superficial injury
- Normal lab, EKG and vital signs
- Small burn area
- Follow up with primary care provider or plastic surgeon within 2–3 days

Discharge instructions for burns

- Wash burn with soap and water qday and change dressing qday for 5–7 days
- Burn aftercare instructions
- Facial burns use triple antibiotic ointment or polysporin ointment 5–7 days
- Antibiotic PO or IM not usually needed
- Pain treatment with NSAID's and/or narcotics prn (hydrocodone, oxycodone)

Consult criteria

- Loss of consciousness
- Neurologic abnormalities
- High voltage burns
- Abnormal lab, EKG or vital signs
- Large burns or suspected deep tissue injury
- Uncertainty of the extent of injury
- Suspected compartment syndrome

Chemical Burns

Considerations

- Alkali cause deeper injury
- Acids cause more superficial injury usually, depending on pH

Evaluation

- Usually all that is needed is history and physical exam for minor chemical burns

Treatment

- Remove chemical from skin
- Clean with soap and water
- Flush or soak with NS if alkali burn
- Pain treatment with NSAID's and/or narcotics prn

Hydrofluoric acid (HFl) burns

- Intense pain and tissue damage

- Use copious irrigation followed by calcium gluconate gel
- Subcutaneous calcium gluconate may be needed to relieve pain
- TBSA (total body surface area) burn > 5% needs admission to monitor for the development of hypocalcemia
    - If HFI concentration > 50% then 1% TBSA burn needs admission

Tetanus prophylaxis

- Tetanus toxoid (ADT) or Tdap 0.5 cc IM if last dose > 5 years
- Tetanus immune globulin 250–500 units IM different site if < 3 or unknown history of previous tetanus immunizations
- Refer to health department or primary care provider to complete tetanus primary vaccination series if < 2 vaccines given in past
    - See Tetanus Protocol

Discharge criteria

- Minor chemical burns

Discharge instructions for burns

- Wash burn with soap and water qday and change dressing qday for 5–7 days
- Burn aftercare instructions
- Facial burns use triple antibiotic ointment or polysporin ointment 5–7 days
- Antibiotic PO or IM not usually needed
- Pain treatment with NSAID's and/or narcotics prn (hydrocodone, oxycodone)

Consult criteria

- Hydrofluoric acid burns
- Abnormal vital signs
- Diabetes or immunosuppression
- Second degree superficial burns ≥ 10% in adults and 5% or greater in children
- Second degree deep and third degree burns
- Burns involving hand, joints, perineum, genitalia
- Comorbid conditions such diabetes, immunosuppression
- Carbon monoxide poisoning

Vital sign and age consult criteria for all burn types

- Hypotension or relative hypotension (SBP < 105 with history of hypertension)
- Inappropriate sinus tachycardia
- Volume depletion

Notes

REFERENCES:

Guyton AC. Combination of Hemoglobin with Carbonmonoxide. In. Textbook of Medical Physiology. 7th ed. W.B. Saunders Co; 1986:500

Thermal Injury Management
Author: Robert L Sheridan, MD; Chief Editor: Jorge I de la Torre, MD, FACS
emedicine.medscape.com/article/1277941

Thermal Burns Author: Richard F Edlich, MD, PhD, FACS, FASPS, FACEP; Chief Editor: Jorge I de la Torre, MD, FACS
emedicine.medscape.com/article/1278244

Extremity Disorders

Section Contents

When using any protocol, always follow the Guidelines of Proper Use (page 12).

Extremity Medical Disorder Protocol

Differential Diagnosis

Painful extremity swelling

- Deep venous thrombosis
- Arterial insufficiency
- Tendonitis, bursitis, and arthritis
- Cellulitis
- Abscess
- Septic arthritis
- Gout
- Radiculopathy
- Peripheral neuropathy

Nonpainful extremity swelling

- Congestive heart failure
- Hepatic cirrhosis
- Post-phlebitic syndrome

General Evaluation

- Complete history and physical exam
- Symptom(s) onset and exacerbating factors
- Associated symptoms
- Neurovascular exam
- Document whether Homan's sign and calf tenderness is positive or negative — Homan's sign not clinically useful, but decreases litigation if documented and is negative regardless of ultimate diagnosis of PE

Deep Venous Thrombosis (see VTE chapter)

Well's DVT criteria

- One point each:
  - Active cancer
  - Paralysis/recent cast immobilization
  - Recently bedridden > 3 days or surgery < 4 weeks
  - Deep vein tenderness
  - Entire leg edema
  - Calf swelling > 3 cm over other leg
  - Pitting edema > other calf
  - Collateral superficial veins
- Two points — alternative diagnosis less likely

High probability: ≥ 3 points

Moderate probability: 1–2 points

Low probability: 0 points

Evaluation

D-dimer

- Useful if negative at cutoff value to rule out DVT or PE
- Negative D-dimer with low to moderate probability Well's DVT score largely excludes venous thromboembolic disease
- Well's criteria high probability: order ultrasound scan regardless of D-dimer result
- Positive — not as useful as negative result which usually rules out VTE disease
  - Frequently positive with hospitalization in past month
  - Chronic bedridden or low activity state
  - Increasingly positive with age without significant acute disease process
    - CHF
    - Chronic disease processes
    - Edematous states
  - D-dimer increases 10 mcg/L for every year over 50 years of age if the upper cutoff is 500 mcg/L (80 year old with d-dimer 700 mcg/L would be in the normal range)
  - If another assay used, then 2% increase/year over age 50 may be used to adjust upper normal limit for age

Well's DVT criteria ≥ 1–2 with painful or swollen extremity

- Order D-dimer test (unless patient likely to have positive result regardless of DVT potential)
- Venous Doppler ultrasound of extremity (unless D-dimer negative)
- Venography if needed
- MRI if needed
- Coumadin (warfarin) therapy can cause falsely negative D-dimer

Discharge criteria

- Well's DVT criteria low probability
- Negative D-dimer (can be falsely negative with warfarin therapy)
- Negative ultrasound (may need to be repeated in 1 week if symptoms persist)

Discharge instructions

- Leg pain aftercare instructions

- Follow up with primary care provider in 3–5 days if pain persists
- Return if worse

Consult criteria

- DVT diagnosis
- Suspected DVT diagnosis
- Severe pain

Peripheral Arterial Disease

- Pain worse with activity
- Risk factors same as with coronary disease

Ankle brachial index (ABI)

- Systolic blood pressure at ankle divided by systolic blood pressure in arm
- Normal 0.9–1.1
- Worsening PAD yields decreasing ABI
- Diabetes can interfere with test due to calcinosis

Discharge criteria

- Stable claudication
- Pain resolved
- ASA 81–325 mg PO each day
- Smoking cessation
- Refer to surgeon

Discharge instructions

- PAD aftercare instructions
- Follow up with PCP or general surgeon within 3–5 days

Consult criteria

- Continuous pain
- Severe pain as presenting complaint
- Limb discoloration
- Heart rate > 100
- Hypotension
- Absent pulse
- Decreased temperature to touch

Cellulitis and Abscess

- See Cellulitis and Abscess Protocols

Septic Arthritis

Differential diagnosis

- Cellulitis
- Gout
- Bursitis
- Osteomyelitis
- Rheumatoid arthritis
- Soft tissue injury
- Pseudogout

Considerations

- Rapid onset
- Usually one joint infected
- Joint is very painful; hot; red; fluctuant
- Signs of acute systemic illness may be present
- Fever, chills and sweats frequently present
- See Synovial Fluid Analysis if joint fluid obtained

Prosthetic joint infections

- Usually needs surgery and prolonged antibiotic treatment
- Early symptoms
  - Erythema, pain, swelling and delayed wound healing may be present
- May occur years after surgery
  - May present with chronic pain and prosthesis looseness
- Suspect if
  - Sinus tract present
  - Drainage from joint
  - Acute onset of pain
  - Chronic pain that develops after prosthetic surgery especially if there was a pain free period after surgery
  - History of wound healing problems or infection after surgery

Evaluation

- History and physical examination
  - Evaluate knee for range of motion as tolerated
- ESR or C-reactive protein (CRP) when diagnosis not clinically evident (significant false positive rate and is nonspecific)

- Combination of ESR and CRP has better sensitivity and specificity
- CBC
- BMP if diabetic
- Knee films
  - May show other reasons for pain and can be used as a baseline after procedures
- Ultrasound can be considered
- Joint aspiration if provider experienced
- Joint fluid analysis — see specific protocol

Treatment

- Admission to hospital for drainage and antibiotics

Discharge criteria

- Only with physician consent

Consult criteria

- All septic joint or suspected septic joint patients

Gout

Differential diagnosis

- Cellulitis
- Septic arthritis
- Bursitis
- Osteomyelitis
- Rheumatoid arthritis
- Soft tissue injury
- Pseudogout

Considerations

- Crystal uric acid deposits in joints and tissues
- Most common cause of monoarticular arthritis age > 60
- Increased warmth, redness and joint swelling
- First metatarsophalangeal joint of foot 75% of cases — most common
- Joint fluid: 20,000–100,000 WBC; poor string and mucin clot test; no bacteria (pseudogout similar)
- Risk factors
  - Age > 40
  - Hypertension
  - Diuretics
  - Ethanol intake
  - Obesity
- Initially with urate lowering therapy there is an increase in acute gout attacks
  - Patients should be reassured that this is expected and they should not discontinue their new medications

Evaluation

- Clinical evaluation usually all that is needed
- If diagnosis uncertain: CBC, C-reactive protein,
  x-rays, joint aspiration

Treatment options (monotherapy)

- NSAID's high dose 5–10 days
  - Narcotics IM or PO prn
- Prednisone 40–60 mg PO qday × 3–7 days

OR

- Dexamethasone 6 mg PO daily × 3–7 days

OR

- Depomedrol (methylprednisolone acetate) 80–120 mg IM
- Can consider intra-articular steroids if attack involves 1–2 large joints – if experienced with joint injections
- Colchicine 2 tablets (1.2 mg) with a third tablet (0.6 mg) an hour later, then qday–bid until attack resolves
  - Only for acute attacks < 36 hours
  - Do not use if patient used colchicine within last 14 days
- Allopurinol 50–300 mg PO qday: adjusted for renal function; start after acute episode resolved

Severe attacks use combination of treatments

- Do not stop urate lowering therapy during an acute attack - symptoms would only worsen if it is stopped or adjusted

- Switch to another treatment or add a second treatment if < 20% improvement in pain score within 24 hours, or < 50% improvement in pain score > 24 hours

Discharge criteria

- Uncomplicated acute gout attack

Discharge instructions

- Gout aftercare instructions
- Follow up with primary care provider within 2–3 days if pain persists

Consult criteria

- Uncertain diagnosis
- Fever history or toxicity
- Tachycardia

Radiculopathy

Lumbar radiculopathy (sciatica)

- Complete history and physical examination
- Check reflexes, SLR (straight leg raise), and neurovascular exam
- Spinal cord compression signs
  - Urinary retention with overflow incontinence or voiding
  - Fecal incontinence, decreased rectal tone and perineal sensation (i.e., cauda equina syndrome — see Back Pain Protocol)
  - Unilateral sciatica more common than bilateral sciatica in cauda equina syndrome
- Healthy non-elderly patients without direct blunt trauma usually need no tests
- Elderly frequently need spine films due to higher incidence of vertebral fractures
- Plain back/pelvic films may be needed in falls, MVC's, direct blunt trauma, depending on severity of injury mechanism
- U/A if renal disease suspected or significant injury mechanism
- D-dimer or CTA if aortic dissection considered
- CBC, C-RP (or ESR) for fever with isolated vertebral back pain only without associated symptoms or findings

CT scan of spine

- Compression fracture > 30%
- Burst fracture
- Posterior vertebral involvement
- For back pain out of proportion on exam

- MRI for spinal cord findings or symptoms

Treatment options

- NSAID's prn
- Dexamethasone 6 mg PO qday for 5–10 days prn pain (caution if diabetic)
- Gabapentin 100 mg qHS, may increase slowly over 2 days up to 300 mg to 600 mg tid as needed and tolerated
- Short narcotic course prn for severe pain — avoid Demerol (meperidine)
- Preferable to minimize bed rest (limit bed rest to no more than 1–2 days if possible, unless a fracture is present)
- Avoid heavy lifting
- Muscle relaxants of questionable usefulness
- Refer as needed to Pain Management (anesthesiologist or neurosurgeon or orthopedic spine surgeon

Piriformis syndrome

- Neuritis of the proximal sciatic nerve, results from compression or irritation of the sciatic nerve by the piriformis muscle due to spasm and/or contracture
- Thought to be the cause of 5–6% of sciatic nerve radicular symptoms
- Piriformis muscle spasm often is detected by careful, deep palpation
- Reproduction of sciatica-type pain with weakness results from resisted abduction/external rotation (Pace test)

- Freiberg test is a diagnostic sign that elicits pain upon forced internal rotation of the extended thigh
- Beatty maneuver reproduces buttock pain by selectively contracting the piriformis muscle
- Point tenderness at the lateral margin of the sacrum may be present
- Difficulty sitting due to an intolerance of weight bearing on the buttock

Evaluation

- Diagnostic ultrasound imaging of the piriformis muscle for abnormalities
- Imaging of the lumbar spine may be helpful in excluding associated diskogenic and/or osteoarthritic contributing pathology
- MR neurography to evaluate for piriformis muscle asymmetry and sciatic nerve hyperintensity at the sciatic notch with 93% specificity

Treatment

- Home stretching program
  - Involved hip flexed and passively adducted/internally rotated
- Piriformis muscle may be injected with steroids and/or local anesthetics using a 3.5-inch (8.9-cm) spinal needle after piriformis muscle localized avoiding direct injection of the sciatic nerve
  - Manually by digital rectal examination or palpating the buttocks
  - Fluoroscopic or ultrasonographic imaging guidance can significantly enhance the effectiveness of the piriformis muscle injection
  - Best performed by specialist
- Physical therapy
- Botulinum toxin
- NSAID's
- Muscle relaxants
  - Dexamethasone 6 mg PO qday for 5–10 days prn pain (caution if diabetic)
  - Gabapentin 100 mg qHS, may increase slowly over 2 days up to 300 mg to 600 mg tid as needed and tolerated

Discharge Criteria for sciatica

- Uncomplicated presentation and findings with ability to control pain and ambulate

Discharge instructions

- Back pain aftercare instructions
- Refer to primary care provider
- If HNP suspected: neurosurgery or orthopedic or pain management (anesthesiology) referral
- Orthopedic referral for fractures

Consult Criteria

- Severe pain with inability to ambulate
- Progressive neurologic deficits
- Signs of cauda equina syndrome
  - Urinary retention is most common finding in cauda equina syndrome
  - Patients without urinary retention have an approximately 1/10,000 chance of having cauda equina syndrome
  - Normal rectal tone usually excludes cauda equina syndrome
  - Saddle numbness
  - Extreme weakness
  - Unilateral sciatica more common than bilateral sciatica in cauda equina syndrome
- Signs of spinal cord impairment
- Evidence of infectious, vascular, or neoplastic etiologies
- Nontraumatic pediatric back pain
- Fracture
- New onset renal insufficiency or worsening renal insufficiency

Cervical Radiculopathy

Definition

- Compression on cervical spine nerve roots

Considerations

- C7 compression involved 60% of cases
- C6 compression involved 25% of cases
- Younger patients have HNP or injury causing foraminal impingement on nerve root
- Elderly have degenerative changes causing foraminal narrowing and nerve compression

Physical findings

Motor deficits

- C5 — weakness of shoulder abduction
- C6 — weakness of elbow flexion and wrist extension
- C7 — weakness of elbow extension and wrist flexion
- C8 — weakness of thumb extension and wrist ulnar deviation

Sensory dermatomes

- C6 — thumb
- C7 — middle finger
- C8 — little finger
- T1 — inner forearm
- T2 — upper inner arm

Deep tendon reflexes (DTR)

- Biceps DTR tests C5–C6
  - Antecubital fossa
- Brachioradialis reflex test C5–C6
  - Distal radius
- Triceps DTR tests C7–C8
  - Distal triceps tendon posterior and slightly above elbow

Evaluation

- History and physical examination
- Check reflexes, hand grip, shoulder strength and neurovascular exam
- Cervical spine films may be obtained
- Healthy non-elderly patients without direct blunt trauma usually need no tests immediately

Treatment options

- Local ice therapy
- NSAID's
- Dexamethasone 6 mg PO qday for 5–10 days prn pain (caution if diabetic)
- Gabapentin 100 mg qHS, may increase slowly over 2 days up to 300 mg to 600 mg tid as needed and tolerated
- Hydrocodone or oxycodone prn severe pain short course
- Semirigid cervical collar for 3–6 weeks prn
- Physical therapy
- Home exercises

Discharge criteria

- Most patients can be discharged home

Discharge instructions

- Cervical radiculopathy aftercare instructions
- Referral to Pain Management (anesthesiologist) or neurosurgeon or orthopedic spine surgeon within 7–14 days as needed

Consult criteria

- Incapacitating pain
- Central spinal cord compression symptoms
  - Loss of anal sphincter tone
  - Loss of bladder control
  - Weakness of arms and legs
- Central cord syndrome
  - Arms weaker than legs

Peripheral Neuropathy (PN)

Definition

- Disorder of peripheral nerves

Causes

- Usually as a complication of diabetes or alcoholism
- HIV

- Lyme disease
- Guillain–Barre' syndrome
- Cancer (paraneoplastic syndromes)
- Hypothyroidism
- Herpes zoster
- Acute nerve root compression
- Renal failure
- Heavy metal poisoning (lead, etc.)
- Nutritional deficiency
- Idiopathic

Evaluation

- Complete history and physical exam
- Motor and sensory exam
  - Gross light touch and pinprick sensation
  - Vibratory sense; deep tendon reflexes
  - Strength testing and muscle atrophy
  - Dorsal pedal and posterior tibial pulses
  - Skin assessment
  - Tinel testing
  - Cranial nerve testing
- Usually no lab testing needed in chronic neuropathy
- Acute neuropathy warrants tests directed at possible causes
  - CMP
  - C-reactive protein
  - CBC
  - Lyme titers if indicated
  - TSH if indicated
  - Lead levels if suspected
  - Chest x-ray if sarcoidosis or lung cancer suspected
  - LP if Guillain–Barre' syndrome suspected

Treatment options

- Symptomatic pain treatment
  - NSAID's
  - Capsaicin cream (depletes and prevents reaccumulation of substance P)
  - Lidocaine tape
  - Gabapentin 900 mg/day initially, then increase as needed every 3 days up to 1800–3600 mg qday
  - Carbamazepine 100–200 mg qday, and may increase slowly up to 1200 mg/day as needed, if above does not work
  - Phenytoin (Dilantin)
  - Amitriptyline
  - Pregabalin
  - Duloxetine (Cymbalta) 60 mg qday
  - Citalopram (Celexa) 20–40 mg qday
- Treatment directed at underlying cause if possible

Discharge criteria

- Stable chronic peripheral neuropathy

Discharge instructions

- Peripheral neuropathy aftercare instructions
- Follow up with PCP or neurologist as needed for chronic PN
- Follow up for acute neuropathy within 1 day

Consult criteria

- Acute neuropathy from a high comorbidity disease process or from an unknown cause

Fibromyalgia

- Widespread chronic musculoskeletal pain and tenderness
- Associated with fatigue, sleep and mood disturbances
- Noninflammatory
- Cause unknown
- Females most commonly
- Lab testing used to rule out other disorders

Treatment choices

- Mirtazapine 15–30 mg daily
- Amitriptyline 10 mg qHS, increase 5 mg q2weeks
- Desipramine (fewer anticholinergic side effects)
- Duloxetine 20–30 mg qAM, increase to 60 mg if needed (treat exhaustion)

- Pregabalin 30 mg qHS, may increase as tolerated
- Gabapentin 100 mg qHS, may increase slowly over 2 days up to 300 mg to 600 mg tid as needed and tolerated

Nonpainful Extremity Swelling

- Treat underlying condition if feasible
- Elevation
- Compression hose
- Follow up with primary care provider
- Judicious diuretic short term use with caution

General Consult Criteria for Extremity Conditions

- Severe pain
- Acute and progressive arterial insufficiency
- Rapidly spreading rash or cellulitis
- Pain out of proportion to exam
- Crepitus or gas in tissues
- Systemic toxic appearance
- Hypotension or relative hypotension SBP < 105 in patient with hypertension history
- Necrotizing fasciitis or gas gangrene
- Large abscess
- Suspected bony involvement
- Immunocompromised

Vital signs and age consult criteria

- Fever ≥ 101°F (39°C) in cellulitis
- Adult heart rate ≥ 110
- SBP < 90 or relative hypotension (SBP < 105 with history of hypertension)
- Orthostatic vital signs
- O_2 Sat ≤ 94% on room air
- Moderate dyspnea

Lab consult criteria

- Adult: WBC > 15,000 or < 1,000 neutrophils
- Bandemia ≥ 15%
- Acute thrombocytopenia
- Acute anemia

Notes

REFERENCES:

Osmon DR, et al. Clin Infect Dis 2013 Jan;56(1):1–10

Khanna D, et al. Arthritis Care Res 2012 Oct;64 (10):1447–61

Harrold L. Curr Opin Rheumatol 2013 May;25(3):304–9

Diabetic Neuropathy Author: Helen C Lin, MD;
Chief Editor: Romesh Khardori, MD, PhD, FACP
emedicine.medscape.com/article/1170337

Age-Adjusted D–Dimer Cutoff Levels to Rule Out Pulmonary Embolism: The Adjust–PE Study JAMA 2014;311(11):1117– 1124
doi:10.1001/jama.2014.2135

FRACTURE PROTOCOL

Considerations

- Complications
  - Neurovascular injury
  - Open fracture
  - Joint involvement
  - Ligament/tendon injury
  - Displaced and angulated
  - Compartment syndrome
  - Fat emboli — long bones
  - Avascular necrosis
  - Osteomyelitis

- Nondisplaced, closed simple long bone fractures usually can be splinted and discharged with orthopedic follow-up
  - Discuss with orthopedic physician (except for simple nondisplaced torus fractures)

Compartment syndrome

- From increased pressure in a muscle or other internal compartment
- Not all signs and symptoms are needed to make diagnosis
- High pressures > 8 hours leads to tissue damage
- Normal tissue pressure is < 10 mm Hg
- Capillary blood flow is compromised at > 20 mm Hg
- Intracompartmental pressures > 30 mm Hg or within 10–30 mm Hg of DBP
- Elevated CPK >1,000U/mL confirms diagnosis
- Elevated LDH

Signs and symptoms (not diagnostic)

- Pain
  - Out of proportion to injury
  - On passive stretch of muscles
- Pallor
- Paresthesia
- Paralysis
  - Sensory and motor findings are late signs
- Poikilothermia — decreased temperature
- Pulselessness
  - Usually not lost until muscle necrosis has occurred
  - Last sign to develop
- Tense muscle compartment on palpation

Treatment

- Consult if suspected
- Keep extremity at level of heart
- Do not use ice if suspected
- Remove cast and padding
  - Surgery fasciotomy is usually necessary

Evaluation

- History of injury
- Past history
- Medication history
- Associated symptoms and complete physical exam
- X-rays of affected areas
- Neurovascular/tendon/ligament exam
- Assess for compartment syndrome
- Assess for open fracture or joint
- Splint as needed for comfort or stability

Vertebral Fractures

Considerations

- Compression fractures commonly seen in the elderly secondary to osteoporosis
- Can be pathologic from cancer
- Point tenderness common at fracture site
- May be caused by high impact

Evaluation

- History and physical examination
- Plain films
- CT scan of affected area may be needed for diagnosis
- CT scan for compression fractures ≥ 30% or any posterior element spinal canal involvement
- CT scan of entire spine for acute neurologic complaints or deficits
- Assess for other injuries
- CBC and U/A for significant mechanism of injury

Treatment options

- Pain control with narcotics usually — PO, IM or IV
- May try ibuprofen 400–600 mg with acetaminophen 650–1000 mg qid PO prn (more pain relief than hydrocodone 5 mg PO)

- Spine immobilization for neurologic complaints or findings
- Elective vertebroplasty
- Early ambulation as tolerated

Discharge criteria recommendation

- Uncomplicated vertebral compression fractures < 30% in osteoporosis patients without significant mechanism of injury
- Patient able to ambulate with or without walker or crutches

Discharge instructions

- Vertebral compression aftercare instructions
- Follow up with neurosurgeon or orthopedic surgeon within 7 days

Consult criteria recommendation

- Consult orthopedic or spine surgeon for compression fractures > 30%
- Acute neurologic deficits or complaints
- Unable to ambulate
- Uncontrollable severe pain
- Posterior element or spinal canal involvement
- Noncompression–type vertebral fractures
- Significant mechanism of injury

Clavicle Fractures

Considerations

- Most common fracture in children
- 80% middle third
- 15% distal third
- 5% proximal third
- May need CT scan for sternoclavicular injuries
- Patients older than 12 years with more than 2 cm of displacement of fracture fragments should be referred to orthopedics for consideration of operative repair
- Younger children are excluded due to having more effective remodeling

Treatment

- Sling for middle and distal end fractures for 4–8 weeks; and for acromioclavicular sprain and separation prn
- Proximal sternoclavicular fractures and dislocations, consult thoracic surgeon
- Posterior sternoclavicular dislocation — notify thoracic surgery promptly if available
- May have stridor or respiratory distress
- May have venous congestion of head or neck or affected arm
- NSAID's (very effective in children); narcotics prn

Posterior sternoclavicular dislocation treatment

- CT scan definitive diagnosis if there is uncertainty
- 3–4 inch roll between scapula and spine to extend or open up affected sternoclavicular joint
- Abduct affected shoulder to 90° and extend shoulder to 15° and apply traction with assistant holding trunk still
- If above fails, maintain traction and manually grasp clavicle and pull forward
- Consult orthopedic surgeon for sternoclavicular dislocations

Discharge criteria recommendation

- Uncomplicated clavicle fracture

Discharge instructions

- Clavicle fracture aftercare instructions
- Referral to orthopedics or PCP within 7–10 days

Consult criteria recommendation

- Immediate consultation for suspected posterior

sternoclavicular joint dislocation
- Neurovascular injury

Scapular Fractures

Considerations

- Can occur with significant trauma to trunk and other injuries
- Evaluate for associated injuries
- Type 1: body of scapula
- Type 2: coracoid and acromion
- Type 3: neck and glenoid
- Shoulder x-rays needed
- CT may be needed if going to surgery for repair

Treatment options

Type 1

- Sling
- Analgesics

Type 2 and 3

- Per orthopedic consultation

Discharge criteria recommendation

- Uncomplicated Type 1 scapular fracture

Discharge instructions

- Scapular fracture aftercare instructions
- Follow up with trauma or thoracic surgeon within 5–10 days

Consult criteria recommendation

- Type 2 and 3 scapular fractures
- For any significant associated injuries

Humerus Fractures

Considerations

- Fall on outstretched hand frequent cause
- Usually elderly
- Younger patients with epiphyseal injuries of growth plate
- Shoulder tense and swollen
- Obtain AP and lateral shoulder x-rays
- Evaluate for neurovascular injury
- Proximal humerus: axillary nerve (test deltoid sensation)
- Humeral shaft: radial nerve (test for wrist drop and 1st web space sensation loss)

Treatment

- Sling
- Physical therapy
- Narcotics prn
- May try ibuprofen 400–600 mg with acetaminophen 650–1000 mg qid PO prn (more pain relief than hydrocodone 5 mg PO)
- Children can take Tylenol with or without ibuprofen prn

Discharge criteria recommendation

- Uncomplicated and minimally displaced proximal closed humerus fracture

Discharge instructions

- Humerus fracture aftercare instructions
- Orthopedic referral within 7 days

Consult criteria recommendation

- Orthopedic consultation for severely angulated or comminuted fracture
- Orthopedic consult for pediatric humerus fractures

Shoulder, Hip, Knee, Wrist, Elbow, and Ankle Dislocations

- Analgesics
- Evaluate for associated injuries
- Reduce if indicated for significant dislocations or concern regarding neurovascular compromise
- Splint as needed for compromise or stability
- Consult orthopedic surgeon

Rib Fractures – Isolated

Considerations

- First and second rib fractures associated with high impact and significant mechanism of injury

Evaluation

- Complete history and physical examination
- Chest x-ray
- Rib films
- Chest CT scan needed for significant mechanism of injury and/or abnormal vital signs or hypoxia
- Ultrasound can detect subtle rib fractures
- U/A to check for kidney injury in low posterior rib fractures
- Evaluate for associated injuries

Treatment options

- Narcotics prn
- NSAID's prn
  - May try ibuprofen 400–600 mg with acetaminophen 650–1000 mg qid PO prn (more pain relief than hydrocodone 5 mg PO)
- Rib belt not recommended due to causing atelectasis and pneumonia

Discharge criteria recommendation

- Simple 1 or 2 rib fractures
- No pulmonary abnormality (pulmonary contusion or pneumothorax)

Discharge instructions

- Rib fracture aftercare instructions
- Follow up with PCP or trauma surgeon within 7–10 days

Consult criteria recommendation

- If more than 2 ribs fractured
- 1st or 2nd rib fractures
- Pulmonary abnormality on chest imaging
- Hypoxia or respiratory distress

Forearm Fractures

Torus fractures of distal forearm

- Splint and sling
- Analgesics
- Torus fracture aftercare instructions
- Orthopedic referral within 10 days

Colles, Smith and Barton's fractures

- Consult orthopedic physician
- Respective fracture aftercare instructions
- OCL sugar tong splint and sling for Colles fracture if discharged
- Reduce if requested by orthopedic surgeon or neurovascular compromise concerns
- Analgesics

Radius and ulnar midshaft fractures

- Consult orthopedic physician
- Splint for comfort as needed

Elbow Fractures

Considerations

- X-ray may or may not show radial head fractures
- Anterior (can be normal) or posterior fat pad sign on x-ray is from joint effusion from fracture or sprain
- Posterior fat pad associated more frequently with fracture

Evaluation

- Elbow x-ray
- Neurovascular examination
- Assess for associated injuries

Treatment options

- Sling
- OCL posterior splint may be needed
- Analgesics prn

- May try ibuprofen 400–600 mg with acetaminophen 650–1000 mg qid PO prn (more pain relief than hydrocodone 5 mg PO)

Discharge criteria recommendation

- Nondisplaced simple proximal radius fracture
- X-ray reveals fat pad sign without obvious fracture

Discharge instructions

- Elbow fracture aftercare instructions
- Inform patient and family that the x-ray shows a fat pad sign that may indicate a fracture present, even if no fracture seen at that time
- Follow up with orthopedic surgeon within 10 days

Consult criteria recommendation

- Proximal ulnar fracture
- Midshaft or distal humerus fracture
- Supracondylar fracture
- Neurovascular deficits
- Neurologic complaints

Metacarpal Fractures

Nondisplaced, nonangulated transverse fracture

Evaluation

- X-ray
- Neurovascular exam

Treatment

- Dorsal splint for 3–4 weeks
- Sling
- Analgesics prn

Discharge criteria recommendation

- Simple closed fracture

Discharge instructions

- Metacarpal fracture aftercare instructions
- Follow up with orthopedic or hand surgeon within 7–10 days

Consult criteria recommendation

- Open fracture
- Neurovascular deficit or complaint

Transverse, angulated and/or displaced fracture

- Consult orthopedic physician

Spiral or oblique fracture

- Consult orthopedic physician

Hip and Femur Fractures

- Consult orthopedic physician
- Pain control

Patella

Fracture

Nondisplaced with extensor function intact

Evaluation

- Knee x-ray with sunrise view
- Assess neurovascular status

Treatment

- Knee immobilizer
- Analgesics
- Crutches

Discharge criteria recommendation

- Closed simple patella fracture with intact extensor function

Discharge instructions

- Patella fracture aftercare instructions
- Orthopedic referral

Consult criteria recommendation

- Displaced > 3 mm or extensor function loss

Dislocation

Evaluation

- Same as patella fracture

Treatment

- Reduce dislocation
- Knee immobilizer
- Analgesics

Discharge criteria recommendation

- Closed simple reduced patella dislocation

Discharge instructions

- Patella dislocation aftercare instructions
- Orthopedic follow-up within 10 days

Consult criteria recommendation

- Nonreducible patellar dislocation

Tibial Plateau and Midshaft Fractures

Considerations

- Tibial plateau fractures may be difficult to see on plain x-ray
- CT scan of knee frequently reveals a more extensive fracture than plain film

Evaluation

- Knee or tibial/fibula x-ray
- CT scan of knee may be needed or requested for tibial plateau fractures
- Neurovascular examination
- Assess for associated injuries

Treatment

- Pain control IM or IV
- Splint knee in extension for tibial plateau fracture
- Splint lower leg if needed

Consult criteria recommendation

- Discuss with orthopedic physician all tibial fractures

Tibial tubercle avulsion

- In adolescents
- Quadriceps contraction causes avulsion
- Type III injuries, the fracture extends through the articular surface
  - May cause anterior compartment syndrome with rupture of anterior tibial tubercle which has been shown to occur in 4 – 20% of patients
  - Frequent serial examinations should be performed
- Nondisplaced fractures may be treated in extension with a brace, cylinder cast, or a long leg cast for 4-6 weeks
- Displaced fractures require operative treatment

Consult criteria

- Discuss with orthopedic physician

Displaced Proximal, Midshaft and Distal Fibula Fractures

Evaluation

- X-ray
- Neurovascular examination
- Assess for associated injuries

Treatment

- Pain control IM or IV
- Splint as needed

Consult criteria recommendation

- Discuss these fractures with orthopedic physician

Nondisplaced Distal Fibula Fracture

Evaluation

- X-ray
- Neurovascular examination
- Assess for associated injuries
- Ligament examination as tolerated

Treatment

- Walking boot
- Crutches
- Analgesics

Discharge criteria recommendation

- Simple closed nondisplaced fibular fracture
- Normal neurovascular examination

Discharge instructions

- Ankle sprain and distal fibular fracture aftercare instructions
- Follow up with orthopedic surgeon within 7–10 days

Consult criteria recommendation

- Neurovascular injury
- Open fracture
- Displaced fracture

Knee Strain

- See Knee Soft Tissue Injury Protocol

Foot Fractures and Dislocations

Tarsal or midfoot

- Consult orthopedic physician
- Analgesics
- Splint for comfort and stability as needed

Metatarsal fractures

Nondisplaced

- Boot
- Crutches
- Analgesics
- Orthopedic referral

Displaced

- Consult orthopedic physician

Calcaneus fractures

- Posterior splint
- Analgesics prn
- Consult orthopedic physician

Toe fractures

- Buddy tape to adjacent toe with padding between toes
- Cast shoe
- Significantly displaced fractures consult orthopedic surgeon

General Orthopedic Consult criteria recommendation

- Acute neurovascular deficits or injury
- Suspected compartment syndrome
- Nonreducible dislocations
- Open fractures, joints or dislocations

Notes

______

______

______

REFERENCES:

Orthopaedics Primary Care by Chinni Pennathur Ramamurti

Am J Emerg Med 2012;30: 606–614

J Pediatr Orthop 2010;30:307–312

Sternoclavicular Joint Injury Treatment & Management
Author: John P Rudzinski, MD, FACEP; Chief Editor: Rick Kulkarni, MD
emedicine.medscape.com/article/828642

Rib Fracture Treatment & Management
Author: Sarah L Melendez, MD; Chief Editor: Rick Kulkarni, MD
emedicine.medscape.com/article/825981

Foot Fracture Treatment & Management
Author: Robert Silbergleit, MD; Chief Editor: Rick Kulkarni, MD
emedicine.medscape.com/article/825060

Surgical versus conservative interventions for treating fractures of the middle third of the clavicle
Mário Lenza, Rachelle Buchbinder,Renea V Johnston, João Carlos elloti,, Flávio Faloppa Cochrane Library 10 MAR 2013
DOI: 10.1002/14651858.CD009363.pub2

Pretell-Mazzini J, et al. *Journal of Pediatric Orthopedics*. 2016;36(5):440-446

Salter Harris Fracture Protocol

Definition

- Disruption of the cartilaginous plates of the physeal area or growth plate that may or may not involve a fracture of the adjacent bone in children

Salter Pneumonic

- Salter 1 — **S**lip of growth plate
- Salter 2 — **A**bove (fracture extends above growth plate)
- Salter 3 — **L**ow (fracture extends below growth plate)
- Salter 4 — **T**hrough (fracture above and below plate)
- Salter 5 — **E**ntire (crush fracture of growth plate area)
- Salter 6 — **R**ing (injury to the perichondral ring or periosteum)

Considerations

- The cartilage growth plate can be weaker than ligaments in children
- Sprains in children can actually be Salter 1 fractures that are not evident on initial x-ray
- Plain x-rays may depict widening of growth plate as only sign of a fracture
- Comparison x-rays of uninjured opposite extremity can be helpful with Salter 1 fractures
- CT scans may be necessary to delineate degree of injury in severely comminuted Salter fractures
- Growth acceleration (uncommon) or growth arrest can occur with Salter fractures
- Long term follow-up at 6 and 12 months important
- Salter 1 fracture of the great toe with subungual hematoma represents an open fracture

Growth plate (physeal) fractures at increased risk of growth arrest are

- Distal femur
- Distal tibia
- Distal radius and ulna
- Proximal tibia
- Triradiate cartilage — acetabulum in children

Evaluation

- History of injury
- Examination for neurovascular and tendon injuries
- Examination for remote undisclosed injuries
- X-ray of injured area
- Comparison x-rays if needed of opposite uninjured extremity

Treatment

- Most Salter 1 and 2 fractures can be treated, if mildly displaced, with reduction if needed, and splinting and follow-up in 7–10 days
- Salter 3 and 4 usually require open reduction and fixation
- Salter 5 fractures are rarely diagnosed acutely and treatment is usually delayed because of the delay in diagnosis
- Antibiotics for great toe Salter fractures with subungual hematoma that are discharged — amoxicillin/clavulanate or cephalosporin
  - Considered an open fracture (preferable to discuss with physician)
- Pain medications as needed

Discharge Criteria

- Nondisplaced Salter 1 and 2 fractures
- Reduced Salter 1 and 2 fractures

Discharge instructions

- Salter Harris fracture aftercare instructions
- Follow up in 7–10 days preferably with orthopedic surgeon

- Instructions in various pediatric "sprains" that there could be a nondisplaced Salter 1 fracture

Consult Criteria

- Displaced Salter fractures
- Open Salter fractures
- Neurovascular deficits
- Tendon deficits
- Salter 3–6 fractures

Notes

REFERENCES:

Salter R, Harris W. Injuries involving the epiphyseal plate. J Bone Joint Surg. 1963 45A: p. 587–621

Orthopaedics Primary Care by Chinni Pennathur Ramamurti

SYNOVIAL FLUID ANALYSIS

Normal

- Transparent clarity
- Clear color
- WBC < 200/ml
- PMN's < 25%
- Culture negative
- No crystals
- Mucin clot firm
- Glucose approximates blood levels

Noninflammatory

- Transparent clarity
- Yellow color
- WBC 200–2000/ml
- PMN's < 25%
- Culture negative
- No crystals
- Mucin clot firm
- Glucose approximates blood levels
- Associated conditions: rheumatic fever, trauma, osteoarthritis

Inflammatory

- Cloudy clarity
- Yellow color
- WBC 200–50,000/ml
- PMN's > 50%
- Culture negative
- Crystals can be present if gout or pseudogout are etiology
- Mucin clot friable
- Glucose decreased
- Associated conditions: SLE, Lyme disease, gout, pseudogout, spondyloarthropathies

Septic

- Cloudy clarity
- Yellow color
- WBC 25,000/ml to often > 100,000/ml
- PMS's > 50%
- Culture often positive
- No crystals
- Mucin clot friable
- Glucose very decreased
- Fever
- C-reactive protein elevated

Notes

REFERENCES:

Septic Arthritis Surgery Author: Gabriel Munoz, MD; Chief Editor: Harris Gellman, MD
medicine.medscape.com/article/1268369

Shoulder Protocol

Shoulder conditions

Impingement syndrome encompasses

- Supraspinatus tendonitis
- Bicipital tendonitis
- Subacromial bursitis

Supraspinatus tendonitis

- Middle aged
- Subacute or chronic pain in shoulder
- Top of shoulder tender distal to acromion
- Abduction beyond 80–120 degrees limited by pain
- X-rays may be normal or show erosions and calcifications in tendon

Bicipital tendonitis

- Pain in anterior shoulder
- Tenderness along long head of biceps and bicipital groove
- Flexion painful with elbow extended
- Rotation restricted by pain
- Flexion against resistant causes pain

Subacromial bursitis

- Least common of shoulder musculotendinous cuff disorders
- Most painful and acute of the 3 impingement disorders
- Any movement of shoulder causes pain
- Shoulder diffusely tender
- May have fever and elevated ESR

Treatment Options

- Severe pain — rest in sling short-term
- Ice packs with severe pain
- NSAID's prn
- Gravity-assisted range of motion pendulum exercises started in hours to days
- Physical therapy
- 1 cc of Depomedrol (methylprednisolone acetate) 40–80 mg/cc or Kenalog (triamcinolone) 10–20 mg/cc mixed with 1 cc of 1–2% plain lidocaine, injected through normal skin if Provider is experienced performing shoulder intraarticular injections
- Dexamethasone 4–6 mg PO qday for 5–10 days prn (caution in diabetic patients)

Discharge Criteria

- Uncomplicated case

Discharge instructions

- Shoulder tendonitis and bursitis aftercare instructions
- Referral to primary care provider or orthopedics if pain persists in 7–10 days

Consult Criteria

- Suspected septic shoulder joint

Thoracic outlet syndrome

- Compression of the neurovascular bundle as it passes out of the thoracic outlet above first rib and behind the clavicle
- May be associated with a cervical rib

3 types of thoracic outlet syndrome

Neurologic (most common)

- C8 and T1 roots most commonly affected
- Pain is in medial arm, forearm, and ring and fifth fingers
- Nocturnal paresthesias
- Weakness
- Cold intolerance
- Neck pain (trapezius)
- Occipital headache
- Anterior chest wall pain

- Raynaud's phenomenon

Venous

- Extremity
  - Swelling
  - Cyanosis
  - Paresthesias

Arterial (most serious and least common)

- Pain
- Coldness
- Numbness
- Pallor
- Seen in young patients with vigorous activity history
- Seen with emboli

Examination

- Provocative tests not reliable

Elevated arm stress test (EAST)

- Most reliable for all three types
- Arms at 90° to body and elbow flexed 90°
  - Hands opened and closed for 3 minutes
- Symptom reproduction is a positive test

Adson's test

- Palpate both radial arteries while patient turns head side to side
- Loss of pulse positive for arterial type

Testing options

- Chest x-ray for cervical rib and pulmonary disease
- Cervical spine
- Duplex scan of arm

Treatment outpatient options

- NSAID's with or without acetaminophen
- Narcotics prn
- Tricyclic antidepressants for chronic pain

Vascular (arterial and venous) outlet obstruction

- Immediate heparinization
- Emergent vascular surgery consultation

Discharge criteria

- Benign presentation

Discharge instructions

- Thoracic outlet aftercare instructions
- Refer to thoracic surgeon

Consult criteria

- Arterial and venous insufficiency
- Severe pain
- Severe neurologic deficit
- Suspected spinal cord etiology

Rotator Cuff Tear (RCT)

Considerations

- 90% with minimal or no injury
- Tenderness of middle third of shoulder
- Unable to abduct shoulder in massive tears
- Weak abduction and pain with minor tears
- Palpable crepitus with movements
- Painless or tolerable passive abduction
- Atrophy with long standing RCT

Treatment options

- Severe pain — rest in sling short term
- Ice packs with severe pain
- NSAID's prn with or without acetaminophen
- Narcotics prn
- Gravity-assisted range of motion pendulum exercises started in hours to days
- Physical therapy
- Local lidocaine injection 2 cc prn through normal skin (if Provider has experience with shoulder injections)
- No steroid injections

Discharge criteria

- Uncomplicated injury

Discharge instructions

- Rotator cuff tear aftercare instructions
- Referral to orthopedics for major RCT tear within 7 days

Consult criteria

- Discuss major tears with physician

Acromioclavicular (AC) Injuries

Acromioclavicular sprain (Type I)

- Partial tear of capsule of AC joint
- Usually in young or middle aged with injury to AC joint
- AC joint tender and may be slightly swollen
- Attempted abduction > 60 degrees causes pain
- X-rays show normal AC joint
- Full function usually achieved after healing

Treatment

- Sling initially
- Early motion encouraged
- Avoid hyperabduction for 3 weeks
- Avoid heavy lifting for 6 weeks
- Ice packs
- NSAID's prn; narcotics prn

Discharge criteria

- Uncomplicated injury

Discharge instructions

- AC sprain aftercare instructions
- Primary care provider or orthopedic follow up within 10–14 days

Acromioclavicular subluxation

- Complete tear of AC joint ligaments with intact coracocalvicular ligaments intact
- Slight widening of AC joint (Type II)
- AC joint markedly swollen
- Outer end of clavicle may protrude slightly upward
- Attempted abduction > 60 degrees causes pain
- X-rays without weights may be normal
- X-rays with 10–lb. weights show widened AC joint

Treatment

- Sling initially 1–2 weeks, unless AC joint displacement of 25–50% (Type III), then wear up to 6 weeks as needed for pain
- Early motion encouraged
- Avoid hyperabduction > 90 degrees for 3–4 weeks
- Avoid heavy lifting for 2 months
- Ice packs
- NSAID's prn; narcotics prn
- Surgery indicated for cases not responding to conservative therapy in 3–6 months
- Surgery indicated for most cases if distal clavicle displaced posterior/superior to acromion and coracoid (Type IV) or AC joint displacement of 100–300% (Type V), or AC joint displacement inferiorly (Type VI)

Discharge criteria

- Uncomplicated injury

Discharge instructions

- AC injury aftercare instructions
- Primary care provider or orthopedic follow up within 10–14 days

Consult criteria

- Complicated injury
- Neurovascular injury or complaints

Notes

REFERENCES:

Orthopaedics Primary Care by Chinni Pennathur Ramamurti

Rotator Cuff Disease Author: André Roy, MD, FRCPC; Chief Editor: Rene Cailliet, MD emedicine.medscape.com/article/328253

Thoracic Outlet Syndrome in Emergency Medicine Clinical Presentation Author: Andrew K Chang, MD; Chief Editor: David FM Brown, MD medicine.medscape.com/article/760477

Shoulder and Arm Trauma Protocol

General Evaluation

- History of injury; past history; medication history
- Associated symptoms and complete physical exam
- X-rays
- Neurovascular/tendon/ligament exam
- Assess for compartment syndrome
- Assess for open fracture or open joint

Acromioclavicular (AC) Injuries

Acromioclavicular sprain

- Partial tear of capsule of AC joint
- Usually in young or middle aged with injury to AC joint
- AC joint tender and may be slightly swollen
- Attempted abduction > 60 degrees causes pain
- X-rays show normal AC joint

Treatment

- Sling initially
- Early motion encouraged
- Avoid hyperabduction for 3 weeks
- Avoid heavy lifting for 6 weeks
- Ice packs
- NSAID's prn; narcotics prn

Discharge criteria recommendation

- Uncomplicated injury

Discharge instructions

- AC sprain aftercare instructions
- Primary care provider or orthopedic follow-up within 10–14 days

Acromioclavicular subluxation

- Complete tear of AC joint capsule
- AC joint markedly swollen
- Outer end of clavicle may protrude slightly upward
- Attempted abduction > 60 degrees causes pain
- X-rays without weights may be normal
- X-rays with 10–lb. weights show widened AC joint

Treatment

- Sling initially
- Early motion encouraged
- Avoid hyperabduction > 90 degrees for 3–4 weeks
- Avoid heavy lifting for 2 months
- Ice packs
- NSAID's prn; narcotics prn

Discharge criteria recommendation

- Uncomplicated injury

Discharge instructions

- AC injury aftercare instructions
- Primary care provider or orthopedic follow-up within 10–14 days

Consult criteria recommendation

- Complicated injury
- Neurovascular injury or complaints

Clavicle Fractures

Considerations

- Most common fracture in children
- 80% middle third
- 15% distal third
- 5% proximal third
- May need CT scan for sternoclavicular injuries

Treatment

Sling

- Middle and distal end fractures for 4–8 weeks
- Acromioclavicular sprain and separation
- Patients older than 12 years with more than 2 cm of displacement of fracture fragments should be referred to orthopedics for consideration of operative repair
  - Younger children are excluded due to having more effective remodeling
- Proximal sternoclavicular fractures and dislocations — consult thoracic or trauma surgeon
- Posterior sternoclavicular dislocation
- Needs immediate reduction to prevent life threatening complications
- May have stridor or respiratory distress
- May have venous congestion of head or neck or affected arm

Posterior sternoclavicular dislocation treatment

- 3–4 inch roll between scapula and spine to extend or open up affected sternoclavicular joint
- Abduct affected shoulder to 90° and extend shoulder to 15° and apply traction with assistant holding trunk still
- If above fails, maintain traction and manually grasp clavicle and pull forward
- Consult thoracic surgeon for sternoclavicular dislocations
- NSAID's (very effective in children); narcotics prn
- CT scan definitive if needed

Discharge criteria recommendation

- Uncomplicated clavicle fracture

Discharge instructions

- Clavicle fracture aftercare instructions
- Follow up with PCP or orthopedic surgeon within 10 days

Consult criteria recommendation

- Immediate consultation for suspected posterior sternoclavicular joint dislocation

Scapular Fractures

Considerations

- Can occur with significant trauma to trunk and other injuries
- Evaluate for associated injuries
- Type 1: body of scapula
- Type 2: coracoid and acromion
- Type 3: neck and glenoid

Evaluation

- Shoulder x-rays
- Chest x-ray
- CT may be needed if going to surgery for repair

Treatment

Type 1

- Sling
- Analgesics

Type 2 and 3

- Orthopedic consultation

Discharge criteria recommendation

- Uncomplicated Type 1 scapular fracture

Discharge instructions

- Scapular fracture aftercare instructions
- Follow up with trauma or thoracic surgeon within 5–10 days

Consult criteria recommendation

- Type 2 and 3 scapular fractures
- For any significant associated injuries
- Discuss all scapular fractures with orthopedic physician prior to discharge

Humerus Fractures

Considerations

- Fall on outstretched hand
- Usually elderly
- Younger patients with epiphyseal injuries of growth plate
- Shoulder tense and swollen
- Obtain AP and lateral shoulder x-rays
- Evaluate for neurovascular injury
- Proximal humerus: axillary nerve (test deltoid sensation)
- Humeral shaft: radial nerve (test for wrist drop and 1st web space sensation loss)

Treatment

- Sling
- Physical therapy
- Narcotics prn
- May try ibuprofen 400–600 mg with acetaminophen 650–1000 mg qid PO prn (more pain relief than hydrocodone 5 mg PO)
- Children can take Tylenol with or without ibuprofen prn
- Orthopedic referral within 7 days

Discharge criteria recommendation

- Uncomplicated and minimally displaced proximal closed humerus fracture

Discharge instructions

- Humerus fracture aftercare instructions
- Orthopedic referral within 7 days

Consult criteria recommendation

- Orthopedic consultation for severely angulated or comminuted fracture
- Orthopedic consult for pediatric humerus fractures

Shoulder (Glenohumeral) Dislocation

Considerations

Anterior dislocation

- Most common: 95–97%
- Patient holds arm adjacent to body
- Any motion causes severe pain
- Rounded shoulder contour is lost
- Hill-Sachs humeral head deformity present in 50%: no treatment
- Bankart fracture — glenoid rim fracture
- Axillary nerve most common neurovascular injury
  - Assess with pinprick over lateral shoulder
- Median and ulnar injuries rare
  - Median nerve
    - Decreased sensation to thumb

- Index and middle finger sensation impaired
- Thumb opposition weak

- Ulnar nerve
  - Decreased sensation and weakness of 4th and 5th fingers
  - Abduction and adduction of 4th and 5th fingers very weak or impossible to perform
  - Flexion of the 4th and 5th metacarpophalangeal joints with interphalangeal joints extended is weak or impossible to perform

Posterior dislocation

- 2–4% of dislocations
- Occurs with seizures, direct anterior shoulder trauma and falls on outstretched hand
- Arm held across chest
- External rotation blocked
- X-ray can be deceptive — less overlap of humeral head and glenoid on AP view

Luxatio Erecta (inferior dislocation)

- 0.5% of glenohumeral dislocations
- Arm held over head
- High complication rate
- 60% neurological injury — most commonly axillary nerve
- Rotator cuff tear > 50%

Evaluation

- Neurovascular exam
- Shoulder x-ray AP and lateral (or Y-view)

Treatment options

- Conscious sedation frequently needed
- Sling for 3–6 weeks in younger patients
- Sling for 1–2 weeks in age > 40 years
- Faster healing and decreased recurrence if arm in 15 degrees external rotation (may be hard to accomplish)
- Aspiration of hemarthrosis and instillation of lidocaine 1% for return visit in 24–48 hours from painful hemarthrosis

Anterior dislocations

External Rotation method

- Patient supine
- Adduct arm and flex 90° at elbow
- Slowly rotate arm externally
- Reduce shoulder before reaching coronal plane

Scapular rotation

- Patient prone
- 5–15 pounds of hanging weights on affected arm
- Rotate inferior scapula medially and superior scapula laterally

OR

- Patient sitting
- Assistant provides traction on wrist with other hand pushing against chest
- Rotate inferior scapula medially and superior scapula laterally

Traction-counter traction (Modified Hippocratic Technique)

- Sheet over flexed forearm and tied around Provider's waist with counter traction with sheet around axilla by assistant
- Be careful of injuring brachial plexus
- Gentle internal and external rotation with traction by Provider

Stimson technique

- Patient in prone position and secured from falling off table
- Arm hanging off table with axilla and brachial plexus protected
- 20 lb. weights taped or attached to forearm or wrist/hand
- Wait 20 minutes
- Shoulder will usually reduce or will need minimal traction at the 20 minute time point

- Can be done without sedation or pain treatment occasionally

Cunningham technique

- Does not require conscious sedation
- Raise bed higher than physician's seated position
- Rest relaxed patient's hand of injured shoulder on physician's shoulder so patient's forearm is horizontal
- Physician places hand on patient's elbow using the arm that patient is resting on
- Have patient shrug shoulders backward
- Patient breathe slowly in and out concentrating on relaxing shoulder
- Physician's other hand massages patient's deltoid and biceps
- Physician's hand on elbow applies no more than 5 pounds of pressure while adducting elbow against patient's side
- An assistant is behind patient helping to rotate shoulders backward while massaging both trapezius muscles at the same time

Posterior dislocations

- Traction along long axis of arm with anterior pressure on posterior shoulder

Luxatio Erecta (inferior dislocation)

- Overhead traction in upward and outward direction on arm with counter traction towards feet with sheet on injured shoulder

Discharge criteria recommendation

- Uncomplicated dislocation

Discharge instructions

- Shoulder dislocation aftercare instructions
- Refer to orthopedic surgeon within 7–10 days
- Wear sling for 3 weeks
- Patients > 50 years need early follow up for early mobilization and to avoid shoulder stiffness

Consult criteria recommendation

- Neurovascular injury
- Compartment syndrome
- Orthopedic consult if irreducible dislocation
- Orthopedic consult if associated fracture excluding Hill-Sachs deformity

Notes

REFERENCES:

Ufberg J, McNamara R. Management of common dislocations. *Clinical Procedures in Emergency Medicine*, 4th ed. pp 946–963

Sternoclavicular Joint Injury Treatment & Management

Author: John P Rudzinski, MD, FACEP; Chief Editor: Rick Kulkarni, MD emedicine.medscape.com/article/828642

Surgical versus conservative interventions for treating fractures of the middle third of the clavicle

Mário Lenza, Rachelle Buchbinder,Renea V Johnston, João Carlos elloti" Flávio Faloppa Cochrane Library 10 MAR 2013

DOI: 10.1002/14651858.CD009363.pub2

Orthopaedics Primary Care by Chinni Pennathur Ramamurti

Itoi E, Hatakeyama Y, Kido T, et al: A new method of immobilization after traumatic anterior dislocation of the shoulder: a preliminary study, J Shoulder Elbow Surg 2003;12:413–415

Handoll HH, Gibson JN, Madhok R. Interventions for treating proximal humeral fractures in adults. Cochrane Database Syst Rev 2004;4:CD000434. (Systematic review)

Trimmings NP. Haemarthrosis aspiration in treatment of anterior dislocation of the shoulder. *J R Soc Med*1985;78:1023–7

ELBOW PROTOCOL

Considerations

- Tendonitis is usually from overuse
- "Tennis elbow" is most common elbow complaint orthopedists see

Lateral Epicondylitis ("Tennis Elbow")

- Chronic overuse syndrome
- Occupations that require a rotary motion at the elbow
- Increased with grasping motions (handshake) or twisting motions
- Point tenderness over lateral epicondyle
- X-rays usually normal
- Ice or heat — whichever provides the greatest relief

Treatment options

- Elimination of offending activity
- Ice pack for 15-20 minutes or ice water bath for 10-15 minutes several times a day as needed
- Rest
- Physiotherapy
- NSAID's prn
- Tylenol prn
- Splinting or "tennis elbow bands"
- May consider steroid injection if recalcitrant

Discharge criteria

- All uncomplicated cases

Discharge instructions

- Elbow tendonitis aftercare instructions
- Follow with PCP or orthopedic surgeon as needed

Consult criteria

- Orthopedic referral for refractory cases

Medial Epicondylitis

- Less common than lateral epicondylitis
- Tenderness over medial epicondyle
- May be associated ulnar neuritis with loss of sensation over palmar 5th finger and lateral palmar surface of 4th finger

Treatment options

- Elimination of offending activity
- Ice pack for 15-20 minutes or ice water bath for 10-15 minutes several times a day as needed
- Rest
- Physiotherapy
- NSAID's prn
- Tylenol prn
- Splinting or "tennis elbow bands"
- May consider steroid injection if recalcitrant

Discharge criteria

- All uncomplicated cases

Discharge instructions

- Elbow tendonitis aftercare instructions
- Follow with PCP or orthopedic surgeon as needed

Consult criteria

- Orthopedic referral for refractory cases

Olecranon Bursitis

- Usually a painless cystic swelling
- Can be painful from trauma, infection or cryptogenic cause
- Transudate fluid if aspirated is from chronic inflammation

Treatment options

Nonpainful bursitis

- Sterile lateral bursal aspiration if experienced (avoid bone and joint) — may be as effective with less complications than steroid injection
- 1 cc of 1–2% plain lidocaine mixed with 1 cc Depomedrol (methylprednisolone acetate) 40–80 mg/cc or Kenalog (triamcinolone) 10–20 mg/cc prn if Provider experienced with injections (do not introduce needle into bursa through cellulitis)
- Elbow ace wrapping

Painful bursitis

- Fluid needs evaluation (culture and gram stain)
- Heat if infectious etiology
- Heat or ice if cryptogenic etiology — whichever provides the greatest relief

Traumatic bursitis

- Ice packs frequently × 2 days
- Elbow ace wrapping
- NSAID's prn; narcotics prn

Discharge criteria

- Nonpainful or minimal painful bursitis
- Not infected

Discharge instructions

- Olecranon bursitis aftercare instructions

Consult criteria

- Infected olecranon bursitis

Nursemaid Elbow

- Peak age 1–4 years
- Toddler pulled up by arm or similar type traction on arm
- Cries for a few minutes and stops usually
- Arm appears normal
- No other history; occasionally no helpful history
- Usually does not need x-ray if history and exam consistent with nursemaid elbow
- X-ray if performed is negative for acute process
- Perform x-ray if unsure of diagnosis

Treatment

- Elbow flexed 90 degrees
- Fully pronate elbow and then supinate
- If performed correctly will feel or hear click
- Patient cries transiently
- Provider leaves room and returns in 5–10 minutes
- Hold an object for toddler to grasp with affected arm to demonstrate resolution or patient moving arm normally

Discharge criteria

- All patients without other concerns (abuse) or other injuries

Discharge instructions

- Nursemaid elbow aftercare instructions

Consult criteria

- If child abuse suspected

Notes

REFERENCES:

Lateral Epicondylitis
Author: Bryant James Walrod, MD; Chief Editor: Sherwin SW Ho, MD
emedicine.medscape.com/article/96969

Orthopaedics Primary Care by Chinni Pennathur Ramamurti

Plancher KD, Halbrecht J, Lourie GM. Medial and lateral epicondylitis in the athlete. *Clin Sports Med.* Apr 1996;15(2):283–305

Nursemaid Elbow Author: Wayne Wolfram, MD, MPH; Chief Editor: Richard G Bachur, MD emedicine.medscape.com/article/803026

Weinstein PS, Canoso JJ, Wohlgethan JR. Long-term follow-up of corticosteroid injection for traumatic olecranon bursitis. *Ann Rheum Dis.* Feb 1984;43(1):44–6

HIP PROTOCOL

Septic Hip

Considerations

- Most common cause of painful hip in infants
- Rapid onset of pain
- Fever
- Elevated ESR and C-reactive protein
- Hip flexed
- All motion of hip resisted
- X-rays show externally rotated hip soft tissue outline

Evaluation

- Neurovascular exam
- Hip and pelvis x-rays
- Hip joint aspiration by specialist if indicated
- Synovial fluid analysis (see Synovial Fluid Analysis as needed)

Treatment

- Orthopedic admission for hip lavage and antibiotics

Consult criteria recommendation

- Suspected septic hip joint

Transient Synovitis

Considerations

- Self-limited disease of children age 3–10 years
- Etiology unknown (viral infection etiology postulated)
- Males twice as likely as females to have
- Crying at night in very young
- Antalgic gait or limp
- Usually afebrile; may have low-grade fever
- Hip held in flexion and slight abduction with external rotation
- 1/3 has no decreased hip motion
- Hip may be tender to palpation and painful to passive motion

Evaluation options

- Neurovascular exam
- CBC
- ESR
- Aspiration of hip by specialist if fever > 99.5; ESR > 20; or there is severe pain with movement
- Hip and pelvis x-rays
- Ultrasound as needed

Treatment

- Local heat and massage
- Bed rest for 7–10 days
- No weight bearing
- Close follow-up

Discharge criteria recommendation

- Diagnosis firm
- Provide transient hip synovitis aftercare instructions

Consult criteria recommendation

- Uncertain diagnosis
- Septic hip suspected

Legg-Calve´-Perthes Disease (Avascular Necrosis of Femoral Head)

Considerations

- Caused by loss of blood supply to hip
- Insidious onset
- Limp often presenting complaint
- Aching in groin and thigh
- Tender over anterior hip joint

- Age 4–10 years most common; range 2–18 years of age
- Male > female prevalence
- 20% bilateral
- Leg externally rotated

Evaluation

- Neurovascular exam
- CBC
- ESR
- Hip and pelvis x-rays
- Ultrasound helpful
- Bone scan diagnostic

Treatment

- NSAID's prn; Tylenol prn
- Non-weight bearing
- Physical therapy twice a week
- Crutches

Discharge criteria recommendation

- Most patients
- If adequate pain control is achievable

Discharge instructions

- Legg-Calve'-Perthes Disease aftercare instructions
- Referral to orthopedic surgeon

Acute consult criteria recommendation

- Severe pain not controlled by medications
- Poor social situation not allowing non-weight bearing

Slipped Capital Femoral Epiphysis (SCFE)

Considerations

- Most patients obese
- Male peak age 13–15 years
- Female peak age 11–13 years
- More common in males
- Bilateral hips in 1/3 of cases
- Present with limp
- Pain referred to knee, thigh, groin or hip
- Commonly with leg externally rotated
- Flexion is restricted
- Do not ambulate if SCFE suspected

Evaluation

- Neurovascular exam
- CBC
- ESR
- C-reactive protein
- AP and frog leg lateral views of both hips
- Klein line is a line drawn parallel to lateral femoral neck that does not transect epiphysis; normally it does transect epiphysis in healthy hips

Treatment

- Immobilization
- Non-weight bearing

Consult criteria recommendation

- Immediate orthopedic consult

Hip Fracture

Considerations

- Elderly fall most common reason
- Affected leg externally rotated

Evaluation

- Hip and pelvis x-rays
- CT scan if plain hip x-ray without definite fracture but there is high suspicion of hip fracture
- Neurovascular exam
- Assess for other injuries
- Evaluate for acute medical condition if the cause of injury

Treatment

- Pain control
- Femoral nerve block

Consult criteria recommendation

- All hip fracture patients
- All suspected hip fracture patients

Hip Dislocation

Considerations

- Posterior dislocation most common

- Frequently seen with total hip replacement

Evaluation

- Hip and pelvis x-rays
- Neurovascular exam
- Assess for other injuries or conditions

Treatment

- Pain control
- May reduce under conscious sedation with propofol or ketamine
- Captain Morgan technique for hip dislocation usually effective
  - Bend your knee 90 degrees with foot on patient's stretcher
  - Drape patient's affected knee bent over physician's knee
  - Tie patient's pelvis to stretcher (best) or assistant holds pelvis against stretcher (backboard helpful)
  - Physician raises heel off stretcher with ball of foot on stretcher (plantar flex), holding patient's knee flexed fully with a hand pushing down on patient's ankle
  - Hip usually reduces
- Apply knee immobilizer
- Many other techniques are available
-

Consult criteria recommendation

- Consult orthopedic physician if needed
- Prosthetic hip dislocations may be discharged without consulting orthopedic surgeon and follow up in office

Notes

REFERENCES:

Orthopaedics Primary Care by Chinni Pennathur Ramamurti

Hip Dislocation in Emergency Medicine
Author: Stephen R McMillan, MD; Chief Editor: Barry E Brenner, MD, PhD, FACEP
emedicine.medscape.com/article/823471

Slipped Capital Femoral Epiphysis
Author: Kevin D Walter, MD, FAAP; Chief Editor: Craig C Young, MD
emedicine.medscape.com/article/91596

Evidence-based care guideline for conservative management of Legg-Calve-Perthes disease in children aged 3 to 12 years 2010 Oct. NGC:008174

Transient Synovitis
Author: Christine C Whitelaw, MD; Chief Editor: Lawrence K Jung, MD
emedicine.medscape.com/article/1007186

KNEE SOFT TISSUE INJURY PROTOCOL

Differential Diagnosis

- Knee strain
- Anterior cruciate ligament tear or strain
- Posterior cruciate ligament tear or strain
- Medial meniscus tear
- Lateral meniscus tear
- Medial collateral tear or strain
- Lateral collateral tear of stain
- Patellar dislocation
- Iliotibial Band Syndrome

Considerations

- Effusions occurring within 6 hours suggest ligament or cartilage injury

- Grade 1: microscopic ligament injury
- Grade 2: severe stretch with partial tear
- Grade 3: complete ligament disruption

Ottawa Knee Rule for obtaining x-rays (any of the following) for injuries < 24 hours and age > 18

- Inability to bear weight (walk 4 steps) immediately and presently
- Patellar tenderness
- Fibular head tenderness
- Age > 55 years
- Unable to flex knee > 90 degrees

Examination

- Palpate for areas of tenderness
- Check for knee effusion
- Neurovascular exam
- Knee x-ray if indicated
  - Evaluate for fracture, dislocation and effusion

Lachman's test

- Knee held in 15–30 degree flexion and move tibia forward
- Positive if motion visible; motion more than in uninjured knee
- Suggests anterior cruciate ligament (ACL) tear

McMurray's test

- Flex knee fully
- Rotate externally or internally and extend the knee
- Painful click on extension suggests meniscus injury
  - Internal rotation: lateral meniscus
  - External rotation: medial meniscus

Apley's test

- Patient in prone position
- Knee flexed
- Compression of foot into knee while rotated causes pain — suggests meniscus injury
- Distraction of foot from knee while rotated causes pain — suggests ligament injury

Treatment Options

- Ice
- Elevation
- Knee immobilizer prn
- Crutches prn
- Analgesics: NSAID's, narcotics prn
- Reduce patellar dislocation

Discharge criteria recommendation

- Uncomplicated injury

Discharge instructions

- Knee injury aftercare instructions
- Referral to orthopedic surgeon for grade 2–3 ligament injury or suspected meniscus injury suspected within 7–10 days
- Primary care provider follow-up for grade 1–2 sprains and contusions within 7–10 days

Consult criteria recommendation

- Neurovascular injury
- Open joint injury
- Grossly unstable joint

Notes

REFERENCES:

Orthopaedics Primary Care by Chinni Pennathur Ramamurti

The Ottawa Knee Rule: Examining Use in an Academic Emergency Department West J Emerg Med. Sep 2012; 13(4): 366–372

Knee Examination

Author: Bert Boonen, MD; Chief Editor: Erik D Schraga, MD
emedicine.medscape.com/article/1909230

Knee Disorders Protocol

Considerations

- Most nontraumatic knee conditions are degenerative or inflammatory
- Blood cultures may be positive in septic arthritis
- Consult physician for acute neurovascular deficits

Synovial fluid analysis

Normal

- Transparent clarity
- Clear color
- WBC < 200/mL
- PMN's < 25%
- Culture negative
- No crystals
- Mucin clot firm
- Glucose approximates blood levels

Noninflammatory

- Transparent clarity
- Yellow color
- WBC 200–2000/mL
- PMN's < 25%
- Culture negative
- No crystals
- Mucin clot firm
- Glucose approximates blood levels
- Associated conditions: rheumatic fever, trauma, osteoarthritis

Inflammatory

- Cloudy clarity
- Yellow color
- WBC 200–50,000/mL
- PMN's > 50%
- Culture negative
- Crystals can be present if gout or pseudogout present
- Mucin clot friable
- Glucose decreased
- Associated conditions: SLE, Lyme disease, gout, pseudogout, spondyloarthropathies

Septic

- Cloudy clarity
- Yellow color
- WBC 25,000/mL to often > 100,000/mL
- PMS's > 50%
- Culture often positive
- No crystals
- Mucin clot friable
- Glucose very decreased
- Fever
- C-reactive protein elevated

Osgood-Schlatter's Disease

Considerations

- Childhood disorder
- Males 10–15 years of age
- Aseptic necrosis within tibial tuberosity
- Pain, swelling and erythema over anterior tibial tuberosity
- Pain during resisted extension
- Pain on kneeling
- Slow onset
- Lateral knee x-ray may or may not show fragmentation of the tibial tubercle
- Clinical diagnosis

Treatment options

- Avoid climbing, running, kicking until pain has resolved
- Initially ice pack 20 minutes every 2–4 hours
- Quadriceps/hip extension exercises once acute episode has resolved
- May use NSAID's for pain
- No steroid injections

Discharge criteria

- All patients usually

Discharge instructions

- Osgood–Schlatter's disease aftercare instructions

Consult criteria

- Orthopedic referral if condition persistent

Prepatellar and Superficial Infrapatellar Bursitis

Considerations

- "Housemaid knee"
- Swelling of involved area

Treatment options

- Avoid kneeling
- Aspirate fluid if experienced with procedure
- May inject 1 cc of triamcinolone 40/cc with 1 cc lidocaine if experienced (do not inject if cellulitis present)
- Ace wrap

Discharge criteria

- Noninfected bursitis

Discharge instructions

- Patellar bursitis aftercare instructions

Consult criteria

- Infected bursitis suspected

Deep Infrapatellar and Anserine Bursitis

Considerations

- Excessive weight bearing may cause
- Pain at rest
- Increased pain with resisted extension
- Pain is felt in knee and may refer to hip, thigh or lower leg
- Swelling may occur
- Tenderness deep to patellar tendon

Treatment options

- Minimize weight bearing
- Avoid climbing, jumping, running, squatting
- Ice packs
- Quadriceps exercise when pain allows
- Range of motion exercises
- Corticosteroid injection prn (if Provider is experienced)
- NSAID's prn; narcotics prn

Discharge criteria

- Noninfected bursitis

Discharge instructions

- Knee bursitis aftercare instructions

Consult criteria

- Infected bursitis
- Orthopedic referral if not resolving

Baker's Cyst

Considerations

- Effusion of semimembranosus bursa
- Predisposes to chronic knee effusion
- Mass behind knee up to 5 × 5 cm
- X-rays may or may not show DJD

Treatment options

- May aspirate if experienced
- Ace wrap prn
- NSAID's prn

Discharge criteria

- Nonseptic joint
- Orthopedic referral

Discharge instructions

- Baker's cyst aftercare instructions

Consult criteria

- Uncertain diagnosis

Iliotibial Band Syndrome

- Most common cause of lateral knee pain among athletes
- Inflammation of the bursa surrounding the iliotibial band
- Lateral knee pain approximately 2 cm above the lateral joint line
- Pain may eventually radiate to the distal tibia, calf, and up to the lateral thigh

Ober test

- Patient lying on unaffected side, examiner stabilizes hip and lower the leg posteriorly to stretcher
- Knee cannot be lowered less than a fist width space from stretcher

Treatment

- Ultrasound
- Ice
- NSAIDs
- Physical therapy and stretching
- Avoid provoking activities

Disposition recommendation

- Orthopedic referral prn
- Physical therapy prn

Chondromalacia Patella

Considerations

- Degeneration of the patellar cartilage
- Any age
- Usually no injury
- Positive Patellar Grind Test — pushing on patella while moving knee into extension causes pain

Treatment options

- Avoid climbing, jumping, running, squatting

Discharge criteria

- Usually most patients

Discharge instructions

- Chondromalacia patella aftercare instructions

Consult criteria

- Orthopedic or primary care provider referral if not resolving

Osteoarthritis (DJD)

Considerations

- Related to increasing age
- Can result from previous injuries or knee surgery
- Knee effusion may be present
- Knee feels like it "gives way" occasionally
- Range of motion limited

Treatment options

- Minimize wear and tear activities
- NSAID's prn; narcotics prn for severe pain — short course
- Oral steroids for 7 days prn if not diabetic
- Knee immobilizer prn
- Crutches or walker prn

Discharge criteria

- Nonseptic knee joint

Discharge instructions

- Knee osteoarthritis aftercare instructions

Consult criteria

- Orthopedic referral for severe knee pain

Gout

Differential diagnosis

- Cellulitis
- Septic arthritis
- Bursitis
- Osteomyelitis
- Rheumatoid arthritis
- Soft tissue injury
- Pseudogout

Considerations

- Crystal uric acid deposits in joints and tissues
- Most common cause of monoarticular arthritis age > 60
- Increased warmth, redness and joint swelling
- First metatarsophalangeal joint of foot involved 75% of the time — most common involved joint
- Joint fluid: 20,000–100,000 WBC; poor string and mucin clot; no bacteria (pseudogout similar)
- Risk factors
  - Age > 40
  - Hypertension
  - Diuretics
  - Ethanol intake
  - Obesity

Evaluation
- Clinical evaluation usually all that is needed
- If diagnosis uncertain may order
  - CBC
  - C-reactive protein
  - X-rays
  - Joint aspiration if experienced Provider

Treatment options (monotherapy)
- NSAID's high dose 5–10 days
- Narcotics IM or PO prn
- Prednisone 40–60 mg PO qday × 3–7 days

OR

- Dexamethasone 6 mg PO daily × 3–7 days

OR

- Depomedrol (methylprednisolone acetate) 80–120 mg IM
- Can consider intra-articular steroids if attack involves 1–2 large joints – if experienced with joint injections
- Colchicine 2 tablets (1.2 mg) with a third tablet (0.6 mg) an hour later, then qday–bid until attack resolves
  - Only for acute attacks < 36 hours
  - Do not use if patient used colchicine within last 14 days
- Allopurinol 50–300 mg PO qday: adjusted for renal function; start after acute episode resolved

Severe attacks use combination of treatments
- Do not stop urate lowering therapy during an acute attack - symptoms would only worsen if it is stopped or adjusted
- Switch to another treatment or add a second treatment is < 20% improvement in pain score within 24 hours, or < 50% improvement in pain score > 24 hours
- Follow up with primary care provider within 2–3 days if pain persist

Discharge instructions
- Gout aftercare instructions

Consult criteria
- Uncertain diagnosis
- Fever or toxicity
- HR ≥ 110

Septic Arthritis

Differential diagnosis
- Cellulitis
- Gout
- Bursitis
- Osteomyelitis
- Rheumatoid arthritis
- Soft tissue injury
- Pseudogout

Considerations
- Onset is rapid
- Usually one joint infected
- Joint is very painful; hot; red; fluctuant
- Signs of acute systemic illness may be present
- Fever, chills and sweats frequently
- C-reactive protein elevated
- Pain and swollen prosthetic knee joint assume septic arthritis until proven otherwise
- See **Synovial Fluid Analysis**

Treatment
- Admission to hospital for drainage and antibiotics

Discharge criteria
- Only with physician consent

Consult criteria
- All septic joint patients

Notes

REFERENCES:

Orthopaedics Primary Care by Chinni Pennathur Ramamurti

Pommering TL, Kluchurosky L. Overuse injuries in adolescents. *Adolesc Med State Art Rev*. May 2007;18(1):95–120, ix

Osgood-Schlatter Disease Author: J Andy Sullivan, MD; Chief Editor: Craig C Young, MD emedicine.medscape.com/article/1993268

ANKLE SPRAIN PROTOCOL

Definition

- Stretching or tearing of the ankle's ligaments

Differential Diagnosis

- Ankle fracture
- Ankle dislocation

Considerations

- 85–90% involves lateral ligaments
- Age < 10 years with traumatic ankle pain and no fracture on x-ray may have Salter type 1 fracture
- Stress testing acutely often limited by pain
- Nonweight bearing for several days has been shown to improve long-term outcomes for all sprains
- Ankle sprain grades
  - Grade 1: Ligament stretching without tearing or instability on exam
  - Grade 2: Some ligament tearing without instability, but more swelling and ecchymosis than grade 1
  - Grade 3: Complete tearing of ligaments with gross instability, marked swelling and ecchymosis and pain

Ottawa Rule (Can defer x-ray if no criteria present below)

- Bony tenderness distal 6 cm of posterior edge or tip of tibia or fibula, or either malleolus
- Bony tenderness base of 5th metatarsal or navicular bone
- Inability to take 4 unassisted steps at time of injury and when being evaluated
- Performed within 10 days of injury
- Not validated in children

Evaluation

- Assess ankle for instability
- Drawer test — anterior
- Assess inversion and eversion for instability
- Neurovascular exam
- Examine for associated ipsilateral leg injuries
- Examine for other remote injuries
- Evaluate as needed for the cause of injury

Treatment Options

- Ice and elevation
- Mild to moderate sprains can be treated with elastic wrap, air splint or plastic boot.
  - Can be weight bearing or nonweight bearing per Provider's discretion
- Severe sprains (ligament laxity) or severe pain — plastic boot or OCL posterior splint and crutches
- Consider nonweight bearing for 5–10 days to improve long-term outcome
- Nondisplaced distal fibula fractures can be treated with OCL posterior splint or plastic boots and crutches
- NSAID's, Tylenol, or narcotics prn

- May combine NSAID's and acetaminophen prn
- Strengthening exercises
- Aggressive pain-free ROM is recommended

Return-to-play criteria during the recovery phase (3 days to 2 wks. post injury) include the following:

- Full, pain-free active and passive ROM
- No pain or tenderness
- Strength of ankle muscles 70–80% of that on the uninvolved side
- Ability to balance on leg for 30 seconds with eyes closed

Return-to-play criteria during the functional phase (2–6 weeks post injury) include the following:

- Normal ROM of the ankle joint
- No pain or tenderness
- Satisfactory clinical examination
- Strength of ankle muscles 90% of the uninvolved side
- Ability to complete functional examination

Discharge Criteria

- Sprains with intact ankle mortise, closed, with no acute neurovascular deficits
- Potential Salter 1 fractures

Discharge instructions

- Ankle sprain aftercare instructions
- Refer to grade 1 and 2 sprains to primary care provider
  - Permissible to refer to orthopedics
- Refer grade 3 or severe sprains to orthopedics within 7–10 days
- Nonweight bearing for 3 weeks improves outcomes
- Refer potential Salter 1 fractures to PCP or orthopedic surgeon for recheck in 10 days

Consult Criteria

- Grossly unstable ankle joint or disrupted ankle mortise
- Potential open ankle joint
- Acute neurovascular deficits
- Fractures (excluding nondisplaced distal fibula fractures)

Notes

REFERENCES:

Dowling S, Spooner CH, Liang Y, Dryden DM, Friesen C, Klassen TP, et al. Accuracy of Ottawa Ankle Rules to exclude fractures of the ankle and midfoot in children: a meta-analysis. *Acad Emerg Med.* Apr 2009;16(4):277–87

Ivins D. Acute ankle sprain: an update. *Am Fam Physician.* Nov 15 2006;74(10):1714–20

Ankle Sprain Author: Craig C Young, MD; Chief Editor: Sherwin SW Ho, MD emedicine.medscape.com/article/1907229

Hand, Wrist, and Distal Forearm Injury Protocol

General Recommendations

Evaluation

- X-ray all orthopedic hand and wrist injuries with mechanism of injury that could cause fractures or dislocations
- Assess neurovascular status and for tendon/ligament deficits

Complications

- Neurovascular injury
- Open fracture
- Joint involvement
- Ligament/tendon injury
- Displaced and angulated
- Compartment syndrome
- Fat emboli — long bones
- Avascular necrosis
- Osteomyelitis

Treatment

- Reduce dislocations if experienced
- NSAID's with or without acetaminophen, or narcotics prn for pain
- Tetanus prophylaxis prn (see Tetanus Guideline)

Discharge criteria

- Simple, nondisplaced, nonrotated closed long bone fractures can be splinted and discharged with orthopedic follow-up usually
  - Discuss with physician (except simple nondisplaced torus fractures)
- Simple dislocations that have been reduced

Consult criteria

- Wrist or proximal metacarpal dislocations
- Open injuries
- Acute neurovascular deficits
- Tendon/ligament injuries
- Nondisplaced, closed simple long bone fractures can be splinted and discharged with orthopedic follow-up usually
  - Discuss with physician (except simple nondisplaced torus fractures)

Compartment syndrome complication

- From increased pressure in a muscle or other internal compartment
- Not all signs and symptoms are needed to make diagnosis
- High pressures > 8 hours leads to tissue damage
- Normal tissue pressure is < 10 mm Hg
- Capillary blood flow is compromised at > 20 mm Hg
- Intracompartmental pressures > 30 mm Hg or within 10–30 mm Hg of DBP

Signs and symptoms (not diagnostic)

- Pain
  - Out of proportion to injury
  - On passive stretch of muscles
- Pallor
- Paresthesias
- Paralysis
  - Sensory and motor findings are late signs
- Poikilothermia — decreased temperature
- Pulselessness
  - Usually not lost until muscle necrosis has occurred
  - Last sign to develop
- Tense muscle compartment on palpation

Treatment

- Consult physician if suspected
- Keep extremity at level of heart
- Do not use ice if suspected
- Remove cast and padding
- Surgery fasciotomy is usually necessary

Human Bite or Clenched Fist Injury

- Amoxicillin/clavulanate preferred antibiotic x 10–14 days
- Need operative irrigation and surgical exploration emergently unless very superficial
- Usually presents late
- Do not perform primary repair of laceration
- Consult physician

- See Human and Animal Bite Protocol

Boxer's Fracture (4th and/or 5th Metacarpal Shaft) and other Metacarpal Fractures

Considerations

- Boxer fractures usually from punching with a closed fist
- No more than 10-15° of angulation in the second and third metacarpals should be accepted without reduction
- No rotational deformity is acceptable

Evaluation

- X-ray
- Assess for neurovascular and tendon injury
- Assess for human teeth injury

Treatment

- Treat with OCL ulnar gutter or boxer's splint
- Most splints leave on for 3–4 weeks
- Sling
- Analgesics
- Fracture splints should be forearm-based and should allow for motion of the interphalangeal (IP) joints
- Splints should extend over the dorsal and palmar aspect of the entire metacarpal being treated
- Generally, the wrist should be placed in 20-30° of extension
  - The metacarpophalangeal (MCP) joints should be immobilized in 70-90° of flexion, with the dorsal aspect of the splint extending to the IP joints; and the volar aspect should end at the distal palmar crease
- Buddy taping the fingers of the involved metacarpal can aid in maintaining rotational control
- After a short period of immobilization, patients may be encouraged to use the fingers on the affected hand to maintain motion

Discharge criteria

- Simple closed Boxer's fracture with < 40 degrees angulation
- Second and third metacarpal fractures ≤ 10–15° of angulation
- No rotational deformity

Discharge instructions

- Boxer's fracture aftercare instructions
- Metacarpal fracture aftercare instructions
- Refer to orthopedic or hand surgeon within 7 days

Consult criteria

- 40 degrees or more of angulation needs reduction (consult physician)
- Greater than 10-15° of angulation in the second and third metacarpals
- Nonreducible dislocations
- Neurovascular compromise
- Loss of ligament or tendon function
- Metacarpal head displaced fractures usually need surgery
- Salter fractures consult physician
- Open fracture
- Human bite

High Pressure Injection Injuries

- Consult physician immediately
- Do not discharge
- Needs surgery

Dislocations of the MP Joint

Evaluation

- X-ray
- Assess for neurovascular and tendon injury
- Assess for human teeth injury if in fist fight

Treatment

- May reduce if seen right after injury without x-ray if there is no doubt to diagnosis
- Metacarpal block may not be needed if seen immediately after injury
- Push your thumb on dorsal surface of hand and distally on proximal phalanx to reduce
- Splinting may not be necessary

Discharge criteria

- Closed simple MP joint dislocations that are reduced

Discharge instructions

- MP joint aftercare instructions
- Refer to orthopedic or hand surgeon within 7–10 days

Consult criteria

- Unable to reduce
- Open joint
- Associated fracture

Scaphoid Fracture (or Suspected Scaphoid Fracture)

Considerations

- Most common carpal fracture
- Snuffbox tenderness (with negative x-ray, 25% of these patients will have a fracture)
- Complication of avascular necrosis may occur
- High malpractice awards when fracture missed

Evaluation

- X-ray — may need special views
- Assess for neurovascular and tendon injury

Treatment

- Thumb spica splint and sling if fracture diagnosed or suspected
  - Cast for 12 weeks placed by outpatient referral provider

Discharge criteria

- Closed simple scaphoid fracture
- See Shoulder and Arm Trauma Protocol

Discharge instructions

- Scaphoid fracture aftercare instructions
- Orthopedic or hand surgeon referral within 7–10 days if diagnosed or suspected

Consult criteria

- Open fracture
- Neurovascular, tendon or ligament deficit

Carpal Bone Fractures or Dislocations

- Consult physician (see Scaphoid Fracture above)

Colles and Smith Fractures

Considerations

- Involves distal forearm
- Colles is a dorsal angulation and Smith fracture volar angulation of fracture
- Angulation ≤ 10 degrees can be treated without reduction anatomically
- Intra-articular step-off > 1–2 mm needs orthopedic consultation
- Ulna is usually within 2 mm of radius at wrist
- Treatment varies depending on age and activity level

Evaluation

- X-ray (lateral, AP and oblique)
- Neurovascular examination
- Ligament and tendon examination

Treatment

- Sugar tong splint
- Sling
- Reduction of significant angulation
- Surgery needed commonly

Discharge criteria

- Consult criteria not met
- Simple closed fracture

Discharge instructions

- Colles or Smith fracture aftercare instructions

- Follow up with orthopedic surgeon within 7 days

Consult physician or orthopedics

- Intra-articular step-off > 1–2 mm
- Dorsal tilt ≥ 10%
- Volar tilt > 20%
- Radial shortening > 3 mm
- Loss of radial angle
- Neurovascular injury
- Open fracture
- Ligament disruption
- Lunate and perilunate wrist dislocations

Notes

____

____

____

REFERENCES:

Orthopaedics Primary Care by Chinni Pennathur Ramamurti

Wrist Fracture in Emergency Medicine
Author: Bryan C Hoynak, MD, FACEP, FAAEM; Chief Editor: Rick Kulkarni, MD emedicine.medscape.com/article/828746

Ann of EM, 2015;65:308

Metacarpal Fractures Treatment & Management
Updated: Aug 27, 2018 Author: Thomas Michael Dye, MD; Chief Editor: Harris Gellman, MD

FINGER INJURY PROTOCOL

General Evaluation and Considerations

- X-ray all finger injuries with mechanism of injury with potential to cause fractures or dislocations
- Assess neurovascular status and for tendon/ligament deficits
- Consult on all open fractures or with acute neurovascular deficits
- Consult on tendon/ligament injuries except as discussed below
- NSAID's or narcotics prn for pain
- Consult for proximal and middle phalanx fractures
- Nondisplaced distal phalange fractures may be splinted in extension and referred to orthopedic or hand surgery

Mallet Finger

- Avulsion of the DIP extensor tendon
- Distal 1 inch foam aluminum splint with joint in full extension for 6 weeks
  - Aluminum padded strip can be applied either dorsally or volarly
- Can initiate splinting up to 6 weeks post injury
- Surgery only option if injury 2 months old (Refer to orthopedic or hand surgeon)
- Refer to primary care provider, orthopedic or hand surgeon for recent injury

Avulsion of the Flexor Profundus Tendon DIP Joint

- Jamming injury (usually children)
- Palmar middle phalanx and dorsal DIP joint swollen and tender
- Unable to actively flex distal phalanx

- Splint in position of function (normal resting position of an uninjured finger)
- Orthopedic referral for surgery

PIP Joint Dislocation

- Usually from hyperextension injury
- May reduce if seen right after injury without x-ray if there is no doubt about the diagnosis
- Local digital anesthesia may not be needed if seen immediately after injury
- Push distal phalanx back into alignment and x-ray
- Splint in full extension for 3 weeks
- Buddy tape with padding between fingers to adjacent finger
- Refer to orthopedic or hand surgeon

Avulsion of the Central Extensor Slip

- Difficult to diagnose at time of injury because of swelling
- Boutonniere deformity of the PIP joint is frequently a late finding
- Due to forceful PIP joint flexion
- Splint in full extension for 3 weeks if suspected or diagnosed
- Refer to orthopedic or hand surgeon within 7 days

Avulsion of the Volar Carpal Plate PIP Joint

- Hyperextension injury or a recently reduced PIP joint dislocation
- Joint movements very painful and limited
- Palmar surface very tender
- Abnormal extension of joint possible on exam
- Splint in full extension for 3 weeks if suspected or diagnosed
- Refer to orthopedic or hand surgeon within 3–7 days

Tear or Avulsion of the Collateral Ligament

- Instability of lateral PIP joint in either direction
- Splint in 15–20 degrees at PIP joint and 70 degrees at MP joint for 3 weeks
- Refer to orthopedic or hand surgeon

Gamekeeper Thumb

- Tenderness over first metacarpal phalangeal joint of thumb
- Rupture of ulnar collateral ligament
- Joint opens up with radial stress > than uninjured thumb
- Associated avulsion fracture is common
- Thumb spica
- Refer to orthopedic or hand surgeon within 3–7 days

Notes

____

____

____

REFERENCES:

Orthopaedics Primary Care by Chinni Pennathur Ramamurti

Mallet Finger Author: Roy A Meals, MD; Chief Editor: Harris Gellman, MD emedicine.medscape.com/article/1242305

Phalangeal Fractures Author: Jay E Bowen, DO; Chief Editor: Craig C Young, MD emedicine.medscape.com/article/98322

Mallet Finger Treatment & Management Updated: Aug 27, 2018 Author: Roy A Meals, MD; Chief Editor: Harris Gellman, MD

Pediatrics

Section Contents

When using any protocol, always follow the Guidelines of Proper Use (page 12).

Pediatric Fever Protocol

Definition

- Rectal temperature > 100.4°F (38°C)

Differential Diagnosis

- Viral infections
- Localized bacterial infections
- Bacteremia
- Sepsis
- Urinary tract infection
- Heat illness

Considerations

- Risk of occult bacteremia has declined markedly with pneumococcal and HIB vaccines
- Males < 6 months without a source of fever have a UTI 7% of the time
- Females < 12 months without a source of fever have UTI 8% of the time
- 0–8 weeks of age are at higher risk of bacterial infection — especially 0–4 weeks of age
- Serious bacterial infection (SBI) can occur without fever
- Hypothermia during infection portends a higher risk
- Fever is not dangerous in of itself unless ≥ 105°F (40.6°C)

- Viruses are the most common cause of fever
- Treating fever has no effect on decreasing febrile seizures
- Pneumonia frequently has a normal pulmonary auscultatory exam

Evaluation

Neonates 0–28 days of age

- CBC count, urinalysis, blood culture, urine culture, chest radiography, and diagnostic LP

Children 5–8 weeks of age

- CBC and U/A
- CXR may be obtained especially if respiratory symptoms present
- Lumbar puncture may be omitted if patient appears well, close follow up within 12–24 hours and no antibiotics have been previously given
  - Maintain low threshold for obtaining lumbar puncture

Children 2–24 months of age

- Complete history of fever, any prior treatments and associated symptoms
- Baseline dehydration assessment, see Pediatric Dehydration Protocol
- Assess interaction, feeding and alertness
- Nontoxic patients with viral source of fever may need no further evaluation
- Fully immunized patients including pneumococcal and hemophilus influenza B will not usually need CBC or blood cultures
- CXR
  - O_2 saturation < 95% on room air
  - Tachypnea or respiratory distress
  - WBC ≥ 15,000 with cough
- Fever ≥ 102°F (38.9°C) without source and patient is immunized to pneumococcal disease
  - Consider CXR
  - Cath U/A in males < 6 months; uncircumcised male < 12 months; females < 24 months
- Dehydration > 5% order BMP (See Pediatric Diarrhea Protocol for baseline dehydration assessment and treatment)
- Urinary complaints — order U/A
  - U/A for fever without a clinical source in girls and uncircumcised boys < 2 years of age
  - Final diagnosis of UTI requires a urine culture
- Decreased alertness, toxic appearance or in distress
  - CBC, chest x-ray, blood culture × 1, cath U/A, urine culture — discuss performance of a lumbar puncture with physician

Children > 24 months of age

- Evaluation based on history and physically exam primarily (if fully immunized)
- Specific workup based on clinical findings and suspicion of disease

Pediatric sickle cell disease (SCD) and fever

Admission criteria

- Age < 2 years with hemoglobin SS (HbSS) disease or hemoglobin S–β° (HbS–β°)
  - HbSC or HbS–β+ less likely to have bacteremia and age alone not an admission criteria
- Temperature > 104°F (40°C)
- WBC > 30,000 or < 5,000
  - Both associated with increased bacteremia risk
  - Bandemia > 1,000 with bacterial infection
- Hemoglobin ≥ 2 gms below baseline in HbSS or HbS–β°
- Hemoglobin ≤ 6 gms
- Previous bacteremia or invasion infection
- Indwelling vascular lines

- Signs of systemic toxicity, vital sign instability or serious infection
- Previously treated with clindamycin or vancomycin instead of ceftriaxone
- Presence of SCD manifestations that require inpatient management
  - Acute chest syndrome
  - Painful crisis
  - Aplastic crisis
  - Splenic sequestration
- Concerns about family not able to recognize changes in patient's condition or inability/difficulty for follow–up (Need clear method to contact family if cultures are positive)

Outpatient management

- Patients that do not meet admission criteria can be considered for outpatient management
- Clinically stable
- Specific plan for follow–up the next day
- Recorded working telephone number recorded in chart
- Ceftriaxone 50–75 mg/kg IM or IV daily unless discontinued by medical provider
- Stress oral hydration
- If vomiting occurs then return for further evaluation
- Adequate PO pain medications

General Fever Treatment Options

(May not apply to specific clinical scenarios noted above)

- Fever may be treated; if patient not uncomfortable, it may not need to be treated unless ≥ 104°F (40°C)
- Alternating Tylenol with ibuprofen not officially recommended and may confuse parents increasing toxicity risk through medication error (may lengthen fever control more than a single antipyretic medication alone though)
- Fever ≥ 102°F (38.9°C) without a source and patient is nontoxic and feeding normally (age 2–24 months) who is fully immunized including pneumococcal and hemophilus influenza B
  - Can be treated with Rocephin (ceftriaxone) 50 mg/kg IM
  - Can have no treatment, but needs close follow up within 12–24 hours
- Fever with a source in patient without toxicity or distress
  - Viral: treat symptoms
  - Suspected bacterial infection: appropriate antibiotic
  - May use Sanford Guide or antibiotic database
- Fever with or without a source and patient toxic or in distress
  - Consult physician promptly

Discharge Criteria

- Healthy prior to fever onset
- No significant risk factors (prematurity or age < 3 months or comorbid conditions)
- Nontoxic and healthy appearance
- Less than 5% dehydration (serum CO_2 ≥ 18 if checked)
- Feeding well
- Reliable caregivers and access to follow-up
- WBC < 18,000 and patient appears well

Discharge instructions

- Pediatric fever aftercare instructions
- Return if patient becomes less active or appears worse
- Follow up with primary care provider in 2–3 days if fever persists

Consult Criteria

- Appears toxic, has poor alertness, decreased interaction or in distress
- Fever ≥ 104.5°F (40.3°C)
- Greater than 5% dehydration
- Poor feeding
- No source of fever
- Immunosuppression
- Splenectomy
- Seizure

- Petechiae

Vital signs and age consult criteria

- Fever ≥ 104.5°F (40.3°C)
- Age ≤ 60 days
- O_2 saturation < 95% on room air
- Pediatric heart rate
  - 0–4 months ≥ 180
  - 5–7 months ≥ 175
  - 8–12 months ≥ 170
  - Hypotension

Lab and x-ray consult criteria

- WBC ≥ 18,000 or < 3,000; absolute neutrophils < 1,000
- Bandemia ≥ 15%
- Acute thrombocytopenia
- New onset anemia
- Serum CO_2 < 18 mEq/L
- Metabolic acidosis
- Glucose ≥ 200 mg/dL
- Significant pneumonia
- Pleural effusion

Notes

REFERENCES:

Rudinsky SL, Carstairs KL, Reardon JM, Simon LV, Riffenburgh RH, Tanen DA. Serious bacterial infections in febrile infants in the post-pneumococcal conjugate vaccine era. *Acad Emerg Med.* Jul 2009;16(7):585–90

Emergent Management of Pediatric Patients with Fever

Author: John W Graneto, DO, FACOEP, FACEP; Chief Editor: Russell W Steele, MD
medicine.medscape.com/article/801598

Management of fever in sickle cell disease Author: Zora R Rogers, MD

Benign Febrile Seizure Protocol

Definition

- A seizure event in infancy or childhood usually occurring between 3 months and 5 years of age, associated with fever, but without evidence of intracranial infection or other defined seizure cause

Differential Diagnosis

- Meningitis
- Encephalitis
- Subdural and epidural infections
- Bacteremia and sepsis
- Epilepsy

Considerations

- Affects 2–4% of all children < 5 years of age
- Occurs in early childhood
- Usually occurs in children with systemic viral infection
- Majority last < 5 minutes
- Rate of serious infections are equivalent to febrile patients without seizures
- Increased rate of febrile seizures on day of DTP vaccination and 8–14 days after MMR vaccination
- Patients with febrile seizure have slightly higher rate of developing epilepsy
- No evidence that treatment with seizure medications decreases future febrile seizures
- No evidence of future cognitive differences in patients with febrile seizures
- Fever treatment does not alter developing febrile seizures
- Mild postictal phase usual
- Occurs in families to some extent
- Febrile seizure is the most common cause of status epilepticus

- Recurrence of seizure during same febrile illness within 24 hours of 1st febrile seizure is 14–24%

Types

Simple febrile seizure

- Lasts < 15 minutes
- Generalized (not focal)
- Occurs only once in 24 hours

Complex febrile seizure

- Lasts > 15 minutes
- Focal features at any time
- Recurs within 24 hours

Evaluation

- Complete history and physical exam
  - Lateral tongue bites more specific than distal tongue bites for seizure
- Serum glucose
- Routine labs usually not indicated
- Lab and x-rays if significant comorbid disease suspected (bacterial infection suspected)
- CT head for focal findings
- Lumbar puncture considered for age < 18 months for any of the following
  - History of irritability, decrease feeding, or lethargy
  - Abnormal appearance or mental status after postictal period
  - Signs of meningitis; severe headache or nuchal rigidity
  - Complex febrile seizure
  - Slow postictal clearing of mentation
  - Pretreatment with antibiotics

Treatment Options

- No specific treatment for simple febrile seizure
- Reassure parents
- Treat any serious underlying cause of fever (see Pediatric Fever Protocol or other appropriate Protocols)

Complex febrile seizures

- Intubation if airway not secure
- IV NS KVO
- Oxygen as needed
- Lorazepam 0.05–0.1 mg/kg IV prn; may repeat q10–15 minutes prn (NMT 4 mg)
- Diastat (diazepam rectal gel) if no IV available
  - Age up to 5 years: 0.5 mg/kg
  - Age 6–11 years: 0.3 mg/kg
  - Age > 12 years: 0.2 mg/kg
  - Round up to higher available dose: 2.5, 5, 7.5, 10, 12.5, 15, 17.5, 20 mg/dose
- Midazolam IV/IM/PR/ET/intranasal 0.1–0.2 mg/kg/dose; not to exceed a cumulative dose of 10 mg)
- If no IV available, give midazolam 10 mg IM if patient's weight ≥ 40 kg and 5 mg IM if ≥ 13 kg

Status epilepticus (beware of "too slow and too low" treatment)

- Lorazepam 0.1 mg/kg IV — **first line drug choice** (NMT 10 mg total dose or 4 mg/dose)
- Cerebyx (fosphenytoin) 15–20 mg/kg IV at 100 mg/minute if no response in 5 minutes to lorazepam or midazolam (Versed)
- Keppra (Levetiracetam) 30-40 mg/kg IV
  - 2-5 mg/kg/minute
  - NMT 2000 mg

Drugs that can be used if lorazepam, midazolam or Cerebyx (fosphenytoin) fail

- Pentobarbital 1 mg/kg boluses IV to maximum 5 mg/kg
- Valproic acid 15 mg/kg over 1–5 minutes (NMT 40 mg/kg)
  - IV infusion 5 mg/kg/hr.
- Phenobarbital 20 mg/kg IV at 100 mg/hr.
- Propofol 2 mg/kg IV bolus (patient intubated), may repeat if needed and start 5 mg/kg/hr. infusion if necessary

- Ketamine 1–4.5 mg/kg IV over 60 seconds or 4–5 mg/kg IM
- Lidocaine 1 mg/kg IV, may repeat x 2 prn (NMT 3mg/kg)

Management of refractory status epilepticus

- Referral to an intensive care unit
- Anesthetic agents such as midazolam, propofol or barbiturates (thiopental, pentobarbital) for generalized convulsive status epilepticus
- Non-anesthetic anticonvulsants such as phenobarbital or valproic acid for nonconvulsive status epilepticus

Discharge criteria recommendation

- Normal neurologic exam
- Simple febrile seizure
- Source of fever can be treated as an outpatient
- Refer to primary care physician or provider
- Discharge instructions
  - Benign febrile seizure aftercare instructions
  - Return if seizure recurs
  - Return if patient appears worse
  - Close follow-up within 1 day preferable

Consult criteria recommendation

- Complex febrile seizure
- Suspected or diagnosed serious underlying infection
- Neurologic abnormality
- History of irritability
- Poor feeding
- Lethargy
- Abnormal appearance or mental status after postictal period
- Signs of meningitis
- Severe headache
- Slow postictal clearing of mentation
- Very recent or concurrent treatment with antibiotics
- Appears toxic, has poor alertness, decreased interaction or distress
- Greater than 5% dehydration
- No source of fever
- UTI — follow UTI Protocol

Vital signs and age consult recommendations

- Age < 3 months
- Pediatric heart rate
  - 0–4 months ≥ 180
  - 5–7 months ≥ 175
  - 8–12 months ≥ 170
- Fever ≥ 104.5°F (40.3°C)
- Hypotension

Lab and x-ray consult recommendations

- WBC ≥ 15,000 or < 3,000; absolute neutrophils < 1,000
- Bandemia ≥ 15%
- Thrombocytopenia
- New onset anemia
- Metabolic acidosis
- Glucose ≥ 200 mg/dL
- Hyperglycemia with metabolic acidosis (decreased serum CO_2 or elevated anion gap)
- Significant pneumonia
- Pleural effusion

Notes

____

____

____

REFERENCES:

Brooks M. Intranasal Midazolam Works for Seizure Emergencies in Kids. Medscape Medical News. Nov 5 2013

Pediatric Febrile Seizures Author: Robert J Baumann, MD; Chief Editor: Amy Kao, MD emedicine.medscape.com/article/1176205

Clinical practice guideline – febrile seizures: guideline for the neurodiagnostic evaluation of the child with a simple febrile seizure. *Pediatrics.* 2011;127;389–394

Pediatric Status Epilepticus Treatment & Management

Updated: Oct 06, 2014

Author: Rajesh Ramachandrannair, MBBS, MD, FRCPC; Chief Editor: Timothy E Corden, MD

Effectiveness of lidocaine infusion for status epilepticus in childhood: a retrospective multi-institutional study in Japan Brain Dev . 2008 Sep;30(8):504-12

Brain Dev, epub, 3/25/21

Crying Infant Protocol

Definition

- Crying child that presents without discernible cause of distress

Differential Diagnosis

- Otitis media
- Infant colic
- Viral illness with anorexia
- Dehydration
- UTI
- Corneal abrasion
- Ocular foreign body
- Oropharynx foreign body
- Hair tourniquet syndrome (hair wrapped around toe or penis)
- Brown recluse spider bite
- Clavicle or tibial fracture
- Gastrointestinal prodrome
- GERD
- Intussusception
- DTP reaction
- PSVT
- Intracranial abnormality or infection
- Congenital cardiac disease (check for decreased femoral pulses)
- Child abuse (nonaccidental trauma)

Considerations

- Crying stimulated by
  - Unmet need: hunger; thirst; desire for attention
  - Distress: anger; discomfort; pain
- Often defined by parental perceptions
- Healthy infants: crying levels increase from birth and peaks at 6–8 weeks of life
- Crying follows circadian rhythm — clusters late afternoon or early evening
- Infants that won't stop crying in the exam area is more predictive of serious illness
- Most serious common cause of explained crying is urinary tract infections
- Clinician intuition about severity of illness is important
- Parental concern is a red flag in identifying serious illness
- Normal physical exam and the patient stops crying usually indicates that a serious illness is likely not present
- Colic (29.5%), acute otitis media (15.5%) and constipation (5.5%) are the most common causes of unexplained crying
- Observational period important to determine if serious illness is present
- Close follow up is important when cause of crying not determined
- Avoid medicating unknown or unclear diagnosis for crying

Colic — recurrent paroxysmal attacks of crying lasting several hours

- Drawing up legs
- Abdomen may appear distended
- Bowel sounds increased
- Flatus may be passed

Colic rules of 3

- Lasting 3 or more hours
- Occurring 3 or more days per week
- Lasting minimum of 3 weeks
- No specific cause identified

Treatment options

- Short trial of hypoallergenic formula
- Stop cow's milk
- Treatments that are not effective
  - Simethicone
  - Lactase enzymes
  - Soy based formula
  - Fiber enriched foods
  - Carrying infant more
  - Car ride stimulators
  - Chiropractic manipulation

Evaluation

- History and physical exam reveals the majority of causes (71%)
- Consider rectal and genital exam if cause not evident
- Urinalysis and culture is the most helpful screening lab test, especially in the very young
- Tests are aimed at suspected causes of excessive crying
- Evaluate for child abuse and order testing as indicated by exam and history

Treatment Options

- Observe for up to 2–3 hours to see if crying ceases
- Aimed at cause of crying

Discharge Criteria

- Patient stops crying in exam area
- Normal vital signs
- O_2 saturation > 95%
- No serious illness detected
- Cause of crying determined to be benign and can be treated as outpatient
- Contact primary care physician or provider to alert of visit and arrange follow-up

Consult Criteria

- Patient will not stop crying
- O_2 saturation ≤ 94%
- Toxic appearance; poor interaction and activity
- Dehydration
- Poor response to treatment
- Worrisome abdominal tenderness
- Petechial rash
- Altered mental status
- Significant disease as cause of crying
- Clinician gut feeling that patient has a serious illness
- Parental concern that a serious illness is present
- Suspected nonaccidental abuse/trauma

Vital signs consult criteria

- Pediatric heart rate
  - 0–4 months ≥ 170
  - 5–7 months ≥ 160
  - 8–12 months ≥ 155
  - 1–3 years ≥ 135
- Hypotension

Lab consult criteria

- WBC ≥ 15,000 or < 3,000
- Bandemia ≥ 15%
- Thrombocytopenia
- Serum CO_2 < 18 mEq/L post rehydration
- Initial serum CO_2 < 17 mEq/L

Notes

REFERENCES:

Barr RG, Paterson JA, MacMartin LM, et al. Prolonged and unsoothable crying bouts in infants with and without colic. J Dev Behav Pediatr. 2005;26(1):14–23

Fahimi D, Shamsollahi B, Salamati P, et al. Excessive crying of infancy; a report of 200 cases. Iran J of Pediatr.

2007;17(3):222–226.

Poole SR, The infant with acute, unexplained, excessive crying. Pediatrics 1991;88(3):450–455

Van den Bruel A, Thompson M, Buntinx F, et.al. Clinician's gut feeling about serious infections in children: observational study. BMJ 2012;345:e6144 (Observational study 3369 children)

URI and Sinusitis Protocol

Definition

- Infection of the nasopharynx, larynx, or sinuses

Differential Diagnosis

- Rhinitis
- Sinusitis
- Laryngitis
- Bronchitis
- Bronchiolitis
- Pneumonia
- Gastroesophageal reflux
- Candidiasis

Considerations

- Sinusitis (rhinosinusitis) is usually viral
- Viral sinusitis difficult to differentiate from bacterial sinusitis early in the course
- Children are 20–100 times more likely to have viral rhinosinusitis then bacterial sinusitis
- Viral rhinosinusitis
  - Congestion
  - Cough
  - Nasal discharge up to 14 days
- Acute bacterial sinusitis is associated with prolonged symptoms lasting more than 10–14 days
- Diagnosis of acute bacterial sinusitis should be made on clinical grounds
- Prescribe antibiotics for worsening sinusitis symptoms or symptoms > 10 days
- Offer observation for an additional 3 days if symptoms not worsening
- CT scan may help in unclear cases. Plain films are rarely helpful
- Antibiotics should not be used to treat nonspecific URI symptoms in previously healthy patients
- Acute bacterial sinusitis does not require antibiotic treatment, especially if symptoms are mild or moderate
- Up to 75% of sinusitis resolves in 1 month without antibiotic treatment
- Severe or persistent moderate symptoms of bacterial sinusitis should receive antibiotic treatment
- Fever not common
- Acute invasive fungal rhinosinusitis
  - Can be caused by Candida, Aspergillus and Phycomycetes species — found in patients with:
    - Diabetes (especially with very high serum glucose levels)
    - Cancer
    - Hepatic disease
    - Renal failure
    - Other immunosuppressive conditions or diseases
- Sinusitis has same pathogens as otitis media

Signs of sinusitis

- Mucopurulent rhinorrhea
- Nasal congestion
- Facial pain, pressure or fullness
- Decreased sense of smell
- Severe headache, malaise, fever
- Pain exacerbation with head movement
- Retro-orbital pain (ethmoid sinus)
- Dental pain (maxillary sinus)
- Ear fullness

Evaluation

- Nasal exam

- Percussion of sinuses for tenderness
- Transillumination for frontal and maxillary sinus opacification
- CBC: severe sinusitis

CT scan indications

- Facial swelling
- Orbital or periorbital swelling
- Visual or mental status changes
- Consider for severe headache

Treatment Options

- Nasal saline for young children
- Antipyretic treatment prn
- Warm compresses to face prn
- Nasal steroids can be considered and is more effective alone versus amoxicillin alone
- Mucolytic (guaifenesin) can be used to thin secretions — efficacy unknown
- Nasal/sinus saline irrigation
- Systemic steroids may be used in sinusitis that has failed multiple rounds of antibiotics

Antihistamines and decongestants

- Without benefit frequently
- Can worsen congestion and sinus pain by thickening of mucus and decreasing drainage
- Can use antihistamines only for allergic rhinosinusitis without viral or bacterial infection
- Can use PO decongestants only for nonbacterial sinusitis

Antibiotics — for persistent moderate symptoms or severe symptoms and are the same as for otitis media

Severe symptoms defined as

- Systemic toxicity with fever of at least 102°F and threat of suppurative complications, daycare attendance, age <2 or >65 years, recent hospitalization, antibiotic use within the past month, or immunocompromised state

- Prescribe antibiotics for worsening sinusitis symptoms or symptoms > 10 days
- Offer observation without antibiotics for an additional 3 days if symptoms not worsening
- Amoxicillin/clavulanate 875 mg PO bid 10–14 days (preferred)
  - Pediatrics 90 mg/kg/day BID for 10 days (NMT 875 mg BID)
- Amoxicillin 80–90 mg/kg/day PO divided q8–12hr
- Cefdinir 300 mg PO BID for 10–14 days or 7 mg/kg bid PO for pediatrics (NMT 600 mg a day)
- Start antibiotics for fever ≥ 102°F (38.9°C) and diagnosis of bacterial sinusitis
- Penicillin allergy can use doxycycline or levofloxacin or moxifloxacin
- May use Sanford guide or antibiotic database

Discharge Criteria

- Uncomplicated rhinosinusitis
- Nontoxic

Discharge instructions

- URI and/or sinusitis aftercare instructions
- Follow up within 10–14 days if symptoms persist

Consult Criteria

- Toxic patients
- Abnormal vision
- Severe headache
- Altered mental status
- Facial swelling
- Vomiting
- Sphenoid sinusitis

Vital signs and age consult criteria

- Fever ≥ 102°F (38.9°C) if felt to be solely from sinusitis
- Age < 2 months
- Hypotension
- O_2 saturation < 95% on room air or respiratory distress

Lab consult criteria

- WBC ≥ 18,000 or < 3,000

- Bandemia ≥ 15%
- Acute thrombocytopenia

Notes

REFERENCES:

American Academy of Pediatrics. Subcommittee on Management of Sinusitis and Committee on Quality Improvement. Clinical Practice Guideline: Management of Sinusitis. Pediatrics 2001;108(3):798–808. (Consensus guideline)

Wald ER, Applegate KE, Bordley C, Darrow DH, Glode MP, Marcy SM, et al. Clinical Practice Guideline for the Diagnosis and Management of Acute Bacterial Sinusitis in Children Aged 1 to 18 Years. *Pediatrics*. Jun 24 2013

Acute Sinusitis Author: Itzhak Brook, MD, MSc; Chief Editor: Burke A Cunha, MD emedicine.medscape.com/article/232670

Clin Infect Dis 2012 Apr;54(8):e72–e112

N Engl J Med 2012; 367:1128–1134

Clin Infect Dis, Vol. 54:e72

OTITIS MEDIA PROTOCOL

Definition

- Infection of the middle ear with acute onset, presence of middle ear effusion, and signs of middle ear inflammation

Differential Diagnosis

- Bell's palsy
- Dental pain
- TMJ pain
- URI
- Mastoiditis
- Ear canal foreign body
- Barotitis media
- Herpes zoster
- Pharyngitis
- Sinusitis
- Serous otitis media

Considerations

- Viruses 35%; S. pneumoniae 25%; H. influenzae 23%; M. catarrhalis 15%; mixed bacteria 10%
- Most commonly occurs 6–36 months of age
- One-half of patients have fever
- Usually associated with URI
- History can include: earache, irritability, rhinitis, GI symptoms, poor feeding, fever, pulling at ear
- Mild cases resolve without antibiotics 80% of the time within 1 week
- Fever is defined as rectal temperature > 38 °C or 100.4°F; axillary temperature is unreliable

Treatment considerations

- Antibiotics increases resolution by another 13%
- 50% of patients will have residual middle ear fluid 1 month after antibiotic treatment so rechecking ears in 10–14 days may be unwarranted unless symptoms continue
- Antihistamines, decongestants, and steroids have no proven effectiveness
- High dose amoxicillin overcomes drug resistance
- Red TM's (tympanic membrane) can also be from fever and crying
- Pneumatic otoscopy most accurate method in diagnosing otitis media

- Otitis media with bulging TM's warrant immediate antibiotic treatment
- Otitis media without bulging TM's will likely clear spontaneously — can delay antibiotics 48–72 hours to see if spontaneous resolution of symptoms occurs
- Antibiotic treatment warranted for age < 6 months or older children > 36 months
- Mastoiditis is the same antibiotic treatment PO as otitis media

Evaluation

- Rectal temperature for age < 3 years unless patient cooperates with oral measurement to nurse's satisfaction
- Feeding, irritability, urine output and fever history
- CBC, chest x-ray, and U/A for fever ≥ 101°F (38.3°C) without a source (no URI symptoms for example)
- BMP for > 5% dehydration
- WBC ≥ 15,000 without a source for fever — get chest x-ray and one blood culture
- Obtain history of recent antibiotic treatment
- Evaluate for TM (tympanic membrane) perforation
- Complete H&P, including nuchal exam

Treatment Options

American Academy of Pediatrics recommendations (February 2013)

- AOM (acute otitis media) management should include pain evaluation and treatment.
- Antibiotics should be prescribed for bilateral or unilateral AOM in children aged at least 6 months with severe signs or symptoms (moderate or severe otalgia or otalgia for 48 hours or longer or temperature 39°C or higher) and for nonsevere, bilateral AOM in children aged 6 to 23 months
- On the basis of joint decision-making with the parents, unilateral, nonsevere AOM in children aged 6 to 23 months or nonsevere AOM in older children may be managed either with antibiotics or with close follow-up and withholding antibiotics unless the child worsens or does not improve within 48 to 72 hours of symptom onset
- Amoxicillin is the antibiotic of choice unless the child received it within 30 days, has concurrent purulent conjunctivitis, or is allergic to penicillin. In these cases, clinicians should prescribe an antibiotic with additional β-lactamase coverage.
- Clinicians should reevaluate a child whose symptoms have worsened or not responded to the initial antibiotic treatment within 48 to 72 hours and change treatment if indicated.
- In children with recurrent AOM, tympanostomy tubes, but not prophylactic antibiotics, may be indicated to reduce the frequency of AOM episodes.
- Clinicians should recommend pneumococcal conjugate vaccine and annual influenza vaccine to all children according to updated schedules
- Clinicians should encourage exclusive breastfeeding for 6 months or longer

Antibiotic options

- Amoxicillin 80 mg/kg divided BID–TID for 10 days — preferred first line drug (NMT 875 mg per dose)
- Amoxicillin/clavulanate 80 mg/kg divided BID for 10 days — NMT 875 mg per dose
  - May be for 5–7 days in mild/moderate AOM for age > 6 years
- Zithromax (azithromycin) 10 mg/kg day 1, then 5 mg/kg qday for following 4 days
- Rocephin (ceftriaxone) 50 mg/kg IM × 1 dose (NMT 1,000 mg)

  - Treat qday for 3 days if resistance is suspected
- Trimethoprim/sulfamethoxazole 0.4 mg/kg BID PO or 0.5 cc/LB BID PO for 10 days
  - Contraindicated in ages < 2 months
- Cefuroxime 30 mg/kg BID for 10 days
- Cefdinir 300 mg bid PO for adult or 7 mg/kg bid PO for pediatrics (NMT 600 mg a day)

Otitis media with draining PE tubes more effectively treated with otic HC/bacitracin/colistin 5 drops tid for 7 days than oral antibiotics

  - May use Ciprodex otic 4 drops bid for PE tubes or TM perforation — age > 6 months
  - May use ofloxacin otic 5 drops bid for 10 days for PE tubes or TM perforation
- May use Sanford Guide or other drug databases

Mastoiditis

Complications

- Hearing loss
- Facial nerve palsy
- Cranial nerve involvement
- Osteomyelitis
- Petrositis
- Labyrinthitis
- Gradenigo syndrome – otitis media, retro-orbital pain, and abducens palsy
- Intracranial extension – meningitis, cerebral abscess, epidural abscess, subdural empyema
- Sigmoid sinus thrombosis
- Abscess formation
- May occur secondary to cholesteatoma

Evaluation

- PE and history may be all that is needed
  - Mastoid area erythema, proptosis of the auricle, and fever
  - Common symptoms of mastoiditis are otalgia, otorrhea, and hearing loss, and the physical signs of mastoiditis (i.e., swelling, erythema, tenderness of the retroauricular region) are usually present
  - Persistent otorrhea beyond 3 weeks is the most consistent sign that a process involving the mastoid has evolved
  - Most patients (>80%) have no history of recurrent otitis media
  - Virtually all otitis media patients have some component of mastoiditis
- CBC
- Plain x–rays may show clouding
- CT scan most accurate — standard for evaluation of mastoiditis

Treatment

- Acute mastoiditis without osteitis or periosteitis treated same as otitis media — should resolve in 2 weeks
  - Refer to ENT
- Acute mastoiditis with periosteitis
  - Parenteral antibiotics, high-dose steroids, and tympanostomy tube insertion
  - Choices:
    - Ceftriaxone (3rd generation) + vancomycin IV
      - Ceftriaxone pneumococcus nonsusceptibility seen in 30% (vancomycin needed)
    - Cefepime (4th generation)
    - Meropenem
    - Zosyn
    - Linezolid (Zyvox)
  - Consult ENT
- Acute mastoiditis with osteitis
  - Surgically treated
  - Consult ENT

Discharge Criteria

- Uncomplicated otitis media and mastoiditis

Discharge instructions

- Otitis media or mastoiditis aftercare instructions
- Follow up in 7–10 days if symptoms persist

Consult Criteria

- Toxic patient
- Dehydration > 5% who have not responded to ORT (oral rehydration therapy — see Pediatric Dehydration Protocol)
- Pneumonia
- Age < 2 months
- Fever of unknown etiology

Notes

____

____

____

REFERENCES:

Pediatrics Vol. 131 No. 3 March 1, 2013

Otitis Media Treatment & Management: Muhammad Waseem, MD, MS; Glenn C Isaacson, MD, FACS, FAAP; Muhammad Aslam, MD; Orval Brown, MD, Daniel Rauch, MD, FAAP; Glenn C Isaacson, MD, FACS, FAAP, et.al.

Emedicine.medscape.com

PEDIATRIC ASTHMA PROTOCOL

Definition

- Reversible acute bronchospasm and airway resistance secondary to infectious, allergic, environmental or internal stimuli

Differential Diagnosis

- Panic disorder
- Pneumonia
- Bronchitis
- Bronchiolitis
- Aspiration
- CHF
- COPD
- Anaphylaxis
- URI
- Vocal cord dysfunction
- Laryngospasm
- Epiglottitis
- Croup
- Retropharyngeal abscess

Considerations

- Cough is commonly the first symptom
- Viral URI or allergens or environmental stimuli most common causes of asthma
- Severe episode may have decreased breath sounds without wheezing
- There is evidence that dexamethasone is preferable to prednisone/prednisolone for pediatric patients presenting to the ED with an acute asthma exacerbation
  - A single PO dose of dexamethasone plus PO dose on day 3 to take at home is as effective as 5 day course of prednisone/prednisolone
    - Onset of action IV is 1 hour
    - PO onset of action is 1–2 hours
    - Duration of action is 36–54 hours
  - Dexamethasone causes less vomiting (has antiemetic properties), has improved compliance, and higher parental preference

Peak flow % of predicted (age > 5 yrs. old)

- Mild asthma ≥ 70
- Moderate 40–69%
- Severe < 40%

Principles of Asthma Management

- Recognizing severity of exacerbation
- Using correct therapy
- Identify and treat any precipitants
- Make correct disposition

Evaluation

- Complete history and physical exam
- Assess respiratory effort
- Assess hydration status
- CBC and/or BMP for significant tachycardia and fever
- O_2 saturation measurement
- Consider peak flows before and after aerosols for age 5 years or higher
- Check radiology interpretations if completed prior to discharge if chest x-ray performed

Chest x-ray if

- Pneumonia suspected
- Significant respiratory distress
- Respiratory distress not responsive to aerosols

Treatment Options

- Supplemental oxygen for O_2 Sat < 94% on room air or significant respiratory distress
- Albuterol (with or without ipratropium) aerosols up to 3 treatments total every 15–20 minutes prn
    - Nebulized lidocaine solutions 1cc of a 1% solution in 4mL of saline to give 0.25% solution after albuterol treatment for intractable cough may be tried

Additional treatment options if needed for severe exacerbations

- Continuous Albuterol with or without atrovent (ipratropium)
- Terbutaline 0.25 mg SQ prn q15–20 minutes up to 3 as needed for age ≥ 12 years
- Terbutaline 0.005–0.01 mg/kg SQ q15–20 minutes up to 3 — age < 12 years (NMT 0.4 mg per dose)
- Epinephrine 0.01 mg/kg SQ in children usually not to exceed 0.3 mg per dose up to 3 doses (if extremely severe may give IV or IM)
- $MgSO_4$ (magnesium sulfate) 25–75 mg/kg IV over 10–20 minutes (NMT 2 gm) for children
- $MgSO_4$ (magnesium sulfate)125–250 mg in 0.3 ml NS aerosol q 20 minutes up to 4 doses as needed (off label use)
    - May combine with albuterol
- May use BiPAP if needed

Steroid treatment options useful for moderate to severe exacerbations (caution with diabetes)

- Onset of action IV is 1 hour. PO onset of action is 1–2 hours
- Duration of action is 36–54 hours
- Dexamethasone 6mg =prednisone 40 mg PO qday x 5–7 days
- Prednisolone 1 mg/kg PO
- OR
- Decadron (dexamethasone) 0.6 mg/kg PO, IV or IM (NMT 10 mg)

Discharge treatment options

- Albuterol MDI with spacer prn at home (or nebulizer) – give up to 7 puffs in spacer for each treatment as needed
- Albuterol syrup per weight for patients unable to use MDI
- Antibiotics not needed usually
- If bacterial infection suspected, use Sanford Guide or antibiotic database

Discharge systemic steroid treatment (caution if diabetic)

- Prednisolone or prednisone 1 mg/kg PO x 3 days (NMT 60 mg/dose)
- Decadron (dexamethasone) 0.6 mg/kg PO and again on day 3 (NMT 20 mg per dose)

— if PO route not usable then IM — preferred over prednisone/prednisolone (see above comment)

Practitioners should consider 2-dose regimen of dexamethasone on day 1 and day 3 as a viable alternative to a 5-day course of prednisone/prednisolone for pediatric asthma

Other discharge medications

- Albuterol MDI 2 puffs q4hr. prn (add spacer if desired)
- Montelukast (Singulair)
  - 5 mg PO qHS chewable tab age 6–14 years
  - 10 mg PO qHS age ≥ 15 years
  - 4 mg PO chewable tab or oral granules qHS age 12 months–5 years
- Consider inhaled steroid Rx only after acute exacerbation has resolved for **uncontrolled asthma**
  - Prescribe double dose if already on single strength dose

    OR
  - Advair diskus bid – age > 3 years (combination of long acting beta-agonist and steroid) to be used only after acute exacerbation has resolved
    - Use 100/50 1 puff bid for age 4–11 years
    - Use adult strength for age ≥ 12 years (NMT 1000mcg/100 mcg/ day)
  - Advair HFA 45/21 or 115/21 2 puffs bid — age ≥ 12 years

Discharge criteria recommendation

- Good response to therapy
- Peak flow ≥ 70% predicted if checked (age 5 years or higher)
- O_2 saturation ≥ 94% on room air
- < 5% dehydrated post ORT (oral rehydration therapy) if needed
- Good follow-up and compliance

Discharge instructions

- Follow up in 1–5 days depending on severity of illness and response to treatments
- Provide pediatric asthma aftercare instructions

Consult criteria recommendation

- Insufficient response to treatment
- Work of breathing moderate to severe post Rx
- Wheezing not resolving adequately
- Patient or family of child feels patient is too dyspneic to go home
- Peak flow < 70% predicted if checked
- Moderate respiratory distress
- Age < 2 months
- > 5% dehydration post rehydration
- Poor feeding
- Unable to self-hydrate
- O_2 saturation < 93% on room air post treatment
- Significant comorbid conditions

Notes

____

____

____

REFERENCES:

Redman E, et al. Arch Dis Children 2013; 98: 916

Williams KW, Â et al. Clin Pediatr 2013;52:30

Keeney GE, et al. Pediatrics March 1, 2014, 133:493–499

Pediatr Emerg Care. 2018 Jan:34:53

Udezue E Lidocaine inhalation for cough suppression *Am J Emerg Med* 2001;19(3):206-7

Pediatric Pneumonia Protocol

Definition

- Infection of pulmonary parenchymal tissue

Differential Diagnosis

- Asthma
- CHF
- Bronchitis
- Bronchopulmonary dysplasia in children with history of prematurity

Considerations

- Community acquired causes
  - Strep pneumoniae
  - Mycoplasma pneumoniae
  - H. influenzae
  - Legionella pneumophilia
  - Klebsiella pneumoniae
  - Influenza
- Comorbid conditions
  - Diabetes
  - CHF
  - HIV
  - Immunosuppression
- Signs and Symptoms
  - Cough
  - Sputum production
  - Fever
  - Chills
  - Rigors
  - Dyspnea
  - Chest pain
- ***Newborns with pneumonia***
  - Rarely cough
  - More commonly present with poor feeding and irritability, as well as tachypnea, retractions, grunting, and hypoxemia
  - Grunting in a newborn suggests a lower respiratory tract disease
- WBC ≥ 15,000 suggest bacterial infection
- Very high or very low WBC predicts increased mortality

Criteria for Respiratory Distress in Children with Pneumonia (WHO)

Signs of Respiratory Distress

- Age 0–2 months: respiratory rate 60/minute
- Age 2–12 months: 50/minute
- Age 1–5 Years: 40/minute
- Dyspnea
- Retractions (suprasternal, intercostal, or subcostal)
- Grunting
- Nasal flaring
- Apnea
- Altered mental status
- Pulse oximetry measurement 90% on room air

Evaluation

- CBC
- Chest x-ray — may not be needed for suspected CAP in patients that will have outpatient treatment (30% negative even if pneumonia is present)
  - Obtain chest x-ray if patient in respiratory distress or hypoxic and has failed outpatient antibiotic therapy
- ABG if severe respiratory distress or fatigue
- Blood cultures if toxic or hypotensive and/or patient is to be admitted

Treatment Options

- Oxygen for O_2 saturation < 93% or in respiratory distress
- Viral pneumonia, which is most common type in preschool patients, usually needs no antibiotic treatment unless immunosuppressed
- IV NS/LR or oral rehydration if dehydrated (see Gastroenteritis Protocols for rehydration therapy)

Nontoxic patient treatment that is to be discharged

No chronic cardiopulmonary disease

Age 1–3 months

- Azithromycin 10 mg/kg/1st day PO, then 5 mg/kg/day for 5 days PO

Age 4 months – 5 years

- Amoxicillin 45 mg/kg/day PO divided q12hr or 40 mg/kg/day PO divided q8hr x 10–14 days (first line drug)
  - Or amoxicillin/clavulanate dosed the same

OR

- Second line azithromycin 10 mg/kg PO on day 1, followed by 5 mg/kg PO on days 2 through 5 (do not exceed adolescent dosing) for suspected atypical pneumonia

Age 5-15 years

- Amoxicillin <40 kg: 45 mg/kg/day PO divided q12hr or 40 mg/kg/day PO divided q8hr
  - > 40kg: 875 mg PO q12hr or 500 mg PO q8hr for 10-14 days) if bacterial pneumonia suspected

    OR

  - Amoxicillin/clavulanate dosed the same

OR/PLUS

- (may combine if clinically needed)
- Azithromycin 10 mg/kg PO on day 1, followed by 5 mg/kg PO on days 2 through 5 for atypical suspected pathogens like mycoplasma (do not exceed adolescent dosing) — not first line
  - May instead use doxycycline age > 7 years of age
- Cefdinir (Omnicef) may be used
  - 7 mg/kg PO q12hr for 10 days or 14 mg/kg PO q24hr for 10 days (second line antibiotic choice)
- **Off label** for community acquired pneumonic empiric treatment: amoxicillin 90 mg/kg/day PO divided q12 hr for 10 days; not to exceed 4,000 mg/day

Age ≥ 16 years

- Levaquin 750 mg PO qday X 10 days or azithromycin (Z-pak)
  - Caution using quinolones in children due to possible arthropathy complications

For patients with significant respiratory distress, hypoxemia, toxicity, or are to be admitted:

- IV NS
- IV Zithromax and Rocephin (ceftriaxone)
- Age ≤ 28 days give ampicillin + gentamicin or cefotaxime IV and admission
- Consult pediatrics

Discharge criteria recommendation

- Nontoxic patient
- No respiratory distress
- O_2 saturation >93%
- No O_2 desaturation on exertion

Discharge instructions

- Pneumonia aftercare instructions
- Follow up with primary care provider within 1–3 days
- Return if worse

Consult criteria and/or admission recommendation

- Significant pneumonia
- Patients that the provider feels need admission
- Significant respiratory distress
- O_2 saturation < 94%
- O_2 desaturation on exertion

- Pleural effusion (diagnostic and therapeutic thoracentesis recommended)
- Significant pneumonia
- High fever ≥ 104°F (40°C) with suspected bacterial etiology
- Temperature < 96°F (35.5°C)
- Appears ill or toxic
- Metabolic or respiratory acidosis
- Immunosuppression
- Age < 2 months
- No significant improvement in 48-72 hours
- Failure of outpatient treatment
- Immunizations not up to date

Vital signs and age consult criteria recommendation

- O_2 Sat < 94% on room air
- Significant tachypnea or respiratory distress
- Lab and x-ray consult criteria
- New onset renal insufficiency or worsening renal insufficiency
- WBC ≥ 18,000 or < 4,000; Neutrophil count < 1,000
- Bandemia ≥ 15%
- Acute thrombocytopenia
- Anion gap > 18
- Significant electrolyte abnormally and hyperglycemia
- Hyperglycemia with metabolic acidosis (decreased serum CO_2 or elevated anion gap)

Notes

____

____

____

REFERENCES:

Bradley JS, Byington CL, Shah SS, et al. The management of community-acquired pneumonia in infants and children older than 3 months of age: clinical practice guidelines by the pediatric infectious diseases society and the infectious diseases society of america. *Clin Infect Dis.* 2011 Oct. 53(7):e25-76

Aujesky D, Auble TE, Yealy DM, et al. Prospective comparison of three validated prediction rules for prognosis in community-acquired pneumonia. *Am J Med* 2005; 118:384-92

Mandell LA, Wunderink RG, Anzueto A, et al. Infectious disease society of America/American Thoracic Society consensus guidelines on the management of community-acquired pneumonia. *Clin Infect Dis* 2007: 44(2):S27-72

Bacterial Pneumonia Author: Nader Kamangar, MD, FACP, FCCP, FCCM, FAASM; Chief Editor: Zab Mosenifar, MD emedicine.medscape.com/article/300157

Pediatric Pneumonia Medication Author: Nicholas John Bennett, MBBCh, PhD; Chief Editor: Russell W Steele, MD emedicine.medscape.com/article/967822

Pediatric Pneumonia Clinical Presentation

Updated: Nov 05, 2018 Author: Nicholas John Bennett, MBBCh, PhD, MA(Cantab), FAAP; Chief Editor: Russell W Steele, MD

BRONCHIOLITIS PROTOCOL

Definition

- Bronchiolitis is an acute infectious disease process of the lower respiratory tract that occurs primarily in young infants, most often in those aged 2–24 months, that may result in obstruction of small airways

Differential Diagnosis

- Asthma
- Pneumonia
- Bronchitis

- Congenital heart disease
- Aspiration
- Foreign body obstruction
- Congestive heart failure
- Bronchopulmonary dysplasia (prematurity history)

Considerations

- Age < 2 years usually
- Fall and spring peaks
- RSV usual cause
- Wheezing and tachypnea usually present
- Hypoxia best predictor of severity of illness
- Variable response to bronchodilators
- Steroids not effective
- Dehydration and poor feeding not uncommon
- Fever usually low grade
- Rhinorrhea and cough frequent
- Apnea more commonly seen in infants < 2 months of age or premature infants
- Hydration treatment possibly helpful

Higher risk

- Prematurity
- Bronchopulmonary dysplasia history
- Cardiac history

Evaluation

- Complete history and physical
- O_2 saturation measurement
- Work of breathing assessment
- Dehydration assessment
- Chest x-ray not routinely be needed unless ill appearing, respiratory distress or underlying cardiopulmonary conditions
- CBC and BMP if moderate to severe respiratory distress or > 5% dehydration
- RSV testing usually not needed unless antibiotics are being considered — positive RSV may stop antibiotic treatment
- RSV testing if admitted, history of prematurity or cardiopulmonary disease history

Treatment Options

- Supplemental oxygen if O_2 saturation < 93%
- Trial with Albuterol aerosol with or without atrovent — may repeat × 2 as needed
  - Controversy whether it is effective
- Oral or IV hydration for dehydration
  - Refer to Pediatric Diarrhea Protocol
- No steroids unless history of asthma

Discharge Criteria

- Feeding well
- Absence of significant respiratory distress
- O_2 saturation ≥ 94% on room air
- < 5% dehydrated post ORT (oral rehydration therapy) if given
- Good follow-up and compliance
- Contact primary care physician or provider to alert of visit if in acute care facility and arrange follow-up

Discharge instructions

- Bronchiolitis aftercare instructions
- Follow up with primary care provider within 1–2 days if seen initially in acute care facility
- Return if symptoms worsen
- Return if activity or feeding decreases

Consult Criteria

- Age < 6 months — discuss with physician
- Significant respiratory distress post treatment or respiratory rate > 60/minute
- Significant chest x–ray infiltrates
- O_2 saturation < 94% on room air post treatment
- Family feels patient is too dyspneic to go home
- > 5% dehydration after any rehydration treatment
- Poor feeding
- Unable to self–hydrate
- Persistent vomiting

- History of apnea
- Significant comorbid conditions
- Toxic appearance
- Respiratory fatigue
- Hypotension
- Heart rate
  - 0–4 months ≥ 180
  - 5–7 months ≥ 175
  - 8–12 months ≥ 170
  - 1–3 years ≥ 160

Notes

REFERENCES:

Kristjansson S, Lodrup Carlsen KC, Wennergren G, et al. Nebulised racemic adrenaline in the treatment of acute bronchiolitis in infants and toddlers. *Arch Dis Child* 1993;69(6):650–4

Bronchiolitis Author: Lucian Kenneth DeNicola, MD, MS, FAAP, FCCM; Chief Editor: Russell W Steele, MD emedicine.medscape.com/article/961963

Gadomski AM, Scribani MB. Bronchodilators for bronchiolitis. Cochrane Database of Systematic Reviews 2014, Issue 6. Art. No.: CD001266. DOI: 10.1002/14651858.CD001266.pub4

Al-Ansari K, Sakran M, Davidson BL, El Sayyed R, Mahjoub H, Ibrahim K. Nebulized 5% or 3% hypertonic or 0.9% saline for treating acute bronchiolitis in infants. *J Pediatr.* Oct 2010;157(4):630–4, 634.e1

CROUP PROTOCOL

Definition

- Infection of the upper respiratory tract (trachea) that is usually of a viral etiology and causes varying degrees of obstruction and is usually self-limited

Differential Diagnosis

- Epiglottitis
- Retropharyngeal abscess
- Foreign body in trachea
- Foreign body in esophagus
- Peritonsillar abscess
- Subglottic stenosis
- Tracheomalacia
- Vocal cord paralysis

Considerations

- Most common in 6 months to 6 years of age
- Peak is 2 years of age
- Parainfluenza virus most common, followed by RSV and influenza
- Seal-like barking cough
- Stridor at rest indicates increased risk
- Can be life threatening
- Drooling may indicate epiglottitis
- Lab tests usually not needed unless patient appears dehydrated or in significant distress
  - Defer blood tests initially when respiratory distress is present
- Imaging not required in mild cases that respond to treatment
- Neck AP & lateral for stridor at rest or significant respiratory distress
  - Extreme caution before obtaining films if in significant distress
  - Steeple sign indicative of croup on neck film
  - Thumb sign or vallecula sign (loss of vallecula) indicative for epiglottitis
  - Retropharyngeal swelling for retropharyngeal abscess

Severity assessment

Mild severity

- Occasional barking cough
- No audible stridor at rest
- Either no or mild suprasternal or intercostal retractions

Moderate severity

- Frequent barking cough
- Easily audible stridor at rest
- Suprasternal and sternal retractions at rest, with little or no agitation

Severe severity

- Frequent barking cough
- Prominent inspiratory and occasionally expiratory stridor
- Marked sternal retractions
- Agitation and distress

Impending respiratory failure

- Barking cough (often not prominent)
- Audible rest stridor
- Sternal retractions may not be marked (fatigue)
- Lethargy or decreased mentation
- Often dusky appearance if no supplemental oxygen given

Evaluation

- Complete history and physical exam
- Patients can sit on parent's lap for exam
- O_2 saturation measurement
- Assess respiratory effort and for respiratory distress
- Assess for dehydration
- BMP if > 5% dehydrated clinically
- CBC if toxic — hold blood draw if severe respiratory distress
- Avoid actions that agitate patient

Imaging studies

- Not required in mild cases or that respond to treatment
- Chest x-ray and soft tissue neck films in cases without adequate response to treatment or moderate or greater severity if clinical situation safely permits

Treatment Options

- Humidified oxygen if O_2 saturation < 95%
- Racemic epinephrine if stridor at rest — observe for 2 hours for recurrence of stridor at rest
- Decadron (dexamethasone) 0.6 mg/kg IM/IV (do not exceed 10 mg)

OR

- Decadron (dexamethasone) 0.15–0.6 mg/kg PO (NMT 10 mg) or prednisolone 1–2 mg/kg PO (NMT 60 mg)
  - Single dosing effective for mild to moderate croup
  - Dexamethasone 0.15 mg/kg as effective as 0.3–0.6 mg/kg
- Consider prednisolone 1–2 mg/kg PO × 5 days
- Avoid steroids in varicella (chickenpox)
- Cool mist vaporizer (or night air) may help
- Antibiotics rarely needed
- Follow up with within 24 hours
- Check radiology interpretations prior to discharge if completed

Discharge criteria recommendation

- Mild croup
- Moderate or severe croup with good response to therapy

Discharge instructions

- Croup aftercare instructions
- Refer to primary care provider
- Return if symptoms worsen

Consult criteria recommendation

- Stridor at rest unresponsive to treatment
- Moderate to severe croup post treatment
- "Severe" severity assessment or impending respiratory failure
- Dehydration > 5% unresponsive to oral hydration
- Epiglottitis
- Pharyngeal or retropharyngeal abscess
- Suspected foreign body

- O_2 saturation ≤ 95% on room air after treatments
- Moderate to severe respiratory distress
- Significant chest x–ray infiltrates
- Depressed sensorium
- Poor oral intake
- Poor home situation

Vital signs consult recommendations

- Pediatric heart rate
    - 0–4 months ≥ 180
    - 5–7 months ≥ 175
    - 8–12 months ≥ 170
    - 1–3 years ≥ 160
    - 4–5 years ≥ 150
    - 6–8 years ≥ 135
        - Hypotension
        - Age > 7 years or < 5 months

Lab consult recommendations

- WBC ≥ 18,000 or < 3,000
- Acute thrombocytopenia
- Bandemia ≥ 15%
- Metabolic acidosis

Notes

REFERENCES:

Croup Author: Germaine L Defendi, MD, MS, FAAP; Chief Editor: Russell W Steele, MD emedicine.medscape.com/article/962972

Russell KF, Liang Y, O'Gorman K, Johnson DW, Klassen TP. Glucocorticoids for croup. Cochrane Database of Systematic Reviews 2011, Issue 1. Art. No.: CD001955. DOI: 10.1002/14651858.CD001955

Pediatr Emerg Care. 2018 Jan:34:53

PEDIATRIC DEHYDRATION AND GASTROENTERITIS PROTOCOL

Definition

- Acute inflammatory or infectious process of the stomach and intestines

Differential Diagnosis

- Colitis
- Appendicitis
- Cholecystitis
- Pancreatitis
- Peptic ulcer disease
- GERD
- Biliary colic
- Renal colic
- Bowel obstruction
- Inflammatory bowel disease
- Pyloric stenosis in infants
- Volvulus in infants
- Diabetic ketoacidosis

Considerations

- Degree (%) of acute weight loss indicates degree of dehydration
- Decreased serum CO_2 and increased anion gap are early indicators of dehydration
    - BUN and creatinine rise later
- Vomiting may occur in early gastroenteritis prior to diarrhea
- Vomiting by itself may indicate mechanical obstruction if without fever or diarrhea
- Vomiting with fever only may be from upper tract UTI
- Viral infections are the usual etiology
- Antibiotics not usually indicated
    - Use Sanford guide or antibiotic database prn

- Oral rehydration therapy (ORT) preferred over IV in mild to moderate dehydration

Dehydration assessment

Mild < 5%

- Alert
- Mucous membranes variable dry
- Skin turgor normal
- Fontanel flat
- Blood pressure normal
- Heart rate normal
- Capillary refill < 2 seconds
- Urine output decreased

Moderate 6–9%

- Irritable
- Mucous membranes dry
- Skin turgor variably reduced
- Fontanel depressed
- Blood pressure variably orthostatic
- Heart rate tachycardic
- Capillary refill 2–3 seconds
- Urine output decreased — oliguria

Severe ≥ 10%

- Lethargic
- Mucous membranes dry
- Skin turgor reduced
- Fontanel depressed
- Blood pressure orthostatic or hypotensive
- Heart rate markedly tachycardic
- Capillary refill ≥ 4 seconds
- Urine output decreased — oliguria/anuria

Evaluation

- Detailed history and PE
- Assess patient activity and interactions
- Perform baseline dehydration assessment
- BMP if appears moderate to severely dehydrated
- Lactic acid level and venous pH if in shock or severely dehydrated
- Blood cultures if septic 10 minutes apart
- CBC and BMP if patient appears less active

OR FOR

  - Pediatric heart rate without fever
    - 0–4 months ≥ 180
    - 5–7 months ≥ 175
    - 8–12 months ≥ 170
    - 1–3 years ≥ 160
    - 4–5 years ≥ 145
    - 6–8 years ≥ 130
    - 9–11 years ≥ 125
    - 12–15 years ≥ 120
    - 16 years or older ≥ 110
- Check U/A if vomiting and fever are only symptoms
- Consider imaging if obstruction suspected
- Stool studies prn

Treatment Options

- See Diarrhea Protocol
- < 5% dehydration by weight (or serum CO_2 > 18 mEq/L) small frequent feedings with pedialyte/rehydrate, etc. up to 24 hours
- Zofran (ondansetron) oral chewable tablet for frequent vomiting
  - 2 mg for 8–15 kg; 4 mg for 14–30 kg; 8 mg for > 30 kg
  - Zofran (ondansetron) 2–4 doses can be prescribed for home if indicated

Oral Rehydration Therapy (ORT) for mild to moderate dehydration

- Oral rehydration formula (WHO formula, Rehydralyte or Pedialyte) for above vital signs; mild to moderate dehydration or serum CO_2 14–18 mEq/L
  - 5 cc every 1–2 minutes for small children by caretaker for < 4 hours — start 20 minutes after Zofran (ondansetron) given

  - 5–10 cc every 1–2 minutes for larger children by caretaker for 1–4 hours
  - Hold ORT 10 minutes if vomiting occurs then resume
  - Reassess for urine production, weight gain, improved heart rate and alertness, and absence of severe vomiting
  - Recheck serum CO_2 if initially < 17 mEq/L
  - Mild dehydration give 50 cc/kg in < 4 hours
  - Moderate dehydration give 50–100 cc/kg within 1–4 hours
- Severe dehydration give IV NS or LR bolus 20 cc/kg; may repeat x 2

Exclusion criteria for Oral Rehydration Therapy

- Age < 6 months of age
- Hematemesis
- Bilious vomiting
- Bloody diarrhea
- VP shunt
- Head trauma
- Focal RLQ tenderness (possible appendicitis)
- Severe dehydration
- Patient vomits 3 or more times after starting ORT

IV therapy criteria and treatment for moderate to severe dehydration

- IV NS or LR hydration for CO_2 < 14 mEq/L
- ORT failure
- IV NS/LR 20 cc/kg bolus, may repeat × 2
- Consult physician
- Up to 2 times maintenance IV D5NS after any vigorous NS rehydration therapy is completed if patient is to be further observed (dextrose clears ketosis faster and decreases return visits)

Home rehydration formula

- In 1 L of water, add 2 level tablespoons of sugar or honey, a quarter teaspoon of table salt (NaCl), and a quarter teaspoon of baking soda (bicarbonate of soda)—add 0.5 cup of orange juice (taste to make sure not too salty)

Discharge Criteria

- Nontoxic patients with mild dehydration
- Patients responding to rehydration with significantly improved vital signs, normal alertness and interaction
- CO_2 ≥ 18 mEq/L if rechecked
- Improved urine output in mild to moderate dehydration

Discharge instructions

- Pediatric dehydration, gastroenteritis, vomiting or diarrhea aftercare instructions
- Frequent small feedings of 10 cc of pedialyte or rehydrate every 10 minutes at home as needed for continued symptoms
- Resume regular diet (except milk initially) as soon as symptoms start resolving
  - May need to change to soy formula in infants
- Follow up with primary care provider within 1 day if symptoms not improving sufficiently at home
- May use dilute apple juice for outpatient treatment of mild gastroenteritis and minimal dehydration

Consult Criteria

- Toxic appearance
- Greater than 5% dehydration post rehydration
- Poor response to treatment
- Persistent vomiting
- Worrisome abdominal tenderness
- Petechial rash
- Seizure

Vital signs consult criteria

- **Pediatric heart rate —** post rehydration therapy
  - 0–4 months ≥ 180
  - 5–7 months ≥ 175

- 8–12 months ≥ 170
- 1–3 years ≥ 160
- 4–5 years ≥ 145
- 6–8 years ≥ 130
- 9–12 years ≥ 125
- 13–15 years ≥ 120
- 16 years or older ≥ 110
- Hypotension develops or orthostatic vital signs

Lab consult criteria

- Serum CO_2 < 18 mEq/L post rehydration or elevated anion gap
- Initial serum CO_2 < 17 mEq/L
- WBC ≥ 15,000 or < 3,000
- Bandemia ≥ 15%
- Acute thrombocytopenia

Notes

REFERENCES:

King CK, Glass R, Bresee JS, Duggan C. Managing acute gastroenteritis among children: oral rehydration, maintenance, and nutritional therapy. *MMWR Recomm Rep*. Nov 21 2003;52:1–16

[Best Evidence] Spandorfer PR, Alessandrini EA, Joffe MD, Localio R, Shaw KN. Oral versus intravenous rehydration of moderately dehydrated children: a randomized, controlled trial. *Pediatrics*. Feb 2005;115(2):295–301

Freedman, S. B et al. Effect of dilute apple juice and preferred fluids versus electrolyte maintenance solution on treatment failure among children with mild gastroenteritis: a randomized clinical trial. JAMA 315, 1966–1974 (2016)

PEDIATRIC DIARRHEA PROTOCOL

Definition

- Increased fluid content of stool and frequency of bowel movements usually secondary to viral or bacterial infection

Differential Diagnosis

- Inflammatory bowel disease
- Irritable bowel syndrome
- Malabsorption syndromes

Considerations

- Degree (%) of acute weight loss indicates degree of dehydration
- Serum CO_2 and increased anion gap early indicators of dehydration
- BUN and creatinine rise later
- Viruses 70–80% — Bacteria 10–20% — Parasites 5% — Use Sanford Guide or other drug databases prn
- Can be from allergy, food intolerance, malabsorption or inflammatory causes.
- Oral rehydration therapy (ORT) preferred over IV in mild to moderate dehydration.

Dehydration assessment

Mild < 5%

- Alert
- Mucous membranes variable dry
- Skin turgor normal
- Fontanel flat
- Blood pressure normal
- Heart rate normal
- Capillary refill < 2 seconds
- Urine output decreased

Moderate 6–9%

- Irritable
- Mucous membranes dry
- Skin turgor variably reduced

- Fontanel depressed
- Blood pressure variably orthostatic
- Heart rate tachycardic
- Capillary refill 2–3 seconds
- Urine output — oliguria

Severe ≥ 10%

- Lethargic
- Mucous membranes dry
- Skin turgor reduced
- Fontanel depressed
- Blood pressure orthostatic or hypotensive
- Heart rate markedly tachycardic
- Capillary refill ≥ 4 seconds
- Urine output decreased — oliguria/anuria

Evaluation

- Detailed history and PE
- Assess patient activity/interaction
- Perform baseline dehydration assessment
- BMP for moderate to severe dehydration
- Venous pH and lactic acid level if in shock or severe dehydration
- CBC and patient appears less active

  OR

Pediatric heart rate is

- 0–4 months ≥ 180
- 5–7 months ≥ 175
- 8–12 months ≥ 170
- 1–3 years ≥ 160
- 4–5 years ≥ 145
- 6–8 years ≥ 130
- 9–12 years ≥ 125
- 13–15 years ≥ 120
- 16 years or older ≥ 110

- Check U/A if vomiting and fever only symptoms
- Consider imaging if obstruction suspected
- Stool studies prn (consider rotavirus antigen)

Oral Rehydration Therapy (ORT) for Mild to Moderate Dehydration

- Oral rehydration formula (WHO formula, Rehydralyte or Pedialyte) for above vital signs; mild to moderate dehydration or serum CO_2 14–18 mEq/L
  - 5 cc every 1–2 minutes for small children by caretaker for < 4 hours
  - 5–10 cc every 1–2 minutes for larger children by caretaker for 1–4 hours
  - Hold ORT 10 minutes if vomiting occurs then resume
  - Reassess for urine production, weight gain, improved heart rate and alertness, and absence of severe vomiting
  - Recheck serum CO_2 if initially < 17 mEq/L
  - Mild dehydration give 50 cc/kg in < 4 hours
  - Moderate dehydration give 50–100 cc/kg within 1–4 hours

Severe dehydration give IV NS bolus 20 cc/kg; may repeat × 2 prn

Exclusion criteria for Oral Rehydration Therapy

- Age < 6 months of age
- Hematemesis
- Bilious vomiting
- Bloody diarrhea
- VP shunt
- Head trauma
- Focal RLQ tenderness (possible appendicitis)
- Severe dehydration
- Patient vomits 3 or more times after starting ORT

IV Therapy Criteria and Treatment for Moderate to Severe Dehydration

- IV NS or LR hydration for CO_2 < 14 mEq/L

- ORT failure
- IV NS or LR 20 cc/kg bolus, may repeat × 2 prn
- Consult physician
- Maintenance IV with D5NS (Dextrose decreases return visits)

Home rehydration formula

- In 1 L of water, add 2 level tablespoons of sugar or honey, a quarter teaspoon of table salt (NaCl), and a quarter teaspoon of baking soda (bicarbonate of soda)—add 0.5 cup of orange juice (taste to make sure not more salty than tears)

Antibiotic therapy for bloody diarrhea

- World Health Organization currently recommends empiric antimicrobial therapy in the setting of febrile acute bloody diarrhea in young children
  - Infections by enteropathogenic *E coli*, when running a prolonged course — septra or ceftriaxone
  - Enteroinvasive *E coli*, based on the serologic, genetic, and pathogenic similarities with *Shigella* — septra or ceftriaxone
  - *Yersinia* infections in subjects with sickle cell disease — septra or cipro (may cause arthropathy and musculoskeletal disorders) or ceftriaxone or doxycycline (avoid doxycycline in age <8 years)
  - *Salmonella* infections in very young infants, if febrile or with positive blood culture findings — ceftriaxone
    - Most salmonella infections do not require antibiotics and they may prolong the illness

Discharge Criteria

- Nontoxic patients with mild dehydration.
- Patients responding to rehydration with significantly improved vital signs, normal alertness and interaction
- $CO_2 \geq 18$ mEq/L, with weight gain and improved urine output in mild to moderate dehydration

Discharge instructions

- Pediatric dehydration or diarrhea aftercare instructions
- Frequent small feedings of 10 cc of pedialyte or rehydrate every 10 minutes at home as needed for continued symptoms
- Resume regular diet (except milk initially) as soon as symptoms start resolving
  - May need to change to soy formula in infants
- Follow up with primary care provider within 1–2 days if symptoms not improving sufficiently at home
- May use dilute apple juice for outpatient treatment of mild gastroenteritis and minimal dehydration

Consult Criteria

- Toxic appearance
- Greater than 5% dehydration post rehydration
- Poor response to treatment
- Worrisome abdominal tenderness
- Petechial rash
- More than 1 visit for same episode of diarrhea

Vital signs consult criteria

- **Pediatric heart rate** — post rehydration therapy
  - 0–4 months ≥ 180
  - 5–7 months ≥ 175
  - 8–12 months ≥ 170
  - 1–3 years ≥ 160
  - 4–5 years ≥ 145
  - 6–8 years ≥ 130
  - 9–11 years ≥ 125
  - 12–15 years ≥ 115
  - 16 years or older ≥ 110
- Hypotension develops or orthostatic vital signs

Lab consult criteria

- Serum $CO_2 < 18$ mEq/L post rehydration
- Initial serum $CO_2 < 17$ mEq/L

- Elevated anion gap
- WBC ≥ 15,000 or < 3,000
- Bandemia ≥ 15%
- Acute thrombocytopenia

Notes

REFERENCES:

King CK, Glass R, Bresee JS, Duggan C. Managing acute gastroenteritis among children: oral rehydration, maintenance, and nutritional therapy. *MMWR Recomm Rep*. Nov 21 2003;52:1–16

[Best Evidence] Spandorfer PR, Alessandrini EA, Joffe MD, Localio R, Shaw KN. Oral versus intravenous rehydration of moderately dehydrated children: a randomized, controlled trial. *Pediatrics*. Feb 2005;115(2):295–301

Pediatric Dehydration Author: Alex Koyfman, MD; emedicine.medscape.com/article/801012

Diarrhea Author: Stefano Guandalini, MD; Chief Editor: Carmen Cuffari, MD medicine.medscape.com/article/928598

Freedman, S. B et al. Effect of dilute apple juice and preferred fluids versus electrolyte maintenance solution on treatment failure among children with mild gastroenteritis: a randomized clinical trial. JAMA 315, 1966–1974 (2016)

Brief Resolved Unexplained Event (BRUE) Protocol

Definition

- Episode that is characterized by some combination of following in patient <1 year of age
  - Apnea (central or obstructive) or altered respiration
  - Color change (cyanotic, pallid, erythematous or plethoric)
  - Change in muscle tone (usually diminished)
  - Choking or gagging
  - Altered level of consciousness
- No other explanation for event
- No other symptoms such as fever, respiratory etc. that could cause the event
- Was labeled in past as Apparent Life Threatening Event

Considerations

- No proven correlation with SIDS
- Average age is 8–14 weeks
- Is a description of an event and not a diagnosis
- Morbidity is low
- If patient did not move when picked up after event suggests event was significant
- If duration of event < 20 seconds, could be respiratory pause
- Was CPR provided or spontaneous or stimulation resolution
- Fluid or vomit present on bed or clothes suggest GERD

Differential diagnosis

- Gastroesophageal reflux disease – 26%
- Pertussis – 9%
- Lower respiratory tract infection – 9%

- Seizure – 9%
- Urinary tract infection – 8%
- Factitious illness including medical child abuse – 3%
- Miscellaneous – 11%

Risk factors

- Age < 60 days
- Gestational age < 32 weeks
- Prior BRUE or multiple episode requiring CPR
- Post–conceptual age < 45 weeks
- Concerning history or physical findings
- Feeding problems
- Respiratory conditions
- Family history of sudden cardiac death

BRUE inclusion criteria

- Duration < 1 minute
- Patient appearance and vital signs returned to normal after event
- Not explained by an identifiable medical condition
- Cyanosis or pallor
- Apnea or irregular breathing
- Change in muscle tone
- Loss or consciousness, lethargy, postictal phase and somnolence

BRUE exclusion criteria

- Duration > 1 minute
- At time of examination
    - Fever or recent fever
    - Tachycardia
    - Tachypnea
    - Low blood pressure
    - Altered mental status
    - Abnormal weight or growth
    - Abnormal head circumference
    - Abnormal muscle tone (hyper or hypotonia)
    - Bruising
    - Abnormal airway sounds
    - Repeat unexplained events
    - Event consistent with a medical condition
    - Acrocyanosis or perioral cyanosis
    - Rubor
    - Breath holding spells
    - Breath holding spells with altered responsiveness
    - Periodic breathing of newborn
    - Seizure activity
    - Muscle tone changes with crying or gagging
    - Eye deviation or nystagmus
    - Infantile spasms

Evaluation

- Patients that appear healthy may only need observation before discharge
- As needed for presenting signs and symptoms
    - CBC, CMP, U/A, urine culture (cath specimen), chest x–ray, LP, and ABG

Disposition

Admitting or consulting criteria

- High risk factors patient
- Patient not returned to baseline
- Cardiorespiratory monitoring needed
- Parents not wanting to take patient home
- Discuss with physician all events

Discharge criteria

- Low risk patient
- After observation period, patient with normal appearance and vital signs
- Outpatient close follow up
- Engage in shared decision making with parents

Notes

____

____

____

REFERENCES:

Brief Resolved Unexplained Events (Apparent Life-Threatening Events)

Updated: Nov 07, 2018

Author: Patrick L Carolan, MD; Chief
Editor: Girish D Sharma, MD, FCCP,
FAAP

Geriatrics

Section Contents — one protocol

Geriatrics Protocol

When using any protocol, always follow the Guidelines of Proper Use (page 12).

GERIATRICS PROTOCOL

Basic Ethical Principles

- Beneficence – act in the patient's best interest
- Autonomy – treatment guided by patient's wishes
- Family responsibility – plays a central role in care of the geriatric patient
- Advance directives – follow wishes of patient and family in care

General Considerations of Elderly

- Live in high density population environments
- May have poor nutritional status
- May have altered immune function
- Have multiple medical problems
- Take multiple medications
- May delay seeking medical evaluation
- Subtle alterations in appearance or behavior may be only indication of serious infections

Pharmacology in the Elderly

Risk factors for adverse drug reactions

- Advanced age and living alone
- Female gender
- Chronic use of medications
- Polypharmacy
- Institutionalization
- Multiple medical problems (especially hepatic or renal insufficiency)

Adverse drug presentations

Confusion

- Anticholinergics
- Antihistamines
- Antidepressants
- Antihypertensives
- Antipsychotics
- Narcotics
- Sedatives
- Digoxin (digitalis)
- Steroids
- NSAID's
- Diuretics

Dementia

- Antihistamines
- Phenothiazines
- Tricyclic antidepressants

Depression

- Sedatives

- Steroids
- Oral diabetic medications
- Ethanol
- NSAID's
- Narcotics

General weakness

- Digoxin (digitalis)
- Diuretics

Nausea

- Digoxin (digitalis)
- Theophylline
- Macrolide antibiotics (erythromycin)
- Iron
- Narcotics
- Steroids
- L-dopa
- ASA

Postural hypotension

- Angina medications
- Hypertension drugs
- Antidepressants
- Antihistamines
- Sedatives
- Beta–blockers

Renal insufficiency

- Digoxin (digitalis)
- Diuretics

Syncope/Near Syncope

- Cardiac drugs
- Hypertension drugs

Urinary incontinence

- Antipsychotics
- Diuretics
- Beta–blockers
- Medications causing fecal impaction
- Sedatives

Urinary retention

- Anticholinergics
- Antihistamines (especially in elderly men with BPH)

Hallucinations

- Anticholinergics

Drugs causing falls

- Antidepressants
- Antihistamines
- Antipsychotics
- Sedatives
- Nitroglycerin

Principles of safe medication usage

- Consider medications as a potential cause for presenting for medical care
- Educate patient about potential adverse reactions
- Obtain drug levels or monitoring tests of medications where appropriate
- Determine compliance and noncompliance of drug use
- Exercise care in prescribing medications that may have an adverse reaction to drugs the patient is currently taking
- Keep refills and number of pills small if appropriate
- Start low and go slow with dosing
- **Do not prescribe atypical antipsychotic medication to dementia patients — use first generation antipsychotic medication such as haloperidol if indicated**

Common Lab Findings in Elderly

- Frequently normal
- Fasting blood glucose: 135–150 mg/dL
- Normal creatinine with evidence of decreased creatinine clearance
- Hemoglobin – women 11 gm/dl; men 11.5 gm/dl
- BUN – up to 28–35 mg/dL

Delirium in the Elderly

- Acute organic brain syndrome manifested by impaired thinking, confusion, deficits in attention, fluctuating course, impaired speech and other symptoms and signs of impaired cognition

Causes of delirium

Medications and substances

- Ethanol
- Anticholinergics
- Antihistamines
- Sedatives
- Narcotics
- Antidepressants
- Lithium
- Neuroleptics
- Tagamet (cimetidine)

Withdrawal

- Ethanol
- Benzodiazepines
- Narcotics

Metabolic

- Electrolyte abnormalities (Na^+ and Ca^{++})
- Hypoglycemia and hyperglycemia
- Acid-base disturbance
- Dehydration
- Hypoxia
- End organ insufficiency – liver, kidney and lungs
- Vitamin deficiency — thiamine, folate
- Fever or hypothermia

Infectious

- Urinary tract infection (most common cause)
- Pneumonia (second most common cause)
- Encephalitis or meningitis
- Sepsis
- Influenza

Neurologic

- Brain tumor
- Subdural hematoma
- Intracerebral hemorrhage
- Seizure disorder
- CVA

Endocrine

- Hyperthyroidism
- Hypothyroidism
- Parathyroid — hyper and hypoparathyroidism

Cardiovascular

- Congestive heart failure
- Arrhythmia
- Acute myocardial infarction

Conditions that mimic delirium

- Dementia
- Depression
- Schizophrenia
- Mania
- Wernicke's aphasia

Evaluation of delirium

- CBC
- BMP
- LFT's
- U/A
- Chest x-ray
- EKG

Ordered as indicated

- Drug levels
- Thyroid studies
- Urine drug screen
- Blood alcohol
- Blood cultures
- CT brain scan
- Lumbar puncture for CSF analysis
- Urine culture

Treatment of delirium

- Treat underlying illness
- Restore any fluid or electrolyte imbalances
- Discontinue unnecessary medication that is contributing to delirium (discuss with physician)

Consult criteria for delirium

- Discuss all cases with physician
- Physician should examine all delirium or acute altered mental status patients

Temporal Arteritis

- True emergency of the elderly
  - Age of onset 50–70 years of age
  - Six times more common in females than in males

- Headache localized over eye or scalp
- Fever, malaise and weight loss are associated symptoms
- Jaw claudication is important associated symptom
- Frequently associated with polymyalgia rheumatica (joint and muscles aches)
- ESR 50–100
- Normal ESR should not dissuade from making the diagnosis of TA as > 15% of biopsy-proven cases have a normal ESR
- C-reactive protein elevated usually
- Vision loss can occur early in course of disease

Treatment

- Prednisone 40–80 mg PO qday or divided bid for several months to one year
  - In suspected temporal with normal ESR, treat with steroids

Disposition

- Minimal symptoms can be treated as outpatient
- Severe symptoms or question of eye involvement should be admitted with IV high dose steroid treatment and ophthalmology consultation

Discharge instructions

- Temporal arteritis aftercare instructions
- Follow up with PCP within 1 day
- Return for visual changes

Consult criteria

- Discuss all temporal arteritis cases with physician

Falls in Elderly

Causes

- Environmental or accidental: 30–50% of patients
- Gait, balance, weakness or deconditioning: 10–25% of patients
- Sensation of dizziness: 5–20% of patients
- Syncope: 2–10% of patients
- Orthostatic hypotension: 2–15% of patients
- Drop attacks: 1–10% of patients
- Other: 1–10% of patients

Physical examination

- Orthostatic blood pressures
  - Definition
    - SBP drop 20 mm Hg or DBP 10 mm Hg with assumption of upright posture
    - Sustained HR increase 30 bpm within 10 min of moving from recumbent to nonexertional standing position (or 40 bpm if 12-19 yrs. of age)
    - Postural blood pressure changes can occur after standing for 10 minutes and so blood pressure should be checked again at 10–15 minutes if low orthostatic blood pressure is suspected as cause of the fall
    - Orthostatic measurements do not, in isolation, reliably diagnose or exclude orthostatic syncope, nor do they exclude life-threatening causes of syncope
    - Orthostatic vital signs are present in up to 40% of asymptomatic patients older than 70 years, and 23% of those younger than 60 years
- Core body temperature
- Skin for evidence of trauma, pallor
- HEENT for vision loss, hearing deficits, cranial nerve deficits, nystagmus
- Neck for carotid bruit, meningeal signs
- Chest auscultation for rales
- Heart for aortic stenosis murmur, arrhythmias
- Extremities for fractures, motion limitations, DJD findings
- Neurologic for altered mental status, focal neurologic deficits, loss of position sense

Lab and x-ray evaluation options as indicated

- CBC
- CMP
- Chest x-ray
- X-ray of injured areas
- U/A
- UDS and blood alcohol
- EKG
- Medication levels
- CT brain scan

Discharge criteria

- Cause of fall benign and no serious injury
- Good social and home support systems if needed

Consult criteria

- Cause of fall requires admission
- New medical condition causing fall
- Significant abnormal lab or imaging study
- Fracture
- See General Patient Criteria Protocol (page 15)

Notes

REFERENCES:

Delirium Author: Kannayiram Alagiakrishnan, MD, MBBS, MHA, MPH; Chief Editor: Iqbal Ahmed, MBBS, FRCPsych (UK)
emedicine.medscape.com/article/288890

American Psychiatric Association. *Diagnostic and Statistical Manual of Mental Disorders, Fifth Edition*. 5th ed. Washington, DC: American Psychiatric Association; 2013

Birkhead NC, Wagener HP, Shick RM. Treatment of temporal arteritis with adrenal corticosteroids: Results in 55 cases in which the lesion was proved at biopsy. *JAMA*. 1975;163:821.

Giant Cell Arteritis Author: Mythili Seetharaman, MD; Chief Editor: Herbert S Diamond, MD
emedicine.medscape.com/article/332483

Ann of EM, Vol.655:622

JEM. 2018;55:780

Annals of EM, Vol. 49, pg. 431

Circulation, epub, 3/9/17

Gynecology

Section Contents

When using any protocol, always follow the Guidelines of Proper Use (page 12).

Vaginal Bleeding Protocol

Definition

- Abnormal vaginal bleeding

Differential Diagnosis

- Abnormal Uterine Bleeding (AUB)
- Spontaneous abortion
- Threatened abortion
- Atrophic endometrium (postmenopausal)
- Systemic disorders
- Hypothyroidism
- Vaginal Laceration
- STD's/Cervicitis
- Rectal Bleeding
- Carcinoma

Structural Causes (PALM)

- Polyp (AUB-P)
- Adenomyosis (AUB-A)
- Leiomyoma (AUB-L)
    - Submucosal myoma (AUB-LSM)
        - Other myoma (AUB-Lo) Malignancy
    - Hyperplasia (AUB-M)

Nonstructural Causes (COEIN)

- Coagulopathy (AUB-C)
- Ovulatory dysfunction (AUB-O)
- Endometrial (AUB-E)
- Iatrogenic (AUB-I)
- Not yet classified (AUB-N)

Considerations

- See Pregnancy Complications Protocol if pregnant
- Usually from a benign etiology
- Rule out pregnancy — prior tubal ligation, negative menstrual and sexual histories do not rule out pregnancy
- Causes of bleeding besides pregnancy need evaluation
- Average tampon holds 5–15cc of blood; average pad holds 15–30 cc of blood
- Postmenopausal vaginal bleeding needs to be evaluated for cancer
- Menorrhagia (days of heavy bleeding) may be treated with tranexamic acid 1300 mg PO TID (Max 5 days)

History

- Gestational history
- Last normal menstrual period noted

- Current medications (anticoagulants, hormones)

Evaluation Options

- Pelvic exam (delay for pregnancy > 20 weeks)
- CBC if tachycardia or hypotension present, or worrisome history for significant hemorrhage
- UCG as indicated
- Serum quantitative HCG if known to be pregnant
- Rh type if pregnant
- Type and screen if tachycardic
- PT/PTT/INR if indicated
- Type and cross match if hypotensive and notify physician promptly
- Consider transvaginal ultrasonography

Estimated Blood and Fluid losses (adults)

	Class I	Class II	Class III	Class IV
Blood loss (cc)	Up to 750	750–1000	1500–2000	> 2000
Blood loss %	Up to 15%	15–30%	30–40%	> 40%
Pulse rate	< 100	> 100	> 120	> 140
Blood pressure	Normal	Normal	SBP < 90	SBP < 70
Capillary refill	Normal	Normal	Delayed	Absent
Pulse pressure	Normal/incr	Decreased	Decreased	Decreased
Respiratory rate	14–20	20–30	30–40	> 35
Urine output (cc/hr.)	> 30	20–30	5–15	Negligible
Mental status	Anxious	Anxious	Confused	Lethargic

(Derived from Advanced Trauma Life Support)

Treatment Options

Dysfunctional uterine bleeding (DUB) with stable vital signs 85 % anovulation

- 85% anovulation
- Most common cause of AUB
- Estrogen 2.5 mg PO QID: add Provera 10 mg qday for 7-10 days when bleeding subsides
- Combination oral contraceptives
  - Nortrel 1/35 one PO bid × 7 days until bleeding stops, then 1 PO qday × 2 weeks
- Provera 10 mg PO qday × 10-30 days
  - Bleeding will resume when hormone therapy is finished
- NSAID's can be used to decrease bleeding and pain

IV NS 250–500cc bolus

- If heart rate ≥ 120
- If SBP < 90
- Avoid > 1 liter of isotonic fluids for acute blood loss before blood products transfusion started if possible
- PRBC's/FFP/platelets 1:1:1 ratio (recommendations range from 4:1:1 to 1:1:1)
- Uncrossed match blood for hemorrhagic shock if needed emergently
- Avoid hypertension
- Target systolic blood pressure of 80-90 mm Hg until major bleeding stopped
- Target Hgb of 7-9 g/dl after termination of major bleeding
  - Tranexamic acid 1 gm/10 minutes IV then 1 gm over 8 hours (no faster than 100 mg/minute)
- If SBP < 105 and heart rate ≥ 110 with history of hypertension
- Notify physician promptly

Bleeding profuse and unresponsive to IV fluid management

- Conjugated estrogen (Premarin) 25 mg IV every 4–6 hours until the bleeding stops

Discharge Criteria

- Pregnancy — see Pregnancy Complications Protocol
- Benign vaginal bleeding such as DUB or irregular menses with heart rate ≤ 100, SBP > 90, and SBP ≥ 105 in patients with hypertension history and no signs of hypovolemia from blood loss

Discharge instructions

- Vaginal bleeding aftercare instructions
- Referral to OB/GYN within 1–10 days depending on severity of symptoms

Consult Criteria

- Pregnancy or postpartum bleeding — see Pregnancy Complications Protocol
- Ectopic pregnancy or possible ectopic pregnancy
- Fever
- Severe abdominal or pelvic pain
- Purulent vaginal discharge
- Continued heavy vaginal bleeding
- Return visit for same vaginal bleeding episode
- Postmenopausal vaginal bleeding
- Notify physician promptly for significant bleeding

Vital signs and age consult criteria

- Age ≥ 55
- SBP < 90 or relative hypotension (SBP < 105 with history of hypertension)
- Adult heart rate > 100
- Orthostatic vital signs

Lab consult criteria

- Hemoglobin decrease > 1 gm
- Hemoglobin < 10 gms unless stable
- WBC ≥ 15,000
- Bandemia ≥ 15%
- Increased anion gap or metabolic acidosis
- Thrombocytopenia
- Elevated coagulation studies
- Creatinine increase > 0.5 from baseline
- Elevated LFT's

Notes

REFERENCES:

Dysfunctional Uterine Bleeding in Emergency Medicine

Author: Amir Estephan, MD; Chief Editor: Pamela L Dyne, MD emedicine.medscape.com/article/795587

Tranexamic Acid Treatment for Heavy Menstrual Bleeding: A Randomized Controlled Trial Lukes, Andrea S. MD, MHSc; Moore, Keith A. PharmD; Muse, Ken N. MD;

Obstetrics & Gynecology:

October 2010 Volume 116 - Issue 4 - pp 865-875

doi: 10.1097/AOG.0b013e3181f20177

Management of abnormal uterine bleeding associated with ovulatory dysfunction. Practice Bulletin No. 136. American College of Obstetricians and Gynecologists. Obstet Gynecol 2013;122:176–85

Hemorrhagic Shock in Emergency Medicine Guidelines

Updated: May 06, 2016 Author: William P Bozeman, MD; Chief Editor: Trevor John Mills, MD, MPH

Pelvic Pain Protocol

Definition

- Female pelvic pain

Differential Diagnosis

- Pelvic inflammatory disease (PID)
- Ectopic pregnancy
- Normal pregnancy
- Ovarian cyst
- Endometriosis
- Ovarian torsion
- Uterine fibroids
- Chronic pelvic pain syndrome
- UTI
- Renal colic

Considerations

- Must be differentiated from GI or urologic causes of pain
- Bilateral tubal ligation does not always prevent pregnancies — order UCG on all BTL patients that would be fertile otherwise

Evaluation

- Pelvic and abdominal exam
- UCG on fertile females
- U/A
- CBC for
  - Fever
  - Tachycardia
  - Hypotension
  - Moderate to severe pain
- BMP for
  - Dehydration
  - Tachycardia
  - Hypotension
  - Diabetes
- C-reactive protein may be helpful for inflammatory disease or PID

Pelvic ultrasound when

- Pregnant
- Suspected ovarian torsion
- Suspected ruptured ovarian cyst with tachycardia
- Suspected tubo-ovarian abscess (TOA)

Pelvic Inflammatory Disease (PID)

Definition

- Spectrum of the female genital tract infection to include uterus, tubes, ovaries and peritoneum

Differential diagnosis

- Ectopic pregnancy
- Normal pregnancy
- Ovarian cyst
- Endometriosis
- Ovarian torsion
- Uterine fibroids
- Chronic pelvic pain syndrome
- UTI
- Renal colic

Considerations

- Common in females of reproductive age
- Gonorrhea and chlamydia are most common causes
- Important to treat sexual partners
- Can lead to tubo-ovarian abscess
- Can lead to infertility, ectopic pregnancy and tubo-ovarian abscess
- Consider admission if patient has never been pregnant
- Usually caused by gonorrhea or chlamydia, but approximately 15% are due to respiratory or enteric organisms that have colonized the lower genital tract

Symptoms and findings

- Can cause peritonitis
- Usually bilateral pelvic pain and tenderness
- Associated with vaginal discharge frequently
- Dyspareunia
- Cervical motion tenderness usually bilateral
- Fever and chills
- Nausea and vomiting

Evaluation

- Pelvic and abdominal exam
- CBC

- UCG (unless hysterectomy history)
- U/A
- ESR and/or C–reactive protein
- Consider RPR
- LFT's if right upper quadrant tenderness for Fitz-Hugh-Curtis syndrome
- Cultures or DNA probes for gonorrhea and chlamydia; wet prep
- Consider pelvic ultrasound if TOA suspected
- CT abdominal/pelvis scan if appendicitis suspected

Treatment options

Outpatient

- Rocephin (ceftriaxone) 500 mg IM
  - Cefixime 800 mg PO as a single dose if IM route or ceftriaxone not available

  +

- Doxycycline 100 mg PO BID × 14 days

  +/-

- Flagyl (metronidazole) 500 mg PO BID × 14 days (avoid ethanol)
  - Add Flagyl if evidence or suspicion of vaginitis

    OR

  - The patient underwent gynecologic instrumentation in the preceding 2–3 weeks
- Treatment for sexual partners or refer for treatment for STD
- NSAID's and/or narcotics prn
- Phenergan (promethazine) or Zofran prn
- May use Sanford Guide or antibiotic database
- Follow CDC recommendations
- All sexual partners in the previous 60 days should be tested and treated.
- Patients should have no sexual contact until treatment is completed, or 7 days after single-dose treatment
- Testing is repeated 3 months after treatment

Inpatient

- Ceftriaxone 1 g IV every 24 hours + Doxycycline 100 mg PO or IV every 12 hours + Metronidazole 500 mg PO or IV every 12 hours

  OR

- Cefotetan 2 g IV every 12 hours + Doxycycline 100 mg PO or IV every 12 hours

  OR

- Cefoxitin 2 g IV every 6 hours + Doxycycline 100 mg PO or IV every 12 hours
- Clindamycin plus gentamicin relegated to an alternative regimen
- Consult physician

Discharge criteria

- Mild to moderate pain
- Does not meet consult criteria

Discharge instructions

- PID aftercare instructions
- Follow up in 3 days to monitor treatment effectiveness
- Return if pain or fever worsens

Consult criteria

- Uncertain diagnosis or toxic appearance
- Suspected pelvic abscess
- Fitz-Hugh-Curtis syndrome (RUQ tenderness and elevated LFT's)
- Pregnancy
- Severe illness (severe pain and vomiting)
- Unable to tolerate PO intake
- Immunodeficiency
- Failure of outpatient therapy
- Return visit for same acute complaint
- Likely noncompliance with outpatient treatment
- Poor follow-up
- Never has been pregnant
- IUD present (needs admission)

Vaginitis

Definition

- Inflammation of the vagina

Differential diagnosis

- 90% of all cases of vaginitis
  - Bacterial vaginosis 40-50%
  - Vulvovaginal candidiasis 20-25%
  - Trichomonas vaginalis infection 15-20%

Other less common causes

- Atrophic vaginitis
- Cervical polyp
- Contact dermatitis
- Entamoeba histolytica infection
- Excessive desquamation of normal vaginal epithelium
- Large cervical ectropion
- Lichen sclerosis
- Lichen simplex chronicus
- Vaginal adenosis
- Vaginal cancer
- Vaginal intraepithelial neoplasia
- Vaginal ulcers
- Cervicitis
- Child sexual abuse
- Cystitis, nonbacterial
- Cytomegalovirus (CMV)
- Rectal foreign Bodies
- Herpes simplex
- Pinworms
- Postpartum infections
- Salmonella infection
- Sexual assault
- Ureaplasma infection
- Varicella-zoster virus
- Urinary Tract Infection, Female

Considerations

- Prognosis very good
- Cultures not very useful
- Bacterial vaginosis is not a STD, but can increase susceptibility to STD's
- Avoid irritants in the vaginal area
  - Perfumes, soaps, and panty liners
  - After swimming or exercise, air the area or change the underwear
- Always clean from front to back

History

- Previous episodes
- Sexually transmitted infection
- Sexual activities
- Birth control method
- Last menstrual period
- Douching practice
- Use of personal hygiene products
- Antibiotic use
- General medical history
- Systemic symptoms (e.g., lower abdominal pain, fever, chills, nausea, and vomiting)

Bacterial vaginosis

- May be asymptomatic in 50% of women
- Treat symptomatic patients
- Associated with preterm birth in pregnancy
  - Always treat pregnant females
- Painless usually (pruritus may be present)
- Thin malodorous discharge, pH 5–6

Amsel's Diagnostic Clinical Criteria (wet prep)

- 3 of following
  - Thin white discharge homogenous that coats vaginal walls
  - Clue cells (>20%)
  - pH > 4.5
  - Whiff test of fishy odor before and after adding KOH

Treatment (select one)

- Metronidazole 500 mg orally twice a day for 7 days (no alcohol during and up to 24 hours after)
- Metronidazole gel 0.75%, 1 full applicator (5 gm) intravaginally, daily for 5 days

- Clindamycin cream 2%, 1 full applicator (5 g) intravaginally at bedtime for 7 days
- Clindamycin 300 mg orally twice a day for 7 days
- Clindamycin ovules 100 mg intravaginally once at bed time for 3 days
- Relapse within 3 months use 10–14 days of treatment
- Tinidazole 2 gm PO daily for 2 days or 1 gm PO daily for 5 days

Pregnancy

- Metronidazole 500 mg orally twice a day for 7 days (no alcohol during up to 24 hours after)
- Metronidazole 250 mg orally 3 times a day for 7 day
- Clindamycin 300 mg orally twice a day for 7 day
- Pregnant women should have a follow-up visit 1 month after completion of treatment

Disposition

- Usually discharge
- Consider admission in severely ill patients
- Consult OB/GYN or physician as needed
- Follow up with OB/GYN as needed

Vaginal candidiasis (vulvovaginosis)

Yeast normal part of vaginal flora that if overgrows causes symptoms

- Well-demarcated erythema of the vulva
- Satellite lesions (discrete pustulopapular lesions) surrounding the redness
- Vulva, vagina, and surrounding areas may be edematous and erythematous, possibly accompanied by excoriations and fissures
- Adherent cottage cheese–like vaginal discharge may be seen
- Cervix usually appears normal

Treatment uncomplicated disease

- Clotrimazole 1% cream 5 g intravaginally for 7-14 days
- Clotrimazole 100 mg vaginal tablet for 7 days
- Clotrimazole 100 mg vaginal tablet, 2 tablets for 3 days
- Miconazole 2% cream 5 g intravaginally for 7 days
- Miconazole 100 mg vaginal suppository, 1 suppository for 7 days
- Miconazole 200 mg vaginal suppository, 1 suppository for 3 days
- Miconazole 1200 mg vaginal suppository, 1 suppository for 1 day
- Nystatin 100,000 unit vaginal tablet, 1 tablet for 14 days
- Fluconazole 150 mg oral tablet once

Recurrent vaginal candidiasis

- ≥4 episodes in 1 year
- 7-10 days of topical therapy

OR

- 150 mg oral dose of fluconazole every third day for a total of 3 doses (days 1, 4, and 7)
- Maintenance is oral fluconazole 100 mg or 150 mg weekly for 6 months
- **Other medications** that may be used up to 6 months include
  - Clotrimazole 500 mg vaginal suppositories once per wk.

Severe vulvovaginal candidiasis

- 7-14 days of topical azole therapy or 150 mg of oral fluconazole repeated in 72 hours; adjunctive use of nystatin cream or low-potency steroid cream may be beneficial

Pregnant patients

- 7 days of topical agents
  - Fluconazole is contraindicated

Disposition

- Discharge usually
- Admission for signs or symptoms of systemic infection (consult physician)
- Sexual partners should be advised for diagnosis and treatment if symptomatic

Trichomonas vaginitis

Considerations

- Asymptomatic in 50% of females and 75% of men
- Discharge malodorous
- Vaginal or vulvar irritation or itching
- Cervix friable (bleeds easily to swab)
- pH >5.5
- WBC's and mobile trichomonads noted 60–80%
- 20% reinfected within 3 months
- Sexual partners need treatment

Treatment

- Metronidazole 2 gm orally in a single dose for men if needed and females 500 mg orally twice a day for 7 days
  - No alcohol during up to 24 hours after treatment
  - No breast feeding during and up to 24 hours after
- Tinidazole 2 gm orally in a single dose is alternative

Treatment failure

- Metronidazole 2 gm PO daily for 3–5 days
- Tinidazole 500mg PO qid and intravaginal 500mg bid for 14 days if metronidazole resistant

Disposition

- Discharge
  - If signs or symptoms of systemic disease consult physician

Chlamydial infection

Urethritis or cervicitis

- Azithromycin 1gm PO x 1 dose

  OR
- Doxycycline 100mg PO bid x 7-10 days

  OR
- Levofloxacin 500 mg orally once daily for 7 days
- All sexual partners in the previous 60 days should be tested and treated. Patients should have no sexual contact until treatment is completed, or 7 days after single-dose treatment. Testing is repeated 3 months after treatment

Ovarian Cysts

Definition

- Fluid filled sac in ovary

Differential diagnosis

- PID
- UTI
- Ovarian torsion
- Appendicitis
- Diverticulitis
- Endometriosis
- Inflammatory bowel disease
- Ovarian cancer

Considerations

- Most asymptomatic and benign
- Cysts < 5 cm usually resolve
- Cysts > 5 cm need referral and follow-up

Evaluation

- Pelvic and abdominal exam
- UCG
- U/A
- CBC for
  - Fever
  - Tachycardia
  - Hypotension
  - Moderate to severe pain
- BMP for

- Dehydration
- Tachycardia
- Hypotension
- Diabetes

Treatment options

- Pain control if not hypotensive
- Notify physician promptly for bleeding from hemorrhagic cysts or signs of hemorrhagic volume loss
  - Heart rate ≥ 110; SBP < 90; orthostatic vital signs or hypotension
    - IV NS 250–500 cc bolus prn
  - See Bleeding Protocol
- Severe pain order pelvic ultrasound
- Oral contraceptives not effective

Discharge criteria

- Simple ovarian cysts
- Stable vital signs

Discharge instructions

- Ovarian cyst aftercare instructions
- Return if pain worsens or dizziness develops

Consult criteria

- Severe pain
- Fever
- Heart rate ≥ 110; SBP < 90; orthostatic vital signs or hypotension

Endometriosis

Definition

- Endometriosis is the presence of endometrial-like tissue outside the uterine cavity, which induces a chronic inflammatory reaction

Differential diagnosis

- Appendicitis
- Ectopic pregnancy
- Diverticulitis
- Inflammatory bowel disease
- UTI
- PID
- Ovarian cysts
- Ovarian torsion
- Primary dysmenorrhea

Considerations

- Dysmenorrhea
- Heavy or irregular vaginal bleeding
- Pelvic, lower abdominal and lower back pain locations
- 15% of all pelvic pain
- Similar evaluation as ovarian cyst if diagnosis in doubt
- UCG if fertile
- 30–40% of women with be subfertile

Treatment options

- Pain control with NSAID's and/or narcotics
- Provera 10–20 mg qday
- Ortho-Cyclen for one month

Discharge criteria

- Pain controlled
- Stable vital signs

Discharge instructions

- Endometriosis aftercare instructions
- Follow up with primary care provider or gynecologist within 7 days if possible

Consult physician if diagnosis uncertain

- Heart rate ≥ 110
- Orthostatic vital signs
- Fever
- Severe pain

Ectopic Pregnancy

Definition

- Pregnancy outside of uterus

Considerations

- ß-hCG can be < 100 mIU/mL

Differential diagnosis

- Threatened abortion
- Inevitable abortion
- Incomplete abortion
- Missed abortion
- Appendicitis
- Diverticulitis
- Inflammatory bowel disease
- UTI

- PID
- Ovarian cysts
- Ovarian torsion
- Primary dysmenorrhea

Evaluation

- Pelvic and abdominal exam
- Rh type
- CBC
- BMP
- ß-hCG
- Pelvic ultrasound (perform even if ß-hCG < 100 mIU/mL
- Type and screen if vital signs stable
- Type and cross for 2 units PRBC's if hypotensive

Treatment options

- Notify physician promptly
- Notify physician if ectopic pregnancy is possible consideration

IV NS 250–500 cc bolus (avoid > 1000 cc IV bolus if possible)

- Heart rate ≥ 115 and rupture suspected
- Orthostatic vital signs
- Give blood early if SBP < 80 mmHg or HR > 130 and patient is clearly not stable (see Vaginal Bleeding Protocol)
- Hypotension

Pelvic Pain Consult Criteria

- Dehydration
- Significant blood loss
- Ectopic pregnancy or possible ectopic pregnancy
- Suspected or diagnosed appendicitis or diverticulitis
- Acute surgical abdomen
- Moderate to severe pain of uncertain cause
- Severe pain with any diagnosis
- Return ED visit within 14 days for same acute pelvic pain complaint
- Elevated LFT's
- Any of the above subtopics consult criteria

Vital signs consult criteria

- Pelvic pain that develops hypotension or relative hypotension (SBP < 110 with history of hypertension)
- Heart rate ≥ 110

Lab consult criteria

- WBC > 15,000 or < 3,000
- Bandemia ≥ 15%
- Significant electrolyte abnormally
- Hyperglycemia with metabolic acidosis (decreased serum CO_2 or elevated anion gap)
- Worsening anemia; decrease > 1 gm hemoglobin
- Metabolic acidosis

Notes

REFERENCES:

Endometriosis Author: Dharmesh Kapoor, MBBS, MD, MRCOG; Chief Editor: Michel E Rivlin, MD emedicine.medscape.com/article/271899

Davis L-J, Kennedy SS, Moore J, Prentice A. Oral contraceptives for pain associated with endometriosis. Cochrane Database of Systematic Reviews 2007, Issue 3. Art. No.: CD001019. DOI: 10.1002/14651858.CD001019.pub2

Endometriosis: diagnosis and management. 2010 Jul. NGC:007969 Society of Obstetricians and Gynaecologists of Canada - Medical Specialty Society

Workowski KA, Berman S. Sexually transmitted diseases treatment guidelines, 2010. *MMWR Recomm Rep.* Dec 17 2010;59:1–110

Pelvic Inflammatory Disease Author: Suzanne Moore Shepherd, MD, MS, DTM&H, FACEP, FAAEM; Chief Editor: Michel E Rivlin, MD emedicine.medscape.com/article/256448

Grimes DA, Jones LB., Lopez LM, Schulz KF. Oral contraceptives for functional ovarian cysts. Cochrane Database of Systematic Reviews 2014, Issue 4. Art. No.: CD006134. DOI: 10.1002/14651858.CD006134.pub5

Counselman FL, et al. Quantitative B-hCG levels less than 1000 mIU/mL in patients with ectopic pregnancy: pelvic ultrasound still useful *J Emerg Med* 1998;16: 699–703

NEJM, 372:2039

emedicine.medscape.com/article/257141

Vaginitis Treatment & Management

Updated: Dec 04, 2018 Author: Hetal B Gor, MD, FACOG; Chief Editor: Michel E Rivlin, MD

Emedicine medscape

Vulvovaginitis Updated: Jan 19, 2018 Author: Jill M Krapf, MD, FACOG; Chief Editor: Christine Isaacs, MD

CCJM. Vol.86:733

Sexually Transmitted Infections Treatment Guidelines, 2021 Recommendations and Reports / July 23, 2021 / 70(4);1–187

Pregnancy Complications Protocol

Definition

- Processes that interfere with a normal intrauterine pregnancy (IUP) progression

Differential Diagnosis

- Threatened abortion — may present with pain and/or bleeding, closed cervical os, benign exam and no tissue passed
- Inevitable abortion — open cervical os and/or non-viable IUP (such as blighted ovum)
- Incomplete abortion — partial passage of products of conception (POC)
- Missed abortion — fetal death < 20 weeks without passage of POC
- Septic abortion — abortion and infection with pain, fever or foul smelling/purulent discharge
- Preeclampsia — IUP > 20 weeks gestation with hypertension, proteinuria, and/or CNS symptoms or epigastric symptoms and frequently edema with > 1+ pitting edema after 12 hours bedrest; pedal, hands and facial edema and rapid weight gain > 2.7 kg/month (weight gain early sign)
- Eclampsia — preeclampsia with seizures
- Hypertension is 140/90 or rise of SBP 20 and DBP 10 over prepregnancy levels
- HELLP — hemolysis; elevated liver enzymes (twice normal); low platelets (<100K)
- Ectopic pregnancy — occurs 2% of all pregnancies
- Treat all suspected or confirmed influenza pregnant patients up to 2 weeks after delivery with influenza medications

Considerations

- Bleeding occurs in 20–30% of pregnancies in first 20 weeks (50% will have eventual spontaneous abortion)
- Late pregnancy (last 20 weeks) bleeding occurs 3–5%
- 11.5% of patients are pregnant who say it is "not possible" to be pregnant
- 7.5% pregnant with recent "normal period"
- Discrimatory zone where ultrasound usually can visualize the gestation
  - hCG 6000 mIU/mL for transabdominal ultrasound
  - hCG 700–1000 mIU/mL for transvaginal ultrasound
  - Normal pregnancy may be lower than discrimatory zone
  - Ectopic pregnancy may have extremely low hCG of down to 10 mIU/mL

General Evaluation

- Pelvic and abdominal exam
- Complete physical examination
- History of LNMP, amount of bleeding, any POC passed
- CBC
- Serum quantitative HCG
- U/A
- Fetal heart tones – usually 110–160/minute (dependent on gestational age)
- Rh type (if there is vaginal bleeding history or findings)
- Transvaginal ultrasound (usually)
- LFT's if preeclampsia/eclampsia present
- BMP if vomiting and tachycardia present
- Type and screen for significant bleeding or tachycardia
- Type and cross for 2 units PRBC's if hypotensive
- Defer pelvic exam last 20 weeks of gestation if bleeding

Hyperemesis gravidarum and nausea/vomiting of pregnancy

- Hyperemesis gravidarum most severe form of nausea and vomiting in pregnancy, with ketosis and weight loss > 5% of prepregnancy weight

Evaluation options

- Vital signs including orthostatics as needed
- U/A, BMP, magnesium, calcium and serum ketones
- LFT's, amylase/lipase if abdominal pain present
- TSH and T4
- Urine culture
- CBC if abdominal pain/tenderness present
- Hepatitis panel if LFT's elevated
- RUQ ultrasound if gallbladder, liver or pancreas disease suspected
- Pelvic/OB ultrasound if not previously performed to confirm single pregnancy
- CT or MRI abdomen for surgical abdomen

Treatment choices

- First line: Vitamin B-6 10–25 mg 3–4 times daily with doxylamine 12.5–25 mg 3–4 times daily
  - Diclegis (doxylamine/pyridoxine)
- Ginger capsules 250 mg 4 times daily can be added at this point if the patient is still vomiting
- IV D5LR 1 liter over 1–2 hours as needed
- Phenergan 6.25–25 mg IV
- Metoclopramide 10 mg IV
- Small frequent feedings
- Discontinue prenatal vitamins with iron

Consult criteria

- Persistent vomiting and volume depletion despite treatment

- Abdominal pain or tenderness out of proportion to vomiting
- Weight loss > 5–7.5%

Ectopic pregnancy

- Occurs 2% of pregnancies
- Missed > 40% of time on first visit
- 90% with pain and 50–80% with bleeding
- 30% have atypical presentations
- Normal pelvic exam does not rule out ectopic
- Falling β-HCG does not exclude ectopic pregnancy
- β-HCG normally double every 2 days when < 10,000 mIU/ml with normal pregnancy
- No IUP on ultrasound is suspicious for ectopic pregnancy
- Perform ultrasound on indeterminate β-HCG
  - β-HCG can be < 100 mIU/mL in ectopic pregnancy

Preeclampsia and eclampsia

- IUP > 20 weeks gestation with hypertension and proteinuria
- Can occur up to 4–6 weeks postpartum
- Frequently with pedal and hand edema
- Gestational hypertension is not associated with proteinuria
- Low dose aspirin 81 mg is effective and safe in 2–3rd trimesters in preventing preeclampsia in women with risk factors for preeclampsia
- Notify physician

Risk factors for preeclampsia or eclampsia

- Advanced maternal age > 40 years or young maternal age < 20 years
- First pregnancy
- Prior preeclampsia history
- Chronic Hypertension
- Multiple gestation
- Molar pregnancy
- Diabetes
- Obesity
- Chronic renal disease
- Anti-phospholipid antibody syndrome

Preeclampsia with severe features

- SBP > 160 or DBP > 110
- RUQ/epigastric pain
- Hyperreflexia
- Thrombocytopenia (<100K/mL)
- New onset headache or visual disturbances
- Eclampsia
- Dyspnea or pulmonary edema
- Elevated PT and PTT
- LFT's twice normal
- Papilledema
- Creatinine >1.1mg/dL or double from baseline

Eclampsia

- Preeclampsia with seizures

Evaluation

- Cardiac monitoring
- CBC (preeclampsia and eclampsia)
- U/A

CMET (preeclampsia and eclampsia)

- PT and PTT
- DIC panel
- LDH
- Uric acid is elevated early in preeclampsia and eclampsia
- OB ultrasound

Treatment options

- Delivery is definitive treatment
- Blood pressure goal of SBP 140–155 mm Hg and DBP 90–100 mm Hg
  - Labetalol 20 mg IV, increase as needed, 40mg, then 80mg, given q10 min prn (NMT 300 mg)
  - Hydralazine 5–10 mg IV may repeat q20min prn (NMT 60 mg)
  - Immediate release nifedpine 10-20mg PO, may repeat in 20min if needed

Seizure prophylaxis

- Magnesium sulfate 4–6 gms IV over 20 minutes followed by drip of 1–2 gms IV/hr.
  - Stop $MgSO_4$ (magnesium sulfate)
    - If DTR's are lost
    - For respiratory depression (calcium gluconate 1 gm IV over 10 minutes if needed to reverse magnesium toxicity)
  - Monitor magnesium levels (therapeutic serum level 4-8mg/dl)
  - Caution if renal failure is present

Active seizures

- Give magnesium sulfate 6 gms IV over 5–10 minutes — followed by magnesium drip of 1–2 gms IV per hour
- Dilantin (phenytoin or Ativan (lorazepam) can be used for magnesium sulfate failure, avoid polypharmacy (see Adult Seizure Protocol)

Postpartum hemorrhage

Treatment options depending on degree of bleeding (notify physician promptly for significant hemorrhage)

- Oxytocin 20 unit IV at 20-40 mUnit/min (may also be given IM)
- Hemabate 250mcg IM, repeat q15-90 min prn, max 2 mg total dose (caution if patient asthmatic)
- Methergine 0.2 mg IM/IV q2-4hr PRN; not to exceed 5 doses, then 0.2-0.4 mg PO q6-8hr PRN for 2-7 days
  - Administer IV only in emergency because of potential for hypertension and CVA (notify physician before giving IV)
    - Administer over >1 minute and monitor BP
- Tranexamic acid 1 gm/10 minutes IV then 1 gm over 8 hours (no faster than 100 mg/minute)

  OR
- 10 mg/kg IV followed by infusion of 1 mg/kg/hour

Placenta abruption

- Separation of a normally positioned placenta after 20 weeks of gestation and before birth

Signs and symptoms

- Painful vaginal bleeding 80% (dark red commonly)
- No vaginal bleeding 20%
- Abdominal tenderness 70%
- Uterine tenderness 70%
- Uterus has tectonic contractions 35%
- Shock out of proportion to estimated blood loss
- Fetal distress
- Premature labor
- Fetal death 15 %

Risk factors for placenta abruption

- Previous abruption
- Hypertension or preeclampsia — most common cause
- Diabetes
- Chronic renal disease
- Oligohydramnios, PROM
- Chorioamnionitis
- Trauma – abdominal or rapid deceleration (sheering forces)
- Advance maternal age
- Cocaine use
- Cigarette smoking
- Alcohol use

Evaluation

- CBC
- BMP
- LFT's
- DIC panel
- Type and screen if not in shock

- Type and cross 4 units PRBC's if class 2 or greater hemorrhage (see Bleeding Protocol)
- Transabdominal ultrasound for fetal lie, fluid index, and evaluation of placenta
- Continuous fetal monitoring

Treatment

- 2 large bore IV's of NS
- If class 2 hemorrhage or greater give 250–500 cc NS bolus and consider blood/FFP/platelet transfusion
- See Bleeding Protocol

Consult criteria

- Notify physician and obstetrician promptly

Placenta previa

- Implantation of the placenta near or over the cervical os
- Occurs in the second and third trimesters of pregnancy
- Common cause of pregnancy bleeding

Signs and symptoms

- Painless bright red vaginal bleeding
- Fetal heart tones may be normal
- Bleeding may be intermittent
- Shock can occur

Evaluation

- **Do not** perform digital vaginal or rectal exam (may provoke increased bleeding), speculum exam acceptable
- CBC
- Type and screen
- DIC panel
- Bedside transabdominal ultrasound for fetal presentation, placentation, and fluid index
- Transabdominal or transvaginal ultrasound in radiology if vital signs stable and bleeding amounts judged not to be dangerous
- Continuous fetal monitoring

Consult criteria

- Consult physician and obstetrics

UTI

- **Treat all asymptomatic** and simple cystitis urinary tract infections for 7–10 days
  - Increased incidence of premature rupture of membranes and fetal death if not treated
- Send urine for culture
- No trimethoprim first trimester or sulfa antibiotic last trimester
- Consult for admission on all pyelonephritis patients that are pregnant

Bacterial vaginosis

- Most common cause of vaginal discharge
- Gardnerella vaginalis replaces normal flora
- Risk of preterm labor, premature rupture of membranes and postpartum endometritis if not treated

Criteria – has 3 of 4

- Profuse thin white discharge
- Fishy odor
- pH > 4.5
- Clue cells

Treatment

- All pregnant patients
- All symptomatic nonpregnant patients

Antibiotics

- Metronidazole options 250 mg PO tid × 7 days (avoid 1st trimester)
  - Gel 0.75% 5 gm intravaginally qday × 5 days
- Clindamycin 300 mg PO bid × 7 days

Treatment Options

- Rhogam 300 microunits IM if Rh negative and vaginal bleeding has or is occurring

- IV D5NS rehydration as needed for vomiting of pregnancy (D5 decreases ketosis); No infusion with D5NS > 300 cc/hr.
- IV NS bolus and drip for hemorrhagic compromise (notify physician promptly)
  - No more than 1 liter NS before starting blood transfusion and FFP if possible
  - Give blood:FFP at 1:1 or 2:1 ratio
  - Improved mortality when FFP added
  - See Bleeding Protocol
- Phenergan (promethazine) 6.25 mg IV (25–50 mg IM or PO) or Zofran (ondansetron) 4 mg IV or Reglan 10 mg IV prn
- Narcotics prn (Category B, or C if commonly used in pregnancy)
- Methergine (methylergonovine) 0.2 mg IM prn postpartum or abortion (spontaneous or incomplete) related heavy bleeding
- See Preeclampsia and Eclampsia sections above

Discharge Criteria

- Benign causes of pain of pregnancy (round ligament, etc.)
- Benign pelvic pain and threatened abortion with stable vital signs
- Rehydration with heart rate < 100 in vomiting of pregnancy

Discharge instructions

- Pregnancy aftercare instructions
- Threatened abortions aftercare instructions
- Follow up with OB/GYN provider within 1–3 days
- Return if pain persists or increases
- Return if bleeding recurs or increases

Consult Criteria

- Heart rate ≥ 110
- BP ≥ 140/90
- Intractable vomiting
- Anemia
- Preeclampsia or eclampsia
- Placental abruption
- Placenta previa
- Ectopic or possible ectopic pregnancy
- Any spontaneous abortion (threatened, missed, septic, incomplete)
- Fetal demise
- Significant vaginal bleeding or hypotension or orthostasis (notify physician promptly)
- Late pregnancy bleeding (last 20 weeks)
- Significant pelvic/abdominal pain or headache
- Pyelonephritis

Notes

____

____

____

REFERENCES:

Hahn SA, Lavonas EJ, Mace SE, Napoli AM, Fesmire FM, American College of Emergency Physicians. Clinical policy: critical issues in the initial evaluation and management of patients presenting to the emergency department in early pregnancy. Ann Emerg Med. 2012 Sep;60(3):381-90.e28

Counselman FL, et al. Quantitative B-hCG levels less than 1000 mIU/mL in patients with ectopic pregnancy: pelvic ultrasound still useful *J Emerg Med* 1998;16: 699-703

Hyperemesis Gravidarum Author: Dotun A Ogunyemi, MD; Chief Editor: Christine Isaacs, MD emedicine.medscape.com/article/254751

American College of Obstetricians and Gynecologists (ACOG). Nausea and vomiting of pregnancy. Washington (DC): American College of Obstetricians and Gynecologists (ACOG); 2004 Apr. 13 p. (ACOG practice bulletin; no. 52)

Coomarasamy A, Honest H, Papaioannou S, et al. Aspirin for prevention of preeclampsia in women with historical risk factors: a systematic review. *Obstet Gynecol.* Jun 2003;101(6):1319-32

Preeclampsia Author: Kee-Hak Lim, MD; Chief Editor: Ronald M Ramus, MD emedicine.medscape.com/article/1476919

Postpartum Hemorrhage in Emergency Medicine Medication Author: Maame Yaa A B Yiadom, MD, MPH; Chief Editor: Pamela L Dyne, MD emedicine.medscape.com/article/796785

Lancet 2010;376:23-32

BMJ 2012; 344:e3054

Nausea and vomiting of pregnancy. Practice Bulletin No. 153. American College of Obstetricians and Gynecologists. Obstet Gynecol 2015;126:e12–24.

Vicken P Sepilian, MD, MSc; Chief Editor: Michel E Rivlin, MD emedicine.medscape.com/article/2041923-workup#c8

Clin Infect Dis: epub 12/19/18

Infectious Disease

Section Contents

When using any protocol, always follow the Guidelines of Proper Use (page 12).

Sexually Transmitted Disease Protocol

Definition

- Diseases transmitted by sexual contact

Differential Diagnosis

- Gonorrhea
- PID
- Chlamydia
- Epididymitis
- Orchitis
- Syphilis
- Hepatitis B
- Prostatitis
- Herpes
- Trichomoniasis

Considerations

- Gonococcal and chlamydial disease frequently seen together
- Syphilis — 100,000 new cases per year

Presentations

- Pelvic inflammatory disease (PID)
- Prostatitis (usually age < 35 years)
- Epididymoorchitis
- Bartholin cyst
- Anogenital Warts
- Urethritis
- Vaginitis

Gonococcal Disease

Definition

- Disease spectrum caused by Neisseria gonorrhoeae

Differential diagnosis

- Nonspecific urethritis
- Chlamydial infections
- Strep pharyngitis
- Leucocytoclastic vasculitis (rash)
- Septic arthritis

- Meningitis
- Orchitis
- Epididymitis
- UTI
- Cervicitis
- PID
- Proctitis
- Conjunctivitis

Considerations

- May be disseminated
    - Joints — frequently single and migratory (knee most common)
    - Skin
    - Tenosynovitis
    - Meningitis
    - Endocarditis
- Coexists 25–50% of the time with chlamydial infection
- May coexist with trichomonas and syphilis

Females

- Asymptomatic carriers
- PID — 20% has gonorrhea
    - Cervical motion tenderness
    - Usually bilateral adnexal tenderness
    - RUQ tenderness with elevated LFT's may represent Fitz-Hugh-Curtis syndrome
- Cervicitis
- Associated often with chlamydia and trichomonas

Males

- Moderate to severe dysuria
- Purulent urethral discharge
- Proctitis (men having sex with men)
- Pharyngitis

Evaluation

- Reproductive/menstrual and sexual history
- Genital exam usually indicated
- Smear with intracellular gram negative diplococci can be performed
- Culture
- RPR prn
- Urine nucleic amplification test for GC and chlamydia (first catch urine)

Uncomplicated gonococcal infection of the cervix, urethra, or rectum among adults and adolescents

- Follow CDC guidelines
- Analgesics prn
- Rocephin (ceftriaxone) 500 mg
    - Ceftriaxone 1 gm IM if weight > 150 kg
- IM route not available may use 800 mg cefixime dose plus azithromycin 2 gm PO
- Cephalosporin allergy may use 240 mg IM dose of gentamicin plus a single 2 g oral dose of azithromycin
- If chlamydia not excluded for urethral, cervical, rectal and pharyngeal uncomplicated infections
    - Add doxycycline 100 mg PO bid × 7 days if

      OR
    - Azithromycin 1 gm PO one dose (not first line)

      OR
    - Levofloxacin 500 mg PO qday for 7 days
- If concerned about syphilis coinfection then doxycycline 100 mg bid PO for 14 days
- A test-of-cure is unnecessary for persons with uncomplicated urogenital or rectal gonorrhea who are treated with any of the recommended or alternative regimens; however, for persons with pharyngeal gonorrhea, a test-of-cure is recommended, using culture or nucleic acid amplification tests 7–14 days after initial treatment

Discharge criteria

- Nondisseminated gonococcal disease
- Nontoxic patient

Discharge instructions

- STD aftercare instructions

- All sexual partners in the previous 60 days should be tested and treated. Patients should have no sexual contact until treatment is completed, or 7 days after single-dose treatment.
- Return if symptoms persist > 3 days
- Return if worse
- Follow up with health department within 3 days

Consult criteria

- Toxic patient
- Disseminated gonococcal disease (example gonococcal arthritis)
- See General Patient Criteria Protocol (page 15)

Pelvic Inflammatory Disease (PID)

Definition

- Spectrum of the female genital tract infections to include uterus, tubes, ovaries and peritoneum

Differential diagnosis

- Ectopic pregnancy
- Normal pregnancy
- Ovarian cyst
- Endometriosis
- Ovarian torsion
- Uterine fibroids
- Chronic pelvic pain syndrome
- UTI
- Renal colic

Considerations

- Common in females of reproductive age
- Gonorrhea and chlamydia are most common causes
- Important to treat sexual partners
- Can lead to tubo-ovarian abscess
- Can lead to infertility, ectopic pregnancy and tubo-ovarian abscess
- Consider admission if patient has never been pregnant

Symptoms and findings

- Can cause peritonitis
- Usually bilateral pelvic pain and tenderness
- Associated with vaginal discharge frequently
- Dyspareunia
- Cervical motion tenderness
- Fever and chills
- Nausea and vomiting

Evaluation

- Pelvic and abdominal exam
- CBC
- UCG
- U/A
- Wet prep
- Consider RPR
- Consider C-reactive protein
- LFT's if right upper quadrant tenderness for Fitz-Hugh-Curtis syndrome
- Gonorrhea/chlamydia DNA probe
- Consider pelvic ultrasound if TOA suspected
- CT scan if appendicitis also suspected

Treatment options

Outpatient

- Rocephin (ceftriaxone) 500 mg IM

+

- Doxycycline 100 mg PO BID × 14 days

+/-

- Flagyl (metronidazole) 500 mg PO BID × 14 days if vaginitis suspected/diagnosed or gynecologic instrumentation in the preceding 2–3 weeks (avoid ethanol)
- Treatment for sexual partners or refer for treatment for STD
- NSAID's; narcotics prn; Phenergan (promethazine) prn
- Follow CDC recommendations

Inpatient

- Ceftriaxone 1 g IV every 24 hours + doxycycline 100 mg PO or IV every 12 hours +

Metronidazole 500 mg PO or IV every 12 hours

OR

- Cefotetan 2 g IV every 12 hours + Doxycycline 100 mg PO or IV every 12 hours

OR

- Cefoxitin 2 g IV every 6 hours + doxycycline 100 mg PO or IV every 12 hours
- Consult physician

Discharge criteria

- Mild to moderate pain
- Does not meet consult criteria

Discharge instructions

- PID aftercare instructions
- Follow up in 3 days to monitor treatment effectiveness
- Return if pain or fever worsens

Consult and admission criteria recommendation

- Uncertain diagnosis or toxic appearance
- IUD present
- Suspected pelvic abscess
- Fitz-Hugh-Curtis syndrome (RUQ tenderness and elevated LFT's)
- Pregnancy
- Severe illness (severe pain and vomiting)
- Unable to tolerate PO intake
- Immunodeficiency
- Failure of outpatient therapy
- Return visit for same acute complaint
- Likely noncompliance with outpatient treatment
- Poor follow up
- Never been pregnant

Urethritis and Epididymoorchitis

Definition

- Infection or inflammation of the urethra, epididymis or testicle

Differential diagnosis for epididymoorchitis

- Testicular torsion
- Mumps
- Trauma
- Hernia
- Tumor – usually painless

Considerations

- Gonorrhea and chlamydia are the main causes and coexist 25–50% of the time
- Urethral discharge
- Tender and swollen epididymis and/or testicle

Gonorrhea

- Dysuria
- Thick purulent discharge from urethra
- Gram negative intracellular diplococci
- Moderate to severe dysuria

Chlamydia

- Thinner discharge from urethra
- Little to no discomfort

Evaluation

- Sexual history
- Genital exam
- Smear for intracellular gram negative diplococci can be performed
- Urine nucleic amplification test for GC and chlamydia (first catch urine)
- Wet smear
- RPR prn

Treatment options

- Follow CDC guidelines
- May use Sanford Guide or other drug databases
- Analgesics prn

Chlamydia

- Doxycycline 100 mg orally twice a day for 7 days

Alternative Regimens

- Azithromycin 1 g orally in a single dose (not first line)

OR

- Levofloxacin 500 mg PO qday for 7 days

Gonorrhea

- Rocephin (ceftriaxone) 500 mg IM

  +

- Doxycycline 100 mg PO bid × 7–10 days to cover chlamydia
- Cefixime 800 mg PO as a single dose if ceftriaxone not available

  OR

- Cephalosporin allergy or if ceftriaxone not available may use gentamicin 240 mg IM dose of plus a single 2 g oral dose of azithromycin

- **Non-gonococcal urethritis**
  - Doxycycline 100 mg orally twice a day for 7 days

  Alternative Regimens

  - Azithromycin 1 g orally in a single dose (not first line)

    OR

  - Levofloxacin 500 mg PO qday for 7 days
- If concerned about syphilis coinfection then doxycycline 100 mg bid PO for 14 days

Discharge criteria

- Nontoxic patient

Discharge instructions

- Epididymoorchitis aftercare instructions
- Return if worse
- Follow up with PCP or urologist in 3–7 days
- All sexual partners in the previous 60 days should be tested and treated. Patients should have no sexual contact until treatment is completed, or 7 days after single-dose treatment.

Consult criteria

- Systemic toxicity
- Refer to General Patient Criteria Protocol prn (page 15)

Genital herpes

- See Genital Herpes Protocol
- Obtain HSV culture of lesions
- Treatment can be extended if healing is incomplete after 10 days of therapy
- Acyclovir 400 mg orally three times a day for 7--10 days

  OR

- Acyclovir 200 mg orally five times a day for 7--10 days

  OR

- Famciclovir 250 mg orally three times a day for 7--10 days

  OR

- Valacyclovir 1 g orally twice a day for 7--10 days

Prostatitis

Definition

- Infection or inflammation of the prostate gland

Differential diagnosis

- Prostate cancer
- Urethritis
- Mechanical back pain
- UTI

Considerations

- Gonorrhea and chlamydia are the main causes in men age < 35 years and coexist 25–50% of the time
- Prostate tender (caution with vigorous palpation if fever or toxicity present)
- Age > 35 years usual cause is bacterial
- Nonbacterial prostatitis is inflammatory condition without infection
- Chronic prostatitis
  - Increases risk of UTI and BPH

Acute bacterial prostatitis age > 35 years

- Fever
- Chills
- Perineal prostatic pain
- Dysuria
- Obstructive bladder symptoms
- Low back pain
- Low abdominal pain
- Spontaneous urethral discharge

Evaluation options

- U/A
- CBC
- RPR if STD suspected

Treatment options

Age < 35 years

- Follow CDC guidelines
- Analgesics prn
- Rocephin (ceftriaxone) 500 mg IM
    - Cefixime 800 mg PO as a single dose if IM route or ceftriaxone not available

+

- Doxycycline 100 mg PO bid × 10–14 days
- Treatment for sexual partners or refer for treatment for STD
- If concerned about syphilis coinfection then doxycycline 100 mg bid PO for 14 days

Age ≥ 35 years

- Septra DS 1 PO bid × 14–28 days
- Quinolone 14–28 days (not recommended for gonorrhea)
- NSAID's and/or narcotics prn

Discharge criteria

- Nontoxic patient
- Refer to General Patient Criteria Protocol prn (page 15)

Discharge instructions

- Prostatitis aftercare instructions
- Return if worse
- Follow up with PCP or urologist in 3–7 days

Consult criteria

- Systemic toxicity
- Urinary retention

Anogenital Warts

- Usually condyloma acuminata
    - Painless pedunculated or sessile wart
    - From human papillomavirus (HPV)

Can be secondary syphilis (condyloma lata)

- Highly contagious (wear gloves)
- Smooth, moist flat wart
- Secondary syphilis rash is maculopapular and mimics other diseases
- Painless chancre sore history or finding
- Order RPR

Antibiotic choices for syphilis

- Bicillin LA 2.4 IM
- Doxycycline 100 mg PO × 14 days

Treatment for condyloma acuminata

- Podofilox 0.5% gel or solution bid on wart only for 3 days, rest 4 days, and another cycle of 3 days, repeat up to 4–6 cycles
- Imiquimod 3.75% or 5% cream 3x weekly at bedtime until cleared or max 16 weeks
- TCA (trichloroacetic acid) application
- Cryotherapy
- No treatment as warts frequently resolve may be tried

Discharge criteria

- All nontoxic patients

Discharge instructions

- Venereal wart aftercare instructions
- Refer to health department or PCP within 3–7 days

Consult criteria

- Complicating comorbidities

Syphilis

Definition

- Infection caused by Treponema palladium

Differential diagnosis

- Pityriasis rosea
- Chanchroid
- Condyloma acuminata
- Psoriasis

- Lymphogranuloma venereum
- Herpes simplex

Considerations

Primary syphilis

- Painless chancre (sore) at site of infection

Secondary syphilis

- Occurs 2–10 weeks after primary infection
- Widespread mucocutaneous lesions
- Can spread to liver, joints, muscle, lymph nodes and brain

Latent syphilis

- Asymptomatic
- Can last up to 30 years
  - Early phase within one year of primary infection
  - Late phase after one year of primary infection

Tertiary syphilis

- Noninfectious at this stage
- Irreversible
- Can affect
  - Heart (coronary aneurysms)
  - Aorta
  - Eyes
  - Brain
  - Nerves
  - Bones
  - Joints
- Neurosyphilis develops in 5% of tertiary syphilis
  - Meningovascular type most common
  - Tabes dorsalis (post column of spinal cord with loss of position sense)

Treatment options

Antibiotics choices for primary, secondary or early latent syphilis

- Bicillin LA 2.4 IM
- Doxycycline 100 mg BID PO × 14 days

Antibiotic choices for late latent syphilis

- Bicillin LA 2.4 million units IM qweek × 3 weeks

Discharge criteria

- Primary, secondary or early latent syphilis

Discharge instructions

- Syphilis aftercare instructions
- Refer to health department within 3 days

Consult criteria

- Late latent syphilis
- Neurosyphilis
- Tertiary syphilis
- Pregnancy

Notes

REFERENCES:

Workowski KA, Berman S. Sexually transmitted diseases treatment guidelines, 2010. *MMWR Recomm Rep.* Dec 17 2010;59:1–110

Update to CDC's Sexually Transmitted Diseases Treatment Guidelines, 2010: Oral Cephalosporins No Longer a Recommended Treatment for Gonococcal Infections. *MMWR Morb Mortal Wkly Rep.* Aug 10 2012;61:590–4

Gonorrhea Author: Brian Wong, MD; Chief Editor: Burke A Cunha, MD emedicine.medscape.com/article/218059

Prostatitis Author: Paul J Turek, MD; Chief Editor: Robert E O'Connor, MD, MPH emedicine.medscape.com/article/785418

Pelvic Inflammatory Disease

Author: Suzanne Moore Shepherd, MD, MS, DTM&H, FACEP, FAAEM; Chief Editor: Michel E Rivlin, MD
emedicine.medscape.com/article/256448

Centers for Disease Control and Prevention, 2015 Sexually Transmitted Diseases Treatment Guidelines

Update to CDC's Treatment Guidelines for Gonococcal Infection, 2020
Weekly / December 18, 2020 / 69(50);1911–1916

CCJM. Vol.86:733

Sexually Transmitted Infections Treatment Guidelines, 2021 Recommendations and Reports / July 23, 2021 / 70(4);1–187

Human Immunodeficiency Virus (HIV) Protocol

Definition

- Infection by HIV

Differential Diagnosis

- Cytomegalovirus
- Mononucleosis
- Syphilis
- Influenza
- Meningitis
- Encephalitis
- Viral hepatitis
- Idiopathic thrombocytopenic purpura
- Candidiasis

Considerations

- Three month window between acquiring primary HIV infection and seroconversion
- Life expectancy is extended with HIV infection on current treatment regimens
- CD4 count below 200/μL is considered AIDS-defining in the United States
- CD4 T-cell count reference range is 500-2000 cells/μL
- Because CD4 counts vary, serial counts are generally a better measure of significant changes
- After seroconversion, CD4 counts tend to decrease (~700/μL) and continue to decline over time
- In children younger than 5 years, the CD4 T-cell percentage is considered more important than the absolute count (< 25% is considered to warrant therapy)
- Rate of progression to AIDS and death is related to the viral load
    - Patients with viral loads greater than 30,000/μL are 18.5 times more likely to die of AIDS than those with undetectable viral loads
- With therapy, viral loads can often be suppressed to an undetectable level (< 20-75 copies/mL; optimal viral suppression); complete inhibition of viral replication appears impossible and may be unnecessary

HIV testing

- Fourth-generation test that detects HIV in the blood earlier than antibody tests can; it identifies the viral protein HIV-1 p24 antigen, which appears in the blood before antibodies do
- If this test is positive, an immunoassay that differentiates HIV-1 from HIV-2 antibodies should be performed
    - Faster than the Western blot test
    - In patients with positive results on the initial antigen test but with negative or

indeterminate results on the antibody differentiation assay

- HIV-1 nucleic acid testing should be performed to determine whether infection is present

Department of Health and Human Services (DHHS) guidelines

- Antiretroviral therapy should be initiated in all patients with a history of an AIDS-defining illness or with a CD4 count below 350/µL
- Antiretroviral therapy should be initiated regardless of CD4 count in pregnant patients, patients with HIV-associated nephropathy, and those with hepatitis B virus (HBV) coinfection when treatment of HBV infection is indicated
- Panel divided on initiation of therapy with CD4 counts of 350-500/µL; 55% considered this a strong recommendation, 45% considered it a moderate recommendation
- Panel also divided on initiation of therapy with CD4 counts above 500/µL: half favored initiation in this setting, and half considered treatment initiation optional

HAART (highly active antiretroviral therapy) or cART (combination antiretroviral therapy)

- Combination of 2 NRTIs with a NNRTI or Protease Inhibitor or Integrase Inhibitor
- Has significantly increased life expectancy
- Potential for hepatotoxicity
- May cause lactic acidosis
- May cause GI symptoms, rashes, headache and psychiatric disorders
- Pneumonia is usually caused by S. pneumoniae in patients on HAART
- Osteoporosis and osteonecrosis may occur
- Treatment prevents immunosuppressive illnesses and helps prevent CV events, non-HIV related cancers, chronic renal, and chronic hepatic disease

Drug interactions with cART

- Increases concentrations of antiarrhythmia drugs
- Increases levels of anticonvulsants
- Increase concentrations of benzodiazepines
  - Okay to give 1 dose in ED
- Increases rhabdomyolysis risk with statin drugs
- Increases warfarin concentrations

Causes

- Unprotected sexual intercourse
- Anal receptive sexual intercourse is high risk
- Parenteral drug use and needle sharing
- Occupational needle stick
- Contaminated blood product transfusion

Signs, Symptoms, Findings or Processes

- May have no symptoms or physical findings
- Fever
- Fatigue
- Night sweats
- Oral ulcers
- Pharyngitis
- Diarrhea
- Genital ulcers
- Rashes
- Alopecia
- Weight loss
- Headache
- Myalgias
- Lymphadenopathy

- Altered mental status
- Pneumonia
- COPD
- Kidney damage
- Progressive multifocal leukoencephalopathy
- CNS lymphoma
- Anemia
- Sensory neuropathies
- Staph pyomyositis with CD4 < 50 cells/mm^3 (usually in thigh)
- Staph folliculitis
- Psychiatric disorders

Immune reconstitution inflammatory syndrome

- Immune system improves with HAART (cART) and attacks dormant opportunistic infections
- Can worsen autoimmune disorders
- Can manifest as pneumonitis, lymphadenitis, hepatosplenomegaly and hypercalcemia
- Treatment is dependent on opportunistic infection involved
- Discontinuation of HAART is rarely needed

Evaluation

- History of CD4 counts if known
- CD4 count 3 months after cART and then q3–6 months for 2 years, then q12 months if CD4 stable at 300–500 cells/mm^3
  - CD4 > 500 optional testing
- Medication history
- Previous hospitalizations
- Previous infections or cancers

Testing options

- CBC
- LFT's
- U/A if fever or urinary symptoms
- BMP if abnormal vital signs or diabetic
- Stool for ova/parasites and cultures
- STD testing if indicated
- HIV testing offered to patient
- Chest x-ray if respiratory complaints or findings
- CT brain or MRI brain with and without contrast for neurologic complaints or findings

Treatment Options

- Treatment of associated infections
- Discuss AIDS related opportunistic infections or findings with physician
- Antiretroviral treatment per physician or experienced practitioner

Discharge Criteria

- Stable afebrile patient
- Social support systems present
- Pneumonia in HAART patients who are nontoxic, not hypoxic with normal blood pressure and heart rate may be candidates for outpatient treatment
  - Treatment is the same as for typical community acquired pneumonia
  - Discuss with physician

Discharge instructions

- HIV aftercare instructions
- Refer to primary care provider, health department or AIDS clinic for follow-up

Consult Criteria

- Toxic patient
- Altered mental status
- Acute neurologic deficit
- Respiratory distress
- Fever
- Unable to ambulate acutely
- Vomiting
- Unable to self-hydrate
- Pericardial or pleural effusion
- Significant weight loss
- Acute psychiatric symptoms
- Pneumonitis
- Acute dyspnea

Lab consult criteria

- Adult WBC ≥ 13,000 or < 1,000 neutrophils;
- Bandemia

- Acute thrombocytopenia
- Hemoglobin < 10 (unless chronic and stable)
- Onset or worsening of renal insufficiency
- O_2 Sat ≤ 94% on room air if acute

Vital sign and age consult criteria

- Adult heart rate > 100

Notes

REFERENCES:

CDC Laboratory Testing for the Diagnosis of HIV Infection: Updated Recommendations. Centers for Disease Control and Prevention

Canavan N. New HIV Treatment Guidelines to Cut Millions of Deaths. *Medscape Medical News* [serial online]. Jul 1 2013

Panel on Antiretroviral Guidelines for Adults and Adolescents. Guidelines for the use of antiretroviral agents in HIV-1–infected adults and adolescents. Department of Health and Human Services. January 10, 2011; 1–174. aidsinfo.nih.gov/contentfiles/AdultandAdolescentGL

Updated May 1, 2014

[Guideline] Panel on Antiretroviral Guidelines for Adults and Adolescents. Guidelines for the use of antiretroviral agents in HIV-1-infected adults and adolescents. Department of Health and Human Services. October 17, 2017

HIV Infection and AIDS Medication Updated: Sep 12, 2018

Author: Nicholas John Bennett, MBBCh, PhD, MA(Cantab), FAAP; Chief Editor: Michael Stuart Bronze, MD

HIV and Hepatitis B Postexposure Prophylaxis Recommendations

Follow your institution's policies and procedures for postexposure prophylaxis if present. Refer to CDC links at the end of this Protocol.

General Wound Guidelines

- Irrigate and clean wound copiously with flushing 1% betadine solution and wash with soap and water for percutaneous injuries and nonintact skin
- Irrigate mucous membranes with water or saline
- Update tetanus as indicated
- The need for tetanus and/or hepatitis B prophylaxis is based on medical history (see Tetanus Protocol)
- Health care providers should be immunized against hepatitis B
- Hepatitis A prophylaxis may (rarely) need to be considered depending on the source-patient situation
- The need for HIV or chemoprophylaxis (antiretroviral) is based on an assessment of the risk developed by the Centers for Disease Control and Prevention (CDC)
- HIV PEP indicated in pregnancy—no testing needed

Testing of Source and Exposed Person

Exposed person

- Hepatitis profile
- HIV testing
- Liver function tests
- Serum anti-HBs titers on exposed person if there is a hepatitis B vaccination history

Source patient (if available)

- HIV
- Hepatitis B antigen
- Hepatitis C antibody
- AST/ALT and alkaline phosphatase level

Prior to initiating antiretrovirals

- PEP indicated in pregnancy—no testing needed
- CBC count with differential and platelets
- CMP
- Urinalysis with microscopic analysis

Risk of acquiring HIV infection

- 0.3% for percutaneous injuries
- 0.1% for non-intact skin exposure
- 0.09% for mucous membrane exposure
- PEP drops rate of infection 80% if started within 24–36 hours occupational HIV transmission since 1999 in U.S.
- No documented cases of HIV transmission in period between initial HIV infection and formation of detectable HIV antibodies

Higher risk of HIV transmission

- Device has visible blood on it
- Deep injury
- Involving a needle placed in blood vessel
- Hollow bore needle
- Source terminal with HIV infection

Recommended HIV Postexposure Prophylaxis (PEP) for Needlestick Injuries

HIV regimens (Indicated in pregnancy—no pregnancy test needed)

Preferred HIV PEP Regimen for 28 days

- Raltegravir (Isentress) 400 mg PO twice daily plus Truvada, 1 PO once daily (Tenofovir 300 mg and emtricitabine 200 mg)
- Well tolerated usually

Alternative Regimens for 28 days

- May combine 1 drug or drug pair with 1 pair of nucleoside/nucleotide reverse-transcriptase inhibitors

One of these

- Raltegravir (Isentress)
- Darunavir (Prezista) and ritonavir (Norvir)
- Etravirine (Intelence) and Rilpivirine (Edurant)
- Atazanavir (Reyataz) and ritonavir (Norvir)
- Lopinavir/ritonavir (Kaletra)

Combined with 1 of these nucleoside/nucleotide reverse-transcriptase inhibitors

- Tenofovir and emtricitabine; available as Truvada
- Tenofovir and lamivudine (Epivir)
- Zidovudine (Retrovir; AZT) and lamivudine (Epivir); available as
- Combivir
- Zidovudine (Retrovir; AZT) and emtricitabine (Emtriva)

- <u>Prescribers unfamiliar with these agents/regimens should consult physicians familiar with the agents and their toxicities</u>

Regimen toxicity

- Nephrotoxicity
  - Truvada 1 tablet daily (tenofovir 300 mg+ emtricitabine 200 mg) — dose q48hr if creatinine clearance 30–49 ml/min: avoid with creatinine clearance < 30 ml/min
  - Combivir 1 tablet PO bid (zidovudine 300 mg + lamivudine 150 mg) — avoid use with creatinine clearance < 50 ml/minute
- Hepatotoxicity
- Lactic acidosis
- Read literature for all adverse reactions/contraindications of any HIV antireviral drugs used

Treatment recommendations

Source of unknown HIV status

- Generally no PEP
- Can consider PEP regimen for HIV risk factors

Unknown source (needle from sharps container, for example)

- Generally no PEP
- Can consider in areas in which exposure to HIV infected persons is likely

HIV negative source

- No PEP

HIV Postexposure Prophylaxis (PEP) for Mucosal Membrane and Nonintact Skin Exposures

Definitions of exposure type

Source of unknown HIV status

- Generally no PEP
- Can consider treatment regimen for HIV risk factors

Unknown source (needle from sharps container, for example)

- Generally no PEP
- Can consider treatment regimen in areas in which exposure to HIV infected persons is likely

HIV negative source

- No PEP

Other body fluids

- Feces, nasal secretions, saliva, sputum, sweat, tears, urine, and vomitus are not considered potentially infectious unless they are visibly bloody

Consultation criteria

Delayed (> 24–36 hours after exposure)

- Interval in which lack of benefit from PEP is undefined

Unknown source

- Use of PEP on case by case basis

Known or suspected pregnancy in exposed person

- Use of optimal PEP not precluded

Breastfeeding in exposed person

- Use of optimal PEP not precluded

Resistance of source virus to antiretrovirals

Toxicity of initial PEP regimen

- Adverse symptoms common with PEP (nausea and diarrhea)
- Symptoms often manageable without changing regimen with GI medications

Preexposure HIV Prophylaxis (PrEP) For At Risk Individuals

- Acute and chronic HIV infection must be excluded by symptom history and HIV testing immediately before PrEP is prescribed
- If vaginal intercourse represents the risk for HIV acquisition, PrEP should be initiated as a daily regimen 7 days before the likely exposure risk and continued daily for 7 days following the last sexual risk
- PrEP should be discontinued if an HIV test shows a positive result
- On-demand PrEP dosing should not be offered to individuals with chronic HBV infection
- Test for hepatitis B and C prior to therapy
- For adults and adolescents weighing at least 35 kg
- PrEP should be considered part of a comprehensive prevention plan that includes a discussion about adherence to PrEP, condom use, other sexually transmitted infections (STIs), and other risk reduction methods

Medications

- Tenofovir and emtricitabine daily; available as Truvada
  - Do not use if CrCl <60 mL/min

OR

- Emtricitabine/tenofovir alafenamide 200 mg/25 mg daily — excluding those with receptive vaginal sex
  - Not recommended with CrCl 15 to <30 mL/min (exception is may have 1 dose on day of dialysis)

Hepatitis B Postexposure Prophylaxis

Unvaccinated exposed worker treatment window

- < 24 hr post needle stick, ocular, or mucosal exposure
- <14 days post sexual exposure

Source HBsAg positive

- HBIG 0.06 cc/kg IM × 1
- Initiate hepatitis B vaccine series

Source HBsAg negative

- Initiate hepatitis B vaccine series

Source unknown or not available for testing

- Initiate hepatitis B vaccine series

Previously vaccinated

Known responder

- No treatment

Known nonresponder with source HBsAg positive or high risk

- HBIG 0.06 cc/kg IM × 1
- Reinitiate hepatitis B vaccine series

OR

- HBIG × 2 one month apart

Antibody response unknown and source HBsAg positive

- Test exposed person
  - If adequate (serum anti-HBs ≥ 10 mIU/cc)
    - No treatment
  - If inadequate (serum anti-HBs < 10 mIU/cc)
    - HBIG × 1
    - Vaccine booster

Antibody response unknown and source unknown or not available for testing

- Test exposed person
  - If adequate titer (serum anti-HBs ≥ 10 mIU/cc)
    - No treatment
  - If inadequate titer (serum anti-HBs < 10 mIU/cc)
    - Vaccine booster
    - Recheck titer in 1–2 months

Postexposure prophylaxis of hepatitis C not recommended for health care personnel who have occupational exposure to HCV-contaminated blood or body fluids in the workplace

- Risk of transmission is 0.2% for percutaneous exposures and 0% for mucocutaneous exposures

Notes

REFERENCES:

http://www.cdc.gov/mmwr/preview/mmwrhtml/rr5011a1.htm#box2

http://www.cdc.gov/mmwr/PDF/rr/rr5409.pdf

http://aidsetc.org/aidsetc?page=cg-301_occupational_pep

http://nccc.ucsf.edu/wp-content/uploads/2014/03/Updated_USPHS_Guidelines_Mgmt_Occupational_Exposures_HIV_Recommendations_PEP.pdf

The clinician managing the exposed person can call the National Clinicians' Post-Exposure Prophylaxis Hotline (PEPline) at 888–HIV-4911 (888–448–4911) at no charge. Service is available 7 days a week, (More information is available at the PEPline website)

emedicine.medscape.com/article/784812

[Guideline] Panel on Antiretroviral Guidelines for Adults and Adolescents. Guidelines for the use of antiretroviral agents in HIV-1-infected adults and adolescents. Department of Health and Human Services. October 17, 2017

Emedicine Medscape HIV Infection and AIDS Medication Updated: Sep 12, 2018

Author: Nicholas John Bennett, MBBCh, PhD, MA(Cantab), FAAP; Chief Editor: Michael Stuart Bronze, MD

cdc.gov/hiv/clinicians/prevention/prep

MMWR,7/24/20

ENDOCARDITIS PROTOCOL

Definition

- Infection of the endocardial surface of the heart including the heart valves

Considerations

Acute endocarditis

- Usually from Staph aureus or group B strep
- Occurs on normal valves
- More aggressive course
- Related to IV drug abuse
- Valve replacement > 60 days prior

Subacute endocarditis

- Usually from Strep viridans or enterococci
- Less aggressive course
- Valve replacement > 60 days prior

Signs and symptoms

- Fever
- Petechiae
- Heart murmur
- CHF
- Neurologic complaints or findings
- Delirium
- Pericarditis
- Neck pain

- Anemia
- Leukocytosis
- Proteinuria
- Hematuria
- Splenomegaly
- Embolic findings
    - Splinter hemorrhages on nail beds
    - Osler nodes on fingertip pads
    - Roth spots are retinal hemorrhages
    - Janeway lesions are nontender macular rash on palms and soles

Evaluation

- History and physical examination
- Consider in IV drug abuser and fever
- CBC
- Chest x-ray
    - Evaluate for septic emboli, cavitary lesions and infiltrates
- C-reactive protein and ESR (elevated > 90% of patients)
- CMP
- U/A
    - Evaluate for proteinuria and hematuria
- Blood culture q30–60 minutes × 3 sets
- EKG
    - For conduction defects (poor prognostic sign)
- Transesophageal echocardiography

Treatment

- Oxygen prn
- Treat CHF if present
- IV NS as needed

Subacute endocarditis

- Penicillin G 2–3 million units IV q4hr
- Vancomycin for suspected resistant organisms

Acute endocarditis

- Nafcillin 2 gms IV q4hr
- Vancomycin for suspected resistant organisms

Prophylaxis

History of

- Congenital heart disease
- Prosthetic valve
- History of prior endocarditis
- Prophylaxis treatment

Procedural conditions

- Dental procedures
- Abscess I&D
- Incision of respiratory mucosa (tonsillectomy)
- Not recommended for GI or GU procedures

Antibiotic regimens

Adult options

- Amoxicillin 2 gms PO

  OR
- Ampicillin 2 gms IV

  OR
- Cleocin (clindamycin) 600 mg PO or IV

  OR
- Cephalexin 2 gm PO

  OR
- Zithromax (azithromycin) 500 mg PO

  OR
- Rocephin (ceftriaxone) 1 gm IV or IM

Pediatric options

- Amoxicillin 50 mg/kg PO — NMT 2 gms

  OR
- Ampicillin 50 mg/kg IV or IM — NMT 2 gms

  OR
- Cleocin (clindamycin) 20 mg/kg PO — NMT 600 mg

  OR
- Zithromax (azithromycin) 15 mg/kg PO — NMT 500 mg

  OR
- Cephalexin 50 mg/kg PO — NMT 2 gm

  OR
- Rocephin (ceftriaxone) 50 mg/kg IV or IM — NMT 1 gm

Consult criteria

- Discuss with physician all endocarditis or suspected endocarditis patients

Notes

REFERENCES:

Antibiotic Prophylactic Regimens for Endocarditis

Author: Mary L Windle, PharmD; Chief Editor: Rick Kulkarni, MD emedicine.medscape.com/article/1672902

Wilson W, Taubert KA, Gewitz M, Lockhart PB, Baddour LM, Levison M, et al. Prevention of infective endocarditis: guidelines from the American Heart Association: *Circulation*. Oct 9 2007;116(15):1736–54

Adult Severe Sepsis and Septic Shock Protocol

For clinical settings that permit the practitioner to perform adult septic shock management and they are trained and experienced to perform those duties

Definitions

Systemic Inflammatory Response Syndrome (SIRS)

- Core temperature > 38° C or < 36° C
- Heart rate > 90/minute unless on beta–blockers
- Respiratory rate > 20/minute or pCO_2 < 32 mm Hg
- WBC > 12,000 or < 4,000 or > 10–15% bands

Sepsis

- Clinical evidence for infection
- 2 or more SIRS criteria met
- New 2016 definition — life-threatening organ dysfunction from dysregulated host response to infection

Severe Sepsis

- Evidence for sepsis AND sepsis-induced tissue hypoperfusion or organ dysfunction
  - Ex: altered mental status, hypoxemia without overt pulmonary disease, acute lung injury with or without pneumonia, elevated lactate >4, or oliguria (urine output < 30 mL/hour), thrombocytopenia < 100,000 platelets, INR > 1.5, bilirubin > 2 or creatinine > 2 (no prior CKD)

Septic Shock

- Older definition as of 2016 — severe sepsis AND sepsis-induced hypotension despite adequate fluid resuscitation
- New **SOFA** definition — subset of sepsis in which particularly profound circulatory, cellular, and metabolic abnormalities are associated with a greater risk of mortality than with sepsis alone
- ***qSOFA score*** **(Quick Sepsis–related Organ Failure Assessment Score)**
  - Respiratory rate ≥ 22 breaths/minute — 1 point
  - Systolic blood pressure ≤ 100 mm Hg — 1 point
  - Altered level of consciousness (GCS <15) — 1 point
  - < 2 points low risk for sepsis
  - ≥ 2 points high risk for poor outcome in suspected infection
  - Not a diagnostic test to determine sepsis (used for mortality risk assessment)

- Positive qSOFA score ≥ 2 points should be evaluated for organ dysfunction

Multiple organ dysfunction syndrome (MODS)

- Progressive organ dysfunction in a severely ill patient
- Failure to maintain homeostasis without intervention
- End stage in infectious conditions (sepsis, septic shock) and noninfectious conditions (e.g., SIRS due to pancreatitis)
- The greater the number of organ failures, the higher the mortality risk, with the greatest risk associated with respiratory failure requiring mechanical ventilation
- MODS can be classified as primary or secondary
  - **Primary MODS** is the direct result of identifiable injury or insult with early organ dysfunction
    - Such as renal failure due to a nephrotoxic agent or liver failure due to a hepatotoxic agent
  - **Secondary MODS** is organ failure that has no attributable cause and is a consequence of the host's response
    - Such as acute respiratory distress syndrome in individuals with pancreatitis

Sepsis definition comment

- There is ongoing defining and redefining over time of sepsis categories with different specialty groups disagreeing to varying degrees

Differential diagnosis

- Anaphylactic shock
- Adrenal crisis and shock
- Cardiogenic shock
- Hypovolemic shock
- Hemorrhagic shock
- DKA
- Neuroleptic malignant syndrome
- Toxic shock syndrome
- Heatstroke
- Cardiac tamponade
- Massive pulmonary embolism
- Adult respiratory distress syndrome (ARDS)
- Other forms of shock

Considerations

- Culture positive bacteremia occurs in 30–50%
- Not all patients with bacteremia have signs of sepsis
- Serious bacterial infections with or without bacteremia may be associated with changes in all organ systems
  - Change in organ function mediated by host immune system mechanisms against infection
- The continuum of severity is from sepsis to septic shock to multiple organ dysfunction syndrome
- ARDS occurs in 20–40% of septic shock
- Hyperoxia may impair oxygen delivery in patients with sepsis, and hyperoxia decreases whole-body oxygen consumption in critically ill patients. Patients should be weaned to the lowest necessary FiO_2.
- No relationship between the CVP and intravascular volume and between the CVP and fluid responsiveness
- Pseudosepsis is defined as fever, leukocytosis, and hypotension due to causes other than sepsis
- Lactic acidosis in sepsis commonly caused by high sympathetic (adrenergic) state and not always from hypoperfusion

Sepsis Therapy

(Meeting treatment goals is associated with improved survival in patients with severe sepsis and septic shock)

Treatment goals

- Maintain MAP ≥ 65 mm Hg
- Target a central venous O_2 ($ScvO_2$) saturation ≥ 70%

- Target serum lactate ≤ 2 mmol/L
- Maintain urine output ≥ 0.5 ml/kg/hour
- Correcting peripheral capillary refill delay

Monitoring

- Vital signs every 5 minutes until stabilized
- Maintain an O_2 saturation ≥ 90%
- Central line placement for possible vasopressors and CVP measurement
- Foley catheter placement

Testing

- ABG
- Lactic acid (lactate) level
- CBC
- BMP
- LFTs
- PT/PTT/INR
- Blood cultures X 2 using different sites
- Sputum culture & sensitivity and gram stain
- U/A and urine culture
- Chest x-ray
- EKG
- Troponin and BNP or NT–ProBNP
- Type and screen
- Cortisol level
- Accucheck for glucose

Treatment

IV fluid and pressor treatment

- Current recommendations from various entities including Medicare for severe sepsis or septic shock
  - 30 ml/kg bolus with NS or LR (may use ideal body weight if patient obese)
- Bolus crystalloids IV 500–1,000 ml every 30 minutes and re-assess response of HR, MAP, CVP
  - Goal is to achieve MAP ≥ 65 and CVP 8–12 mm Hg
- Give at least 30 ml/kg of fluid, but often patients need ≥ 4 L to achieve adequate volume resuscitation
- Fluid overload is associated with increased mortality so too aggressive IV fluid hydration may be deleterious to the patient
  - Caution in heart failure patients that demonstrate high CVP or pulmonary edema
- End stage renal failure patients frequently do not receive enough IVF in septic shock

- MAP is < 65 mm Hg then start norepinephrine (Levophed) IV if not responsive to IV NS or LR
  - Norepinephrine start at 2–4 mcg/minute IV — usual dosage range 8–12 mcg/minute (may need up to 30 mcg/minute in refractory shock)

  Add vasopressin 0.01–0.04 units/min when an additional agent is needed to maintain MAP
- For patients with refractory shock and an $ScvO_2$ < 70%, consider the following
- Consider using dobutamine IV up to 20 mcg/kg/minute especially if there is evidence of myocardial dysfunction
- If hematocrit < 25% — transfuse packed red blood cells to raise hematocrit > 25%
- Give methylprednisolone 100 mg IV if adrenal sufficiency present or suspected
  - 50 mg IV q6hr until shock resolved

Empiric antibiotic treatment

- Administer antibiotics within one hour of recognition of severe sepsis or septic shock, and after collection of blood cultures when feasible.
- Attempt to achieve source control as soon as the site of infection is identified This may include, but is not limited to,

removing indwelling catheters, draining abscesses, or relieving a source of obstruction (ureteral stone, biliary stone blocking the biliary tree, etc.).

- **Suggested empiric regimens**
  - Vancomycin 1 gm IV q12hr (adjust for renal insufficiency)

PLUS one of the following

- Piperacillin/tazobactam (Zosyn) 3.375–4.5 gms IV q6hr

  OR
- Meropenem (Merrem) 1 gm IV q8hr

  OR
- Imipenem (Primaxin) 0.5–1 gm IV q8hr

  OR
- Cefepime (Maxipime) 2 gm IV q12hr

  OR
- Ceftazidime (Fortaz) 2 gm IV q8–12hr

Consider the addition of an aminoglycoside or fluoroquinolone in patients with:

- Neutropenia
- Pneumonia causing respiratory failure
- Proven resistant infections such as pseudomonas or Acinetobacter

Special considerations

- In addition to the empiric coverage above, patients with suspected or proven intra-abdominal sepsis should receive anaerobic coverage with piperacillin/tazobactam, or a carbapenem —ertapenem (Invanz) or meropenem (Merrem), or clindamycin, and/or metronidazole.
- A macrolide antibiotic (e.g. azithromycin) should be added to patients with bacteremia from Streptococcus pneumonia
- Dose adjustments need to be considered in patients with renal or hepatic dysfunction.

Protective lung strategy in ARDS for intubated ventilated patients

Given the high incidence of ARDS in patients with severe sepsis or septic shock, consider

- Tidal volumes of 6 ml/kg of ideal body weight
- Plateau pressure < 30 cm H_2O

Consult recommendations

- Close management of patient
- Patients with severe sepsis or septic shock should be cared for in an intensive care unit setting

Notes

REFERENCES:

Rossi P, et al. *Clin Physiol Funct Imaging* 2007, 27:180–184

Cornet AD, et al. *Crit Care* 2013 Apr 18;17:313

Rivers E et al. *New Engl J Med* 2001; 345:1368–1377

Raghunathan K et al. Crit Care Med. Mar 26 2014. [Epub ahead of print]

The Surviving Sepsis Campaign Guidelines: 2012 – published in Crit Care Med 2013; 41:580–637

Caironi P et al. *New Engl J Med* 2014; 370:1412–1421

The ProCESS Investigators. *New Engl J Med* 2014; 370: 1683–1693

CHEST, June, 2014; pg.1407

ACEP NOW: New Sepsis Definitions Spark Debate on Twitter
Jeremy Samuel Faust, MD, MS, MA on March 16, 2016

Assessment of Clinical Criteria for Sepsis For the Third International Consensus Definitions for Sepsis and Septic Shock (Sepsis-3)
JAMA. 2016;315(8):762-774. doi:10.1001/jama.2016.0288

Bacterial Sepsis Updated: Feb 05, 2019 Author: Amber Mahmood Bokhari, MBBS; Chief Editor: Michael Stuart Bronze, MD

Am J EM. 2017;35:1946

MENINGITIS PROTOCOL

Definition

- Infection or inflammation of the meninges

Differential diagnosis

- Brain abscess
- Brain neoplasms
- Delirium tremens (DTs)
- Subarachnoid hemorrhage
- Encephalitis
- Febrile seizures
- Herpes simplex encephalitis
- Noninfectious meningitis, including medication-induced meningeal inflammation
- Meningeal carcinomatosis
- Central nervous system vasculitis
- Stroke
- All causes of altered mental status and coma
- Leptospirosis
- Subdural empyema

Most bacterial common causes

- S. pneumoniae 42%
- N. meningitides 25%
- S. agalactiae 12%
- L. monocytogenes 8%
- H. influenzae 7%

Signs and symptoms (that may be present)

- Headache (may be worse with movement)
- Fever
- Nuchal rigidity
- Kernig's sign (Unable to strengthen leg when hip flexed 90°
- Brudzinski's sign (neck flexion causes hip and knee flexion
- Mental status changes
- Petechiae
- Shock
- Seizures
- Photophobia

Testing

Lumbar puncture normal values

- Opening pressure is 80-200 mm H_2O
- WBC 0–5 cells, mostly lymphocytes
- Glucose 50–75 mg/dL (may be elevated in diabetes mellitus)
- Protein 15–40 mg/dL (may be elevated in diabetes mellitus)

- CBC with differential
- CMP +/- coagulation studies
- Blood cultures X 2
- Serum procalcitonin helpful in differentiating bacterial vs aseptic meningitis in children (threshold of 0.5 ng/mL)
- Stool and throat cultures as indicated
- Give antibiotics prior to CT brain scan if bacterial meningitis suspected
- CSF
  - Tube #1 Cell count and differential

- Tube #2 Protein and glucose
- Tube #3 Gram stain, C&S, AFB, cryptococcal antigen, India ink
- Tube #4 Cell count and differential, rapid bacterial antigens, HSV, (VDRL, fungal studies as indicated)

- CT brain prior to lumbar puncture when:
  - Coma
  - Focal neurologic deficits
  - Persistent seizures
  - Known malignancy or HIV

Bacterial meningitis findings

- Opening pressure may be high (200-300 mm/H_2O though may be elevated in any type of meningitis)
- WBC 100–5,000 (mostly PMNs — 80%)
  - CSF WBC count of 500/µL or higher
  - May be altered in partially treated meningitis
  - No cell count result can exclude bacterial meningitis
  - Lymphocytosis with normal CSF chemistries seen in 15-25%, especially when cell counts < 1000 or with partial treatment
- Glucose may be low (<40 mg/dL)
- Protein may be high (>100 mg/dL)
  - CSF glucose–to–blood glucose ratio of 0.4 or lower
- CSF lactate level of 31 mg/dL or higher

Viral meningitis findings

- Opening pressure is 90-200 mm H_2O
- WBC count usually is 10-300/µL
- Common causes
  - HSV
  - HIV
  - Enteroviruses
  - West Nile virus
  - Human herpesvirus (HHV)-2
  - Lymphocytic choriomeningitis virus (LCM)
- Glucose concentration is typically normal
  - Can be below normal in meningitis from lymphocytic choriomeningitis virus (LCM), herpes simplex virus (HSV), mumps virus, and poliovirus
  - Protein concentration tends to be slightly elevated, but can be normal

Other meningitis causes

- Fungus
  - Candida
  - Cryptococcus neoformans
  - Coccidioides immitis
  - Blastomyces dermatitidis
  - Histoplasma capsulatum
- Lyme disease
  - No corticosteroids
  - Ceftriaxone 2 gm IV q24hours X 14–28 days
- N fowleri (amoeba)

Treatment

- ABCs
- IVF as indicated
- Dexamethasone 0.15 mg/kg q6h IV 15–20 minutes before or with antibiotics for suspected bacterial meningitis (indicated in suspected or proven pneumococcal or H. influenza B disease)
- Viral meningitis usually needs supportive care only unless HIV or HSV (consult infectious disease)
  - HSV meningitis/encephalitis — acyclovir 10 mg/kg IV q8h X 10–14 days for meningitis and 14–21 days for encephalitis
- Fungal meningitis needs antibiotics and admission

Antibiotics

- Age 0–4 wk.
  - Ampicillin plus either cefotaxime or an aminoglycoside
- Age 1 month–50 years
  - Ceftriaxone 2 gm IV q12hours or cefotaxime 2–3 gms IV Q6h

    Plus

  - Vancomycin 500–750 mg IV q6h
- Adults > 50 years (and alcoholic or debilitating disease patients)
  - Ampicillin 2 gms IV q4h

    Plus
  - Ceftriaxone 2 gm IV q12hours or cefotaxime 2–3 gms IV Q6h

    Plus
  - Vancomycin 500–750 mg IV q6h
- Penicillin anaphylaxis history
  - Chlamphenicol 50mg/kg/day divided q6h (NMT 4 gm daily)
- Head trauma (basilar skull fracture)
  - Ceftriaxone 2 gm IV q12hours or cefotaxime 2–3 gms IV Q6h

    Plus
  - Vancomycin 500–750 mg IV q6h
- Infected cerebral shunt
  - Usually needs removal
  - Vancomycin 500–750 mg IV q6h

    Plus
  - Cefepime 2 gms IV q8h

Chemoprophylaxis for close contacts of bacterial meningitis

- Suspected or proven meningococcal disease
  - Rifampin (600 mg PO every 12 hours for 2 days
  - Ceftriaxone 250 mg IM in a single dose
    - Recommended for pregnant patients
  - Ciprofloxacin 500-750 mg in a single dose
- H. influenza suspected
  - Rifampin 20 mg/kg PO daily for 4 days (NMT 600 mg daily)

Recommended disposition

- Admit usually
- Viral meningitis with proven benign etiology and mild symptoms can be considered for outpatient therapy
- Consult on all meningitis cases

Notes

REFERENCES:

Meningitis Updated: Jul 16, 2019

Author: Rodrigo Hasbun, MD, MPH; Chief Editor: Michael Stuart Bronze, MD

emedicine.medscape.com/article/232915

[Guideline] Tunkel AR, Hasbun R, Bhimraj A, Byers K, Kaplan SL, Michael Scheld W, et al. 2017 Infectious Diseases Society of America's Clinical Practice Guidelines for Healthcare-Associated Ventriculitis and Meningitis. *Clin Infect Dis*. 2017 Feb 14

Haemophilus Meningitis Updated: Jul 09, 2018 Author: Prateek Lohia, MD, MHA;

emedicine.medscape.com/article/1164916

TETANUS PROTOCOL

Tetanus infection

Definition

- Anaerobic infection caused by Clostridium tetani producing a toxin that causes muscle spasms and pain

Differential diagnosis

- Conversion disorder
- Meningitis
- Encephalitis
- Dystonic drug reaction
- Mandible dislocation
- Hypocalcemia
- Black widow spider bite
- Subarachnoid hemorrhage
- Peritonsillar abscess

- Retropharyngeal abscess
- Rabies

Considerations

- Found in soil, feces, house dust and is ubiquitous
- Tetanus spores can remain in normal tissue for months to years
- Tetanus infection may occur without apparent wound
- Incidence of tetanus infection has decreased markedly secondary to childhood immunizations and current tetanus prophylaxis recommendations
- Medium incubation period is 7 days, but can be less than 4 days or greater than 14 days
- Tetanus booster does not prevent acute tetanus disease occurrence
  - It prevents future infections
  - Tetanus immune globulin prevents acute infections in under-immunized patients
  - Elderly are frequently under-immunized

Signs and symptoms

- 75% have generalized muscle rigidity – "lockjaw"
- Dysphagia
- Fever
- Tachycardia
- Sweating
- Laryngospasms – can cause asphyxia
- Acute abdominal pain mimicking surgical abdomen

Evaluation

- History and physical examination
- No specific lab tests available
- Diagnosis is clinical
- Spatula test
  - Touching tongue with tongue blade causes masseter spasm and biting of the blade
  - Sensitivity 94%
  - Specificity 100%
  - No complications from procedure

Treatment

- Tetanus immune globulin 3,000–5,000 units IM with part of dose injected around infection site
- Rapid sequence intubation if needed acutely
  - Needed in 2/3 of patients
- Wound debridement out to 2 cm from wound edges
- Incision and drainage of any abscesses

Medications

- Valium
  - Adult
  - Mild spasms 5–10 mg PO
  - Moderate spasms 5–10 mg IV
  - Severe spasms 40 mg/hour IV infusion
- Pediatric
  - Mild spasms 0.1–0.8 mg/kg PO divided tid–qid (NMT 10 mg)
  - Moderate to severe spasms 0.1–0.3 mg/kg IV q4–8h (NMT 10 mg)
- Antibiotics
  - Efficacy not proven
  - May try penicillin, Flagyl (metronidazole) or doxycycline
- Vecuronium (if intubated)

Consult criteria

- All tetanus infection cases

Tetanus prophylaxis

- Tetanus prophylaxis
  - High risk = every 5 years
  - Low risk = every 10 years
  - Tetanus IG 250–500 units IM at different site from wound if high risk and less than 3 tetanus or unknown history of immunizations previously in life — usually with the elderly

High risk wound

- More than 6 hours old
- Greater than 1 cm deep
- Exposed to saliva or feces
- Stellate wounds
- Crush wounds
- Puncture wounds

- Ischemic appearance

Tdap

- Recommended by CDC for adults (Boostrix is brand name Tdap)
  - Adults age ≥ 65 years who have not previously received it
  - For adults having close contacts with infants < 12 months of age who have not previously received it
  - Healthcare workers who have not previously received it
- ACIP recommends a single Tdap 0.5 cc IM dose for persons aged 11 through 18 years who have completed the recommended childhood (DTP/DTaP) vaccination series and for adults aged 19 through 64 years
- To ensure continued protection against tetanus and diphtheria, booster doses of either Td or Tdap should be administered every 10 years throughout life
- Tdap contains pertussis in addition to tetanus toxoid and diphtheria toxoid
- Tdap or Td are formulations 0.5 cc IM recommended for adults age ≥ 65 years who have not received it
  - Pediatric Td and Tdap contain 3–4 times more diphtheria toxoid than adult formulation (do not give to adults)
- Recommended in pregnancy after 20 weeks gestation (ideally between 27 and 36 weeks of gestation) regardless of vaccination history and time since prior Td or Tdap

Catch–up tetanus immunization recommendations

- If persons aged 7–18 years have never been vaccinated against pertussis, tetanus, or diphtheria, these persons should receive a series of three tetanus and diphtheria toxoid–containing vaccines, which includes at least 1 Tdap dose
  - The preferred schedule is 1 dose of Tdap 0.5 cc IM, followed by 1 dose of either Td or Tdap ≥4 weeks afterward, and 1 dose of either Td or Tdap 6–12 months later. Persons aged 7–18 years who are not fully immunized against tetanus and diphtheria should receive 1 dose of Tdap, preferably as the first dose in the catch-up series
- If persons aged ≥19 years have never been vaccinated against pertussis, tetanus, or diphtheria, these persons should receive a series of 3 tetanus and diphtheria toxoid–containing vaccines, which includes at least 1 Tdap dose
  - The preferred schedule is 1 dose of Tdap, followed by 1 dose of either Td or Tdap at least 4 weeks afterward, and 1 dose of either Td or Tdap 6–12 months later
  - Persons aged ≥19 years who are not fully immunized against tetanus and diphtheria should receive 1 dose of Tdap, preferably as the 1st dose; if additional tetanus toxoid–containing doses are required, either Td or Tdap may be used.

Discharge instructions

- Wound aftercare instructions
- Refer to health department or primary care provider to complete tetanus primary vaccination series if < 2 vaccines given in past

Notes

REFERENCES:

Tetanus Author: Patrick B Hinfey, MD; Chief Editor: John L Brusch, MD, FACP emedicine.medscape.com/article/229594

reference.medscape.com/drug/adacel-boostrix-tetanus-reduced-diphtheria-toxoids-acellular-pertussis-vaccine-999568

Updated Recommendations for Use of Tetanus Toxoid, Reduced Diphtheria Toxoid and Acellular Pertussis Vaccine (Tdap) in Pregnant Women and Persons Who Have or Anticipate Having Close Contact with an Infant Aged <12 Months --- Advisory Committee on Immunization Practices (ACIP), 2011

Weekly October 21, 2011 / 60(41);1424-1426

cdc.gov/mmwr/volumes/69/wr/mm6903a5.htm

Use of Tetanus Toxoid, Reduced Diphtheria Toxoid, and Acellular Pertussis Vaccines: Updated Recommendations of the Advisory Committee on Immunization Practices — United States, 2019

Weekly / January 24, 2020 / 69(3);77–83

Fiona P. Havers, MD[1]; Pedro L. Moro, MD[2]; Paul Hunter, MD[3]; Susan Hariri, PhD[1]; Henry Bernstein,

Dermatology

Section Contents

When using any protocol, always follow the Guidelines of Proper Use (page 12).

Human and Animal Bite Protocol

Human Bites

- 15–20% infection rate
- Staph aureus most common
- Usually hand wounds are from fist fight

Evaluation

- Wound exploration
- X-ray
- Assess bone, joint, muscle and tendon for injury

Treatment options

- Consider closure only if all 4 criteria present:
  - Cosmetically significant (face wound)
  - Uninfected wound
  - Less than 12 hours old (< 24 hours on face)
  - Not on hand or foot
- Do not close puncture wounds
- Flush with > 250 cc of 1% betadine solution using 18 gauge angiocath (mix 1 cc of 10% betadine with 9 cc of NS)
- May rinse with NS or potable tap water profusely
- Remove devitalized tissue
- ADT or Tdap 0.5 cc IM if more than 5 years from last dose
- Tetanus immune globulin 250–500 units IM different site if < 3 tetanus immunizations in the past
- Refer to health department or primary care provider to complete tetanus primary vaccination series if < 2 vaccines given in past
  - See Tetanus Protocol
- Antibiotics prophylaxis
  - Superficial: none

Deeper wound antibiotic treatment options

- Amoxicillin/clavulanate 875 mg PO bid × 5 days for prophylaxis (adults > 40kg)
- Amoxicillin/clavulanate 15 mg/kg PO bid × 5 days for prophylaxis (pediatrics < 40 kg)
- Doxycycline 100 mg PO bid × 5 days if allergic to penicillin
- Doxycycline 1.5–2 mg/kg PO bid × 5 days if allergic to penicillin (age > 8 years and < 45 kg)
- May refer to Sanford Guide or other drug databases

Discharge criteria

- Superficial wounds without infection
- No bone, joint or tendon involvement

Discharge instructions

- Human bite aftercare instructions
- Return if infection occurs in bite
- Return if pain increases

Consult criteria

- Infected wounds
- Closed fist wounds penetrating to joint, tendon or bone
- Significant bites to hand
- Fever
- Toxicity

Dog Bites

- 15–20% infection rate
- Most common pathogens
  - Aerobes: staph aureus, Pasteurella multocida, streptococcus
  - Anaerobes: enterobacter, pseudomonas, bacillus
- Infection occurring < 24 hours — Pasteurella multocida commonly
- Infection occurring > 24 hours — staph or strep commonly

Evaluation

- Wound exploration

- X-ray
- Assess bone, joint, muscle and tendon for injury
- Assess for foreign body (tooth, etc.)

Treatment

- Flush with > 250 cc of 1% betadine solution (mix 1 cc of 10% betadine with 9 cc of NS using 18 gauge angiocath)
- Rinse with NS or potable tap water profusely
- ADT or Tdap 0.5 cc IM if more than 5 years from last dose
- Tetanus immune globulin 250–500 units IM different site if < 3 tetanus immunizations in the past
- Refer to health department or primary care provider to complete tetanus primary vaccination series if < 2 vaccines given in past
  - See Tetanus Protocol
- Add viricidal 1% benzalkonium chloride if risk of rabies
- Remove devitalized tissue
- Consider closure
  - Bite < 8 hours old
  - Bite < 12 hours old on face
  - Do not close puncture wounds
- Antibiotic prophylaxis
  - Usually not needed
  - Use in high risk wounds; facial wounds
  - Use in immunocompromised or asplenic patients
  - Same antibiotic regimen as for human bites
- Consider rabies prophylaxis
- Notify rabies control (see Rabies prophylaxis section below)

Discharge criteria

- Same as human bites

Discharge instructions

- Dog bite aftercare instructions
- Return if infection occurs in bite
- Return if pain increases

Consult criteria

- Severely infected wounds
- Wounds penetrating to joint, tendon, or bone
- Neurovascular deficit or injury
- Significant bites with large area of injury or to hand or face
- Fever
- Toxicity

Cat Bites

- High infection risk
- 25–50% infection rate
- Pasteurella multocida up to 80% of infections
- Infection after > 24 hours usually streptococcus — can progress rapidly
- May cause
  - Osteomyelitis
  - Septic arthritis
  - Abscess
  - Sepsis
  - Epidural abscess
  - Endocarditis

Evaluation

- Wound exploration
- X-ray
- Assess bone, joint, muscle and tendon for injury
- Assess for foreign body (tooth, etc.)

Treatment

- Flush with > 250 cc of 1% betadine solution using 18 gauge angiocath (mix 1 cc of 10% betadine with 9 cc of NS)
- May rinse with NS or potable tap water profusely
- ADT or Tdap 0.5 cc IM if more than 5 years from last dose
- Tetanus immune globulin 250–500 units IM different site if < 3 tetanus immunizations in the past
- Refer to health department or primary care provider to complete tetanus primary vaccination series if < 2 vaccines given in past
  - See Tetanus Protocol

- Add viricidal 1% benzalkonium chloride if risk of rabies
- Remove devitalized tissue (not puncture wounds)
- Closure not recommended on
  - Puncture wounds or deep bites
  - Infected wounds
  - Wounds > 24 hours

Antibiotics prophylaxis options

- Amoxicillin/clavulanate 875 mg PO bid-tid × 5 days for prophylaxis (adults > 40 kg)
- Amoxicillin/clavulanate 15 mg/kg PO bid-tid × 5 days for prophylaxis (pediatrics < 40 kg)
- Doxycycline 100 mg PO bid × 5 days if allergic to penicillin
- Doxycycline 1.5–2 mg/kg PO bid × 5 days if allergic to penicillin (age > 8 years and < 45 kg)

Mild infections options

- Amoxicillin/clavulanate 875 mg PO bid × 10–14 days (adults > 40 kg)
- Amoxicillin/clavulanate 15 mg/kg PO bid × 10–14 days (pediatrics < 40 kg)
- Doxycycline 100 mg PO bid × 10–14 days if allergic to penicillin
- Doxycycline 1.5–2 mg/kg PO bid × 10–14 days if allergic to penicillin (age > 8 years and < 45 kg)

Moderate infections options

- Amoxicillin/clavulanate 875 mg PO bid × 10–14 days (adults > 40 kg)
- Amoxicillin/clavulanate 15 mg/kg PO bid × 10–14 days (pediatrics < 40 kg)
- Doxycycline 100 mg PO bid × 10–14 days if allergic to penicillin
- Doxycycline 1.5–2 mg/kg PO bid × 10–14 days if allergic to penicillin (age > 8 years and < 45 kg
- Rocephin (ceftriaxone) 1–2 gms IM qday × 10–14 days
- Rocephin (ceftriaxone) 50 mg/kg IM qday × 10–14 days not to exceed adult dose for children

Rabies prophylaxis

- There have been no cases of dog-mediated rabies in the U.S. in the last 2 years (as of March 2021)
- Rabies in the U.S. is primarily transmitted through wild animal vectors such as bats, foxes, raccoons, and skunks.
- If the suspected animal can be safely captured, PEP may be briefly delayed while testing is done (although bites to the head and neck may require earlier intervention)
- Bites from dogs, cats, and ferrets who remain asymptomatic during a 10-day observation period do not require PEP
- Potentially rabid animal that involve licks to intact skin, feeding, touching, or handling blood, urine, or feces, do not constitute an exposure and do not require PEP
- No documented cases of human-to-human rabies transmission
- There have been no rabies PEP failures in Canada or the US since the current biologics have been used
- There are no contraindications to rabies vaccination
- Unless there are signs of bat exposure (i.e., bite/scratch marks), the individual was found crying or upset, or the bat was found in proximity to the person, rabies PEP is not required
- Notify rabies control as needed

Discharge criteria

- Superficial wounds
- Mild to moderate infected wounds

Discharge instructions
- Cat bite aftercare instructions
- Return if infection occurs in bite
- Return if pain increases

Consult criteria
- Severely infected wounds
- Wounds penetrating to joint, tendon, or bone
- Neurovascular deficit or injury
- Significant bites with large area of injury or to hand or face
- Fever
- Toxicity

Wild Animal Bites
- Similar evaluation, treatment and disposition as Dog Bites Protocol
- Notify rabies control (see Rabies prophylaxis section above)

Notes

REFERENCES:

Human Bites Author: Jeffrey Barrett, MD; Chief Editor: John L Brusch, MD, FACP emedicine.medscape.com/article/218901

Animal Bites in Emergency Medicine Author: Alisha Perkins Garth, MD; Chief Editor: Joe Alcock, MD, MS emedicine.medscape.com/article/768875

Ahmad O, et al. *CJEM*. 2021 Mar;23(2):153-155

De Serres G, et al. *Clin Infect Dis*. 2009;48:1493-9

Liu C, et al. *R I Med J*. 2020 Aug 3;103(6):51-53

Spider Bite and Insect Sting Protocol

Brown Recluse Spider Bite
- Found in dark areas
- Envenomation can be mild if spider has recently fed
- Symptoms develop 4–8 hours after bite
- Symptoms and findings that may occur are
  - Local reaction only
  - Tissue necrosis
  - Severe pain
  - Pruritus
  - Fever
  - Nausea/vomiting
  - Headache
  - Myalgias
  - Initial papule which develops central dark area of necrosis over 48–72 hours

Evaluation
- History of bite
- Exam of lesion area

Systemic symptoms
- CBC to check for thrombocytopenia and anemia
- BMP to check for renal involvement
- PT/PTT/INR and DIC panel if DIC suspected
- U/A to check on dipstick for blood for hemolytic anemia

Treatment options
- Clean wound
- Benadryl (diphenhydramine) or other antihistamines for pruritus and rash
- ADT 0.5 cc IM if more than 5 years from last dose or Tdap 0.5 cc IM — see Tetanus Protocol

Antibiotics if secondary infection present and is nonpurulent

- Amoxicillin/clavulanate 875 mg PO bid x 5–7 days
- Amoxicillin/clavulanate 45 mg/kg/day PO divided q12hr or divided q8hr x 5–7 days
- Cephalexin 500 mg q6hr PO x 5–10 days (or other cephalosporins PO/IV)
  - Pediatric 25–50 mg/kg/day PO divided q6hr not to exceed 500 mg/dose
- Clindamycin 300–450 mg q6–8hr PO/IV x 5–10 days
  - Pediatric 20-30 mg/kg/day PO/IV divided q6hr–q8hr × 5– 10 days not to exceed 450 mg/dose

Uncomplicated purulent cellulitis (select one)

- Doxycycline 100 mg PO bid × 6–10 days if allergic to penicillin
- Doxycycline 1.5–2 mg/kg PO bid × 6–10 days if allergic to penicillin (age > 8 years and < 45 kg) — NMT 100 mg per dose
- Trimethoprim/sulfamethox-azole (Septra DS) bid x 6–10 days
- Trimethoprim/sulfamethox-azole (Septra) 8-12 mg TMP/kg/dose or 0.5 cc/LB bid PO for PO q12hr for 6–10 days for children
  - Contraindicated in ages < 2 months
- Clindamycin 300 mg PO tid for 6–10 days
  - Pediatric — clindamycin 20-30 mg/kg/day PO divided tid × 6–10 days (NMT 300 mg/dose usually)

- Follow up with primary care provider or surgeon within 7 days if wound necrotic

Discharge criteria

- Nontoxic patient
- No systemic symptoms

Discharge instructions

- Brown recluse spider bite aftercare instructions
- Return if pain worsens
- Return if fever occurs
- Return for occurrence of systemic symptoms
- Referral to plastic surgery if skin grafting possible need

Consult criteria

- Toxic patient
- Systemic symptoms
- Anemia
- Thrombocytopenia
- DIC
- Acute renal insufficiency
- Significant cellulitis
- Necrotic area > 2 cm

Black Widow Spider Bites

- Red hourglass on abdomen

Grade 1 (mild envenomation)

- Immediate pain at site
- Normal vital signs

Grade 2 (moderate envenomation)

- Muscle pain in bitten extremity
- Muscle pain may extend to abdomen if lower extremity bitten
- Muscle pain may extend to chest if upper extremities bitten
- Diaphoresis at bite site
- Normal vital signs

Grade 3 (severe envenomation)

- Generalized muscular pain
- Generalized diaphoresis
- Nausea/vomiting
- Headache
- Hypertension
- Tachycardia

Evaluation

- U/A for hematuria
- CPK
- Labs and other testing to rule out other acute abdominal process if suspected

Treatment options

- IV NS
- Tetanus prophylaxis (see Tetanus Practice Guide)
- Cool compresses to site
- Benadryl (diphenhydramine) IV 50 mg or weight adjusted for pediatrics if antivenin to be given
- Pain control with narcotics
- Black widow antivenin (consult physician before using)

Consult criteria

- All black widow spider bites
- Before any antivenin given

Bees, Wasps, and Fire Ants

- Refer to Allergy Protocol if needed
- Remove stinger
- Cool compresses
- Can make a Adolph Meat Tenderizer paste with water and apply for 1 hour to break down proteins in venom
- NSAID's prn for pain
- Topical hydrocortisone cream may be used
- Tetanus prophylaxis if > 10 years (see Tetanus Practice Guide)
- Respective aftercare instructions

Local Reactions from Insect Bites or Stings

- 1–5 cm of nontender induration usually
- Light pink or red color
- Antihistamine OTC prn
- Cool compresses prn
- Steroids 1–3 day course can be considered — usually not needed (caution in diabetes)
- If cellulitis present, refer to Cellulitis Practice Guide
- Local reaction aftercare instructions

Notes

REFERENCES:

Brown Recluse Spider Envenomation Author: Thomas C Arnold, MD, FAAEM, FACMT; Chief Editor: Joe Alcock, MD,MS
emedicine.medscape.com/article/772295

Clark RF, Wethern-Kestner S, Vance MV, Gerkin R. Clinical presentation and treatment of black widow spider envenomation: a review of 163 cases. *Ann Emerg Med.* Jul 1992;21(7):782–787

Widow Spider Envenomation Author: Sean P Bush, MD, FACEP; Chief Editor: Joe Alcock, MD, MS
emedicine.medscape.com/article/772196

SNAKE BITE PROTOCOL

Considerations

- 2,000 venomous snake bites per year
- Alcohol intoxication frequently a contributing factor
- Mortality < 0.5% with advent of antivenin
- Venomous snake bites involve pit vipers (Crotalids) or coral snakes
- Eastern coral snake considered deadly
- Arizona coral snake not deadly
- Oozing at fang bite site reliable predictor of envenomation
- **Usual treatment is medical, not surgical**

Pit vipers (are responsible for majority of venomous bites)

- Rattlesnakes
- Cottonmouths
- Copperheads
- Water moccasins

Identification

Pit vipers

- Depressions or pits between eyes and nostrils
- Triangular head
- Elliptical eyes
- 2 fangs
- Subcaudal plates

Coral snake

- Black nose
- Colored rings
- Confused with King snake
  - "Red on yellow, kill a fellow; red on black, venom lack" denoting color rings of Coral and King snakes respectively
- Venom usually either hemotoxic or neurotoxic

Crotalid (Pit Viper) Envenomation Grading

No envenomation

- Snakebite suspected
- Minimal pain
- No systemic symptoms or lab abnormalities in first 12 hours after bite

Mild envenomation

- Local redness, swelling, ecchymosis limited to bite site

Moderate envenomation

- Local redness, swelling, and ecchymosis that extends beyond bite site
- Nausea
- Paresthesias
- Metallic taste in mouth
- Mild hypotension
- Mild tachypnea
- Coagulation factors normal and no active bleeding signs

Severe envenomation

- Rapidly spreading swelling, redness, and ecchymosis to involve entire limb
- Altered mentation
- Respiratory compromise
- Severe hypotension (7%)
- Extreme tachycardia
- Fibrinolysis and coagulopathy
- Active bleeding

Coral Snake Envenomation

- Coral snake bite symptoms can be delayed up to 12 hours
- Ptosis early sign
- Muscle weakness
- Tremors
- Salivation
- Slurred speech
- Dizziness
- Respiratory failure
- Other neurologic abnormalities

Diagnosis of Snake Bites

- Fang marks (pit vipers)
- History of snake exposure
- Local tissue injury
- Coral snake may have tiny punctures and minimal local tissue changes

Evaluation of Snake Bites

- History and physical exam
- Mark edematous area with a pen every 15–30 minutes to assess progression
- CBC
- CMP
- PT/PTT/INR
- U/A

Moderate to severe envenomation

- EKG
- Chest x-ray
- ABG
- Troponin
- DIC panel

Treatment Options

- Clean wound with antiseptic or soap/water
- No arterial constrictive banding, no wound excisions, no ice
- Venous banding can be considered if there is a large snake bite and prolonged delay reaching hospital
- Keep limb immobilized at heart level
- Tetanus toxoid (ADT) 0.5 cc IM if > 5 years since last dose or Tdap 0.5 cc IM
- Tetanus immune globulin 250–500 units IM at different site if < 3 tetanus doses in life
- Refer to health department or primary care provider to complete tetanus primary vaccination series if < 2 vaccines given in past
  - See Tetanus Protocol
- Antibiotics choices if infected — usually not needed otherwise
  - Rocephin, dicloxicillin, septra or doxycycline

Pain and nausea control options prn

- Dilaudid (hydromorphone) 0.5–1 mg IV (double if IM) prn — may repeat prn
- Morphine 2–5 mg IV prn — may repeat prn
  - Stadol (butorphanol) 0.5–1 mg IV (double if IM) — may repeat prn (avoid in opiate addiction)
- Phenergan (promethazine) 6.25 mg IV or 25–50 mg IM prn
- Zofran (ondansetron) 4–8 mg IV prn

Pit viper antivenin (mainstay of treatment) — notify physician

Crofab (less allergic reactions than horse serum)

- Read package insert
- Mild or no envenomation does not require antivenin for pit vipers
- 4–6 vials IV for moderate to severe envenomation initially — give slowly for first 10 minutes at 25–50 cc/hr to observe for allergic reaction
  - 2 vials IV q6hr up to 3 doses if further doses needed after initial dosing

Coral snake (eastern) antivenin

- Read package insert
- Pretreat with diphenhydramine 50 mg IV and famotidine 20 mg IV
- Keep epinephrine at bedside
- 3–6 vials IV over 1–2 hours if definitely bitten
- 10 vials IV initially if systemic manifestations present

Complications of antivenin

Acute allergic reaction – see Allergy Protocol Anaphylaxis sections

- Benadryl (diphenhydramine) 50 mg adult IV; 1.25 mg/kg pediatrics not to exceed 50 mg
- Pepcid (famotidine) 20 mg IV/PO – 40 mg PO for adult
- Pepcid (famotidine) 0.25 mg/kg IV/PO for pediatric (NMT 20mg IV or 40 mg PO)
- Methylprednisolone 125 mg IV for adults
- Methylprednisolone 1 mg/kg IV for children not to exceed 125 mg
- If reaction is severe notify physician immediately
  - Epinephrine 0.3–0.5 SQ/IM/IV for adults depending on severity; pediatrics 0.1 mg/kg SQ/IM/IV depending on severity not to exceed 0.5 mg
- It is preferable to consult on venomous snake bite patients

Serum sickness

- Fever
- Arthralgias

- Rash
- Usually occurs 7–10 days after antivenin; can occur earlier

Treatment

- Antihistamines prn
- Steroids for 7–10 days PO

Discharge Criteria

- Pit viper bite is dry, and is asymptomatic after 8 hours of observation
- Sonoran and Arizona coral snake bite: can be discharged

Discharge instructions

- Snake bite aftercare instructions
- Refer to primary care provider or surgeon

Consult Criteria

- Notify physician promptly for all snake bites
- All eastern coral snake or suspected eastern coral snake bites (need admission)
- Pit vipers with any significant envenomation (usually need admission)
- Abnormal vital signs
- Abnormal lab; chest x-ray; EKG
- Neurologic abnormalities
- Suspected compartment syndrome (consult surgeon)

Notes

REFERENCES:

Snakebite Author: Brian James Daley, MD, MBA, FACS, FCCP, CNSC; Chief Editor: Joe Alcock, MD, MS
emedicine.medscape.com/article/168828

Coral Snake Envenomation
Author: Robert L Norris, MD; Chief Editor: Joe Alcock, MD, MS
emedicine.medscape.com/article/771701

Dart RC. Sequelae of pit viper envenomations. In: Campbel JA, Brodie ED Jr, eds. Biology of the pit vipers. Tyler, Texas.: Selva Publishing, 1992:395–404

Kitchens CS, Van Mierop LHS. Envenomation by the eastern coral snake (Micrurus fulvius fulvius): a study of 39 victims. JAMA 1987; 258:1615–8

CELLULITIS PROTOCOL

Definition

- Local inflammatory reaction of the skin and subcutaneous tissue secondary to bacterial infection

Differential Diagnosis

- Erysipelas
- Osteomyelitis
- Septic arthritis
- Lymphadenitis
- Abscess
- Deep vein thrombosis
- Necrotizing fasciitis

Considerations

- Pain, tenderness, redness, swelling and warmth
- Abscess frequently co-exists
- Associated with outpatient treatment failure
  - Fever 100.4° F or 38°C
  - Chronic leg ulcers
  - Chronic edema
  - Prior cellulitis in the same area
  - Cellulitis at a wound site
  - Cellulitis of the hand
- **Subacute spread or redness and edema may extend beyond drawn margins during the first**

48 hrs. without representing treatment failure

- Decreasing intensity of the erythema is often a more important variable of improvement with antibiotic treatment

Caused by

- S. aureus (MRSA)
- Group A streptococcus
- H. influenzae
- Pseudomonas
- Anaerobes

Complications

- Bacteremia
- Osteomyelitis
- Septic joint
- Cavernous sinus spread

Higher risk

- Diabetics
- Peripheral vascular disease
- Chronic edema
- IV drug abuse
- Immunocompromised

Evaluation of cellulitis

- Complete history and physical examination
- Assess for tissue gas
- Palpate for tenderness

No tests needed

- For small area of involvement
- No fever or systemic signs
- No high risk factors

Testing considerations

- CBC, BMP for high risk factors
- CRP, CPK and CMP for suspected necrotizing fasciitis or gas gangrene
- Blood cultures if toxic or septic appearance or deep seated infection
- Ultrasound useful to evaluate for possible abscess if suspected
- X-ray or CT scan with IV contrast if crepitus noted or tissue gas suspected

Treatment Options

Uncomplicated purulent cellulitis (select one)

- Usually caused by Staphylococcus aureus, aka CA-MRSA
- Septra DS (trimethoprim /sulfamethoxazole), doxycycline (age > 8 years) or clindamycin for community acquired MRSA for 5–10 days
- Clindamycin 20-30 mg/kg/day PO/IV divided q6hr–q8hr × 10 days; not to exceed 450 mg/dose
- Doxycycline 1.5–2 mg/kg PO bid × 10 days (age > 8 years and < 45 kg) not to exceed 100 mg bid

Uncomplicated non–purulent cellulitis (select one)

- Usually caused by Group A streptococcus though S. aureus MSSA is possible which is sensitive to methicillin usually
- Amoxicillin/clavulanate 875 mg PO bid x 5–7 days
- Dicloxicillin 250–500 mg q6hr PO x 5–10 days
  - <40 kg —12.5 –100 mg/kg/day PO depending on severity divided q6hr
- Cephalexin 500 mg q6hr PO x 5–10 days (or other cephalosporins PO/IV)
  - Pediatric 25–50 mg/kg/day PO divided q6hr not to exceed 500 mg/dose
- Cefazolin 1–2 gms IV q8hr x 10 days
  - Pediatric 25-100 mg/kg divided q6hr–q8hr
- Clindamycin 300–450 mg q6–8hr PO/IV x 5–10 days
  - Pediatric 20-30 mg/kg/day PO/IV divided q6hr–q8hr × 5–10 days not to exceed 450 mg/dose

Drain associated abscesses and pack as needed

- Leave pack in usually 2 days

- Bedside ultrasound frequently changes therapy if abscess found with cellulitis (see examples below
- See Soft Tissue Abscess Protocol

Necrotizing fasciitis

- Prompt diagnosis and treatment reduces mortality and amputations
- Early diagnosis missed in almost 75% of cases
  - Misdiagnosed as cellulitis or abscess
  - Mortality > 70% when missed
- Initially fever or pain may be present with malaise, myalgias, diarrhea and anorexia in the first 24 hours
- Pain out of proportion to swelling and erythema most consistent finding
  - Other potential findings or symptoms
    - Tenderness extending beyond the erythema and swelling due to toxins and enzymes spreading along fascia
    - Indistinct margins
    - Lymphangitis rarely seen due to depth of infection
    - Rapidly progressive despite antibiotic treatment
    - Edema 75%, erythema 72%, tenderness 68%, fever 60%, skin bullae or necrosis 38%
    - CRP > 200 with mild increase WBC suggestive of group A streptococcus infection
    - Elevated CPK and creatinine without hypotension suggest severe group A strep infection
    - Leukemoid reactions with WBC's 50k – 150k in C. sordelli infections
    - Serum sodium < 135 mmol/L
    - Diffuse capillary leak (may require 10–12 liters NS qday
    - Gas in tissues consult surgeon immediately

Causes

- Defined port of skin entry
  - Penetrating wounds
  - Chicken pox, insect bites, injection sites etc.
- 50% group A streptococcus without skin penetration
  - Often at sites of nonpenetrating injury such as bruises or strains

Gas gangrene

- Penetrating wounds
- May be caused also by GI portals from adenocarcinoma
- Clostridium perfringens causes 80%
  - May occur at prior gas gangrene sites years before
- C. septicum may cause spontaneous nontraumatic gas gangrene from GI portals from adenocarcinoma in patients with neutropenia
- C. sorgellii from natural childbirth or abortion, or GYN procedures
  - Leukemoid reactions with WBC's 50k – 150k in C. sordelli infections
- **Gas in tissues consult surgeon immediately**

Imaging for necrotizing fasciitis or gas gangrene if needed

- CT scan with IV contrast
- MRI (not as definitive as CT enhanced scan)

Treatment

- Prompt surgical intervention

Antibiotics IV for necrotizing fasciitis

- Polymicrobial infection use vancomycin or linezolid plus Zosyn (piperacillin–tazobactam or Primaxin (imipenem/cilastatin) or ceftriaxone–metronidazole
- Group A streptococcal infections use penicillin plus clindamycin IV for 10–14 days
- A. hydrophilia (usually fresh water) use doxycycline plus ceftriaxone or ciprofloxacin

- V. vulnificus (usually salt water) doxycycline plus ceftriaxone or cefotaxime
- MRSA use vancomycin or linezolid, daptomycin or ceftaroline

Antibiotics for gas gangrene

- Penicillin plus clindamycin IV for 10–14 days

Human, dog or cat bite

- Amoxicillin/clavulanate x 10 days or Sanford guide or antibiotic databases
  - See Cat and Dog bite sections

Preseptal ocular cellulitis

- Amoxicillin/clavulanate x 10 days or Sanford guide or antibiotic database
  - See Preseptal cellulitis section

Waterborne cellulitis

Fresh water

- Commonly aeromonas hydrophilia (or others)

Treatment

- Doxycycline (age ≥ 8 years) plus IV gentamicin etc.)
- Bactrim
- Ceftriaxone
- Quinolone such as ciprofloxacin or levofloxacin (caution in children due to possible arthropathy complications)

Salt water

- Commonly vibrio species
  - May progress rapidly to necrotizing infection, even if initially a superficial infection
- Treatment
  - Third generation cephalosporin such as cefepime, ceftriaxone plus doxycycline (age ≥ 8 years)
  - Quinolone such as ciprofloxacin or levofloxacin (caution in children due to possible arthropathy complications)

Bedside ultrasound can change therapy (see below)

Brown recluse spider bite causing both cellulitis and abscess of proximal anterior thigh

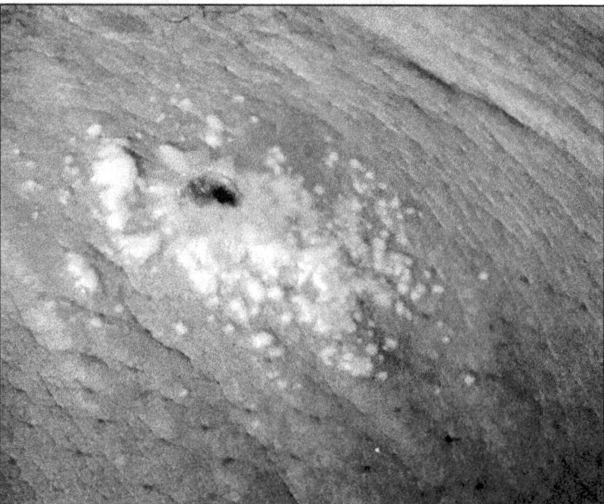

In performing bedside ultrasound for skin soft tissue exams, use the linear high frequency probe

Cobblestone appearance ultrasound image of cellulitis (fat globules with surrounding edema)

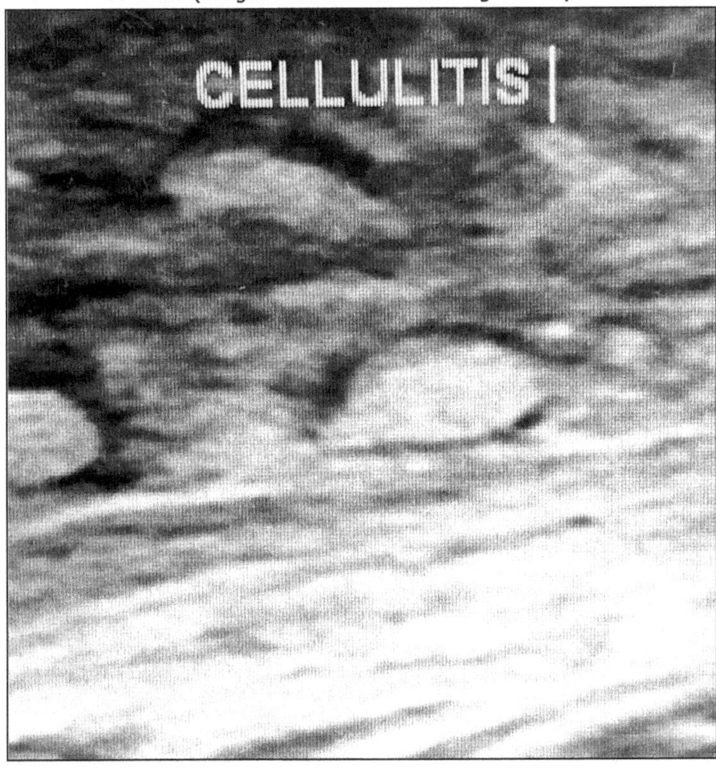

Abscess associated with the cellulitis

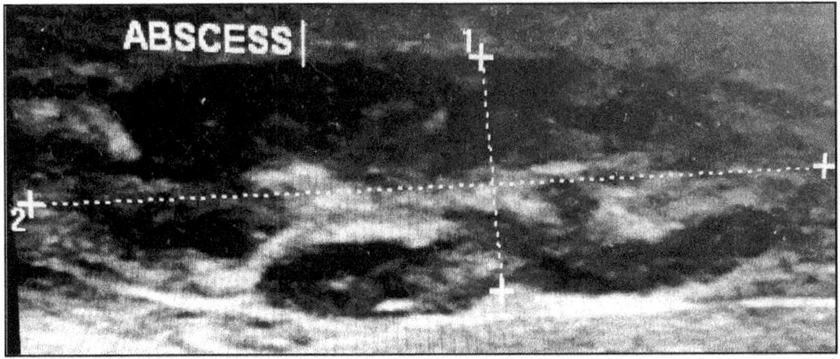

Discharge Criteria

- Mild cellulitis without systemic toxicity
- Available follow up

Discharge instructions

- Cellulitis aftercare instructions
- Follow up with PCP within 3–5 days if not improving

- Return if fever develops or pain increases
- Return for progressive increase in cellulitis

Consult Criteria

- Any documented fever
- Spreading rapidly
- Pain out of proportion to exam
- Crepitus or gas in tissues
- Systemic toxic appearance
- Necrotizing fasciitis or gas gangrene
- Large abscess
- Facial cellulitis
- Orbital cellulitis
- Suspected bony involvement
- Poorly controlled diabetic patients
- Failure of outpatient antibiotics

Higher risk comorbidities

- Diabetics with poor control
- Peripheral vascular disease
- Chronic edema
- IV drug abuse
- Immunocompromised

Vital signs and age consult criteria

- Age < 6 months
- Hypotension
- Any fever

Lab consult criteria

- WBC ≥ 15,000 or < 3,000
- Bandemia ≥ 15%
- Acute thrombocytopenia
- Significant electrolyte abnormally
- Glucose ≥ 350 mg/dL in diabetic patient
- Glucose ≥ 200 mg/dL in non-diabetic patient
- Hyperglycemia with metabolic acidosis (decreased serum CO_2 or elevated anion gap)
- Metabolic acidosis

Notes

____

____

____

REFERENCES:

Goh T, et al. *Br J Surgery* January 2014, Vol. 101, Issue 1, pages e119-e125

Hsiao C, et al. *Am J Emerg Med* 2008; 26: 170-175

Huang KF, et al. *J Trauma* 2011; 71: 467-473

Majeski J, Majeski E. *South Med J* 1997; 90: 1065-1068

Peterson D, et al. *Acad Emerg Med* 2014 May;21(5):526-531

Volz KA, et al. *Am J Emerg Med* 2013 Feb;31(2):360-4

Sabbaj A, et al. *Acad Emerg Med* 2009 Dec;16(12):1290-7

JEM,53(4):485

Soft Tissue Abscess Protocol

Definition

- Collection of purulent material in the soft tissues

Differential Diagnosis

- Cellulitis
- Erysipelas
- Osteomyelitis
- Septic arthritis
- Lymphadenitis
- Deep vein thrombosis
- Necrotizing fasciitis

Considerations

- Incision and drainage usually curative (antibiotics recommended)
- MRSA most common cause
- Cellulitis frequently surrounds abscess
- May be in deep areas like the buttocks
- Ultrasound useful when in doubt of an abscess being present
- Recurrent groin and axillary abscesses suggest hidradenitis suppurativa

Higher risk comorbidities

- Diabetics
- Peripheral vascular disease
- Chronic edema
- IV drug abuse
- Elderly
- Immunocompromised

Evaluation

- Assess for systemic toxicity
- Bedside ultrasound frequently changes therapy
- Examine for deeper structure involvement
- Culture Bartholin cysts for GC and Chlamydia
  - Usually from E coli or vaginal flora more than STD
- Consider abscess culture
- CBC, BMP for high risk factors
- Blood cultures if toxic or septic appearance

In performing bedside ultrasound for skin soft tissue exams, use the linear high frequency probe

Bedside ultrasound of abscess

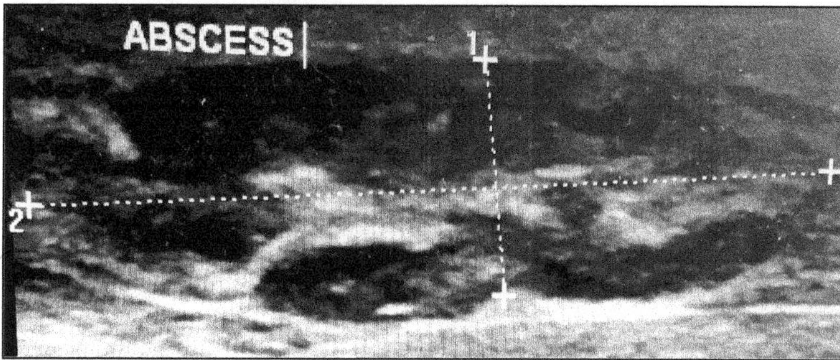

Treatment Options

- Skin prep with betadine
- Local anesthesia with ethyl chloride and/or lidocaine
- May use 18–20 gauge needle to aspirate to confirm an abscess
- Incise with #11 scalpel maximum area of swelling and/or tenderness
- Break any deeper adhesions
- Drain and irrigate pus
- Pack with gauze if large abscess present for 24–48 hours — patient can remove at home or return to see a Provider
- Do not pack facial abscesses
- NSAID's, Tylenol or narcotics short course prn

Loop drainage technique

- Very useful in pediatrics (also used in adults)
- After local anesthesia and skin prep with betadine, incise lateral edge of abscess 3–5 mm with #11 scalpel
- Introduce small curved hemostat in cavity and break up loculations
- With tip of hemostat find other edge of abscess and tent skin and incise down to hemostat bringing tip through skin

- Usually 4 cm or less should separate incised openings. If more distance needed then consider additional loops
- Irrigate pus out
- Draw a vessel loop, sterile rubber band or trimmed Penrose drain back through the abscess from second opening
- Tie loop loosely with enough space to get a finger under the loop
- Keep area clean with gauze
- Can shower or bathe
- Remove loop when drainage had stopped and cellulitis improved, usually within 7–10 days

Has superior results and decreased pain than conventional I&D

Antibiotic choices

- All abscesses > 2 cm by ultrasound treated with MRSA antibiotics 5–10 days (beneficial in smaller abscesses also)
  - Trimethoprim/sulfamethox–azole) DS PO bid
    - Pediatric 0.5 ml/kg bid (max dose 20 ml)
  - Doxycycline (age ≥ 8 years)
  - Clindamycin
- Severe infection
  - Patients who have failed I&D plus oral antibiotics
  - Meet SIRS criteria
  - Immunocompromised patients
  - Vancomycin or Daptomycin or Linezolid or Televancin or Ceftaroline and admission
- Consider antibiotics for higher risk patients

Discharge Criteria

- Uncomplicated abscess without toxicity
- No high risk co-morbidity
- Outpatient follow up available

Discharge instructions

- Abscess aftercare instructions
- Return if pain worsens or involved area increases in size
- Return if fever develops or worsens

Consult Criteria

- Rapidly spreading
- Pain out of proportion to exam
- Crepitus or gas in tissues
- Systemic toxic appearance
- Hypotension
- Necrotizing fasciitis
- Gas gangrene
- Vital signs significantly abnormal
- Facial abscess
- Large abscess
- Perirectal or pilonidal abscess
- Suspected bony or muscle involvement
- Poorly controlled diabetic patient
- Failure of recent I&D treatment

Higher risk comorbidities

- Diabetics with poor control
- Peripheral vascular disease
- Chronic edema
- IV drug abuse
- Elderly
- Immunocompromised

Vital signs and age consult criteria

- Age < 6 months or ≥ 70 years old
- Hypotension or relative hypotension SBP < 105 in patient with hypertension history
- Fever > 101°F (38.3°C)

Lab consult criteria

- WBC ≥ 15,000 or < 3,000
- Bandemia ≥ 15%
- Acute thrombocytopenia
- Significant electrolyte abnormally
- Glucose ≥ 350 mg/dL in diabetic patient
- Glucose ≥ 200 mg/dL in non-diabetic patient
- Hyperglycemia with metabolic acidosis (decreased serum CO_2 or elevated anion gap)
- Worsening anemia
- Metabolic acidosis

Notes

REFERENCES:

Stevens DL, et al. Clin Infect DisÂ July 15, 2014; 59(2): 147–159.

Talan DA, et al. Ann of Emerg Med. October 5, 2017.

Aprahamian CJ1, Nashad HH2, DiSomma NM3, Elger BM4, Esparaz JR5, McMorrow TJ4, Shadid AM4, Kao AM3, Holterman MJ1, Kanard RC4, Pearl RH6. Treatment of subcutaneous abscesses in children with incision and loop drainage: A simplified method of care. J Pediatr Surg. 2016 Dec 30. PMID:

Henoch-Schonlein Purpura Protocol

Definition

- Henoch-Schonlein purpura (HSP) is an inflammatory disorder characterized by a generalized vasculitis involving the small vessels of the skin, kidneys, GI tract, joints, and rarely the lungs and central nervous system

Differential Diagnosis

- Disseminated intravascular coagulation
- Meningitis
- Idiopathic Thrombocytopenic Purpura
- Mononucleosis
- Rocky Mountain spotted fever
- Septic shock
- Acute renal failure
- Intussusception
- Hand-Foot-Mouth disease
- Kawasaki disease
- Acute Glomerulonephritis
- Chicken pox
- Thrombocytopenic Purpura
- Systemic Lupus Erythematosus

Considerations

- Disease of children and young adults
- Diffuse vasculitis of unknown etiology
- Often an antecedent infection history present
- Peak incidence is 4 years of age
- Typical age range 2–11 years of age
- Spring peak
- Renal involvement most serious sequelae
  - Develops within 3 months of rash
  - Renal failure can develop up to 10 years after rash
    - More common in adults
- Generally a benign self-limited condition
- 40% have reoccurrence usually with rash and abdominal pain
- Normal platelet count, PT, and PTT

Signs and Symptoms

- Palpable purpura
- Rash of erythematous papules followed by nonthrombocytopenic purpura
  - Typically on buttocks; lower extremities; can be elsewhere
- Abdominal pain — 2/3 of patients; can mimic acute abdomen
- Low grade fever
- Vomiting
- Diarrhea — can be bloody
- Arthritis — 70% of patients; transient and no permanent deformity
- Nephritis

- End stage renal disease develops in 5% of cases
- Hematuria
- Intussusception
- Intracranial hemorrhage

Evaluation

- CBC
- CMP
- U/A
- PT/PTT/INR
- CT abdomen/pelvis scan if severe abdominal pain or bleeding present

Treatment

- IV NS for signs of hypovolemia
- Ibuprofen per weight
- Prednisone 1 mg/kg qday (NMT 60–80 mg/dose) × 5–7 days if renal or severe GI involvement
  - Long term kidney disease may not be prevented
- Methylprednisolone 0.8–1.6 mg/kg IV qday if unable to tolerate PO steroids (NMT 64 mg/day)
- Discontinue any known precipitants
- Severe disease requires IVIG with immunosuppressants, plasmapheresis and possible renal transplant

Discharge Criteria

- Normal platelet count
- Normal renal function
- Minimal or no abdominal pain
- Discuss with physician prior to discharge

Discharge instructions

- Henoch-Schonlein Purpura aftercare instructions
- Follow up within 24 hours if discharged on prednisone

Consult Criteria

- Severe abdominal pain
- Neurologic abnormalities
- Gastrointestinal bleeding
- Intussusception
- Renal involvement

Notes

REFERENCES:

Henoch-Schonlein Purpura Author: Noah S Scheinfeld, MD, JD, FAAD; Chief Editor: Craig B Langman, MD
emedicine.medscape.com/article/984105

Chartapisak W, Opastirakul S, Hodson EM, Willis NS, Craig JC. Interventions for preventing and treating kidney disease in Henoch-Schönlein Purpura (HSP). Cochrane Database of Systematic Reviews 2009, Issue 3. Art. No.: CD005128. DOI: 10.1002/14651858.CD005128.pub2

ERYTHEMA MULTIFORME PROTOCOL

Definition

- Erythema multiforme (EM) is an acute, self-limited, and occasionally recurring skin condition thought to be a type IV hypersensitivity reaction associated with certain infections, medications, and other various triggers

Differential Diagnosis

- Urticaria
- Herpes simples
- Pityriasis rosea
- Secondary syphilis
- Viral exanthems
- Septicemia
- Drug eruptions
- Collagen vascular disease
- Serum sickness

Considerations

Erythema multiforme (EM) minor

- Target lesions or raised red papules
- No mortality

Erythema multiforme major

- Similar to EM minor with mucous membrane involvement
- Epidermal detachment < 10% total body surface area
- No mortality

Stevens Johnson Syndrome (SJS)

- Widespread blisters/bullae on trunk and face
- Mucous membrane involvement
- SJS — epidermal detachment < 10% BSA (body surface area)
- Mortality approximately 5%

Toxic Epidermal Necrolysis (TEN)

- Widespread blisters/bullae on trunk and face
- Mucous membrane involvement
- TEN — epidermal detachment > 30% BSA
- Mortality approximately 30%

Symptoms and Findings

Erythema multiforme: minor and major

- Burning sensation of rash
- Pruritus usually absent
- Eye involvement up to 10%; bilateral purulent conjunctivitis
- Any mucous membrane involvement is mild
- Viral type prodrome in 50%

Rash

- Target or iris lesions (red papules and macules with central clearing)
- Vesiculobullous lesions can develop in existing rash
- Sudden onset and symmetrical
- Centripetal spread
- Favors palms and soles
- Dorsal hands
- Extensor limb surfaces
- Face

SJS/TEN

- Generalized cutaneous and/or mucocutaneous vesiculobullous lesions
- Hemorrhagic bullae
- Fever
- Vomiting and diarrhea can occur
- Oral pain may be severe
- Eye pain and discharge
- Dyspnea may occur
- Dysuria
- Oral involvement may appear similar to aphthous ulcers
- Nasal pharynx, respiratory tract, GI and GU systems can be involved

Causes

- No identifiable cause in 50%
- Viral
  - Herpes simplex (10%)
  - Chicken pox
  - Various other viruses
- Bacterial
  - Mycoplasma
  - Salmonella
  - Gonorrhea
  - Various others
- Fungal
- Postvaccination
- Drugs
  - Sulfonamides
  - Hypoglycemics
  - NSAID's
  - Anticonvulsants
  - Various antibiotics
  - Malignancy
  - Hormonal
  - Autoimmune disorders

Evaluation

- Erythema multiforme
  - Testing driven by history and physical exam
  - May not need testing
- SJS/TEN

- CBC
- CMP
- LFT's
- Chest x-ray
- Cultures prn

Treatment Options

- Remove offending agents if identified
- Erythema multiforme
  - Symptomatic treatments
  - Narcotics short course prn
  - NSAID's prn
  - Cool compresses with saline or Burrow's solution
  - Saline or Benadryl (diphenhydramine) elixir gargles prn for oral findings/symptoms
  - No oral steroids
  - Acyclovir for herpes associated erythema multiforme
- SJS/TEN
  - IV NS for hydration
  - Cultures prn
  - Burn unit treatment

Discharge Criteria

- Uncomplicated erythema multiforme

Discharge instructions

- Erythema multiforme aftercare instructions
- Return immediately if signs of SJS/TEN develops

Consult Criteria

- Refer to General Patient Criteria Protocol (page 15)
- All suspected SJS/TEN

Notes

REFERENCES:

Erythema Multiforme Author: Jose A Plaza, MD; Chief Editor: William D James, MD emedicine.medscape.com/article/1122915

Sokumbi O, Wetter DA. Clinical features, diagnosis, and treatment of erythema multiforme: a review for the practicing dermatologist. *Int J Dermatol.* Aug 2012;51(8):889–902

Ann of EM, 8/14, pg. 119

ERYTHEMA NODOSUM PROTOCOL

Definition

- Erythema nodosum (EN) is an acute, nodular, erythematous eruption that usually is limited to the extensor aspects of the lower legs, thought to be a hypersensitivity reaction

Differential Diagnosis

- Urticaria
- Nodular vasculitis
- Insect bites
- Erysipelas
- Superficial thrombophlebitis

Considerations

- Delayed hypersensitivity reaction
- Painful red tender 2–6 cm nodules on extensor lower extremities
- Usually acute and self-limited
- May last weeks to years
- More common in females age 30–50 years
- Idiopathic 50% of the time
- Often a marker for systemic disease

Causes

- Idiopathic 50% of the time
- Most commonly secondary to strep infections; sarcoidosis

- Drug reactions
  - Sulfa
  - Penicillin
  - Oral contraceptives
- Systemic infections
  - Tuberculosis
  - Fungal
- Ulcerative colitis
- Malignancy
  - Leukemia
  - Lymphoma

Evaluation

- Strep test of pharynx
- ESR or C-reactive protein (may be very high)

Treatment

- NSAID's prn
- Treat underlying infection or causes if found
- Cool compresses prn
- Elevation of legs
- Bed rest

Discharge Criteria

- All uncomplicated cases

Discharge instructions

- Erythema nodosum aftercare instructions

Consult Criteria

- Refer to General Patient Criteria Protocol (page 15)
- Serious associated comorbidities

Notes

REFERENCE:

Erythema Nodosum Author: Jeanette L Hebel, MD; Chief Editor: Dirk M Elston, MD
emedicine.medscape.com/article/1081633

DYSHIDROTIC ECZEMA PROTOCOL

Definition

- Vesicular eruption with pruritic deep-seated vesicles of the fingers, hands and feet of unknown etiology

Differential Diagnosis

- Scabies
- Contact dermatitis
- Irritant dermatitis
- Erythema multiforme
- Herpes simplex

Considerations

- Related to stress; drugs; illness
- "Id" reaction from variety of stimuli; distant fungal infections
- Lasts approximately 3 weeks
- Is a chronic relapsing palmoplantar dermatitis
- Spring and summer prevalence
- Warm climates
- 50% have childhood atopic dermatitis, asthma or similar conditions
- Symmetric distribution

Treatment Options

- Moisturizing lotions (Eucerin)
- Topical steroids
- Oral steroids such as prednisone 20–40 mg or dexamethasone 4–6 mg daily for a short course up to 7–10 days with taper
- Tacrolimus ointment
- Ultraviolet A light
- Oral antihistamines prn itching
- Ointments beneficial where increased moisture is needed
- Creams preferred in scalp and moist areas
- Avoid precipitating agents

Discharge Criteria

- Uncomplicated process

Discharge instructions

- Dyshidrotic eczema aftercare instructions

Consult Criteria

- Moderate to severe superinfection

Notes

REFERENCES:

National Institute for Clinical Excellence. *Frequency of application of topical corticosteroids for atopic eczema*. London, England: National Institute for Clinical Excellence (NICE); 2004:34

Dyshidrotic Eczema Author: Sadegh Amini, MD; Chief Editor: Dirk M Elston, MD
medicine.medscape.com/article/1122527

Dyshidrotic Eczema Author: Sadegh Amini, MD; Chief Editor: Dirk M Elston, MD
medicine.medscape.com/article/1122527

Dyshidrotic Eczema emedicine medscape
Updated: Jun 29, 2018 Author: Sadegh Amini, MD; Chief Editor: William D James, MD

ATOPIC DERMATITIS/ECZEMA PROTOCOL

Definition

- Poorly defined red patchy plaque-like rash with edema acutely and skin thickening chronically, mostly on flexor surfaces
- Also known as Eczema

Differential Diagnosis

- Seborrheic dermatitis
- Discoid eczema
- Contact dermatitis
- Scabies
- Insect bites
- Psoriasis

Considerations

- Can be acute or subacute
- Chronic relapsing most common
- Pruritic inflammation of epidermis or dermis
- Family history of asthma, hay fever, allergic rhinitis, allergic dermatitis
- Immune modulated
- More frequent in formula fed babies
- Manifests in infancy or early childhood usually and persists into adolescence
- Relationship to food allergies: milk, soy, eggs, wheat
- More frequent in winter
- Increased humidity contribution
- Bathing with hot water removes moisture from skin — worsening the rash

Symptoms

- Dry skin
- Erythematous patches and plaques
- Surrounding erythema and scaling may occur
- Skin excoriations frequent

- Often in skin flexures — antecubital and popliteal fossa
- May be generalized

Treatment Options

- Tacrolimus or pimcrolimus ointment
- Antihistamines
- Topical steroids
- May need oral steroids
- Avoid soap and hot water on rash as much as possible
- Topical or oral antibiotic for staph superinfection
- Eucerin
- Tar containing shampoo for scalp seborrheic dermatitis
- Avoid wool clothing

Discharge Criteria

- Uncomplicated process

Discharge instructions

- Atopic dermatitis or eczema aftercare instructions

Consult Criteria

- Moderate to severe superinfection

Notes

REFERENCES:

Margolis JS, Abuabara K, Bilker W, Hoffstad O, Margolis DJ. Persistence of Mild to Moderate Atopic Dermatitis.*JAMA Dermatol.* Apr 2 2014

Atopic Dermatitis Author: Brian S Kim, MD; Chief Editor: William D James, MD emedicine.medscape.com/article/1049085

Hanifin JM, Cooper KD, Ho VC, Kang S, Krafchik BR, Margolis DJ, Schachner LA, Sidbury R, Whitmore SE, Sieck CK, Van Voorhees AS. Guidelines of care for atopic dermatitis. J Am Acad Dermatol. 2004 Mar;50(3):391–404

PSORIASIS PROTOCOL

Definition

- A chronic, relapsing, multisystem inflammatory condition manifested most commonly with skin rash and arthritis, with a familial predisposition

Differential diagnosis

- Seborrheic dermatitis
- Atopic dermatitis
- Tinea corporis, pedis or capitis
- Contact dermatitis
- Blepharitis
- Syphilis
- Squamous cell carcinoma
- Diaper dermatitis
- Pustular eruptions
- Various skin malignancies

Considerations

- Rash most commonly on elbows, knees, scalp, lumbosacral region, intergluteal clefts and glans penis
- Arthritis occurs in up to 30% of patients
- Plaque-type most common rash
  - Plaques are raised, red, may be inflamed, with silvery white scaly appearance
- Ocular involvement occurs in up to 10% of patients
- Flares may be secondary to recent strep throat or viral infection, immunization or trauma

Guidelines on psoriasis biologic therapy from the British Association of Dermatologists

- Offer biologic therapy to people with psoriasis who require systemic therapy if methotrexate and cyclosporine have failed
- If methotrexate and cyclosporine are not tolerated or are contraindicated

- If psoriasis has a large impact on physical, psychological, or social functioning

Guidelines on the management and treatment of psoriasis with biologics by the American Academy of Dermatology and the National Psoriasis Foundation

- Offer monotherapy with TNF-alpha Inhibitors
- Offer monotherapy Interleukin-17 Inhibitors

Symptoms and Findings

- Scaling red macules, papules and plaques that are frequently pruritic
- Guttate psoriasis are small pink 1–10 mm macules commonly on upper trunk frequently 2–3 weeks after strep throat
  - Rash may be pustular
- Fever, chills, hypothermia and dehydration may occur when most of the body is covered with psoriasis rash
- Pits on the nails
- Arthritis is usually of hands and feet, though may include large joints
- White oral lesions and/or cheilosis
- Geographic tongue
- Blepharitis
- Uveitis
- Conjunctivitis

Evaluation options

- Usually a clinically diagnosis
- Joint x-rays may help with determining type of arthritis
- If immunologic therapy started, obtain baseline CBC, BMP, LFT's and TB screening

Treatment options

- Systemic steroids not effective and may worsen the psoriasis when discontinued
- Minimize soap exposure to rash as much as is practical
- Moisturizing lotions
- Sunlight exposure
- Sea bathing
- Topical corticosteroids for rash (avoid very potent steroids in children)
  - Triamcinolone 0.025–0.1% cream is drug of choice for new treatment (have a break from treatment every 4 weeks for potent steroids)
  - Betamethasone cream 0.025–0.1% for disease resistant to triamcinolone or hydrocortisone creams (have a break from treatment every 4 weeks for potent steroids)
- Ocular corticosteroids for eye involvement
  - Prednisolone 1% (Pred Forte) bid
  - Dexamethasone 1% ophthalmic
- Coal tar 0.5–33% (DHS Tar, Doctar, Theraplex T)
  - Shampoo for scalp lesions
  - Topical corticosteroid in addition to coal tar preparation increases effectiveness
- Salicylic acid preparations help to remove scales
- Calcipotriene (vitamin D analogue)
- Combination therapy with tazarotene (a retinoid) or calcipotriene with a topical corticosteroid more effective than either alone
- Oatmeal baths may help symptoms

Severe cases may need treatment from some of the following

- Systemic retinoids, cyclosporine, methotrexate, azathioprine, a Biologic, or hydroxyurea — **consult dermatologist prior to using and read PDR**
  - Methotrexate patients monitor closely for bone marrow, liver, lung and kidney toxicities
  - Biologics are infliximab (Remicade), etanercept (Enbrel), adalimumab (Humira), and alefacept (Amevive) — **consult**

dermatologist prior to using and read PDR

- Psoralen with ultraviolet A light retinoids PUVA (do not use in skin cancer prone patients or if 150 PUVA treatments already given)
- Ultraviolet B
- Anthralin preparations 0.1–1% (Drithocreme, Anthra-Derm)

Phosphodiesterase-4 inhibitors

- Apremilast (Otezla)

Interleukin inhibitors — Monotherapy treatment option for adults with moderate-to-severe plaque psoriasis

- Ustekinumab (Stelara)
- Secukinumab (Cosentyx)
- Ixekizumab (Taltz)
- Brodalumab (Siliq)

Disease–modifying antirheumatic drugs (DMARD's) methotrexate and azathioprine

Considerations

- Check CBC, creatinine, LFT's and investigate abnormalities before DMARD or Biologics medications used
- Document negative pregnancy test and discussion of contraception in fertile females before treatment
- Consider pneumovax vaccination
- Document PPD results before Biologics therapy
- Be familiar with effects and side effects of medications as listed in the Physician Desk Reference (PDR)

Biologics (tumor necrosis factor inhibitors)

- Infliximab (Remicade)
  - Reserve infliximab for use in people with very severe disease or people in whom other available biologic agents have failed or cannot be used
  - Monotherapy treatment option for adults with moderate-to-severe plaque psoriasis
  - British Association of Dermatologists recommendation
- Etanercept (Enbrel)
  - Monotherapy treatment option for adults with moderate-to-severe plaque psoriasis
- Adalimumab (Humira)
  - Offer adalimumab as a first-line biologic agent to adults with psoriasis, particularly when psoriatic arthropathy is a consideration
- **Avoid TNF antagonist therapy in people with significant heart failure**
  - Stop in the event of new or worsening preexisting heart failure and seek specialist advice

Cautions

- Severe infection risk exists
- Stop all DMARDs and Biologics if infection identified or suspected until treated and resolved
- Malignancy risks may be increased
- Do not use in optic neuritis or multiple sclerosis patients or in a first degree relative of these patients
- Do not use in patients with significant heart failure
- Avoid live vaccines
- Biologics may be used with or without DMARDs
- Be familiar with effects and side effects of medications as listed in the Physician Desk Reference (PDR)

Discharge criteria

- Uncomplicated psoriasis

Discharge instructions

- Psoriasis aftercare instructions
- Referral to PCP or dermatologist

Consult criteria

- Systemic symptoms or findings
- Fever
- Systemic treatment needed for severe disease
- Prescribing Biologics or DMARDs

Notes

REFERENCES:

National Institute for Health and Clinical Excellence (NICE). Psoriasis: the assessment and management of psoriasis. London (UK): National Institute for Health and Clinical Excellence (NICE); 2012 Oct. 61 p. (NICE clinical guideline; no. 153)

Mason AR, Mason J, Cork M, Dooley G, Hancock H. Topical treatments for chronic plaque psoriasis. Cochrane Database of Systematic Reviews 2013, Issue 3. Art. No.: CD005028. DOI: 10.1002/14651858.CD005028.pub3

Psoriasis Author: Jeffrey Meffert, MD; Chief Editor: Robert E O'Connor, MD, MPH emedicine.medscape.com/article/1943419

[Guideline] Smith CH, Jabbar-Lopez ZK, Yiu ZZ, Bale T, Burden AD, Coates LC, et al. British Association of Dermatologists guidelines for biologic therapy for psoriasis 2017. *Br J Dermatol*. 2017 Sep. 177 (3):628-636

[Guideline] Menter A, Strober BE, Kaplan DH, et al. Joint AAD-NPF guidelines of care for the management and treatment of psoriasis with biologics. *J Am Acad Dermatol*. 2019 Feb 13

Psoriasis Updated: Feb 28, 2019 Author: Jacquiline Habashy, DO, MSc; Chief Editor: William D James, MD

Emedicine medscape

CONTACT DERMATITIS PROTOCOL

Definition

- Hypersensitivity reaction manifested by acute or chronic inflammatory reactions to substances that contact the skin

Differential Diagnosis

- Cellulitis
- Scabies
- Atopic dermatitis/eczema
- Psoriasis
- Herpes simplex
- Erythema multiforme

Considerations

- Comprises 90% of workman's compensation dermatologic claims
- Rash limited to exposure area with sharp margins or linear excoriations

Some causes

- Rhus dermatitis (toxicodendron)
  - Poison ivy, poison oak, poison sumac
- Metals: nickel common
- Chemical
  - Hair dyes; paraphenylenediamine

Treatment Options

- Identify and limit exposure
- Soothing moist dressings
- Topical steroids
- Systemic steroids with severe cases up to 10 days
- Toxicodendron or Rhus dermatitis (poison ivy, etc.) use soap and water, especially under nails
- Zanfel over the counter can be used for Rhus dermatitis acutely
- Psoralen plus UVA, azathioprine and cyclosporine are used for steroid-resistant chronic hand dermatitis
    - Azathioprine — chronic immunosuppression with this purine antimetabolite increases neoplasia risk, mutagenic risk, and hematologic toxicities

Discharge Criteria

- Uncomplicated process

Discharge instructions

- Contact dermatitis aftercare instructions

Consult Criteria

- Severe superinfection

Notes

REFERENCES:

Allergic Contact Dermatitis Author: Daniel J Hogan, MD; Chief Editor: William D James, MD
emedicine.medscape.com/article/1049216

Bourke J, Coulson I, English J, British Association of Dermatologists Therapy Guidelines and Audit Subcommittee. Guidelines for the management of contact dermatitis: an update. Br J Dermatol. 2009 May;160(5):946–54

IMPETIGO PROTOCOL

Definition

- Impetigo is a highly contagious gram-positive bacterial infection of the superficial layers of the epidermis that exists in 2 forms which are bullous impetigo and non-bullous impetigo

Differential Diagnosis

- Erythema multiforme
- Fixed drug eruption
- Bullous pemphigoid
- Herpes simplex
- Herpes zoster
- Insect bites
- Stevens-Johnson syndrome
- Toxic Epidermal Necrolysis
- Varicella (Chicken pox)
- Atopic dermatitis
- Scabies

Considerations

- Contagious superficial bacterial infection of epidermis
- Crusted erosions or ulcers
- Most common in children ages 2–5 years
- Clinical diagnosis
- Predisposing factors
- Close contact with infected person
- Warm/humid climates
- Poor hygiene
- Crowding
- Poverty
- Non-bullous form most common
- MRSA most prevalent
- GABHS still occurs

Treatment Options

- Gentle washing of crusts with soap and washcloth
- Mupirocin topical for 5–10 days or until lesions gone for 2 days (as effective as cephalexin and drug of choice)
- Retapamulin bid for 5 days (expensive)

    - Superior to mupirocin and oral antibiotics
    - Not for mucosal membranes
- More widespread and severe cases can give systemic antibiotics — choices

Purulent

(Usually caused by Staphylococcus aureus, aka CA-MRSA)

- Septra DS bid PO adult (trimethoprim/sulfamethoxazole)
    - Septra 8-12 mg TMP/kg/dose or 0.5 cc/LB bid PO q12hr for 10 days for children
- Doxycycline 100 mg PO bid x 7 days
    - Doxycycline (age >8) children < 45 kg: 2–4 mg/kg PO qday x 7 days
- Clindamycin 300–450 mg q6–8hr PO x 10 days
    - Pediatric 20-30 mg/kg/day PO divided q6hr–q8hr x 10 days not to exceed 450 mg/dose

Nonpurulent

(Usually caused by Group streptococcus though S. aureus MSSA is possible which is sensitive to methicillin)

- Dicloxicillin 250 mg q6hr PO x 5–7 days
    - < 40 kg —12.5 –100 mg/kg/day PO depending on severity divided q6hr x 7 days not to exceed adult dosing
- Cephalexin 500 mg q6hr PO x 5–7 days (or other cephalosporins PO)
    - Pediatric 25–50 mg/kg/day PO divided q6hr not to exceed 500 mg/dose x 7 days not to exceed adult dosing
- Cefazolin 1–2 gms IV q8hr x 10 days for inpatient
    - Pediatric 25-100 mg/kg divided q6hr–q8hr not to exceed adult dosing
- Clindamycin 150–300 mg q6–8hr PO x 5–7 days
    - Pediatric 20-30 mg/kg/day PO divided q6hr–q8hr x 7 days not to exceed 450 mg/dose

Discharge Criteria

- Uncomplicated infection

Discharge instructions

- Impetigo aftercare instructions
- Return if fever develops
- Follow up with PCP if rash persists > 10 days

Consult Criteria

- Systemic symptoms
- Immunocompromised

Notes

REFERENCES:

Scheinfeld N. A Primer In Topical Antibiotics For The Skin And Eyes. *J Drugs Dermatol.* 2008;7(4):409–415

Impetigo Author: Lisa S Lewis, MD; Chief Editor: Russell W Steele, MD emedicine.medscape.com/article/965254

Koning S, van der Sande R, Verhagen AP, van Suijlekom-Smit LWA, Morris AD, Butler CC, Berger M, van der Wouden JC. Interventions for impetigo. Cochrane Database of Systematic Reviews 2012, Issue 1. Art. No.: CD003261. DOI: 10.1002/14651858.CD003261

SCABIES PROTOCOL

Definition

- Dermatitis secondary to the mite Sarcoptes scabiei, spread by direct contact with hosts or fomites

Differential Diagnosis

- Insect bites
- Atopic dermatitis

- Contact dermatitis
- Urticaria
- Psoriasis
- Lice
- Secondary syphilis
- Bedbug bites
- Dyshidrotic eczema
- Chicken pox
- Folliculitis

Considerations

- No symptoms for 2–6 weeks after infection, but may still spread the mite
- Marked pruritus especially at night
- Transmission primarily from skin to skin
- Transmission can occur from infected linens or clothing
- Eggs hatch in 3 days
- Mite viable 2–5 days
- Lesions are small excoriations with erythematous papules
- Burrow not always present, but pathognomonic
- Burrow is grey to red to brown thin line 2–15 mm in length
- Does not affect scalp in adults
- Can affect scalp in infants
- Diagnosis is clinical
- Can be confirmed with microscopic visualization of mite
- Itching can last 4 weeks after treatment due to hypersensitivity reaction to dead mite
- Itching lasting > 4 weeks search for another cause of the itching

Distribution

- Intertriginous areas
- Sides and webs of fingers
- Axillary folds
- Flexor wrists
- Extensor elbows
- Waist
- Genital folds
- Buttocks
- Thighs
- Extensor knees
- Posterior feet

Evaluation options if desired

Burrow ink test

- Washable felt tip marker across suspected burrow and ink removed with alcohol
- Remaining ink outlines the burrow

Skin scraping

Treatment

- Permethrin cream 5%
    - Massage cream in from neck to soles of feet
    - Leave on 8–14 hours
    - Second application one week later
- Lindane (Kwell lotion)
    - Massage cream thinly from neck to soles of feet
    - Leave on 8–14 hours
    - Second application one week later
- Oral ivermectin 200 mcg/kg × 1 dose with food
    - Not recommended in pregnant or lactating women
    - Not recommended in children < 15 kg
    - Repeat in 1–2 weeks prn
    - Crusted scabies may treat day 1, 2, 8, 9, 15 along with topical scabicide (also on day 22 and 29 if severe)
- Benadryl (diphenhydramine) prn itching
- Topical steroids prn once mite eradicated
- Treat all family members or close contacts
- Infected linens and clothing washed in hot water and dried with heat or ironing, or seal clothes in large plastic bag for 3–5 days if unable to laundry or dry clean
- Crusted scabies should be removed (warm soaks and then 5% salicylic acid in petrolatum and then scraped off (avoid salicylic acid in large surface areas due to toxicity)

- Crusted scabies have heavy mite burden and may need repeated treatments
- The itch may fade faster if one soaks in a warm tub of water until the fingertips become wrinkled, then scrub the areas that itch. This will remove dead mites and their debris much faster than shedding normally. This may have to repeat once or twice to stop the itch.
- Antihistamines and steroids orally or topically will help make itch more tolerable

Discharge Criteria

- Nontoxic patient with routine symptoms

Discharge instructions

- Scabies aftercare instructions
- Follow up with PCP as needed

Consult Criteria

- Moderate to severe topical or systemic superinfection

Notes

REFERENCES:

Scabies Author: Megan Barry, MD; Chief Editor: William D James, MD emedicine.medscape.com/article/1109204

Strong M, Johnstone P. Interventions for treating scabies. Cochrane Database of Systematic Reviews 2007, Issue 3. Art. No.: CD000320. DOI: 10.1002/14651858.CD000320.pub2

Centers for Disease Control and Prevention (CDC). Ectoparasitic infections. In: Sexually transmitted diseases treatment guidelines, 2010. MMWR Recomm Rep. 2010 Dec 17;59(RR-12):88–90

CUTANEOUS CANDIDIASIS PROTOCOL

Definition

- Infections of the skin caused by the yeast Candida albicans or other Candida species

Considerations

- Present in normal flora in GI tract and vagina
- May colonize skin but not normal flora
- Disease caused by overgrowth
- Tissue damage resulting from trauma, xerostomia, radiation-induced mucositis, ulcerations, skin maceration, or occlusion
- Predisposed in endocrine conditions such as diabetes mellitus, Cushing syndrome, corticosteroid use
- Predisposition in immunocompromised states
- Candida auris is an emerging fungus that presents a global health care threat with severe illness in hospitalized patient and is often resistant to multiple medications

Differential diagnosis

- Intertrigo
- Mucosal candidiasis
- Onychomycosis
- Seborrheic dermatitis

Presentation

- Red moist, occasionally macerated rash, commonly see in skin folds (**Intertrigo**)
- Itching and pain/soreness
- White papules or plaques
- May be present in nails
- In males, on scrotum or penis, in contrast to tinea cruris which usually spares scrotum or penis

Diagnosis

- Usually a clinical diagnosis
- KOH prep is easiest lab test for yeast and pseudohyphae

Treatment

Candidal vulvovaginitis

- Topical antifungal agents including miconazole nitrate (Micatin, Monistat-Derm) or clotrimazole (Lotrimin, Mycelex) creams
- Fluconazole (150 mg) PO x 1
- Itraconazole (600 mg) PO x 1

Oral candidiasis in infant

- Nystatin oral suspension 1 mL (100,000 U) to each side of the mouth 4 times daily for 10–14 days or until symptoms gone for 48–72 hours
  - Preterm infants is half the mg dose with same frequency and length of treatment

Oral candidiasis in adults

- Nystatin (1:100,000 U/mL, 5 mL oral rinse and swallow qid)

Candidal diaper dermatitis

- Air drying
- Frequent diaper changes
- Baby powders and zinc oxide paste are adequate preventive measures

Intertrigo

- Keep skin dry
- Topical nystatin powder, clotrimazole, or miconazole bid for 10–14 days (may need longer term treatment)
- Fluconazole 100 mg PO qd for 1-2 wk. (may need longer term treatment)
- Itraconazole 100 mg PO qd for 1-2 wk.
- May add low potency steroid cream short term treatment for inflammatory relief
- Ketoconazole shampoo with showers or bathing to rash 10–14 days (may need long term treatment)
- Ketoconazole cream bid to rash x 10–14 days or longer
- Ketoconazole 200 mg PO qd for if other treatment unsuccessful 1-2 wk.
  - **Black box warning** for liver toxicity and QT prolongation
  - **Tinea versicolor** may use off label ketoconazole 400 mg PO x 1 every several months as needed

Disposition

Admission or consult criteria

- Severe inflammatory disease
- Immunocompromised state
- Systemic symptoms

Discharge criteria

- Most patients with localized disease

Notes

____

____

____

REFERENCES:

Cutaneous Candidiasis Author: Noah S Scheinfeld, JD, MD, FAAD; Chief Editor: Dirk M Elston, MD

May 22, 2018
emedicine.medscape.com/article/1090632-overview

www.cdc.gov/fungal/diseases/candidiasis

Tinea Capitis Protocol

Definition

- A disease caused by superficial fungal infection of the skin of the scalp

Differential Diagnosis

- Alopecia areata
- Psoriasis
- Drug eruptions
- "Id" reaction
- Contact dermatitis
- Seborrheic dermatitis
- Secondary syphilis
- Impetigo
- Systemic lupus erythematosus

Considerations

- Is a fungal superficial infection of the scalp
- Most common in younger pediatric population
- Spread by person to person contact
- Spread by shared objects such as combs and hair brushes
- Erythematous patch increasing over time
- Alopecia can occur
- May develop painful lymphadenopathy
- Kerion can develop — multiple boggy nodules of pus with associated hair loss
- Diagnosis can be clinical or confirmed with KOH prep

Treatment Options

- Adult
  - Oral griseofulvin 500 mg to 1 gm microsize PO qday for 6–8 weeks, may need 8–12 weeks
  - Sporanox 200 mg PO qday for 2 weeks
  - Terbinafine 250 mg PO qday for 4–6 weeks (monitor for liver disease)
  - Fluconazole at 50–100 mg/day or 150 mg once weekly for 2–4 weeks for more severe infection
- Pediatric
  - Oral griseofulvin 20–25 mg/kg microsize PO qday for 6–8 weeks (do not exceed adult doses)
  - Sporanox 3–5 mg/kg PO qday for 2 weeks (do not exceed adult doses)
- Monitor LFT's due to possible liver toxicity of griseofulvin
- Six weeks or more may be needed for treatment

Discharge Criteria

- Uncomplicated rash
- Children may return to school once appropriate treatment has started

Discharge instructions

- Tinea capitis aftercare instructions
- Follow up within 14 days if no improvement in rash
- Follow up in 3–4 weeks if rash persists

Consult Criteria

- Moderate to severe superinfection
- Systemic symptoms
- Immunocompromised

Notes

REFERENCES:

Shemer A, Plotnik IB, Davidovici B, Grunwald MH, Magun R, Amichai B. Treatment of tinea capitis - griseofulvin versus fluconazole - a comparative study. *J Dtsch Dermatol Ges*. Apr 10 2013

González U, Seaton T, Bergus G, Jacobson J, Martínez-Monzón C. Systemic antifungal therapy for tinea capitis in children. Cochrane Database of Systematic Reviews 2007, Issue 4.

Art. No.: CD004685. DOI: 10.1002/14651858.CD004685

Tinea Capitis Author: Grace F Kao, MD; Chief Editor: Dirk M Elston, MD emedicine.medscape.com/article/1091351

TINEA CORPORIS PROTOCOL

Definition

- Superficial fungal infection of the body

Differential Diagnosis

- Tinea versicolor
- Cutaneous candidiasis
- Seborrheic dermatitis
- Psoriasis
- Impetigo
- Pityriasis rosea
- Secondary syphilis

Considerations

- Commonly called "ring worm"
- Erythematous lesion with central clearing
- Diagnosis usually clinical
- KOH prep will show the fungal hyphae

Treatment Options

- Luliconazole 1% cream qday for 1 week (recent FDA approval)
- Topical Lamisil qday for 1–4 weeks (apply on rash and 2 cm out from rash)
- Lotrimin bid for 2–6 weeks (apply on rash and 2 cm out from rash)
- Treat until no rash visible for 2 days
- Oral griseofulvin or ketoconazole for more severe infection (monitor LFT's)
  - May combine with topical treatment
  - May use in immunosuppressed patients
  - Use in tinea unguium (nails) or tinea Capitis
- Fluconazole at 50–100 mg/day or 150 mg once weekly for 2–4 weeks for more severe infection
- Oral itraconazole in doses of 100 mg/day for 2 weeks for more severe infection
- Avoid sharing infected objects
- Launder all possible infected linens and clothing separately
- Good hand washing
- Topical steroids can be used for initial 1–4 days to relieve symptoms

Tinea unguium treatment options

- Menthol ointment OTC daily for many months (Vicks VapoRub)
- Oral itraconazole 200 mg PO qday for 12 weeks
- Terbinafine 250 mg PO qday for toenail for 12 weeks, for fingernail for 6 weeks (monitor for liver disease)
- Penlac (ciclopirax) without lunula involvement for 48 weeks associated with Trichophyton rubrum

Discharge Criteria

- Uncomplicated rash
- Children may return to school once appropriate treatment has started

Discharge instructions

- Tinea corporis aftercare instructions
- Follow up within 14 days if no improvement in rash
- Follow up in 3–4 weeks if rash persists

Consult Criteria

- Moderate to severe superinfection
- Systemic symptoms
- Immunocompromised

Notes

REFERENCES:

Brooks M. FDA Approves New Topical Antifungal Luliconazole 1%. Medscape Medical News. Nov 15 2013

Tinea Corporis Author: Jack L Lesher Jr, MD; Chief Editor: Dirk M Elston, MD emedicine.medscape.com/article/1091473

Crawford F, Hollis S. Topical treatments for fungal infections of the skin and nails of the foot. Cochrane Database of Systematic Reviews 2007, Issue 3. Art. No.: CD001434. DOI: 10.1002/14651858.CD001434.pub2

Tinea Pedis Author: Courtney M Robbins, MD; Chief Editor: Dirk M Elston, MD emedicine.medscape.com/article/1091684

TINEA CRURIS PROTOCOL

Definition

- A pruritic superficial fungal infection of the groin and adjacent skin

Differential diagnosis

- Acanthosis Nigricans
- Allergic Contact Dermatitis
- Cutaneous Candidiasis
- Erythrasma
- Familial Benign Pemphigus (Hailey-Hailey Disease)
- Folliculitis
- Intertrigo
- Irritant Contact Dermatitis
- Plaque Psoriasis
- Seborrheic Dermatitis

Considerations

- Usually spares scrotum and penis
- Second most common dermatophytosis
- Transmitted by fomites, such as contaminated towels or hotel bedroom sheets, or by autoinoculation from a reservoir on the hands or feet
- 3 times more common in men
- History may include visiting a tropical climate, wearing tight-fitting clothes (including bathing suits) for extended periods, sharing clothing with others, participating in sports, or coexisting diabetes mellitus or obesity
- T rubrum is the most common etiologic agent

Treatment

- Treat all active areas of tinea cruris infection simultaneously
- If unable to use topical treatments consistently, or with extensive or recalcitrant infection, treat as candidates for systemic administration of antifungal therapy
- Terbinafine 1% (Lamisil) topical 1–2 daily for 2 weeks (most effective)
- Butenafine 1% (Mentax) cream topical 1–2 daily for 2–4 weeks
- Clotrimazole 1% (lotrimin) bid–tid for 2–4 weeks

Severe or extensive or multiple dermatophyte infections use topical plus PO

- Terbinafine 250mg PO qday for 2–3 weeks (liver disease contraindicated)
- Itraconazole 200mg PO qday for 1–2weeks (not in CHF patients, has many drug interactions, and prolongs QTc)
- Fluconazole 150–300 mg PO qweek for 3–4 weeks

Consult criteria

- Severe symptoms
- Significant bacterial superinfection
- Recalcitrant infections

Discharge criteria

- Uncomplicated infection

Discharge instructions

- Put on socks before undershorts to reduce the possibility of direct contamination
- Weight loss as indicated
- Dry crural folds completely after bathing and use separate towels for drying the groin and other parts of the body
- Keep the groin region dry to prevent recurrence
- Avoid wearing tight-fitting clothing
- Antifungal powders, which have the added benefit of drying the region, may be helpful in preventing recurrence
- Avoid sharing toys, personal items and close contact
- Launder all linens separately
- Good hand washing
- Wear loose fitting clothes

Notes

____

____

____

REFERENCES

Tinea Cruris Updated: Sep 11, 2020

Author: Michael Wiederkehr, MD; Chief Editor: Dirk M Elston, MD

emedicine.medscape.com/article/1091806

TINEA BARBAE PROTOCOL

Definition

- Ssuperficial dermatophyte infection that is limited to the bearded areas of the face and neck and occurs almost exclusively in older adolescent and adult males
- Tinea faciei is a superficial dermatophyte infection limited to the glabrous skin of the face in pediatric and female patients

Differential diagnosis

- Acne vulgaris
- Allergic contact dermatitis
- Cutaneous candidiasis
- Actinomycosis
- Folliculitis
- Irritant contact dermatitis
- Pediatric syphilis
- Rosacea

Treatment for tinea barbae

- Avoid contact with infected animals
- Shaving or hair depilation is recommended with warm compresses to remove crusts and debris
- Topical formulations with antifungal compounds can be applied, but tinea barbae requires oral antifungal therapy
- Griseofulvin 500 mg microsize PO qday until lesions resolved for 2 weeks (check LFT's)
- Terbinafine 250mg PO qday for 4 weeks (liver disease contraindicated–checks LFT's)
- Itraconazole 200mg PO bid for 1 week or 100 mg PO bid for 4 weeks (NMT 400 mg/day)
- Fluconazole 150 mg PO qweek up to 6 weeks

Treatment for tinea faciei

- Topical therapy may be sufficient if follicular papules are not present

- Topical ciclopirox and terbinafine
- Isolation and treatment of infected pets
- Isoconazole nitrate and diflucortolone valerate combination therapy has been used successfully
- Rarely chronic and/or multiple lesions may require systemic therapy (see above in treatment for tinea barbae)

Consult criteria

- Dermatology as needed

Discharge criteria

- All uncomplicated patients

Notes

____

____

____

REFERENCES

Tinea Barbae Updated: Apr 06, 2021 Author: Robert A Schwartz, MD, MPH; Chief Editor: William D James, MD emedicine.medscape.com/article/1091252

TINEA PEDIS (ATHLETE'S FOOT) PROTOCOL

Definition

- Superficial fungal infection of the foot

Differential Diagnosis

- Cutaneous candidiasis
- Erythema multiforme
- Psoriasis
- Secondary syphilis
- Dyshidrotic eczema
- Pustular psoriasis

Considerations

- Most common superficial dermatophyte fungal infection
- Commonly called "athletes foot"
- Excessive sweating and occlusive footwear predispose to infection
- Acute and chronic states occur
- Inflammatory vesicles and bullae
- Located in toe webs — most common 4th and 5th
- Clinical diagnosis usually
- Can confirm with KOH prep if desired
- Can lead to cellulitis

Treatment Options

- Luliconazole for the treatment of interdigital tinea pedis in adults that requires a 2–week treatment period (expensive)
- Topical Lamisil bid 1–4 weeks and rash gone for 2–4 days
- Oral terbinafine, itraconazole or ketoconazole for more severe infection (monitor for liver disease)
  - May combine with topical treatment
- Avoid sharing infected objects
- Launder all possible infected linens and clothing separately
- Good hand washing
- Avoid tight fitting shoes
- Keep feet dry
- May use topical steroid initial 2–4 days of treatment to relieve symptoms

Discharge Criteria

- Uncomplicated rash
- Children may return to school once appropriate treatment has started

Discharge instructions

- Tinea pedis aftercare instructions
- Follow up with PCP within 14 days if no improvement in rash
- Follow up with PCP in 3–4 weeks if rash persists

Consult Criteria

- Moderate to severe superinfection
- Systemic symptoms
- Immunocompromised

Notes

REFERENCES:

Tinea Pedis Author: Courtney M Robbins, MD; Chief Editor: Dirk M Elston, MD medicine.medscape.com/article/1091684

Crawford F, Hollis S. Topical treatments for fungal infections of the skin and nails of the foot.. Cochrane Database of Systematic Reviews 2007, Issue 3. Art. No.: CD001434. DOI: 10.1002/14651858.CD001434

URTICARIA PROTOCOL

Definition

- Vascular reaction of the skin with transient wheals, soft papules and plaques usually with pruritus

Differential Diagnosis

- Erythema multiforme
- Angioedema
- Serum sickness
- Cutaneous vasculitis
- Toxic epidermal necrolysis
- Leprosy
- Juvenile rheumatoid arthritis
- Thrombophlebitis
- Cellulitis
- Pityriasis rosea
- Drug eruptions

Considerations

- Transient wheals — soft papules and plagues
- Is pruritic
- Acute reaction lasting < 30 days — usually allergic
- Chronic reaction lasting > 30 days — often idiopathic
- Angioedema can occur with chronic urticaria
- Ask about precipitants as in Causes

Causes

- Idiopathic
- Food allergies
- Infections
- Medications
- Insect bites or stings
- Sunlight
- Physical and emotional stressors
- Autoimmune diseases
- Hashimoto's thyroiditis
- Systemic diseases
- Serum sickness
- Transfusion reaction

Treatment Options

Benadryl (diphenhydramine)

- Adult: 25–50 mg PO, IM or IV
- Pediatrics: 1–2 mg/kg PO or IM (NMT 50 mg)
- May continue for 5–7 days PO

Pepcid (famotidine)

- Adult: 20 mg IV or 40 mg PO
- Pediatric: 0.25 mg/kg IV or 0.5 mg/kg PO (not to exceed maximum adult dose)

Epinephrine

- Adult 0.3 mg SQ/IM if urticaria part of anaphylaxis reaction (see Allergy Protocol)

Consider steroids (caution if diabetic)

- Prednisone 40–60 mg PO qday for 5–10 days (> 40 kg)
- Prednisone/prednisolone 1 mg/kg PO qday for 5–10 days (< 40 kg)

- Dexamethasone 4–6 mg qday for 5–10 days
- Avoid offending agent if known

Discharge Criteria

- Good resolution of rash and itching

Discharge instructions

- Urticaria aftercare instructions
- Return if rash persists or worsens
- Follow up with primary care provider within 7 days

Consult Criteria

- Systemic symptoms
- Hypotension
- See General Patient Criteria Protocol (page 15)

Notes

REFERENCES:

Fedorowicz Z, van Zuuren EJ, Hu N. Histamine H2–receptor antagonists for urticaria. Cochrane Database of Systematic Reviews 2012, Issue 3. Art. No.: CD008596. DOI: 10.1002/14651858.CD008596.pub2

Acute Urticaria Author: Henry K Wong, MD, PhD; Chief Editor: Michael A Kaliner, MD medicine.medscape.com/article/137362

Urticaria (Hives) Updated: Jun 13, 2018
Author: Henry K Wong, MD, PhD; Chief Editor: Dirk M Elston, MD

PITYRIASIS ROSEA PROTOCOL

Definition

- Common skin disorder observed in otherwise healthy people, more frequently in children and young adults which manifests as an acute, bilateral, self-limiting, papulosquamous eruption with a 6 to 8 week duration

Differential Diagnosis

- Viral exanthem
- Tinea corporis
- Erythema multiforme
- Secondary syphilis
- Drug eruption
- Tinea versicolor
- Seborrheic dermatitis

Considerations

- More common in late childhood to early adulthood
- Spring and fall prevalence
- Etiology unknown
- Not contagious
- Self-limited
- Typically resolves in 6–8 weeks, but can last 3–4 months
- Differential diagnosis considerations are secondary syphilis or drug eruption

Appearance

- Herald patch — single oval slightly raised plaque 2–5 cm, red color, on trunk usually
- Generalized eruption 1–2 weeks after herald patch
  - Fine scaling plaques and papules
  - Dark pink "Christmas tree" pattern along cleavage lines
  - Most noticeable on back

Treatment Options

- Benadryl (diphenhydramine) prn
- Aveeno or calamine prn

- UV exposure may hasten resolution
- Topical steroids

Discharge Criteria

- Self-limited disease so no consultation usually needed

Discharge criteria

- Pityriasis rosea aftercare instructions
- Follow up within 7–10 days as needed

Consult Criteria

- See General Patient Criteria Protocol as needed (page 15)

Notes

REFERENCES:

Pityriasis Rosea Author: Robert A Schwartz, MD, MPH; Chief Editor: Dirk M Elston, MD emedicine.medscape.com/article/1107532

Chuh AAT, Dofitas BL, Comisel G, Reveiz L, Sharma V, Garner SE, Chu FKM. Interventions for pityriasis rosea. Cochrane Database of Systematic Reviews 2007, Issue 2. Art. No.: CD005068. DOI: 10.1002/14651858.CD005068.pub2

HERPES SIMPLEX GINGIVOSTOMATITIS PROTOCOL

Definition

- Grouped vesicles on erythematous base of the skin or mucous membranes usually causes by herpes simplex−1

Differential Diagnosis

- Aphthous stomatitis
- Hand-Foot-Mouth disease
- Candidiasis
- Chanchroid
- Pharyngitis
- Secondary syphilis
- Urethritis

Considerations

- Regional lymphadenopathy can occur
- Oral lesions are HSV-1 type usually
- HSV-1 type can cause genital herpes
- Recurrent outbreaks in one-third of patients; decreases over time
- Prodrome of tingling, itching or pain approximately 24 hours preceding rash
- Diagnosis clinical
- Can be confirmed with Tzanck smear

Triggers

- Skin infections
- Stress
- UV radiation

Treatment Options

- Avoid skin contact with infected individuals
- Antiviral treatment within 48–72 hours of onset of lesions
- Lysine 1000 mg PO qD-TID x 6-12 months for prevention can be tried
  - Topical: (Super Lysine Plus) applied q2hr x 11days

Antiviral choices

- Acyclovir ointment 5% 5 times a day for 5 days
- Acyclovir 400 mg PO qid × 7 days for severe infection
- Pediatric acyclovir oral dosing 15 mg/kg 5 times a day for 7 days (do not exceed adult doses)
- Valtrex (valacyclovir) 2000 mg PO q12h × 1 day for lip

- Valacyclovir 1,000 mg PO bid for 7–10 days for intraoral lesions
- Abreva cream 10% OTC may help

Aphthous stomatitis

- Unknown etiology
- Many triggers
- May last weeks to months
- Recurrent

Treatment

- Local treatment with lidocaine 2% solution 5 ml swish and swallow qid prn (caution pediatric patients)
- Chlorhexidine, salt water or dilute hydrogen peroxide rinse
- Dexamethasone elixir 0.5mg/5 ml swish and spit qid — NPO for 30 minutes after
- Aphthasol (amlexanox) 0.5 cm to affected area qid after brushing teeth

Discharge Criteria

- Benign local disease

Discharge instructions

- Herpes simplex-1 aftercare instructions
- Follow up with PCP within 7–10 days as needed
- Return if rash increases or spreads

Consult Criteria

- Encephalitis
- Altered mental status
- Disseminated infection
- Severity of symptoms enough to cause dehydration
- Immunocompromised
- Ocular involvement
- Refer to General Patient Criteria Protocol (page 15) as needed

Notes

REFERENCES:

Nasser M, Fedorowicz Z, Khoshnevisan MH, Shahiri Tabarestani M. Acyclovir for treating primary herpetic gingivostomatitis. Cochrane Database of Systematic Reviews 2008, Issue 4. Art. No.: CD006700. DOI: 10.1002/14651858.CD006700.pub2

Herpes Simplex Author: Michelle R Salvaggio, MD, FACP; Chief Editor: Burke A Cunha, MD emedicine.medscape.com/article/218580

HERPETIC WHITLOW PROTOCOL

Definition

- Herpes simplex infection of the digits manifested as painful grouped vesicles

Differential Diagnosis

- Felon
- Paronychia
- Cellulitis

Considerations

- Patients usually less than 20 years of age
- Usually caused by HSV-1 (60%)
- From autoinoculation
- Incision not recommended
- Lesions crust over in 10–14 days and viral shedding stops at this point (heals in another 5–7 days after that)
- May have prodrome of fever and malaise
- Herpetic gingivostomatitis is almost pathognomonic in children
- Process is self-limited

Treatment Options

- Avoid skin contact with uninfected individuals

- Antiviral treatment within 48–72 hours of rash onset
- **Do not incise**

Antiviral choices

- Acyclovir ointment 5% 5 times a day for 5 days
- Acyclovir 400 mg PO qid × 7 days for severe infection
- Pediatric acyclovir oral dosing 15 mg/kg 5 times a day for 7 days (do not exceed adults doses)
- Valtrex (valacyclovir) 500–1000 mg PO bid × 7 days for adults

Discharge Criteria

- Most patients without severe superinfection

Discharge instructions

- Herpetic whitlow aftercare instructions
- Follow up with PCP within 7–10 days

Consult Criteria

- Moderate to severe superinfection
- Immunocompromised

Notes

REFERENCES:

Herpetic Whitlow Author: Michael S Omori, MD; Chief Editor: Steven C Dronen, MD, FAAEM emedicine.medscape.com/article/788056

Nasser M, Fedorowicz Z, Khoshnevisan MH, Shahiri Tabarestani M. Acyclovir for treating primary herpetic gingivostomatitis. Cochrane Database of Systematic Reviews 2008, Issue 4. Art. No.: CD006700. DOI: 10.1002/14651858.CD006700.pub2

GENITAL HERPES PROTOCOL

Definition

- Sexual transmitted disease by skin to skin contact caused by herpes simplex type 2 usually and occasionally by herpes simplex type 1 virus

Differential Diagnosis

- Candidiasis
- Syphilis
- Chanchroid
- Herpes zoster

Considerations

- May be transmitted during asymptomatic periods
- Recurrent outbreaks less frequent over time
- May cause systemic complaints
- Grouped vesicles crusting over in 4–15 days
  - New lesions appears 75% of time forming in 4–10 days
- Viral shedding lasts about 12 days
- Reactivation recurs in 90% of patients in the first year, sometimes multiple times
- May be asymptomatic

Treatment Options

- Avoid sexual contact with infected individuals
- Antiviral treatment within 48–72 hours of rash onset
- Analgesics prn
  - Vaseline or topical lidocaine may be applied to prevent pain during micturition
  - Micturition whilst sitting in a bath can help prevent urinary retention

Antiviral choices

Primary infection

- Acyclovir 400 mg PO tid × 7–10 days for severe infection

- Acyclovir 200 mg orally five times a day for 7–10 days
- Pediatric acyclovir oral dosing 15 mg/kg 5 times a day for 7 days (do not exceed adults doses)
- Valacyclovir 1 g orally twice a day for 7–10 days for adults
- Famciclovir 250 mg orally three times a day for 7–10 days
- Treatment can be extended if healing is incomplete after 10 days of therapy
- Topical acyclovir not recommended

Recurrent herpes

- Acyclovir 400 mg PO bid for 5 days
- Valacyclovir 500 mg PO bid for 3 days or 1,000 mg PO qday for 5 days

Discharge Criteria

- Immunocompetent patient without systemic symptoms

Discharge instructions

- Genital herpes aftercare instructions
- No sexual relations during prodrome and until lesions healed
- Follow up within 7–10 days prn
- Return if unable to void
- Return if rash worsens

Consult Criteria

- Systemic symptoms
- CNS infection
- Severe local symptoms
- Immunocompromised
- Urinary retention secondary to severe pain or sacral nerve involvement
- Refer to General Patient Criteria Protocol (page 15) as needed

Notes

REFERENCES:

Herpes Simplex Author: Michelle R Salvaggio, MD, FACP; Chief Editor: Burke A Cunha, MD emedicine.medscape.com/article/218580

Centers for Disease Control and Prevention (CDC). Diseases characterized by genital, anal, or perianal ulcers. In: Sexually transmitted diseases treatment guidelines, 2010. MMWR Recomm Rep. 2010 Dec 17;59(RR-12):18–39

HERPES ZOSTER (SHINGLES) PROTOCOL

Definition

- Acute dermatomal reactivation of varicella virus (chickenpox) in dorsal nerve roots ganglia

Differential Diagnosis

- Herpes simplex virus infection
- Varicella (chickenpox)
- Impetigo
- Cellulitis
- Folliculitis
- Contact dermatitis
- Prodromal pain thought to be
    - Biliary colic
    - Appendicitis
    - Angina

Considerations

- Seen with increasing age and decreasing immunocompetence
- Many patients have normal immune systems
- 10–20% of the general population will eventually develop herpes zoster
- Can have mild symptoms
- Immunosuppression increases risk of occurrence
- Prodrome of pain 3–5 days before rash occurs in 75% of cases
- Rash may be pruritic
- Rash crusts over in 7–10 days
- Complete healing may take more than 4 weeks
- Prodrome frequently causes medical evaluation for unrelated diseases
- Pain duration is usually < 1 month
- Recurrence is rare
- Herpes zoster can cause varicella (chickenpox) in exposed non-immunized patients
- Increased incidence of stroke and acute MI from cerebral or coronary artery involvement

Findings

- Initially a vesicular patchy dermatomal rash on a red base that may involve 1 or more adjacent dermatomes
- Usually no more than 2–3 adjacent dermatomes involved with normal hosts
- Thoracic dermatomes followed by lumbar dermatomes are the most commonly involved areas
- Fever, malaise, headache and fatigue occur in < 20% of patients
- Can involve cranial nerves and visceral organs
- Pain is usually described as burning, stabbing or throbbing

Post-herpetic neuralgia (PHN)

- Pain > 1 month is defined as post-herpetic neuralgia
- Increases with increasing age, rash severity and severity of pain
- Occurs in 10–15% of cases
- Most debilitating symptom of disease
- May be difficult to control pain
- Antiviral therapy early in disease may help prevent PHN

Postherpetic Neuralgia Treatment Guidelines (American Academy of Neurology 2008)

- Tricyclic antidepressants (TCAs)
  - Amitriptyline
  - Nortriptyline
  - Desipramine
  - Maprotiline(tetracyclic)
- Gabapentin
- Pregabalin
- Opioids
- Topical lidocaine patches are effective in the treatment of PHN
  - Topical lidocaine may be considered first line in elderly patients, especially if there are concerns regarding the adverse CNS effects with oral medications
- Strong opioids and capsaicin cream are second-line choices
  - Capsaicin patches show promise but the long-term effects of repeated applications, particularly on sensation, are unclear
- SSRI's limited usefulness

Treatment Options

- Antiviral treatment started within 72 hours of rash
  - Many experts recommend that if new skin lesions are still appearing or complications of herpes zoster are present, treatment should be started even if the rash began more than 3 days ago
- Valtrex (valacyclovir) 1,000 mg PO tid × 7 days

- Oral antiviral therapy should be considered for patients younger than 50 years with mild pain and rash, and truncal involvement to decrease PHN
  - Brivudin, famciclovir, and valacyclovir show greater efficacy than acyclovir
- Topical antiviral therapy is not recommended
- Consider varicella immune globulin in elderly or pediatric patients
- Shingrix (zoster vaccine recombinant, adjuvanted) for the prevention of shingles in adults aged 50 years and older
- Steroids may help quality of life in patients at risk for PHN — controversial
  - Prednisone 40–60 mg qday × 1 week; taper over following week
- The treatment of choice is high-dose intravenous acyclovir for immunocompromised patients
- Pain management approaches should be individualized based on pain severity, underlying conditions, and prior response to specific medications
- Acetaminophen and/or NSAIDs
  - For mild to moderate pain
    - Alone or in combination with weak opioids such as codeine or tramadol
- For moderate to severe pain, strong opioids such as oxycodone or morphine may be used
- Moderate to severe pain not rapidly responsive to treatment with an opioid analgesic or unable to tolerate opioids
  - Add or use one or some of following
    - Gabapentin or pregabalin
    - Tricyclic antidepressants (TCAs — especially nortriptyline)
    - Corticosteroids (e.g., prednisone or dexamethasone) may be considered
- For patients with pain that is inadequately controlled, refer to a pain specialist to evaluate eligibility for neural blockade

Discharge Criteria

- Uncomplicated infection

Discharge instructions

- Herpes zoster aftercare instructions
- Return for systemic symptom develop
- Follow up within 7–10 days

Consult Criteria

- Immunosuppression
- Severe or disseminated disease
- 3 or more dermatomes affected
- Ophthalmic disease or ophthalmic dermatomal involvement
- Involvement of trigeminal nerve
- Visceral involvement
- Intractable pain
- Ramsey Hunt syndrome (7–8th cranial nerve involvement)
- Acute altered mental status
- Meningitis or encephalitis

Notes

____

____

____

REFERENCES:

Gagliardi AMZ, Gomes Silva BN, Torloni MR, Soares BGO. Vaccines for preventing herpes zoster in older adults. Cochrane Database of Systematic Reviews 2012, Issue 10. Art. No.: CD008858. DOI: 10.1002/14651858.CD008858.pub2

Sampathkumar P, et al. Herpes Zoster (Shingles) and Postherpetic Neuralgia *Mayo Clin Proc*2009;84:274–280

Yawn BP, et al. A population-based study of the incidence and complication rates of herpes zoster before zoster vaccine introduction *Mayo Clin Proc* 2007; 82: 1341–1349.

Herpes Zoster Author: Camila K Janniger, MD; Chief Editor: Dirk M Elston,MD emedicine.medscape.com/article/1132465

NEJM, Vol. 369, pg. 255

Mayo Clin Proc, Vol. 84, pg. 274

[Guideline] Dworkin RH, Johnson RW, Breuer J, Gnann JW, et al. Recommendations for the management of herpes zoster. *Clin Infect Dis*. 2007 Jan 1. 44 Suppl 1:S1-26

[Guideline] Fashner J, Bell AL. Herpes zoster and postherpetic neuralgia: prevention and management. Am Fam Physician. 2011 Jun 15. 83 (12):1432-7

[Guideline] Stevens DL, Bisno AL, Chambers HF, Dellinger EP, Goldstein EJ, Gorbach SL, et al. Practice guidelines for the diagnosis and management of skin and soft tissue infections: 2014 update by the infectious diseases society of America. *Clin Infect Dis*. 2014 Jul 15. 59 (2):147-59.

Herpes Zoster (Shingles) Updated: Jan 25, 2019
Author: Camila K Janniger, MD; Chief Editor: Dirk M Elston, MD; emedicine medscape

Tick Bite Protocol

Definition

- Various disease processes transmitted by tick bites

Differential Diagnosis

- Lyme disease
- Rocky Mountain spotted fever
- Babesiosis
- Ehrlichiosis
- Measles
- Meningococcemia
- Rubella
- Varicella
- Mononucleosis
- Disseminated gonorrhea
- Typhus
- Kawasaki disease
- Toxic shock syndrome
- Secondary syphilis
- Gastroenteritis
- Allergic vasculitis
- Collagen vascular disease
- Juvenile rheumatoid arthritis
- Heat illness

Considerations

- Many patients with tick borne disease do not recall a tick bite
- Degree of tick engorgement is a marker for length of attachment
- Most tick borne illness occurs after attachment for 24–48 hours
  - Low risk of infection within 36 hours of tick attachment
- Antibiotic treatment following a tick bite is not recommended as a means to prevent anaplasmosis, babesiosis, ehrlichiosis, or Rocky Mountain spotted fever
  - In areas that are highly endemic for Lyme disease, a single prophylactic dose of doxycycline (200 mg for adults or 4.4 mg/kg for children of any age weighing less than 45 kg) may be used to reduce the risk of acquiring Lyme disease after the bite of a high risk tick bite
- Hard body ticks cause most disease
- Ticks are found in brushy or wooded areas usually
- Lifecycle over 2–3 years
- Have to brush against where tick is (they do not jump, fly, or drop on to people)
- Spring and summer time when most tick borne diseases are transmitted

- "Summer fever" or "summer virus" check CBC for thrombocytopenia and CMP
- Can cause DIC (disseminated intravascular coagulation)
- Can cause acute renal failure
- Beef and pork allergy thought to occur from Lone Star tick among others

Tick removal

- Grasp head and mouth parts at skin and pull with gentle pressure for several minutes until tick is removed
- Can inject skin at site with lidocaine 1% to see if tick will release on its own
- Any mouth parts left in skin are not infectious

Tick types

Deer tick

- Lyme
- Ehrlichiosis
- Babesiosis

Dog tick

- Rocky Mountain spotted fever (RMSF)

Lone Star tick

- Lyme
- RMSF
- Ehrlichiosis
- Tularemia
- Alpha–gal syndrome is a recently identified type of food allergy to red meat and other products made from mammals.
  - The condition begins when a Lone Star tick bites and transmits the alpha–gal substance that may cause an allergic response in some

Tick-borne diseases

- Lyme disease
- Rocky Mountain spotted fever (RMSF)
- Babesiosis
- Relapsing fever
- Tularemia
- Ehrlichiosis
- Q-fever
- Colorado Tick fever
- Tick paralysis

Lyme Disease

- See Lyme Disease Protocol

Rocky Mountain Spotted Fever

Symptoms and findings

- Fever and chills
- Up to 30–40% of patients report no tick bite within the past 14 days
- Headache
- Photosensitivity
- Nausea and vomiting
- Diarrhea
- Myalgias
- Maculopapular rash on extremities 3–5 days after fever onset spreading to rest of body
  - 10–20% do not get rash
  - 40–60% gets petechial rash 6 days after illness onset

Lab testing for

- CBC
  - Leukopenia
  - Anemia
  - Thrombocytopenia
- CMP
- Single titer of 1:64 supportive; 4 fold rise diagnostic
- PCR can be ordered

Treatment

- Adult: doxycycline 100 mg PO bid for 7 days continuing until afebrile for 2 days
- Children > 45 kg: doxycycline 100 mg PO qday for 7 days continuing for 2 days until afebrile
- Children < 45 kg: doxycycline 2–4 mg/kg PO qday for 7 days continuing until afebrile for 2 days
- Age < 8 consult physician (usually can use doxycycline for the treatment course needed in rickettsial infections)

- Macrolides (erythromycin) or Zithromax (azithromycin) do not work

Babesiosis

Malarial like disease

- Diffuse weakness is hallmark of disease
- Fever and chills
- Nausea and vomiting
- Headache
- Cough
- Diarrhea
- Splenomegaly
- Jaundice
- Petechiae

Lab findings

- Hemolytic anemia
- Thrombocytopenia
- Elevated LFT's
- Organisms can be seen on a slide smear prep

Treatment

- Adults — Zithromax (azithromycin) 500 mg qday for 7–10 days plus Atovaquone 750 mg PO bid for 7–10 days
- Children — Zithromax (azithromycin) 12 mg/kg qday for 7–10 days plus Atovaquone 20 mg/kg PO bid for 7–10 days (do not exceed adult doses)

Ehrlichiosis

Considerations

- Transmitted by Lone Star tick

Symptoms and findings

- Appear toxic
- Fever, chills and rigors
- Headache
- Nausea and vomiting
- Rare maculopapular rash 5–10% of patients
- Arthralgias

Lab testing for

- Leukopenia
- Anemia
- Thrombocytopenia
- Elevated LFT's and creatinine

Treatment

- Adult: doxycycline 100 mg PO bid for 14 days
- Children > 45 kg: doxycycline 100 mg PO qday for 14 days
- Children < 45 kg: doxycycline 3 mg/kg PO qday for 14 days
- Age < 8 consult physician (usually can use doxycycline for the treatment course needed in rickettsial infections)

Discharge Criteria For Tick Diseases

- Mild disease in healthy patient

Discharge instructions

- Tick bite aftercare instructions
- Follow up within 1–2 days
- Return if symptoms worsens or rash develops

Consult Criteria

- Ill appearing patient
- Thrombocytopenia
- Hepatitis
- Splenectomy
- Immunocompromised
- Hemolytic anemia
- Significant comorbidities
- Refer to General Patient Criteria Protocol (page 15)

Notes

____

____

____

REFERENCES:

Rocky Mountain Spotted Fever Author: Burke A Cunha, MD; Chief Editor: Michael Stuart Bronze, MD emedicine.medscape.com/article/228042

Ehrlichiosis Author: Burke A Cunha, MD; Chief Editor: Michael Stuart Bronze, MD emedicine.medscape.com/article/235839

American Academy of Pediatrics. Rocky Mountain Spotted Fever. In: Pickering LK, ed. 2003 Red Book: Report of the Committee on Infectious Disease. Elk Grove Village, IL: American Academy of Pediatrics; 2005:532–533

American Academy of Allergy, Asthma and Immunology (AAAAI) and World Allergy Organization (WAO) 2018 Joint Congress: Abstract 627, presented March 3, 2018; Abstract 721, presented March 5, 2018

cdc.gov/ticks/alpha-gal/index.html

cdc.gov/ticks/tickbornediseases/tick-bite-prophylaxis

Lyme Disease Protocol

Definition

- Infection caused by the spirochete Borrelia burgdorferi

Differential Diagnosis

- Rocky Mountain spotted fever (RMSF)
- Babesiosis
- Relapsing fever
- Tularemia
- Ehrlichiosis
- Q-fever
- Colorado Tick fever
- Rheumatic fever
- Viral meningitis
- Septic arthritis
- Juvenile rheumatoid arthritis
- Brown recluse spider bite
- Fibromyalgia
- Reiter syndrome

Considerations

- Transmitted by bite of infected tick
- Most common tick infection in North America
- Peak April and November prevalence
- Transmitted by deer tick most commonly
- 1/3 of patients recall a tick bite
- In areas that are highly endemic for Lyme disease, a single prophylactic dose of doxycycline (200 mg for adults or 4.4 mg/kg for children of any age weighing less than 45 kg) may be used to reduce the risk of acquiring Lyme disease after the bite of a high risk tick bite
- Can cause hepatitis
- Ocular involvement — keratitis, iritis, optic neuritis
- No person-to-person transmission
- Incubation 3–30 days (3–10 days most common)
- Carditis is admitted for IV antibiotics

Symptoms

Stage 1

Erythema migrans (EM)

- Is initial rash
- "Bull's eye" rash
- Macule with distinct red border that enlarges with central clearing
- Diameter > 5 cm
- Occurs in 90% of patients
- May be multiple in 10–20% of patients
- May have central induration, vesiculation or necrosis

Other symptoms/findings

- Headache
- Regional lymphadenopathy
- Myalgias
- Arthralgias
- Fatigue and malaise

Stage 2

- Days to weeks after tick bite
- Aseptic meningitis
- Cranial neuritis
- Radiculoneuritis

- Bell's palsy most common nerve involvement
- May present without rash
- Prognosis generally good

Cardiac

- Tachycardia
- Bradycardia
- AV block
- Myopericarditis

Stage 3

- Onset > 1 year after tick bite
- Acrodermatitis (resembles scleroderma)
- Arthritis
  - Brief attacks
  - Monoarthritis or oligoarthritis
  - Occasionally migratory
  - Most common joints: knee, shoulder, elbow

Evaluation

- CBC — leukocytosis, anemia, thrombocytopenia
- ESR > 30 seconds
- BMP
- LFT's
- Serology

Treatment

- Remove tick
- NSAID's prn
- ASA for cardiac involvement
- Vaccine (LYMErix) for prevention
- Doxycycline 100 mg PO within 72 hours of a deer tick bite effective in preventing Lyme disease

Stage 1 choices

- Amoxicillin 500 mg TID PO or doxycycline 100 mg BID PO (first choice) or cefuroxime for 21 days
- Zithromax (azithromycin) for 14–21 days

Stage 2 choices

- Amoxicillin with probenecid for 30 days
- Doxycycline for 10–21 days

AV Block

- First choice
  - Ceftriaxone 2 gms IV q24hrx 14–28 days (first choice for AV block)
  - Doxycycline 100 mg BID PO for 14–28 days (Europe)
- Second choice
  - Cefotaxime 2 gms IV q8hr. for 14–28 days
- May need pacemaker for high degree AV block

Neurologic manifestations

- Acute meningitis or radiculopathy
  - Ceftriaxone 2 gms IV q24hrx 14–28 days
  - Doxycycline 200-400 mg/day PO in two divided doses for 10-28 days
  - Cefotaxime 2 gms IV q8hr. for 14–28 days
  - Penicillin G 5,000,000 units IV q6hr. for 14–28 days
  - Lyme meningitis admit
  - Encephalitis IV antibiotics only
- Consult physician

Stage 3

Lyme arthritis

- Amoxicillin 500 mg TID PO or doxycycline 100 mg BID PO (first choice) or cefuroxime for 30–60 days
- Ceftriaxone 2 gms IV q24hr x 14–28 days if oral treatment unsuccessful
- Consult physician

Discharge Criteria

- Patients treated with oral therapy

Discharge instructions

- Tick bite aftercare instructions
- Follow up within 3–7 days
- Return if symptoms worsens

Consult Criteria

- Stage 2 or 3
- Immunocompromised
- Systemic symptoms
- Meningeal/encephalitis signs

Notes

REFERENCES:

Nadelman RB, et. al. Prophylaxis with single-dose doxycycline for the prevention of Lyme disease after an *Ixodes Scapularis* tick bite *NEJM* July 12, 2001

Mayo Clin Proc, 4/10,e13

Final Report of the Lyme Disease Review Panel of the Infectious Diseases Society of America April 22, 2010

emedicine.medscape.com/article/330178

VARICELLA (CHICKEN POX) PROTOCOL

Definition

- Successive crops of pruritic vesicles evolving to pustules and crusts caused by varicella zoster virus primarily in childhood

Differential Diagnosis

- Herpes simplex infection
- Herpes zoster
- Impetigo
- Hand-Foot-Mouth disease
- Henoch-Schonlein Purpura
- Erythema multiforme
- Stevens-Johnson syndrome
- Toxic Epidermal Necrolysis
- Scabies
- Toxic shock syndrome

Considerations

- Fever and malaise may occur
- Primarily childhood disease
- Older patients may have more severe disease — pneumonia or encephalitis
- Transmission by airborne droplets or direct contact
- Infectious period is from 2 days before first vesicle to when all vesicles are crusted
- Epidemics occur in winter and early spring in 3–4 year cycles
- Diagnosis is clinical
- "Dew drop" vesicle is initial finding
- New lesions usually stop appearing by day 5
- Palms and soles spared
- Self-limiting

Treatment and Prevention

- Supportive
- Vaccination
- Antivirals may decrease duration of infection (acyclovir and valacyclovir)
  - Especially useful in adults and immunocompromised
- No aspirin (can cause Reyes syndrome)
- Antibiotic choices for secondary bacterial infection
  - Mupirocin topical for 5–10 days
  - Retapamulin topical bid for 5 days (expensive)

  Purulent
  - Trimethoprim/sulfamethox–azole)
  - Doxycycline
  - Clindamycin

  Nonpurulent
  - Beta–lactams (cephalexin, amoxicillin/clavulanate etc.)
- Varicella zoster immune globulin for post–exposure up to 10 days in high risk individuals (pregnancy, immunocompromised)

Discharge Criteria

- Uncomplicated infection in children
- Trim nails

Discharge instructions

- Varicella aftercare instructions
- Return if systemic symptoms worse

Consult Criteria

- Encephalitis
- Altered mental status acutely
- Pregnancy
- Immunocompromised
- Systemic symptoms
- Moderate to severe secondary superinfection
- Adult infection

Notes

REFERENCES:

Klassen TP, Hartling L. Acyclovir for treating varicella in otherwise healthy children and adolescents. Cochrane Database of Systematic Reviews 2005, Issue 4. Art. No.: CD002980. DOI: 10.1002/14651858.CD002980

Chickenpox Author: Anthony J Papadopoulos, MD; Chief Editor: Dirk M Elston, MD emedicine.medscape.com/article/1131785

HAND INFECTION PROTOCOL

Definition

- Local inflammatory reaction of the skin and/or subcutaneous tissue of the hand secondary to bacteria or viral infection

Paronychia

Definition

- Cellulitis or abscess of nail margins and/or nail bed

Differential diagnosis

- Felon
- Draining osteomyelitis
- Herpetic whitlow
- Neoplasm

Considerations

- Secondary to trauma, nail biting, chemicals, incorrect nail trimming or chronic moist environment (dishwashers, bartenders, etc.)
- Acute infection: staph or strep
- Chronic infection: C. albicans or other fungi
- Vesicles suggest herpes infection
  - Do not incise herpes infection (herpetic whitlow)

Evaluation

- CBC, BMP if signs of systemic infection present
- X-ray if chronic or recurrent to check for osteomyelitis

Treatment

No abscess

- Warm soaks and antibiotics

Subcuticular Abscess

- Local 1% plain lidocaine digital block
- Elevate eponychial fold at the nail plate
- Incise at maximal swelling and tenderness to allow drainage
- If pus extends below nail, remove lateral ¼ – ½ of nail
- Give antibiotics for any associated cellulitis — MRSA coverage (see Soft Tissue Abscess Protocol) or antibiotic database

Discharge criteria

- Noncomplicated paronychia without systemic

symptoms/findings or bony involvement

Discharge instructions

- Paronychia aftercare instructions
- Refer to primary care provider or hand surgeon within 7–10 days as needed

Consult criteria

- Osteomyelitis
- Systemic symptoms/findings
- Associated proximal hand or tendon infection

Felon

Definition

- Infection/abscess of the pulp space of the distal finger

Differential diagnosis

- Paronychia
- Draining osteomyelitis
- Herpetic whitlow

Considerations

- Wooden splinters, minor cuts or diabetic testing methods are the common causes
- Paronychia spreading to pulp
- Staph aureus most common infection
- Can lead to osteomyelitis

Evaluation

- X-ray if osteomyelitis is suspected
- Neurovascular and tendon examination

Treatment

- Discuss with physician unless experienced
- Digital block with 1% plain lidocaine ± Marcaine (bupivacaine)

Longitudinal incision in the midline is effective without serious complications that are observed with other recommended incisions (incise skin only)

OR

- Lateral incision 5 mm distal to DIP joint on the dorsal 1/3 avoiding the neurovascular bundle, extending not past the distal nail corner (incise skin only)
  - Avoid incising the ulnar thumb side, and the radial side of index or middle finger to avoid a scar that interferes with pinching
- Pack with gauze
- Splint and elevate finger

Antibiotics choices

- Cefazolin IV, then cephalexin or dicloxicillin PO × 10 days
- Septra DS bid × 10 days
- Clindamycin 300 mg tid × 10 days

Discharge instructions

- Felon aftercare instructions
- Follow up in 24 hours
- NSAID's or narcotic short course

Consult criteria

- Osteomyelitis
- Flexor tenosynovitis
- Systemic symptoms or findings

Herpetic Whitlow Protocol

Definition

- Herpes simplex infection of the digits manifested as painful grouped vesicles

Differential diagnosis

- Felon
- Paronychia
- Cellulitis

Considerations

- Patients usually less than 20 years of age
- Usually caused by HSV-1
- Do not incise

Treatment options

- Avoid contact with infected individuals
- Antiviral treatment within 48–72 hours

Antiviral medication choices

- Acyclovir ointment 5% 5 times a day for 5 days
- Acyclovir 400 mg PO qid × 7 days for severe infection
- Pediatric acyclovir oral dosing 15 mg/kg 5 times a day for 7 days (do not exceed adult doses)
- Valtrex (valacyclovir) 500–1000 mg PO bid × 7 days for adults

Discharge criteria

- Most patients without severe superinfection

Discharge instructions

- Herpetic whitlow aftercare instructions
- Follow up with PCP within 7–10 days

Consult criteria

- Moderate to severe superinfection
- Immunocompromised

Closed (Clenched) Fist Infection or Injury

Definition

- Laceration or skin injury from a clenched fist striking human teeth

Differential diagnosis

- Cellulitis
- Osteomyelitis
- Abscess

Considerations

- Assumed to be from human teeth in altercations
- High risk for infection
- All bite wounds with evidence of infection require physician consultation
- Usually over the MP dorsal joint

Evaluation

- Neurovascular and tendon examination
- X-ray
- CBC if fever present
- Assess for infection

Treatment

- No suturing of wound
- Irrigate with > 250 cc of 0.1% betadine with 18 gauge angiocath (1% betadine: mix 1 cc of 10% betadine with 99 cc NS)
- May use tap water mixed with soap initially, then flushed with tap water (potable water)
- If no infection present, and no neurovascular or tendon acute deficits or injuries, then prescribe amoxicillin/clavulanate for 5 days or follow Sanford Guide or other drug databases for prophylaxis treatment
- Pain treatment prn
- See Human and Animal Bite Protocol

Discharge criteria

- Noninfected wound
- No bony, tendon or neurovascular acute abnormality
- Reliable follow up

Discharge instructions

- Human bite aftercare instructions
- Return if infection occurs in bite
- Return if pain increases

Consult criteria

- Infected wound
- Bony, tendon or neurovascular acute abnormality
- Hand surgeon preferred if available

Deep Space Infection

- Consult physician

Flexor Tenosynovitis

Definition

- Infection or inflammation of the flexor tendon sheath

Differential diagnosis

- Noninfectious flexor tenosynovitis
- Fracture

- Septic joint
- Tendon rupture
- Gout
- Rheumatoid arthritis
- Endocarditis

Considerations

- Usually penetrating injury history to volar surface; frequently cat bites
- Kanavel's signs
  - Pain on passive extension
  - Finger held in flexed position
  - SEVERE tenderness along tendon sheath
  - Symmetric swelling (sausage finger)
  - May see with ultrasound using linear probe in water bath as dark fluid collections around tendon

Consult criteria

- All patients
- Admission
- Surgical treatment
- IV antibiotics

Notes

REFERENCES:

Herpetic Whitlow Author: Michael S Omori, MD; Chief Editor: Steven C Dronen, MD, FAAEM emedicine.medscape.com/article/788056

Nasser M, Fedorowicz Z, Khoshnevisan MH, Shahiri Tabarestani M. Acyclovir for treating primary herpetic gingivostomatitis. Cochrane Database of Systematic Reviews 2008, Issue 4. Art. No.: CD006700. DOI: 10.1002/14651858.CD006700.pub2

Felon Author: Glen Vaughn, MD; Chief Editor: Steven C Dronen, MD, FAAEM emedicine.medscape.com/article/782537

Common Acute Hand Infections Dwayne C. Clark, CDR, MC, USN, Naval Hospital Jacksonville, Jacksonville, Florida *Am Fam Physician.* 2003 Dec 1;68(11):2167–2176

Hand Infections Author: Rohini J Haar, MD; Chief Editor: Rick Kulkarni, MD emedicine.medscape.com/article/783011

Hematology and Oncology

Section Contents

When using any protocol, always follow the Guidelines of Proper Use (page 12).

Venous Thromboembolic Disease Protocol

Definition

- Formation of thrombus within veins that may or may not propagate toward the central circulation

Differential diagnosis

- Cellulitis
- Hematoma
- Superficial thrombophlebitis
- Varicose veins
- Contusion or muscle strain/tear
- Arterial insufficiency
- Postphlebitic syndrome
- Dependent edema
- Lymphedema
- Baker's cyst

Considerations

- Deep vein thrombosis (DVT) and pulmonary embolism (PE) are manifestations of the same disease process
- DVT involves the legs most commonly, followed by the arms
- Early recognition and treatment are very important in decreasing morbidity and mortality
- Thrombus damages vein valves causing reflux of blood and postphlebitic syndrome — chronic edema and venous stasis ulcers
- Most DVT's develop complete or partial recanalization and collaterals over time
  - More than half of patients with proximal DVT have residual vein thrombosis on ultrasound 6 months - 1 year after completion of therapy
  - Presence of residual DVT has been shown to be a risk factor for recurrent VTE
- Proximal large vein thrombosis can cause pulmonary embolism
- PE occurs in ~ 10% of DVT
- Calf DVT may produce 1/3 of PE (ultrasound not as accurate there)

- Most DVT is occult and resolves spontaneously
- Up to 40% of DVT patients when diagnosed have a silent PE
- CTA should only be performed in the context of clinical suspicion and in patients with an appropriate pre-test probability
- Thrombophilia screening should only be performed after therapeutic management if indicated (usually not indicated)
  - Tests should never be performed in the acute setting: both anticoagulant therapy and the inflammatory state accompanying any thromboembolic event falsify the results and preclude any conclusions
- Paradoxical emboli may pass through an atrial septal defect and cause a CVA or distal arterial occlusion
- D-dimers remain elevated for 7 days after symptomatic thrombus

Risk factors

- Cancer
- Advanced age
- Immobilization > 3 days
- Major surgery in the prior 4 weeks
- Clotting disorders are common risk factors for venous thromboembolism (VTE)
  - 5–10% of VTE is from protein C, protein S or antithrombin III disorders
  - Factor V Leiden mutation
- Most common risk factor is prior VTE
- CHF
- AMI
- CVA
- Sepsis
- Estrogens
- IV drug abuse
- Pregnancy and postpartum period
- Thrombocytosis and polycythemia vera

Virchow triad for formation of thrombus

- Venous stasis
- Activation of the coagulation system
- Vein damage

Goals of DVT treatment

- Reduce morbidity
- Prevent postphlebitic syndrome
- Prevent pulmonary embolism

Signs and symptoms

DVT

- Extremity pain
- Involved area red and swollen
- May be asymptomatic

Severe DVT

Phlegmasia alba dolens

- Blanched leg appearance
- Massive iliofemoral thrombotic occlusion

Phlegmasia cerulea dolens

- Follows phlegmasia alba dolens
- Associated with arterial spasm
- Risk of gangrene
- Shock may occur
- Mortality 20–40% if venous gangrene develops
- Notify or consult promptly a physician for phlegmasia of any type
- May be treated conservatively with heparin and elevation if no ischemia present

Pulmonary embolism (see section in Dyspnea Protocol and below)

- Hypoxemia
- Chest pain
- Shock or hypotension
- May have no symptoms or findings

EKG

- Sinus tachycardia most common

  - Nonspecific STT wave changes or with ischemic appearing biphasic T waves in V2 and V3
  - New right bundle branch block
  - S1Q3T3 pattern in 19%
  - Right axis deviation in 5%
  - Left axis deviation in 10%
  - New onset atrial fibrillation
  - EKG may be normal in 13%

Evaluation options

- Chest x-ray
- CBC if fever or tachycardia present
- BMP if diabetic or tachycardia present
- D-dimer (if negative with Well's criteria 0–1 makes PE unlikely)
- CT chest (see below)
- Apply Well's pulmonary embolism and DVT criteria and chart Well's score as indicated
- Extremity venous ultrasound for moderate to high probability Well's criteria as indicated
  - CT abdominal/pelvis scan for suspected intra-abdominal or pelvic DVT
  - Venography if needed
  - MRI if needed
- Record positive or negative calf tenderness and Homan's sign (for malpractice considerations)

Evaluation with D-dimer

- Useful if negative at cutoff value to rule out DVT or PE
  - Rare exception is cancer (especially hematological cancer) patients with PE may have negative d–dimer in small percentage (0.4%)
- Negative D-dimer with low to moderate probability Well's DVT or PE score largely excludes venous thromboembolic disease
- Well's DVT criteria high probability: order ultrasound scan regardless of D-dimer result
- If positive — not as useful as a negative result which usually rules out VTE (venous thromboembolic) disease
- Frequently positive with
  - Hospitalization in past month
  - Chronic bedridden or low activity state
  - Increasingly positive with age without significant acute disease process
    - D-dimer increases 10 mcg/L for every year over 50 years of age if the upper cutoff is 500 mcg/L (80 year old with d-dimer 700 mcg/L would be in the normal range)
    - If another assay used, then 2% increase/year over age 50 may be used to adjust upper limit for age
    - D–dimer age adjusted calculators available
  - CHF
  - Chronic disease processes
  - Edematous states

Well's DVT criteria

- One point each:
  - Active cancer
  - Paralysis/recent cast immobilization
  - Recently bedridden > 3 days or surgery < 4 weeks
  - Deep vein tenderness
  - Entire leg edema
  - Calf swelling > 3 cm over other leg
  - Pitting edema > other calf
  - Collateral superficial veins
- Two points — alternative diagnosis less likely

High probability: ≥ 3 points

Moderate probability: 1–2 points

Low probability: 0 points

Testing and imaging for DVT

Well's DVT criteria ≥ 1–2 with painful or swollen extremity

- Order D-dimer test (unless patient likely to have positive result regardless of DVT potential)

- Venous Doppler ultrasound of extremity (unless D-dimer negative)
  - May be falsely negative with calf DVT
- Venography if needed
- MRI if needed
- Coumadin (warfarin) therapy can cause falsely negative D-dimer
- Ultrasound may be repeated if negative, and DVT suspicion persists, in 5–7 days

Well's PE criteria score 3 or greater consider D-dimer and CT chest PE protocol

- Suspected DVT = 3
- Alternative diagnosis less likely than PE = 3
- Heart rate > 100 = 1.5
- Immobilization/surgery past 4 wks. = 1.5
- Previous DVT/PE = 1.5
- Hemoptysis = 1
- Cancer past 6 months = 1

Well's score ≥ 6: order CTA chest PE protocol

Document positive or negative Homan's sign or calf tenderness regardless of Well's scores

Document PERC and/or Well's scores when appropriate

Pulmonary Embolism (PE)

Definition

- Blockage of pulmonary artery usually by a migrating blood clot from legs (most commonly) or pelvic veins

Differential diagnosis

- Acute coronary syndrome
- Acute pericarditis
- ARDS
- Panic disorder
- Aortic stenosis
- Atrial fibrillation
- Cardiogenic shock
- Cor pulmonale
- Cardiomyopathy
- COPD
- Fat embolism
- Mitral stenosis
- Acute MI
- Pneumothorax
- Pulmonary hypertension
- Sudden cardiac death
- Superior vena cava syndrome
- Syncope or near syncope

Considerations

- Can be either minimally asymptomatic or catastrophic
- Occurs 1 person per 1,000/year
- Clinical assessment performed by experienced physicians has proven non-inferior to standardized prediction scores and has an important place in everyday clinical practice
- CTA should only be performed in the context of clinical suspicion and in patients with an appropriate pre-test probability
- Commonly a missed diagnosis on initial evaluation
- PE are increasingly observed as incidental findings, i.e., without clinical correlate
- Reliability of detection of PE via CTA decreases significantly in peripheral clots with small filling defects (<6mm) and, overall, the incidence is overestimated
- Present in > 30% of DVT patients even though one half have on PE symptoms
- Common cause of hospitalized patient death
- One year mortality is 24%
  - Mainly due to cardiac disease, recurrent PE, infection or cancer
- NT-proBNP >500 ng/L associated with central PE and possible predictor of increased death risk (pre–existing conditions such renal failure and atrial fibrillation that have chronic increased NT-proBNP

would make this assumption not as useful)

- Elevated troponin is an increased severity risk marker — 19% probability of death during hospitalization
- Massive PE second only to sudden cardiac death as a cause of sudden death
- Majority of deaths from PE occur in the first 1–2 hours of care
- Nonmassive PE defined as a systolic BP ≥ 90 mmHG and accounts for 95.5–96% of patients
- See Well's Pulmonary Embolism Criteria in above section

Pulmonary Embolism Rule-out Criteria (PERC Rule)

(Reportedly decreases significantly the likelihood of pulmonary embolism if all 8 criteria met — not superior to clinical gestalt)

- Age < 50
- Pulse oximetry > 94%
- Heart rate < 100
- No history of DVT or VTE
- No hemoptysis
- No estrogen use
- No unilateral leg swelling
- No recent surgery or trauma hospitalization past 4 weeks

American College of Physicians (ACP) 2015

- Plasma D-dimer tests are more appropriate for those at intermediate risk for a PE, and no testing may be necessary for some patients at low risk
- Use either the Wells or Geneva rules to choose tests based on a patient's risk for PE
- In low risk patients, clinicians should use the 8 Pulmonary Embolism Rule-Out Criteria (PERC), and if negative for all 8 criteria then no testing is needed
- Intermediate risk patients or for those at low risk who do not meet all of the rule-out criteria, use a high-sensitivity plasma D-dimer test initially
- In patients >50 years use an age-adjusted threshold age × 10 ng/mL
  - Normal D-dimer levels increase with age
- D-dimer level below the age-adjusted cutoff should not receive any imaging studies
  - Patients with elevated D-dimer levels should receive imaging
- Patients at high risk skip the D-dimer test and proceed to CT pulmonary angiography
  - Negative D-dimer test does not eliminate the need for imaging in these patients
- Obtain ventilation-perfusion scans in patients with a contraindication to CT pulmonary angiography or if CT pulmonary angiography is unavailable
- Use validated clinical prediction rules to estimate pretest probability in patients in whom acute PE is being considered

American College of Emergency Physicians (ACEP) 2011

- Negative quantitative D-dimer assay results can be used to exclude PE in patients with a **low** pretest probability for PE
- Negative quantitative D-dimer assay results may be used to exclude PE in patients with an **intermediate** pretest probability for PE
- PE unlikely patients (Wells score 4) or low pretest probability for PE who require additional diagnostic testing (positive D-dimer result or highly sensitive D–dimer not available), a negative multidetector CT pulmonary angiogram alone can be used to exclude PE
- Intermediate or high pretest probability for PE and a negative CT pulmonary angiogram result in whom a clinical concern for

PE still exists and CT venogram has not already been performed, consider additional diagnostic testing (e.g., D-dimer, lower extremity imaging, VQ scanning, traditional pulmonary arteriography) prior to exclusion of VTE disease

- Venous ultrasound
  - May be considered as initial imaging in patients with obvious signs of DVT for whom venous ultrasound is readily available
  - Patients with relative contraindications for CT scan (e.g., renal insufficiency, CT contrast agent allergy)
  - Pregnant patients
  - A positive finding in a patient with symptoms consistent with PE can be considered evidence for diagnosis of VTE disease and may preclude the need for additional diagnostic imaging

Risk factors

Virchow triad

- Endothelial injury
- Stasis or turbulence of blood flow
- Blood hypercoagulability

- Immobilization
- Malignancy
- Inherited or acquired thrombophilia states (hypercoagulable states)
- Acute medical illness
- Surgery past 3 months
- Trauma (mostly lower extremities or pelvis) past 3 months
- Oral contraceptives or estrogen
- Pregnancy
- Prior pulmonary embolism
- COPD
- Heart failure
- Stroke, hemiplegia or paralysis
- Central venous lines within past 3 months

Signs and symptoms

- Tachypnea (respiratory rate >16/min) — 96%
- Rales — 58%
- Accentuated second heart sound — 53%
- Tachycardia (heart rate >100/min) — 44%
- Fever>37.8°C (100.04°F) — 43%
- Diaphoresis — 36%
- S_3 or S_4 gallop — 34%
- Clinical signs and symptoms suggesting thrombophlebitis — 32%
- Lower extremity edema: 24%
- Cardiac murmur — 23%
- Cyanosis — 19%

Presenting complaints and findings

- Dyspnea — 73%
- Pleuritic chest pain — 66%
- Cough — 37%
- Hemoptysis — 13%
- Hypoxia
- Delirium in elderly
- Wheezing
- Productive cough
- Syncope or near syncope
- Hypotension or relative hypotension (for the patient with hypertension history)
- Lung infarction
- New onset atrial fibrillation
- Ventricular arrhythmia
- Pleural effusion
- Pulseless electrical activity

Testing options

- Chest x–ray (may be normal or nonspecific)
  - Westermark sign — decreased vascularity
  - Hampton hump — pleural based triangular density from pulmonary infarction (rare)
- CBC
- EKG
  - Sinus tachycardia most common

- Nonspecific STT wave changes or with ischemic appearing biphasic T waves in V2 and V3
- New right bundle branch block
- S1Q3T3 pattern in 20%
- Right axis deviation in 5%
- Left axis deviation in 10%
- New onset atrial fibrillation
- D–dimer (do not use in high clinical PE probability — scan instead)
  - More useful in eliminating younger healthy patients if negative
- ABG (may be normal or have increased A–a gradient or hypoxemia)
- BNP or NT-proBNP
- Troponin
- Echocardiogram RV strain have 10% mortality, 0% mortality with normal RV function
- Chemistries
- CTA chest pulmonary embolism protocol
- V/Q lung scan if CTA chest not available or contraindicated
  - May be performed in healthy low risk patients (if normal then very useful)
  - Low probability scans can have PE from 4–20% depending whether clinical suspicion is low or high
- Leg venous ultrasound

Treatment guidelines

American College of Chest Physicians (ACCP)

- Dabigatran, rivaroxaban, apixaban, or edoxaban are preferred over vitamin K antagonist (VKA) therapy as long-term (first 3 months) anticoagulant therapy for noncancer patients
- Low-molecular-weight heparin (LMWH) is recommended over VKA therapy, dabigatran, rivaroxaban, apixaban, or edoxaban as long-term (first 3 months) anticoagulation therapy for patients with cancer-associated thrombosis
- Aspirin is recommended over no aspirin to prevent recurrent venous thromboembolism (VTE) in patients who are stopping anticoagulant therapy and do not have a contraindication to aspirin
- In most patients with acute PE not associated with hypotension, systemically administered thrombolytic therapy is not recommended
- Selected patients with acute PE who deteriorate after starting anticoagulant therapy but have yet to develop hypotension and who have a low bleeding risk, systemically administered thrombolytic therapy is preferred over no such therapy
- Thrombolytic therapy is suggested in select patients with acute PE not associated with hypotension and with a low bleeding risk whose initial clinical presentation or clinical course after starting anticoagulation suggests a high risk of developing hypotension
- Thrombolytic therapy is not recommended for most patients with acute PE not associated with hypotension
- First episode of VTE and with a low or moderate risk of bleeding should have extended anticoagulant therapy
- First episode of VTE with a high bleeding risk should have therapy limited to 3 months
- Patients who have PE and preexisting irreversible risk factors, such as deficiency of antithrombin III, proteins S and C, factor V Leiden mutation, or the presence of antiphospholipid antibodies, should be placed on long-term anticoagulation

Treatments

- IV NS 250–500 ml bolus if hypotensive and notify physician promptly **(severe PE patients may decompensate with IVF bolus due to acute very high right ventricular pressure and strain from PE — exercise caution and consider norepinephrine drip instead)**
- **Embolectomy** in very unstable patients in centers with CV surgery available and thrombolytics thought not to be adequate therapy or contraindicated
  - Nitric oxide 10ppm inhalation may be tried to temporize condition prior to surgery or thrombolytics — selective dilation of the pulmonary vasculature and antiplatelet activity

Anticoagulation

- Is passive anticoagulation— prevents new thrombus formation while body breaks down existing thrombus
- **Enoxaparin** (LMWH) 1mg/kg q12hour SQ or 1.5 mg/kg q24hours SQ
  - Do not use with creatinine clearance <30
  - Do not use with history of heparin induced thrombocytopenia (HIT)
  - No PTT monitoring
- **Heparin** (unfractionated) load 80units/kg IV and 18 units/kg/hour IV
  - Goal is PTT 1.5–2.5 times normal
  - Creatinine clearance <30 increased bleeding risk

  Do not use with history of heparin induced thrombocytopenia Stop all heparins if platelet count drops to 100,000, or a 50% decrease in baseline platelet count occurs, or 30% decrease in platelet count with new thrombus formation development (heparin induced thrombocytopenia — a life threatening immune process)
- **Warfarin** 15 mg PO load
  - Overlap with heparin until INR 2–3
  - 2–10mg PO daily (start >6 hours after LMWH)
  - **<u>Contraindicated in pregnancy</u>**

Direct oral anticoagulants (DOACs)

- **Apixaban (Eliquis)** 10 mg PO BID x 7 days, then 5 mg BID
  - Not recommended in severe liver disease
- **Rivaroxaban (Xarelto)** 15 mg PO q12hr for 21 days with food, then 20 mg PO qday

Thrombolytics

- **TPA** 100mg IV over 2 hours
- May give 100mg IVP during CPR in PE or suspected PE coding patients and continue code for 1 hour
- Heparin bolus and drip near end of TPA infusion or immediately following

Discharge criteria for pulmonary embolism

Hestia criteria for outpatient PE therapy — A “No” answer to all questions needed to treat outpatient

- Hemodynamically unstable
- Clot busting necessary
- Bleeding issues

- Oxygen required
- Ongoing anticoagulation
- Severe pain
- Inpatient status needed
- Renal failure
- Liver disease
- Pregnancy
- Documented HIT
- Clinical judgment that outpatient therapy is safe for patient
- No tachycardia

Consult criteria

- Discuss all patients with a physician

Admission criteria

- Unstable or severe PE admit to ICU
- Patients not meeting Hestia criteria
- New elevation of troponin and/or NT-proBNP
- Clinical judgment that overrides Hestia criteria

Discharge

- Hestia criteria for outpatient PE therapy — A "No" answer to all questions needed to treat as outpatient
- Clinical judgment that outpatient therapy is safe for patient
- No tachycardia

DVT treatment

May be treated as outpatient if none of the following present

- Pulmonary embolism
- Significant cardiopulmonary comorbidities
- Pregnancy
- Morbid obesity
- Homeless
- Creatinine > 2 mg/dL
- No follow up
- Inherited bleeding disorder
- Iliofemoral DVT
- Contraindications to anticoagulation
- Disorder of coagulation
- Patient does not want to be discharged

- Enoxaparin (Lovenox) 1 mg/kg SQ q12hr (1 mg/kg SQ q24hr if creatinine clearance<30 ml/minute)

OR

- Heparin (unfractionated) 80–100 U/kg IV loading dose and 15–18 U/kg/hour IV (keep PTT 2–2.5 times normal

OR

- Fondaparinux (Arixtra) – no INR or PTT monitoring needed
  - < 50 kg: 5 mg SQ qday
  - 50–100 kg: 7.5 mg SQ qday
  - > 100 kg: 10 mg SQ qday
- Warfarin (Coumadin)
  - 2–10 mg PO qday to achieve INR 2–3
  - Treatment for 3–6 months
  - Can cause initially a transient hypercoagulable state if started without heparin treatment
  - Has a myriad of drug and other substances interactions
  - Can cause life threatening hemorrhage
  - Read drug information before using to determine interactions and patient risks
- Thrombin inhibitors
  - Argatroban for heparin-induced thrombocytopenia
- Thrombolytics
  - Use under direction of physician
  - For severe iliofemoral DVT (Phlegmasia cerulea dolens) — catheter directed

Direct oral anticoagulants (DOACs)

- **Rivaroxaban** 15 mg PO q12hr for 21 days with food, then 20 mg PO qday for 6 months
- **Dabigatran** for prophylaxis and if patient on parenteral anticoagulant 5–10 days already
- **Apixaban (Eliquis)** 10 mg PO BID x 7 days, then 5 mg BID
  - Not recommended in severe liver disease

Mechanical extraction

- Consult vascular surgeon or interventional physician with appropriate skill set

DVT prophylaxis

- Enoxaparin (Lovenox) 40 mg SQ q24hr

OR

- Heparin (unfractionated) 5,000 units SQ q8–12h

For admitted patients with any of the following

- Age > 60 years
- CHF
- Systemic infection
- History of DVT or PE
- Inflammatory disorders
- Cancer
- ICU admission
- Hypercoagulable state
- Immobilization ≥ 3 days or severely compromised ambulation

Discharge criteria

- DVT not meeting exclusionary criteria above
  - Discuss with physician

Consult criteria

- All DVT and PE patients, or suspected DVT/PE diagnosis
  - Tachycardia
  - Hypotension or relative hypotension (SBP < 105 with history of hypertension)
  - Dyspnea

Notes

REFERENCES:

Deep Venous Thrombosis Author: Kaushal (Kevin) Patel, MD; Chief Editor: Barry E Brenner, MD, PhD, FACEP emedicine.medscape.com/article/1911303

Büller HR, Prins MH, Lensin AW, Decousus H, Jacobson BF, Minar E, et al. Oral rivaroxaban for the treatment of symptomatic pulmonary embolism. *N Engl J Med.* Apr 5 2012;366(14):1287–97

Boyles S. Thrombolysis aids PE survival, but ups bleeding risk. *MedPage Today* [serial online]. June 17, 2014; Updated June 18, 2014;Accessed June 22, 2014

Pulmonary Embolism Author: Daniel R Ouellette, MD, FCCP; Chief Editor: Zab Mosenifar, MD emedicine.medscape.com/article/300901

Age-Adjusted D-Dimer Cutoff Levels to Rule Out Pulmonary Embolism: The ADJUST-PE Study *JAMA.* 2014;311(11):1117-1124. doi:10.1001/jama.2014.2135

Circulation;129:917

J Emerg Med. 2017;52:184

Clin Chest Med. 2018;39:539

Myths in the Evaluation of Acute Pulmonary Embolism; emedhome.com clinical pearl

Stussi-Helbling M, et al. Am J Med. 2019

SICKLE CELL ANEMIA PROTOCOL

Definition

- Inherited disorder of hemoglobin synthesis causing sickling and destruction of RBC's with resulting vascular obstruction and tissue ischemia

Differential Diagnosis

- Appendicitis
- Cholecystitis
- Pneumonia
- Pulmonary embolism
- Acute myocardial infarction
- Priapism
- Anemia from other causes
- Hemorrhage
- Pancreatitis
- Osteomyelitis
- CVA
- Meningitis
- Hepatitis

Considerations

- Has increased incidence of life threatening infections
- Functional asplenia
- Chronic hemolysis
- Hand-foot syndrome — ages 6–24 months
  - Dactylitis presenting as bilateral painful and swollen hands and/or feet in children
- Aseptic necrosis of bone (humeral or femoral head) and salmonella osteomyelitis may occur
- Vascular occlusion pain most common presentation
- Stroke common
- Pulmonary embolism increased risk
- Mean survival: females 48 years; males 42 years from SS disease
- WBC elevated; platelet count elevated; reticulocyte count averages > 2–3%
- Precipitants
  - Infection
  - Cold exposure
  - Dehydration

Crises types

Vaso–occlusive crises

- Bones
- Lungs (acute chest syndrome)
- Musculoskeletal pain most common complaint
- Abdominal pain 2nd most common complaint

Acute chest syndrome (ACS)

- Pulmonary infiltrates with one of the following:
  - Chest pain
  - Cough
  - Fever
  - Tachypnea
  - Wheezing
- Leading cause of death
- 50% of ACS cases develop in patients admitted for other sickle cell disease diagnoses
- May need simple or exchange transfusion
- Antibiotics such as azithromycin, ceftriaxone etc., among others pending cultures
- Bronchodilators for bronchospasm

Aplastic Crises

- Severe anemia from cessation of erythropoiesis; can be related to parvovirus B19V infection
- Low reticulocyte count

Acute splenic sequestration crises

- Sudden hemoglobin decrease ≥ 2 gms
- Syncope
- Abdominal distension

Priapism

- Sickle cell patients may need exchange transfusion
- Consult urologist immediately
- See Male Genitalia Protocol

Pediatric sickle cell disease (SCD) and fever

Admission criteria

- Age < 2 years with hemoglobin SS (HbSS) disease or hemoglobin S–β° (HbS–β°)
  - HbSC or HbS–β+ less likely to have bacteremia and age alone not an admission criteria
- Temperature > 104°F (40°C)
- WBC > 30,000 or < 5,000

- Both associated with increased bacteremia risk
- Bandemia > 1,000 with bacterial infection
- Hemoglobin ≥ 2 gms below baseline in HbSS or HbS–β°
- Hemoglobin ≤ 6 gms
- Previous bacteremia or invasion infection
- Indwelling vascular lines
- Signs of systemic toxicity, vital sign instability or serious infection
- Previously treated with clindamycin or vancomycin instead of ceftriaxone
- Presence of SCD manifestations that require inpatient management
    - Acute chest syndrome
    - Painful crisis
    - Aplastic crisis
    - Splenic sequestration
- Concerns about family not able to recognize changes in patient's condition or inability/difficulty for follow–up (Need clear method to contact family if cultures are positive)

Outpatient management

- Patient that do not meet admission criteria can be considered for discharge
- Clinically stable
- Specific plan for follow–up the next day
- Recorded working telephone number recorded in chart
- Ceftriaxone 50–75 mg/kg IM or IV daily unless discontinued by medical provider
    - 100 mg/kg if meningitis present or suspected
- Stress oral hydration
- If vomiting occurs then return for further evaluation
- Adequate PO pain medications

Evaluation of sickle cell anemia

- Complete physical exam
- CBC
- BMP
- U/A
- Reticulocyte count (should be elevated)
- Chest x-ray
- ABG if significant dyspnea
- LFT's for abdominal pain
- Blood cultures if febrile
- O_2 saturation measurement

History for

- Prior episodes
- Transfusion history
- Dyspnea
- Fever
- Cough
- Headache
- Neurologic deficits
- Previous hemoglobin level

Treatment Options

- D5½NS or NS at 1.5–2 times maintenance rate if not hypotensive or hypovolemic — otherwise IV NS as needed for hypovolemia or hypotension
    - D5½NS preferred
- Supplemental oxygen if hypoxic or O_2 saturation < 92% or in respiratory distress
- Albuterol aerosol if dyspneic without CHF
- Folic acid PO as outpatient if not already taking it
- Hydroxyurea outpatient treatment
    - Start: 15 mg/kg PO qday
    - Titrate by 5 mg/kg/d q8–12wk
    - NMT 35 mg/kg/day

Pain control

- Toradol (ketorolac) 10 mg PO or 10–15 mg IV prn (avoid IM)
    - Do not use Toradol (ketorolac) if creatinine is elevated
    - Ketorolac therapeutic ceiling is around 10 mg
- Dilaudid (hydromorphone) 0.5–1 mg IV or 1–2 mg IM — may repeat × 2 prn
- Morphine 2–5 mg IV or 5–10 mg IM — may repeat × 2 prn
- Phenergan (promethazine) or Zofran (ondansetron) with narcotics IV
- Hydrocodone or oxycodone PO prn if discharged

Exchange transfusion indicated for

- Significant cardiopulmonary decompensation
- Priapism
- Acute nervous system event
- Acute chest syndrome

Transfusion indicated for

- Acute ischemic stroke
- Severe acute chest syndrome
- Multiorgan failure syndromes
- Right upper quadrant syndrome
- Priapism that does not resolve after adequate hydration and analgesia
- Severe anemia (hemoglobin < 6 gms or 2 gm/dL below baseline)
- Symptomatic anemia (consult physician)

Discharge criteria recommendation

- Resolution of the painful crises to the satisfaction of provider and patient
- No indications for admission

Discharge instructions

- Sickle cell anemia aftercare instructions
- Return if pain persists or worsens
- Return if fever develops
- Follow up with PCP in 1 day
- See Pediatric sickle cell section above

Consult criteria recommendation

- Refractory pain crises
- Signs of bacterial infection
- Fever
- Acute chest syndrome
- Acute splenic sequestration crises
- Aplastic crises (reticulocyte count not elevated)
- Hemoglobin < 6 gms or 2 gm/dL below baseline
- CVA or TIA
- Refractory priapism
- Symptomatic or significant anemia

Notes

REFERENCES:

Sickle Cell Anemia Author: Joseph E Maakaron, MD; Chief Editor: Emmanuel C Besa, MD

emedicine.medscape.com/article/205926

Benjamin LJ, Swinson GI, Nagel RL. Sickle cell anemia day hospital: an approach for the management of uncomplicated painful crises. Blood. 2000;95:1130–1136

Embury SH, Garcia JF, Mohandas N, et al. Effects of oxygen inhalation on endogenous erythropoietin kinetics, erythropoiesis, and properties of blood cells in sickle-cell anemia. N Engl J Med.1984;311:291–295

(Am J Emerg Med, epub, 7/18/20)

CANCER EMERGENCY PROTOCOL

Definition

- Cancer conditions and treatments resulting in urgent and emergent symptoms and findings

Considerations

- There is an increase in the amount of cancer patients surviving longer
- Cancer is the second most common cause of death in the U.S.

3 most common categories of cancer emergencies

- Neutropenic fever (most common)
- Mechanical complications
- Metabolic derangements

Neutropenic fever

Definition

- WBC (white blood count) < 500 cells/µL
- WBC < 1000 cells/µL with anticipation of WBC < 500 cells/µL
- Temperature > 101°F (38.3°C) on one reading or 100.4°F (38.0°C) > 1 hour

Considerations for neutropenic fever

- May have minimal symptoms besides fever
  - Pneumonia patients may have no infiltrates on chest x-ray and or any cough
  - CT chest may be needed to make diagnosis
- UTI patients may not have much frequency, dysuria or pyuria
- Progression of symptoms may be rapid
- Staphylococcus aureus and coagulase neg. staphylococcus are the most common pathogens

Evaluation

- CBC
- CMP
- Chest x-ray
- Blood cultures 5 minutes apart x 2
- Blood culture from any central venous catheters
- U/A
- Urine culture and sensitivity
- Lactic acid level if hypotensive or evidence of tissue hypoperfusion or sepsis

Treatment

- Early empiric antibiotic monotherapy with
  - Ceftazidime 1 gm IV q8–12hr or cefepime 1 gm IV q12hr

    OR
  - Imipenem-cilastatin 500–1000 mg IV q6hr or meropenem 1 gm IV q6hr

    ADD
- Vancomycin 1 gm IV q12hr for the following
  - Suspected central catheter related infection
  - History of MRSA colonization
  - Preliminary blood culture growth of gram positive bacteria
  - Hypotension or cardiovascular compromise or sepsis
- Neupogen (filgrastim) may be added per physician or oncologist
- Reverse isolation room if admitted and available

Discharge criteria

- Per physician consultation
- Most patients will be admitted

Consult criteria

- All febrile neutropenic patients
- Notify physician promptly if patient is hypotensive (or recent history of hypotension) or appears toxic, or signs/symptoms of hypoperfusion present

Mechanical cancer emergencies

- Spinal cord compression
- Superior vena cava syndrome
- Neoplastic cardiac tamponade
- Hyperviscosity syndrome
- Leukostasis

Spinal cord compression

Definition

- Compression of the spinal cord by tumor

Considerations

- Back pain with history of cancer is a Red Flag
- Patient outcomes improved with rapid detection

- Very important to consider this as a possible diagnosis

Symptoms and findings

- Back pain worsened by cough, worse at night or in supine position
- Numbness and paresthesia
- Loss of proprioception
- Bowel or bladder incontinence
- Bladder retention with overflow incontinence
- Decreased rectal tone or numbness
- New onset radicular pain on occasion may be caused by nerve root compression by tumor
- Back pain and tenderness may or may not be midline

Evaluation

- Complete history and physical exam with detailed neurologic and rectal tone exam
- MRI scan is the preferred imaging modality
- CBC, CMP, U/A as indicated
- Plain spine films for vertebral lesions

Treatment

- Decadron (dexamethasone) 0.1 mg/kg IV when suspected or diagnosed (NMT 10 mg) and then 4 mg qid
- Radiation therapy may be needed

Discharge criteria

- Per physician and/or oncologist

Consult criteria

- All suspected or diagnosed spinal cord compression patients to be discussed with physician or oncologist and neurosurgeon

Superior vena cava syndrome

Definition

- Obstruction of the superior vena cava

Considerations

- More of an urgency than emergency unless
  - Cerebral edema or laryngeal edema present

Common causes are

- Lung cancer
- Lymphoma
- Central line related DVT (deep vein thrombosis) of superior vena cava

Symptoms or findings

- May be vague
- Venous distension of neck, chest or upper extremities
- Facial or neck swelling
- Chronic cough
- Hoarseness
- Supine facial cyanosis (rare but pathognomonic)
- Dyspnea
- Fatigue
- Headache

Evaluation options

- Thorough history and physical exam
- CBC and CMP
- Chest x-ray
- CT scanning with contrast may be considered

Treatment options

- Elevate head of bed
- Radiation therapy
- Corticosteroid therapy with dexamethasone 0.1 mg/kg IV or IM (NMT 10 mg)
- Diuretic therapy
- Outpatient management

Discharge criteria

- No cerebral edema or airway impairments/ concerns
- Diagnosis firm

Discharge instructions

- Follow up with PCP or oncologist within 1–2 days
- Return if worsening symptoms

Consult criteria

- Discuss all patients with suspected or diagnosed superior vena cava syndrome with physician

Neoplastic cardiac tamponade

Definition

- Pericardial effusion with impairment of cardiac filling and function

Considerations

- May present with stable vital signs or hypotension
- Beck's triad of hypotension, muffled heart sounds and jugular venous distension may not present

Symptoms and findings (may or may not be present)

- Beck's triad
- Cardiomegaly on chest x-ray
- Low EKG voltage
- Dyspnea
- Pulsus paradoxus present up to 60% of patients (decrease in blood pressure > 10 mm Hg with inspiration — may be seen with COPD and asthma patients also)
- Volume depletion may mask findings
- Associated malignant pleural effusion may occur

Evaluation

- Chest x-ray
- CBC and CMP
- EKG
- Echocardiogram (diastolic collapse diagnostic)

Treatment

- Needle pericardiocentesis per physician
- Pericardial window per cardiothoracic surgeon

Consult criteria

- All suspected or diagnosed cardiac tamponade patients

Hyperviscosity syndrome

Definition

- Elevation of blood viscosity from increase in plasma proteins or blood component cells causing impaired circulation to tissues

Considerations

- Symptoms related to degree of hyperviscosity

Symptoms and findings (variable)

- Mental status changes (may be only manifestation)
- Unexplained dyspnea
- Headache
- Total serum protein minus albumin > 4
- Vision changes
- Somnolence
- Epistaxis
- Vertical nystagmus
- Hearing impairment
- Ataxia
- Retinal hemorrhages
- Paresthesias
- Congestive heart failure
- Low anion gap may be seen with multiple myeloma
    - Low anion gap may also be seen with lithium treatment or low serum albumin

Evaluation

- Serum viscosity measurement
- CBC and CMP
- Other tests as dictated by symptoms or findings

Treatment options

- Per physician
- Phlebotomy of 2–3 units of blood
- IV NS hydration

Consult criteria

- All suspected or diagnosed hyperviscosity syndrome patients

Leukostasis

Definition

- Tissue hypoperfusion secondary to elevated WBC

Considerations

- Seen with acute leukemias
- Typically seen when WBC > 100,000 cells/µL
- Can be seen with monoblastic leukemia of 25,000–50,000 cells/µL
- Watch out for tumor lysis syndrome with leukemia chemotherapy
    - Hyperkalemia
    - Hyperuricemia
    - Hyperphosphatemia
    - Renal failure

Evaluation

- CBC
- CMP
- Chest x-ray
- Uric acid as needed for tumor lysis syndrome

Treatment

- Chemotherapy
- Tumor lysis syndrome treated with
    - Aggressive IV fluid hydration
    - Allopurinol 300 mg PO
    - Amphojel 30–60 cc PO for hyperphosphatemia
    - Hemodialysis
- Blood transfusion can cause hyperviscosity and rapid patient deterioration
- Supplemental oxygen for dyspnea or O_2 saturation < 92%

Consult criteria

- All patients with leukostasis or tumor lysis syndrome

Immune checkpoint inhibitors

- The potential presence of immune-related adverse events necessitates a new approach to the evaluation of cancer patients if they are on Immune Checkpoint Inhibitors
- Restores immune system function
- Some examples:
    - Pembrolizumab (Keytruda)
    - Nivolumab (Opdivo))
- Patients with dyspnea, in addition to considering pneumonia or pulmonary embolus, consider immune-mediated pneumonitis
- Patients with chest pain, consider myocarditis and pericarditis
- Patients with headache, consider hypophysitis
- Neutropenia is not likely to be present
- Thyroiditis is a common adverse effect
- Hepatitis
- With potentially serious immune-related adverse effects such as neurologic, pulmonary, and cardiac toxicities, systemic glucocorticoids may need to be initiated expeditiously

Evaluation

- CBC, CMP, troponin, chest x-ray, thyroid studies, d–dimer, CTA chest, CT or MRI brain as indicated

Metabolic emergencies

Syndrome of Inappropriate Antidiuretic Hormone Secretion (SIADH)

Definition

- Excess release of ADH (antidiuretic hormone) causing hyponatremia with water retention in euvolemic patient

Considerations

- Less than maximally dilute urine
- Urine sodium > 30
- Normal renal, adrenal and thyroid function
- Absence of diuretic therapy

Symptoms and findings

- Hyponatremia
- As in above Considerations
- Frequently chronic and stable
- Anorexia
- Weakness
- Confusion

Evaluation

- CBC
- CMP
- Urine sodium
- Chest x-ray

Treatment options

- Depends on degree of hyponatremia and associated symptoms or findings
- Demeclocycline 250 mg PO q6hr
- See Hyponatremia Protocol
  - Hypertonic saline 3% IV 100 mg/hr. for 2 hours if needed
    - Or 1–2 cc/kg/hour in order to raise the serum sodium by 2.5 mEq/hour
  - Fluid restriction 500–1,000 cc of water per day
  - Be cautious of rapid hyponatremia correction

Consult criteria

- Discuss all suspected or diagnosed SIADH patients with a physician

Notes

REFERENCES:

Neutropenic Fever Empiric Therapy

Author: Mary Denshaw-Burke, MD, FACP; Chief Editor: Thomas E Herchline, MD

emedicine.medscape.com/article/2012185

Nieto AF, Doty DB. Superior vena cava obstruction: clinical syndrome, etiology, and treatment. Curr Probl Cancer 1986;10:441–484

Hughes WT, Armstrong D, Bodey GP, et al. 2002 Guidelines for the use of antimicrobial agents in neutropenic patients with cancer-IDSA Guidelines. Clin Infect Dis 2002;34:730–751

Kralstein J, Fishman WH. Malignant pericardial disease: Diagnosis and treatment. Cardiol Clin 1987;5:583–589

Gross P, Reimann D, Henschkowski J, et al. Treatment of severe hyponatremia: conventional and novel aspects. J Am Soc Nephrol 2001; 12:S10–14

El Majzoub I, et al. *Ann Emerg Med.* 2019 Jan;73(1):79-87

Bischof JJ, et al. *Ann Emerg Med.* 2019 Jan;73(1):88-90

Psychiatric and Social

Section Contents

When using any protocol, always follow the Guidelines of Proper Use (page 12).

Adult and Adolescent Psychiatric Protocol

Considerations

- Suicide 9th leading cause of death
- Actively suicidal patient or patient dangerous to others are not competent to refuse evaluation and treatment, and may not depart from the department until psychiatrically and medically cleared by an evaluation to do so
- Patients with depression, substance abuse or schizophrenia are at higher risk of suicide
- Evaluation of medical causes of psychiatric symptoms important
- Evaluation for patient being dangerous to self or others very important
- Chemical (medication) restraints preferred, if needed, and if possible

Restraints used when all interventions to reduce patient's dangerous behavior fail

- Placed without discussion or negotiation
- Carries risk of injury and death

Indications

- Prevent harm to patient or staff
- Prevent disruption of treatment
- Decrease stimulation of patient

- Honor patient's request for them to be applied to keep patient from harming themselves

Relative contraindications

- Delirium
- Dementia

General guidelines

- Team of at least 4 persons
- Leather restraints recommended
- Explain to patient need for restraints
- Staff member should be visible to patient at all times
- Placed so an IV is accessible
- Remove potentially dangerous objects from patient
- Raise patient's head to reduce aspiration
- Use verbal or chemical restraints after physical restraints placed if needed
- Check of circulation and limb swelling by nursing staff q15 minutes
- Remove restraints one at a time until 2 left, then last 2 together
- Never leave only one limb restrained
- Place in private area assessable and visible to staff
- Provide bedpan and nursing call light

Contraindications

- Organic brain syndrome
- Sepsis
- Cardiac illness
- Fever or hypothermia
- Metabolic disturbance
- Orthopedic problems

Restraints Time Rules

- Not to exceed 4 hours in adults
- Not to exceed 1 hour for children < 9 years of age
- New order needed when time expires
- Restraint protocols change with time and apply new directives as they occur

Evaluation

- Directed by history and physical examination
- Routine lab tests are low yield and need not to be performed frequently unless indicated by history and physical exam
- Routine drug screens in alert, awake, and cooperative patients need not to be routinely performed
- Consider use of observation period to determine if psychiatric symptoms are from intoxication when substance abuse has occurred

Mental Status Examination

OMI HAT (OMI = organic disease; HAT = psychiatric or functional)

- O = Orientation
- M = Memory
- I = Intellect
- H = Hallucinations
- A = Affect disorder
- T = Thought disorder

Suicidal Ideation or Attempt

- All patients with significant psychiatric symptoms need to be asked about suicidal ideation or attempt
- Need acute psychiatric evaluation
- Cannot leave until cleared of acute suicide risk or a risk of danger to others
- Treat injuries or ingestions as per appropriate protocols

Thought Disorders

- Acute psychosis
- Brief reactive psychosis
- Schizophrenia
- Delusional

Acute psychosis

- Loss of contact with reality
- Hallucinations (usually auditory)
- Fixed delusions (a fixed false belief)

- Rule out organic conditions or drug causes

Treatment

- Treat any organic causes
- No acute treatment besides an outpatient referral if stable, chronic and not dangerous to self or others

Agitation treatment — alone or combination therapy (combination more effective)

- Lorazepam 2–4 mg IM or Versed 3–5 mg IM prn (may be combined with Haldol)
- Haldol 5–10 mg (in elderly use 1–2 mg) IM or Droperidol 5 mg IM (works faster) prn (read droperidol's black box warning about fatal arrhythmias
- Geodon (ziprasidone) 10–20 mg IM (use Haldol if dementia–related psychosis)
- Cooperative patient — Lorazepam 4 mg PO with Risperdal (risperidone) 3 mg PO prn (use Haldol instead of risperidone if dementia–related psychosis)

Brief reactive psychosis

- Acute psychosis caused by a marked stressor
- One day to < 1 month
- Treatment same as acute psychosis

Schizophrenia (present for 6 months)

- Same as acute psychosis
- Disorganized speech and behavior, and a flat affect may be present

Treatment

- No acute medication therapy if not dangerous to self or others
- Outpatient antipsychotics and referral

Delusional disorder

- Non-bizarre delusions (jealousy or persecutory)
- Other schizophrenia symptoms not present
- Assess for organic brain syndrome
- Treatment as outpatient

Mood Disorders

Anxiety disorder

- Evaluate for organic cause
- Benzodiazepines useful if symptoms are severe
- Outpatient referral if not dangerous to self or others

Depression

- Evaluate for organic cause
- Consider antidepressant if symptoms are severe
- Outpatient referral if not dangerous to self or others and can care for self

Personality Disorder

- Outpatient referral if not dangerous to self or others and can care for self

Pain Management in Psychiatric Patients

- Treat with analgesics as indicated in limited amounts prn
- Antidepressants for chronic pain prn
- Pain clinic and psychiatric referral prn
- Refer to primary care provider prn

Discharge Criteria

- Cleared by psychiatric evaluation or provider medical evaluation
- Not dangerous to self or others
- Able to care for self or has support systems to care for self
- No suspected organic cause of psychiatric symptoms
- See General Patient Criteria Protocol (page 15)

Discharge instructions

- Respective psychiatric aftercare instructions
- Return if suicidal or homicidal

Consult Criteria

- Agitated patients requiring chemical or physical restraints
- Dangerous to self or others
- Cannot care for self and no support systems
- Organic causes of symptoms
- Delirium
- See General Patient Criteria Protocol (page 15)

Notes

REFERENCES:

Chemical Restraint Author: Benjamin B Mattingly, MD; Chief Editor: Rick Kulkarni, MD emedicine.medscape.com/article/109717

Emergent Treatment of Schizophrenia Author: Paul S Gerstein, MD; Chief Editor: Pamela L Dyne, MD emedicine.medscape.com/article/805988

Depression Author: Jerry L Halverson, MD; Chief Editor: David Bienenfeld, MD emedicine.medscape.com/article/286759

Alcohol Intoxicated Patient Protocol

Definition

- Blood level over legal limit by State statute
- Causing impairment of cognition or function

Differential Diagnosis

- Subdural hematoma
- CVA
- Coexisting intoxicating substances
- Meningitis
- Encephalitis
- Delirium
- Withdrawal syndromes
- Hepatic encephalopathy
- Postictal state

Considerations and comorbidities

- Alcohol metabolized around 20–30 mg% per hour regardless of blood concentration (zero order kinetics)
- Neurologic disorders
  - Altered mental status
  - Nystagmus
  - Pupillary dilation
  - Ataxia
- Minor head trauma from
  - Seizures
  - Falls
  - Altercations
  - Assaults
- Increased traumatic brain injury (coagulopathy common)
  - Intracerebral hemorrhage
  - Subdural hematoma
  - Epidural hematoma
- Embolic stroke
  - Atrial fibrillation
- Hemorrhagic stroke
- Alcohol related seizures
  - Withdrawal seizures
  - Usually single
  - Treat with Ativan (lorazepam) 1–4 mg IV Q15–30 minutes prn
  - Occur within 6–12 hours of withdrawal
  - No other anticonvulsant treatment besides lorazepam needed usually
  - May continue any existing seizure medication in addition to lorazepam
- Increased infections
  - Altered immune system

  - Fever not uniformly present
  - WBC not necessarily increased
- Hypoglycemia
- Alcoholic ketoacidosis
- Mild lactic acidosis
- Thiamine deficiency
- Hypomagnesemia
  - Contributes to withdrawal symptoms
  - Can be present despite normal blood levels
- Rhabdomyolysis
  - Complication of chronic alcoholism and binge drinking
  - Impaired gluconeogenesis
  - Compartment syndrome incidence increased

Evaluation

- Complete history and physical examination
- CMP; Magnesium level prn
- Bedside glucose check if hypoglycemia suspected
- CBC — if infection suspected
- U/A — ketosis, infection or rhabdomyolysis if suspected
- CPK if rhabdomyolysis or compartment syndrome suspected
- Blood alcohol level
- LFT's and ammonia level if chronic alcoholic and mental status worse than expected from blood alcohol level
- CT head scan
  - Evidence of head trauma with:
    - Significant headache
    - Nausea
    - Vomiting
    - Evidence of skull fracture
    - Neurologic acute abnormalities
    - Altered mental status changes worse than expected from degree of alcohol intoxication
    - New onset seizure
- Chest x-ray
  - Fever
  - Respiratory finding or complaints
  - O_2 saturation decreased from patient's baseline or < 94% if acute
- Evaluation for other injuries or comorbidities as indicated

Osmolol gap > 10–20 suspect substance ingestion (Normal < 10)

- Gap = Osmolality measured – Osmolality calculated (calculation equation: $2(Na^+ + K^+)$ + glucose/18 + BUN/2.8; normal 280–300mOsm/L)
- Ethanol mg%/4.6 is added to osmolol gap equation if present
- Gap > 50 carries high specificity for toxic alcohol such as methanol, ethylene glycol, or isopropyl alcohol
- Normal gap < 10

Treatment Options

- IV D5NS hydration as indicated
- Ativan (lorazepam) IV for seizures
- Feed awake patient without acute neurologic deficits
- Thiamine 100 mg IM or slow IV
- $MgSO_4$ (magnesium sulfate) 2 gms IM or IV unless in renal failure
- Appropriate antibiotic treatment

Discharge Criteria

- Clinically sober or blood alcohol < 300 and decreasing, and patient alert and has a ride home and not driving
- Unlikely to acutely decompensate
- Has support system

Discharge instructions

- Alcohol abuse aftercare instructions
- Follow up with PCP or local alcohol treatment center

Consult Criteria

- Fever
- Significant infectious process
- Acute neurologic deficits
- Acute imaging abnormalities
- Poor support system
- Hypoglycemia

- Acute hepatitis AST>ALT usually
- Mental status changes not attributable to intoxication
- Osmolol gap > 10 if checked
- Alcoholic ketoacidosis
- Metabolic acidosis
- Pneumonia
- Seizure
- Suicidal or dangerous to others
- Refer to General Patient Criteria Protocol (page 15)

Notes

____

____

____

REFERENCES:

Rathlev NK, et al. Alcohol-related seizures J of Emerg Med 2006; 31:157–163

Morton WA, et al. A prediction model for identifying alcohol withdrawal seizures Am J Drug Alcohol Abuse 1994;20:75–86

Withdrawal Syndromes Author: Nathanael J McKeown, DO; Chief Editor: Asim Tarabar, MD emedicine.medscape.com/article/819502

WITHDRAWAL PROTOCOL

Definition

- Acute systemic manifestations of withdrawal from a substance to which the patient is addicted

Differential Diagnosis

- Subdural hematoma
- CVA
- Coexisting intoxicating substances
- Meningitis
- Encephalitis
- Delirium
- Withdrawal syndromes
- Hepatic encephalopathy
- Postictal state

Considerations for Ethanol Withdrawal

- Mild ethanol withdrawal resolves in 1–2 days
- Need to determine cause of altered mental status in alcoholic patients
- Determine degree of intoxication
- Seizures have increased occurrence
    - Postictal state as a cause of altered mental state
- Infection risk increased
- Head trauma incidence increased
- Wernicke's encephalopathy may occur
- Hepatic encephalopathy from chronic alcoholism can be caused by upper gastrointestinal bleeding if hepatic cirrhosis present
- Fluid and electrolyte abnormalities have increased incidence

Ethanol Withdrawal Signs and Symptoms

- Tachycardia
- Fever
- Hypertension
- Diaphoresis
- Tremor
- Anxiety
- Agitation
- Seizures
- Hallucinations
- Delirium tremens
- Each successive withdrawal occurrence can have more severe symptoms

Early withdrawal symptoms

- Occurs within hours after alcohol intake reduction
- Can occur without a total cessation of alcohol intake
- Headache

- Insomnia
- Vivid dreams
- Malaise
- Hand tremor
- Hallucinations
- Tachycardia

Ethanol related seizures

- Can occur from intoxication
- Can occur from ethanol withdrawal
- Lifetime risk is 5–10%
- Withdrawal seizures progress to delirium tremens 30% of the time
- May occur within 7 hours following decreased ethanol intake
- Ativan (lorazepam) seizure prophylaxis may be given as 1–4 mg IV or IM
- Ativan is seizure treatment of choice: 1–4 mg IV prn (NMT 10 mg)
- Dilantin not effective
- Usually there is a single seizure; not focal usually

Delirium tremens

- Severe autonomic dysfunction plus delirium
- Rarely occurs before 48–72 hours of decreased ethanol intake
- Can start magnesium replacement in withdrawal patients with normal or low serum levels

Comorbidities

- Pneumonia
- Pancreatitis
- Hepatitis
- Hepatic cirrhosis
- Intracranial hemorrhage

Wernicke's encephalopathy

- Thiamine deficiency
- Confusion
- Oculomotor abnormalities
- Ataxia
- Korsakoff's psychosis has long term sequelae

Alcoholic ketoacidosis

- Can occur after binge drinking
- Free fatty acids metabolized from adipose tissue as a starvation ketosis
- Suppressed gluconeogenesis and insulin release occurs
- Usually occurs 24–72
- Beta–hydroxybutyrate is most common ketone which is not measured on routine ketone testing
  - Serum ketones may be minimal or negative
  - Acetone is the ketone that is measured in lab

Symptoms and findings

- Nausea and vomiting
- Abdominal pain
- Dehydration
- Confusion
- Tachycardia and tachypnea
- Arterial pH usually > 7.2

Evaluation Options

- Cardiac monitor and O_2 saturation for moderate to severe withdrawal
- Complete history and physical examination
- CMP; magnesium level
- Bedside glucose check
- CBC
- U/A
- CPK
- Blood alcohol level
- CT head scan for
  - Evidence of head trauma with:
    - Headache
    - Nausea
    - Vomiting
    - Evidence of skull fracture
    - Neurologic acute abnormalities
    - New onset seizure
    - Acute altered mental status not attributed to withdrawal
- Chest x-ray
  - Fever
  - Respiratory finding or complaints

- O_2 saturation decreased from patient's baseline
- Evaluation for other injuries or comorbidities as indicated

Treatment Options

- IV D5NS hydration as indicated (rate 50–250 cc/hr.) if not hypotensive
- IV NS or LR 500–1000 bolus if hypotensive (notify physician immediately)
- Lorazepam 1–4 mg IV q 15–30 minutes prn for moderate to severe withdrawal symptoms or findings (monitor for respiratory depression)
- Feed awake patient without acute neurologic deficits besides intoxication
- Thiamine 100 mg IM or slow IV
- $MgSO_4$ (magnesium sulfate) 2 gms IM or IV unless in renal failure
- Potassium as needed PO or IV
- Appropriate antibiotic treatment if infection present
- Avoid antipsychotic medications

Discharge Criteria

- Mild withdrawal
- Good social support
- Next day follow-up preferred
- Consider valium (diazepam) 10 mg qid taper by 25% every 2 days for 7–10 days of treatment

Discharge instructions

- Withdrawal aftercare instructions
- Return if withdrawal symptoms worsen
- Referral to addiction program

Consult Criteria

- Symptoms do not respond to 3 doses of benzodiazepines
- Moderate to severe withdrawal
- Alcoholic ketoacidosis
- Vomiting
- Delirium tremens
- Fever
- Pneumonia
- Significant infectious process
- Acute neurologic deficits
- Acute imaging abnormalities
- Poor acute support system
- Hypoglycemia
- Acute hepatitis
- Mental status changes not attributable to intoxication or withdrawal
- Osmolol gap > 10 if checked
- Metabolic acidosis
- Refer to General Patient Criteria Protocol (page 15)

Opioid Withdrawal

- Symptoms
  - Restlessness
  - Dilated pupils
  - Lacrimation
  - Nausea and vomiting
  - Abdominal cramps
  - Diarrhea
  - Muscle cramps
- Mental status remains normal
- Not life threatening except in neonates

Evaluation

- Complete history and physical examination
- CBC optional
- CMP or BMP optional
- U/A optional
- Other testing as indicated by history, examination or findings

Treatment Options

- Supportive
- Clonidine 0.1 mg q8hr for 3–10 days prn withdrawal if not hypotensive
- Consider lorazepam 1–2 mg PO q4–6h prn for 3–5 days
- Loperamide 2 mg PO tid prn diarrhea (NMT 8 qday)
- Rehydration if needed
- Inpatient treatment program if available and patient agreeable

Discharge Criteria

- Stable patient without significant comorbidities

- Support systems available

Discharge instructions

- Withdrawal aftercare instructions
- Return if withdrawal symptoms worsen
- Referral to addiction program

Consult Criteria

- Refer to General Patient Criteria Protocol (page 15)
- Suicidal ideation
- Significant comorbidities

Notes

REFERENCES:

Rathlev NK, et al. Alcohol-related seizures J of Emerg Med 2006; 31:157–163

Morton WA, et al. A prediction model for identifying alcohol withdrawal seizures Am J Drug Alcohol Abuse 1994;20:75–86

Withdrawal Syndromes Author: Nathanael J McKeown, DO; Chief Editor: Asim Tarabar, MD emedicine.medscape.com/article/819502

SEXUAL ASSAULT PROTOCOL

Definition

- Defined as carnal knowledge of victim with force or threat against will of patient and varies state to state

Considerations

- Assess for nonsexual injuries
- 5–6% of victims are male
- Preexisting STD rate of victims are higher than the rate of what is acquired from the sexual assault
- Sexual assault exam and evidence collection is up to 72–96 hours post assault
- Notify police
- HIV PEP is indicated in all HIV-negative patients following significant exposure to a substantial-risk bodily fluid
  - Substantial risk fluid to vagina, rectum, eye, mouth, nonintact skin (including dermatitis), or percutaneously is considered a significant exposure
    - Blood
    - Semen
    - Vaginal secretions
    - Rectal secretions
    - Breast milk
    - Any fluid visibly contaminated with blood
  - Negligible-risk fluids (if no visibly blood) are as follows:
    - Urine
    - Tears
    - Saliva
    - Nasal secretions
    - Sweat
- HIV PEP is recommended only in patients who present to care 72 hours or sooner since the last exposure

Infection and pregnancy risks

- Gonorrhea: 4%
- Chlamydia: 1.5%
- Trichomonas: 12%
- Syphilis: 0.1%
- HIV: 0.1% if assailant HIV positive
- Pregnancy: 1–5%

Evaluation

- Be compassionate
- Evaluate for other injuries

- UCG or serum pregnancy tests in fertile female patients

HIV testing

- Ag/Ab combination (alternative, Ab only) upon presentation and then at 4-6 weeks and 3 months
- Testing at 6 months indicated if patient recently infected with hepatitis C

Hepatitis B testing

- Hepatitis B surface antigen (HBsAg) upon presentation and then at 6 months, if susceptible
- Hepatitis B surface antibody (HBsAb) upon presentation and then at 6 months, if susceptible
- Hepatitis B core antibody (HBcAb) upon presentation and then at 6 months, if susceptible

Hepatitis C testing

- Surface antibody upon presentation and then at 6 months, if susceptible

Other tests, if applicable

- Syphilis serology upon presentation and then at 4-6 weeks and 6 months
- Gonorrhea (nucleic acid amplification) from all exposed sites (genital, pharyngeal, anal)
- Chlamydia (nucleic acid amplification) from all exposed sites (genital, pharyngeal, anal)

Baseline laboratory tests for PEP medications

- Urine human chorionic gonadotropin (HCG), if applicable, upon presentation and then at 4-6 weeks
- Complete blood cell (CBC) count
- Aspartate transaminase (AST) and alanine transaminase (ALT)

Source testing

- HIV Ab/Ag (and quantitative polymerase chain reaction [PCR], if applicable), hepatitis B, hepatitis C, and STI screening as above.
- Individual state laws on source testing have substantial variability, and legal ramifications that should be known for each jurisdiction
  - cdc.gov/hiv/policies/laws/states/

PEP is not 100% effective

History

- Date, time and location of event?
- Areas of body involved?
- Number of assailants?
- Is assailant known to victim?
- Weapons, threats, restraints and foreign bodies used?
- Type of sexual acts?
- Did ejaculation occur?
- Was condom used?
- What clean-up occurred by victim: shower, defecation, or douche?
- Were clothes changed?
- Conception prophylaxis used?
- Last menstrual period?
- Date of last consensual sexual intercourse?

Examination

- Performance of "rape kit" by provider or SANE personnel
- Activate SANE nurse program if available to perform "rape kit" and protocols
- Pelvic exam
- Rectal exam
- GC and chlamydial cultures
- RPR
- Hepatitis B testing
- Offer HIV testing
- X-rays as indicated by comorbid trauma
- Document trauma to genital and rectal areas, along with rest of body

Treatment Options

Sexual transmitted disease (STD) prophylaxis options

Antibiotics

- Ceftriaxone 500 mg IM in a single dose

PLUS

- Metronidazole 2 g orally in a single dose

PLUS

- Doxycycline 100 mg orally twice a day for 7 days
- Offer hepatitis B vaccination if none previously; repeat in 1 and 6 months if no history of prior hepatitis B vaccination

Pregnancy prophylaxis if patient agreeable

- Ovral 2 tablets PO now and 2 tablets PO in 12 hours

OR

- Preven 2 tablets PO now and 2 tablets PO in 12 hours
- Offer sexual assault counseling by trained counselor

CDC Postexposure Assessment 2010

- Assess risk for HIV infection in the assailant
- Evaluate characteristics of the assault event that might increase risk for HIV transmission
- Consult with a specialist in HIV treatment, if PEP is being considered
- If the survivor appears to be at risk for HIV transmission from the assault, discuss antiretroviral prophylaxis, including toxicity and lack of proven benefit
- If the survivor chooses to start antiretroviral PEP, provide enough medication to last until the next return visit; reevaluate the survivor 3–7 days after initial assessment and assess tolerance of medications
- If PEP is started, perform CBC and serum chemistry at baseline (initiation of PEP should not be delayed, pending results)
- Perform HIV antibody test at original assessment; repeat at 6 weeks, 3 months, and 6 months.

Discharge Criteria

- No comorbid conditions needing admission
- Safe home environment or shelter

Discharge instructions

- Sexual assault aftercare instructions
- Refer to primary care provider and counseling resources
- Notify DHS as indicated
- Notify police if not aware of incident

Consult Criteria

- Comorbid conditions needing admission
- Refer to General Patient Criteria Protocol (page 15)

Notes

REFERENCES:

CDC Sexually Transmitted Disease Guidelines, 2010 Sexual Assault and STDs, updated January 28, 2011

Sexual Assault Author: William Ernoehazy Jr, MD, FACEP; Chief Editor: Pamela L Dyne, MD
emedicine.medscape.com/article/806120

Centers for Disease Control and Prevention, 2015 Sexually Transmitted Diseases Treatment Guidelines

HIV Prophylaxis in Sexual Assault Updated: Dec 04, 2018
Author: Derek T Larson, DO; Chief Editor: Michael Stuart Bronze, MD

Domestic Violence Protocol

Definition

- Pattern of assaultive or coercive behaviors including physical, sexual, and/or psychological attacks

Considerations

- Intimate partner abuse (IPV) occurs not infrequently in pregnancy
- Economic coercion occurs
- Barriers exist to leaving a relationship — economic; religious; children
- Reported statistic of 7 attempts to leave before actually leaving
- IPV patients often present with injuries — frequently central body or defensive areas (arms and feet used for protection)
- History can be vague and evasive
- Can present with a STD from abuser
- Increased incidence of depression, anxiety and PTSD
- 60% increase in physical disorders
- 4–6 times increase in depression
- Children also frequently abused
- Most dangerous time for the abused is in disclosure of abuse and in attempting to leave relationship

Evaluation

- Evaluation for injuries
- Establish IPV diagnosis
- For emotional disorders

SAFE questions

S = Stress/safety: Do you feel safe in your relationship? What stress do you experience?

A = Afraid/abused: Have you or your children been abused? Have you ever felt afraid in your relationship?

F = Family: Does your family or friends know of your abuse? Can you tell them? Will they help?

E = Emergency plan: Do you have one? Do you have a safe place to go? Enough money available?

Treatment

- Provide safe environment
- Develop a safety plan
- Referral to abuse counseling and shelter
- Provide community IPV/domestic violence resources and contact numbers
- Do not prescribe sedatives (can interfere with ability to flee)

Discharge instructions

- Domestic abuse aftercare instructions

Consult Criteria

- Patients that need admission for injuries
- Patient that need admission for safety
- Suicidal or homicidal ideation
- Refer to Psychiatric Protocol
- Refer to General Patient Criteria Protocol (page 15)

Notes

REFERENCES:

Domestic Violence Author: Lynn Barkley Burnett, MD, EdD, LLB(c); Chief Editor: Barry E Brenner, MD, PhD, FACEP

emedicine.medscape.com/article/805546

CDC Injury Prevention and Control: Intimate Partner Violence updated June 24, 2014

cdc.gov/violenceprevention/intimatepartnerviolence

CHILD ABUSE PROTOCOL

Definition

- Physical and/or psychological abuse of children, or neglect of children

Considerations

- Types of child abuse
  - Physical
  - Psychological
  - Sexual
  - Neglect
- Bruises most common abuse finding
- Bruises may be in various stages of healing
- Nonambulatory infants rarely bruise themselves
- Inflicted visceral injury usually is of hollow viscera
- Head injury most common cause of mortality
- More common where mother is also abused
- Mother's boyfriend who is not the father is common suspect
- Injuries with no plausible explanation

Head injury symptoms or findings in abused infants (increasing in seriousness)

- Extreme fussiness
- Inconsolable crying
- Irritability
- Lethargy
- Hypotonia
- Poor feeding
- Vomiting
- Tachypnea
- Bradycardia
- Hypothermia
- Seizures
- Gaze preferences
- Unequal pupils
- Unreactive pupils
- Stupor
- Coma
- Death

Shaken baby syndrome

- Usually < 1 year of age
- Retinal hemorrhages commonly present

Triad — some or all may be present

- Subdural or subarachnoid hemorrhage
- Cerebral edema
- Retinal hemorrhages

CT head scan best diagnostic approach for brain injury

Fractures with higher abuse association

- Posterior rib fractures
- Metaphyseal fractures
- Bilateral or multiple fractures
- Multiple fractures in various stages of healing
- Digit fractures
- Scapular fractures
- Complex skull fractures

Evaluation

- Maintain high index of suspicion
- Is directed toward injuries

- CBC
- U/A
- CMP
- Skeletal survey
- CT head if suspected head or brain injury
- Cervical spine protection until cleared by imaging if altered mental status and suspected head injury

Treatment

- Aimed at injuries
- Child protection actions

Disposition

- Discuss with physician
- Contact Child Protective Services or DHS if abuse diagnosed or suspected
- Do not discharge patient until cleared to do so by physician
- Admission if patient safety is in question
- Report to police if a crime has occurred
- Contact primary care physician to discuss case for similar previous concerns and if discharged to arrange close follow up

Notes

REFERENCES:

CDC Injury Prevention and Control: Child Maltreatment Prevention updated May 23, 2014

cdc.gov/violenceprevention/childmaltreatment

Child Abuse Author: Julia Magana, MD; Chief Editor: Richard G Bachur, MD emedicine.medscape.com/article/800657

ELDER ABUSE PROTOCOL

Definition

- Pattern of assaultive or coercive behaviors including physical, sexual, psychological attacks

Considerations

- 3% of elderly have been abused
- Increased incidence of cognitive impairment

Signs may include

- Injuries in various stages of healing
- Unexplained injuries
- Delay in seeking treatment
- Injuries inconsistent with history
- Contradictory explanations given by the patient and caregiver
- Laboratory findings indicating under dosage or over dosage of medications
- Bruises, welts, lacerations, rope marks, burns
- STD's
- Dehydration, malnutrition, decubitus ulcers, poor hygiene
- Signs of withdrawal, depression, agitation, or infantile behavior
- Abuser may not leave medical provider alone with patient
- Abuser more concerned about medical bill
- Abuser displays anger or indifference toward patient

Evaluation

- High index of suspicion
- Complete history and physical exam
- Pelvic exam for STD (may need "rape kit")
- Aimed at injuries and home situation
- CBC prn
- CMP prn
- U/A prn

- Drug levels of medications prn
- UDS (urine drug screen) prn
- Blood alcohol prn
- Relevant x-rays
- CT head, abdomen or chest as indicated

Treatment

- Directed toward injuries and comorbidities
- Protection of patient

Disposition

- Discuss with physician
- Contact DHS if abuse diagnosed or suspected
- Do not discharge patient until cleared to do so by physician
- Admission if patient safety is in question
- Report to police if crime occurred

Notes

REFERENCES:

CDC Injury Prevention and Control: Elder Abuse

cdc.gov/violenceprevention/elderabuse

Elder Abuse Author: Monique I Sellas, MD; Chief Editor: Barry E Brenner, MD, PhD, FACEP
emedicine.medscape.com/article/805727

Environmental

Section Contents

When using any protocol, always follow the Guidelines of Proper Use (page 12).

HEAT ILLNESS PROTOCOL

Definition

- Heat induced metabolic derangements with possible tissue injury

Differential Diagnosis

- Meningitis
- Encephalitis
- Serotonin syndrome
- Thyroid storm
- Thyrotoxicosis
- Sepsis and septic shock
- Neuroleptic malignant syndrome
- Tetanus
- Delirium
- Delirium tremens
- Heat stroke
- Infection in elderly without sepsis
- Malignant hyperthermia
- Intracerebral hemorrhage
- CVA
- Drugs

Considerations

- Normal temperature range is 97°F–100.4°F or 36.1°C–38°C
- Prior heat illness increases risk of developing future heat illness

Excessive heat causes damage to multiple organ systems

- Heart
- Liver
- Kidneys
- Lungs
- Muscles
- Central nervous system

Heat regulation mainly by

- Radiation
- Evaporation
- Conduction
- Convection

Risk Factors for heat illness

Age

- Elderly
- Neonates

Medical Illness

- Alcoholism
- Hyperthyroidism
- Obesity

Medications

- Anticholinergics
- Beta–blockers
- Diuretics
- MOA inhibitors
- Phenothiazines
- Tricyclic antidepressants

Illicit drugs

- Amphetamines
- Cocaine

Social

- Bedridden
- Living alone
- Lack of air conditioning
- Unable to care for self

Mild Forms of Heat illness

Heat edema

- Swollen hands and feet after prolonged sitting/standing in hot temperatures

Heat rash ("prickly heat")

- Sweat glands become blocked

Heat cramps

- Electrolyte imbalance; volume depletion; hyperventilation
- May be hyponatremic and hypochloremic
- No rhabdomyolysis

Heat tetany

- Carpopedal spasm from hyperventilation secondary to hyperthermia

Heat syncope

- Benign syncope from prolonged standing in hot environment

Severe Forms of Heat illness

Heat exhaustion

- Water or salt depletion
- Fatigue
- Weakness
- Hyperventilation
- Headache
- Dizziness
- Vertigo
- Nausea
- Vomiting
- Muscle cramps
- No CNS dysfunction
- Temperature usually < 104°F (40°C)
- Sweating present

Heat stroke

- Hyperthermia with CNS dysfunction:
  - Confusion
  - Delirium
  - Ataxia
  - Seizures
  - Coma
- Temperature usually > 104.5°F (40.5°C)
- May or may not have sweating present
- Mortality 30–80%
- Fatigue
- Weakness
- Hyperventilation
- Headache
- Dizziness
- Vertigo
- Nausea
- Vomiting
- Muscle cramps
- Rhabdomyolysis
- Compartment syndrome
- Multi-organ dysfunction
- Lactic acidosis

Evaluation

Heat illness excluding heat stroke

- CBC prn
- BMP prn
- U/A in elderly; diabetics; immunocompromised

Heat stroke

- CBC

- BMP
- LFT's
- Lactic acid level
- CPK
- Chest x-ray
- EKG

Treatment

Mild forms of heat illness

- Oral or IV rehydration and sodium replacement
- Cool environment

Heat exhaustion

- Remove from hot environment
- No antipyretic medication (may impair heat dissipation)

Rapid cooling as needed

- Remove clothing
- Ice packs to axilla, groin and/or behind neck all prn
- Spray with tepid water and fanned prn
- IV NS or LR rehydration prn

Heat stroke

- Remove from hot environment
- No antipyretic medication (may impair heat dissipation)
- Place foley

Rapid cooling

- Remove clothing
- Ice packs to axilla; groin; behind neck
- Spray with tepid water and fanned (lower temperature to 38.3°C (101°F) to avoid overshoot
- Lorazepam or diazepam to control shivering, treat seizures and sedate patient prn
- IV NS or LR rehydration
  - NS 500–1000 cc bolus if hypotensive in adults
  - NS 20 cc/kg bolus if hypotensive in children
    - Avoid too rapid IV NS replacement — may cause cerebral edema (free water deficit corrected over 48 hours)
- Water deficit in liters = Total body water [0.6 × Kg] – Total body water [desired Na+ / measured Na+] (For hypernatremia patients)
- Free water deficit should be replaced slowly over 48 hours

Discharge Criteria

- All heat illness patients without heat stroke or severe heat exhaustion with good response to therapy
- Not hypotensive
- Refer to General Patient Criteria Protocol

Discharge instructions

- Heat illness aftercare instructions
- Return if symptoms worsen

Consult Criteria

- Heat stroke
- Severe heat exhaustion
- Significant electrolyte disturbances
- Refer to General Patient Criteria Protocol (page 15)
- Age ≥ 70 years

Notes

REFERENCES:

Inter-Association Task Force on Exertional Heat Illness. Consensus Statement 2002. (Guidelines)

Heatstroke Author: Robert S Helman, MD; Chief Editor: Joe Alcock, MD, MS emedicine.medscape.com/article/166320

Environmental Emergencies: Heat Illness in Emergency Medicine David A. Townes, MD, MPH, FACEP emedhome.com/features cdc.gov/niosh/mining/userfiles/work/pdf/2017-125.pdf

Hypothermia Protocol

Definition

- Pathologic state in which core body temperature falls below 35°C (95°F)

Differential Diagnosis

- Cerebrovascular accident
- Toxicity
- Alcohols
- Barbiturates
- Benzodiazepines
- Carbon monoxide
- Narcotics
- Ethylene glycol
- Gamma-hydroxybutyrate
- Sedative hypnotics

Considerations

- Core temperature regulated in thermoneutral zone of 36.5°C and 37.5°C (97.7°F and 99.5°F)
- Heat production is a function of metabolism
- Hypothermia affects all organ systems
- Afterdrop in core temperature can occur after rewarming started due to peripheral cold blood return perfusing the body
- Most hypothermia patients will by dehydrated

Heat loss occurs by

- Radiation – most rapid (50% of heat loss)
- Conduction
- Convection
- Evaporation

Hypothermia severity

- Mild = 32–35°C or 89.6–95°F
- Moderate = 28–32°C or 82.4–89.6°F
- Severe = 20–28°C or 68–82.4°F
- Profound < 20°C or 68°F

Risk Factors

- Burns
- Environmental cold exposure or immersion
- Toxicological causes
- Extremes of age
- Hypoadrenalism
- Hypothyroidism
- Hypoglycemia
- Hypopituitarism
- Malnutrition
- Spinal cord injury
- Sepsis
- Uremia

Findings as Temperatures Decrease

Mild hypothermia progression

- Shivering, impaired judgment, confusion
- Tachycardia, tachypnea, cold diuresis
- Bradycardia, respiratory depression, hyperglycemia, ataxia, dysarthria

Moderate hypothermia progression

- Stupor, lethargy, arrest of shivering
- Atrial arrhythmias, Osborn J-waves on EKG (upward deflection of terminal S wave), increased bradycardia
- Insulin ineffective, decreased oxygen utilization
- Progressive decreased level of consciousness, bradycardia, and respiratory rate

Severe hypothermia progression

- Ventricular fibrillation susceptibility increased
- Pulse decreased by 50%

- Oxygen consumption decreased by 50%
- Loss of reflexes and voluntary movement
- Acid-base abnormalities
- No pain response
- Decreased cerebral perfusion by 2/3
- Pulmonary edema
- Apnea
- Hypotension

Profound hypothermia progression

- Lowest level for resumption of cardiac activity, pulse 20% of normal
- Asystole

Evaluation

- Complete history and physical examination (auscultate up to 60 seconds if needed)
- CBC
- BMP
- LFT's
- Chest x-ray
- EKG
- ABG (temperature correction not needed)
- PT/PTT/INR (coagulation panel)
- CPK
- Blood alcohol and toxicology panel as indicated
- Cardiac, oxygen saturation and vital sign monitoring

Treatment Considerations and Options

- IV fluid resuscitation as needed with NS or D5NS (avoid lactated ringer's solution)
  - Do not give D5 IV containing fluids as a bolus (too high tonicity)
- Immunocompromised patients should receive empiric antibiotics
- Intubation as needed
- NG tube if intubated
- Most cardiac dysrhythmias correct with rewarming alone
- Malignant ventricular dysrhythmias use amiodarone (avoid lidocaine and procainamide)
- Defibrillation likely ineffective with core temperature < 30°C (86°F)

Passive rewarming

- Increases temperature 0.3–1.2°C/hour
- For mild hypothermia where shivering is present and patient is healthy
- No external heat added
- Patient covered with blankets
- Remove wet garments
- Cover patient's head except face

Active external rewarming

- Increases temperature 0.3–1.2°C/hour
- For mild hypothermia with impaired thermogenesis due to illness, intoxication, medications or comorbidities
- For moderate hypothermia
- Forced warmed air systems used
- Warmed blankets
- Heat packs
- Heat lamps

Active core rewarming

- Increases temperature approximately 3°C/hour
- For severe hypothermia
- Warmed IV fluids (44°C or 111°F) — warm 1 liter for approximately 2 minutes in microwave
- Warmed humidified air or oxygen in addition to passive and active external rewarming

Extracorporeal rewarming

- Increases temperature approximately 1–18°C/hour
- Indicated for severe or profound hypothermia
- Hypothermia unresponsive to other rewarming methods
- Completely frozen extremities
- For no signs of perfusion
- Hemodialysis (can increase temperature 1–4°C/hour)
- Cardiopulmonary bypass (can increase temperature 18°C/hour)

Discharge Criteria

- Mild hypothermia that responds to passive rewarming in healthy patient

Discharge instructions

- Hypothermia aftercare instructions

Consult Criteria

- Discuss all hypothermia patients with physician

Admission Criteria

- Hypothermia < 32°C or 89.6°F

Notes

REFERENCES:

N Engl J Med 2012;367(20):1930–8 Accidental Hypothermia Douglas J.A. Brown, M.D., Hermann Brugger, M.D., Jeff Boyd, M.B., B.S., and Peter Paal, M.D.

emedicine.medscape.com/article/770542

Frostbite and Exposure Skin Injury Protocol

Definition

- Cold related injury or death of tissue from freezing secondary to prolonged cold exposure

Differential Diagnosis

- Hypothermia
- Frostnip
- Trench foot
- Pernio
- Chilblains (3–6 hours of cold moist exposure without freezing)

Frostbite

Considerations

- Extremities, head, and nose most commonly affected
- Initial appearance of injury often fails to predict depth or eventual outcome

Degrees of Injury

First-degree injury

- Erythema, edema, waxy appearance, hard white plaques, and loss of sensation

Second-degree injury

- Erythema, edema, and formation of blisters filled with clear or milky fluid
- Form within 24 hours of injury

Third-degree injury

- Blood-filled blisters
- Progressing to a black eschar in several weeks

Fourth-degree injury

- Full-thickness damage affecting muscles, tendons, and bone, with necrosis of tissue

Evaluation

- Assess for hypothermia
- No lab needed in mild cases
- Assess for severe frostbite
  - CBC
  - CMP
  - U/A for evidence of myoglobin
  - CPK
  - Cultures if infection suspected
  - Technetium-99 scintigraphy 2–7 days after injury is helpful in decision making about amputation

Treatment

- Remove wet clothing
- Ibuprofen 400 mg PO prior to rewarming to improve tissue salvage
- Protect from refreezing

- Rapid rewarming for more severe cases
- Put affected area in warm water (40–42°C or 104–108°F) for 20–30 minutes
- Elevate extremity after rewarming
- Separate damaged digits with dry gauze
- Apply aloe vera (without alcohol, salicylates or other additives) after thawing
    - May be used for debridement also
- Tetanus prophylaxis (see Tetanus Protocol)
- Antibiotics not indicated unless infection present
- Liberal use of analgesics up to 7–10 days
- Leave hemorrhagic blisters intact
- Debride clear fluid filled blisters
- Physical therapy post discharge or admission
- Avoid massaging frostbite area (may increase injury)
- Splinting prn
- Cycloplegia, artificial tears and eyelid closure with dressing for corneal cold injury

Discharge Criteria

- First degree injury

Discharge instructions

- Frostbite aftercare instructions

Consult Criteria

- Second, third and fourth degree frostbite injuries
- Eye injury

Admission Criteria

- Greater than first degree frostbite
- Risk of refreezing exists

Non-freezing Environmental Injuries

Trench foot

- Non-freezing injury from prolonged exposure to cold, wet environment
- May cause gangrene
- Rewarm in water if needed
- Elevate to reduce edema
- Keep warm and dry
- Ibuprofen prn
- Tetanus prophylaxis (see Tetanus Protocol)

Pernio

- 12–hour to 3–day exposure to cold moist environment without freezing
- Scaling skin and edema
- Cyanotic and red skin lesions
    - Occasionally deep seated
- Use protective clothing for prevention and emollient creams for treatment
- Tetanus prophylaxis (see Tetanus Protocol)

Chilblains

- 3–6 hours of cold moist exposure without freezing
- Chronic form from recurrent Pernio
- Swelling, tender SQ vesicles with or without bluish discoloration
- Hemorrhagic bullae and skin ulcers in severe cases
- Gently rewarm, dress with dry protective bandages
- Tetanus prophylaxis (see Tetanus Protocol)

Frostnip

- Superficial and reversible ice crystal formation without tissue destruction
- Transient numbness and paresthesia that resolves after rewarming

Disposition

- Discuss with physician trench foot, pernio and chilblains patients

Discharge instructions

- Respective aftercare instructions

Notes

REFERENCES:

Cold Injuries Author: Richard F Edlich, MD, PhD, FACS, FASPS, FACEP; Chief Editor: Lars M Vistnes, MD, FRCSC, FACS emedicine.medscape.com/article/1278523

Frostbite Author: C Crawford Mechem, MD, MS, FACEP; Chief Editor: Dirk M Elston, MD medicine.medscape.com/article/926249

ALTITUDE ILLNESS PROTOCOL

Definition

- Syndromes resulting from lack of oxygen

Differential Diagnosis

- Anxiety
- Encephalitis
- Diabetic ketoacidosis
- Meningitis
- Migraine
- Hyponatremia
- Hypoglycemia
- Hypothermia
- Cerebrovascular accident
- Transient ischemic attack
- Transient global amnesia
- Subarachnoid hemorrhage
- Subdural hemorrhage
- Carbon monoxide poisoning
- Reyes syndrome
- Nonspecific headache
- Brain tumors
- Dehydration
- Viral syndrome

Syndromes

- Acute mountain sickness (AMS)
- High-altitude cerebral edema (HAPE)
- High-altitude pulmonary edema (HACE)

Considerations

Hypoxia is primary insult

- Degree of injury dependent on rate of hypoxia onset and magnitude
- Increase minute ventilation occurs acutely with a resultant respiratory alkalosis
- Renal compensation to respiratory alkalosis occurs more slowly than compensation to respiratory acidosis
- Increased cerebral perfusion occurs
- Symptoms occur 4–10 hours after ascent
- Incidence affected by sleeping altitude
- Physical fitness not protective
- Occurs more commonly in age < 50 years

Acute Mountain Sickness (AMS)

Definition

Headache plus one of following:

- Nausea/vomiting
- Fatigue
- Dizziness
- Insomnia

Considerations

- Mild form of high altitude illness
- Generally benign

- Occurs around 6,000 feet altitude or higher with incidence of 10–40%, increasing as altitude increases
- Usually self-limited and improves over 1–3 days if no further ascent is undertaken
- Continued ascent will worsen AMS and can result in HACE
- O_2 saturation not helpful in diagnosing or managing AMS or HACE

Findings and symptoms

- Patients appear ill
- Normal neurologic examination
- Heart rate and blood pressure can vary
- May have rales, but oxygen saturation normal or near normal
- Fever is absent
- May have retinal hemorrhages
- Peripheral edema may be present

Treatment options

- Halt ascent
- Acetazolamide 250 mg PO q12hr
  - Prophylaxis — 125 mg PO q12hr starting 24 hours before ascent and continuing during ascent to at least 48 hours after arrival at highest altitude (or descent)
- Dexamethasone 4 mg PO/IM q6hr for treatment and prophylaxis (not more than 10 days)
- Ibuprofen or Tylenol for headache
- Phenergan (promethazine) prn for nausea
- Oxygen for more severe cases (4L/min to keep O_2 saturation > 92%)
- Descent for more severe symptoms

Discharge criteria

- Usually discharged

Discharge instructions

- Acute mountain sickness aftercare instructions

Consult criteria

- Discuss high altitude illness with physician

High-altitude Cerebral Edema (HACE)

Definition

- Acute Mountain Sickness with gait ataxia and altered mental status

Considerations

- Usually normal exam except for gait ataxia
- Focal neurologic deficits rare
- Continued ascent with AMS can lead to HACE
- Papilledema can occur
- Retinal hemorrhages occur
- Coma can occur

Evaluation options

- CBC
- CMP
- ABG
- CT brain
- MRI brain

Treatment

- Immediate evacuation to lower altitude
- Oxygen 4L/min to keep O_2 saturation > 92%
- Dexamethasone 8 mg PO/IM, followed by 4 mg PO/IM q6hr
- Elevate head of bed 30 degrees

Discharge criteria

- Dependent on severity
- Re–evaluate in 24 hours to assure symptom clearance

Discharge instructions

- High-altitude cerebral edema aftercare instructions if discharged
- Average full recovery is 2.4 weeks

Consult criteria

- Discuss with physician

High-altitude Pulmonary Edema

Definition

- Noncardiogenic pulmonary edema from increased capillary hydrostatic pressure and pulmonary hypertension

Considerations

- Exercise at high altitude increases risk
- Fever common
- Orthopnea common
- Frothy pink sputum is a late finding
- Cyanosis can occur
- May occur with HACE

History and physical examination criteria

2 of the following:

- Weakness or decreased exercise tolerance
- Cough
- Dyspnea at rest
- Chest tightness or congestion

PLUS

2 of the following:

- Rales or wheezing
- Central cyanosis or O_2 saturation is lower than expected from elevation
- Tachycardia
- Tachypnea

Evaluation

- Chest x-ray
- Ultrasound of lungs show comet tail artifacts (B–lines)
- CBC
- CMP
- BNP or NT–ProBNP
- EKG
- Troponin

Treatment options

- Oxygen 6–8 liters by mask until improved then 5L/min to keep O_2 saturation > 92%
- Albuterol aerosol prn
- Immediate descent
- Bed rest
- Nifedipine 10 mg PO q6hr if oxygen not available and not hypotensive
- Cialis (tadalafil) 10 mg bid to decrease pulmonary hypertension
- Dexamethasone 8–10 mg PO/IM/IV initially then 4 mg PO/IM/IV q4hr
- Narcotic or non-narcotic cough suppressants prn
- Phenergan (promethazine) prn nausea or vomiting

Discharge criteria

- Normal O_2 saturation (> 90%) breathing room air
- Significant clinical improvement and improved chest x–ray
- No dyspnea at rest

Discharge instructions

- High-altitude Pulmonary Edema aftercare instructions

Admission criteria

- O_2 saturation < 95%
- Dyspnea at rest
- Inability to descend

Consult criteria

- Discuss all HAPE and high altitude illness patients with physician

Notes

REFERENCES:

Altitude-Related Disorders Author: Rahul M Kale, MD, FCCP; Chief Editor: Ryland P Byrd Jr, MD
emedicine.medscape.com/article/303571

Milledge JS, Beeley JM, Broome J, Luff N, Pelling M, Smith D. Acute Mountain Sickness Susceptibility, Fitness and

Hypoxic Ventilatory Response. Eur Respir J 1991;4:1000–3

Near Drowning Protocol

Definition

- Survival from a submersion occurring within the past 24 hours of sufficient submersion duration to warrant medical attention or survival beyond 24 hours of a submersion

Differential Diagnosis

- Child abuse
- Child neglect
- Suicide attempt
- Hypothermia
- Seizure
- Drug or toxin ingestion
- Hypoglycemia
- Head and neck trauma

Considerations

- Classified either cold water (< 20°C or 68°F) or warm water (≥ 20°C or 68°F) injury
- Very cold water injury is with water temperature ≤ 5°C (41°F)
- Most patients have an aspiration of water < 4 cc/kg
- Blood imbalances occur with aspiration > 11 cc/kg
- Electrolyte imbalances occur with aspiration > 22 cc/kg
- PO ingestion more likely to cause electrolyte imbalances
- Primary injury is hypoxemia
- Survival mainly determined by amount of brain hypoxemia and injury
- Laryngospasm can prevent aspiration
- Heimlich maneuver not effective in removing aspirated water
- Differences between freshwater and salt water submersions not clinically significant

Orlowski score — 1 point for each item

- Age 3 years or older
- Submersion time of more than 5 minutes
- No resuscitative efforts for more than 10 minutes after rescue
- Comatose on admission to the emergency department
- Arterial pH of less than 7.10
- Score of 2 or less = 90% complete recovery
- Score of 3 or more = 5% survival

History of event includes

- Submersion time
- Water temperature
- Symptoms
- Associated injuries
- Type of rescue
- Response to treatment
- Cough or shortness of breath
- Concomitant drug or alcohol use
- Past medical history (seizures, cardiac, diabetes, etc.)

Physical findings categories

- Asymptomatic
- Symptomatic
  - Abnormal vital signs
  - Dyspnea
  - Neurologic deficit
  - Altered level of consciousness
  - Anxiety
- Cardiopulmonary arrest
- Expired

Evaluation Options Depending on Severity of Presentation

- Remove wet clothing
- Chest x-ray – all patients
- O_2 saturation – all patients
- ABG
- CBC
- BMP

- LFT's
- U/A
- PT/PTT/INR
- Fibrinogen, D-dimer, fibrin split products
- Troponin useful in severe presentations for prognosis
- Toxicology evaluation as indicated
- C-spine imaging as indicated
- CT head as indicated for trauma or altered mental status
- Evaluate for associated injuries
- Core temperature
- Cardiac and O_2 saturation continuous monitoring prn

Treatment Options

- Notify physician immediately for altered mental status, neurologic abnormalities, hypoxia or hypotension
- Oxygen up to 100% FiO_2 depending on symptoms and findings
- Albuterol inhalations prn
- Correct any hypothermia (see Hypothermia Protocol)
- IV NS prn hypotension
- Vasopressors prn hypotension
- Intubation prn severe respiratory distress
- Extracorporeal cardiopulmonary resuscitation after active chest compressions may improve survival
- Steroids are of no benefit
- Hypothermia patients should be resuscitated while aggressive attempts to restore normal body temperature ensue
- Antibiotics can be given for submersion in sewage or contaminated water

Discharge Criteria

- Patients with normal examination, normal vital signs and normal chest x-ray and lab, and trivial history may be discharged after 6 hours observation
- Immersion history with mild symptoms, normal lab and chest x-ray, may be discharged after 6–12 hours of observation

Discharge instructions

- Near drowning aftercare instructions
- All discharged patients should be rechecked in 24–48 hours
- Return or see primary care provider promptly if cough, fever or shortness of breath occurs

Admission Criteria

- Hypoxia
- Acute neurologic findings
- Symptomatic patients
- Acute chest x-ray findings
- Prolonged submersion history

Consult Criteria

- Discuss all near drowning patients with physician

Notes

REFERENCES:

Topjian AA, Berg RA, Nadkarni VM. Pediatric cardiopulmonary resuscitation: Advances in science, techniques, and outcomes. Pediatrics. 2008;122:1086–1098

Prognostic factors in pediatric cases of drowning and near-drowning. Orlowski JP JACEP 1979 May;8(5):176–9

Drowning Author: G Patricia Cantwell, MD, FCCM; Chief Editor: Joe Alcock, MD MS emedicine.medscape.com/article/772753

Medications

Section Contents

Pain Management Protocol

Drug Interactions

When using any protocol, always follow the Guidelines of Proper Use (page 12).

Pain Management Protocol

Considerations

- Pain is the most frequent complaint for seeking care in the emergency department or acute care settings
- Many studies have demonstrated the under-treatment of pain by Providers
- Abuse of prescription narcotics has increased in the recent past
- Under-treatment of pain can lead to pseudoaddiction — a condition where the patient actively seeks, over time, pain control
  - This is frequently perceived by Providers as drug seeking behavior
- JCAHO has standards regarding pain assessment and the right of the patient to adequate control of pain
  - This can cause the perception that the policy contributes to abuse of opioid prescriptions
- Chronic pain is not managed well in the acute care settings
- Degree of chronic pain is not always reflected in the Provider's observation of the patient's degree of discomfort or in abnormal vital signs
  - Acute pain is reflected more so in patient's signs of discomfort and abnormal vital signs

Opioid Risk Tool

Low risk 0 Moderate risk 4–7 High risk ≥ 8

	Add up points	Female patient	Male patient
Family history of substance abuse	Alcohol Illegal drugs Prescription drugs	1 point 2 points 4 points	3 points 3 points 4 points
Personal history of substance abuse	Alcohol Illegal drugs Prescription drugs	3 points 4 points 5 points	3 points 4 points 5 points
Age 16–45 years		1 point	1 point
History of preadolescent sexual abuse		3 points	0 point
Psychological disease	Attention deficit disorder OCD Bipolar Schizophrenia Depression	2 points 2 points 2 points 2 points 1 points	2 points 2 points 2 points 2 points 1 point

Analgesic medication facts

- Analgesics do not alter the ability to diagnose the cause of undifferentiated abdominal pain, and they may even improve diagnostic accuracy
- Antiemetics do not enhance the analgesic effects of opioids at the commonly used doses
- There is no evidence that any NSAID provides any better analgesia than another. The analgesic effect from ketorolac is similar to other NSAIDs
- Ibuprofen 600 mg plus acetaminophen 1,000 mg has better pain relief than hydrocodone 5 mg
- Codeine has limited utility due to its low potency and frequent side effects
- **Addiction or abuse potential significantly increases if opioids prescribed more than 3 days or >180 MME/day in opioid naïve patients**
- Use of short-acting opioids such as heroin or oxycodone several times daily for at least 2 weeks is needed before opioid dependence develops
- It is more effective to give pain medication on a regular dosing schedule rather than waiting for the pain to be uncontrolled
- The increase in intrabiliary pressure with morphine is of no clinical significance
- Opioid analgesics can be an important part of pain management in patients with chronic or recurrent pain syndromes that is best treated by a pain clinic or patient's medical provider
- When narcotics are prescribed in short courses to treat acute pain, iatrogenic addiction is rare (≤3 days or ≤ 180 MME/day)
- In most studies, the analgesic effect of tramadol is equivalent or only slightly better than placebo

Best to prescribe opioids acutely 3 days or less at q4hr max dosing intervals that are ≤ 180 mg Morphine Equivalents (MME)

Oxycodone 10 mg	12 tablets	180 MME
Oxycodone 7.5 mg	16 tablets	180 MME
Oxycodone 5 mg	18 tablets	135 MME
Hydrocodone 10 mg	18 tablets	180 MME
Hydrocodone 5 mg	18 tablets	90 MME
Hydrocodone 10 mg per 5ml elixir	90 ml	180 MME
Morphine 15 mg	12 tablets	180 MME
Morphine 30 mg	6 tablets	180 MME
Hydromorphone 2 mg	18 tablets	144 MME
Hydromorphone 4 mg	11 tablets	176 MME
Tramadol 25 mg	18 tablets	45 MME
Tramadol 50 mg	18 tablets	90 MME

Evaluation

- Urine and serum drug screens are not particular routinely useful in evaluating patients
  - Drug screens may be useful if patient states they have not used controlled substances for the past 10 days to determine truthfulness
  - Drug screens may be useful if patient states they are taking prescription narcotics currently and the drug screen is negative, perhaps indicating that they are selling the opioid
- If a pattern of abuse is suspected and/or required by law, check controlled substance prescription databases where available
- Take a history of pain treatment
- Patients who request a specific controlled substance may be more suspect for abuse behavior

Treatment Options

- Patients with chronic pain that come to the emergency department or urgent care setting should be tactfully informed that chronic pain is best managed long term by one Provider in the clinic setting
- Preferable to manage pain if reasonable with non–opioid therapy
  - Check to see if non–opioid therapy has been tried and optimized where appropriate
- Use multimodal pain control methods, such as NSAID with acetaminophen, gabapentin, topical preparations, antidepressants, heat or ice, physical therapy etc. where appropriate
  - Prescribe opioids only when necessary and for most intense pain that is likely to require opioids
- Older patients should receive lower opioid dosing and extended dosing intervals
- If the Provider assesses a reasonable need to prescribe controlled pain medications, it should be of a short course and limited number of pills (≤ 180 MME/day) without refills usually, with shortest acting and lowest dose used where appropriate
  - Exceptions are situations where a terminal cancer patient or other similar type patients with significant pain considerations that will have a delay in treatment in the outpatient office setting
- Pain amenable to local injections, such as dental pain etc., in patients with frequent repeat visits, can be treated with Marcaine (bupivacaine) local blocks depending on skill level of Provider and referred to an outpatient settings for further care
- It is appropriate to express concern for the patient's dependence on controlled substances where the Provider feels it may be productive and appropriate
- There are situations where a noncontrolled substance is more effective, such as in migraine therapy, and it should be used instead
- It may be necessary to decline controlled substance treatment of pain in patients with a history of

troublesome behavior of controlled substances use where appropriate

- Effective chronic pain treatment decreases visits, use of resources, improves patient care and improves patient satisfaction
- Antiemetic medication should not be used routinely with PO narcotics
- Oxycodone may be preferred over hydrocodone for patients that routinely take acetaminophen

Starting Dose for Opioid Naïve Patent		Immediate Release Half-life
Hydromorphone	2–4 mg q4–6 hours PO prn	2–3 hours
Morphine	10–-30 mg q hours PO prn	2–3 hours
Oxycodone	5–10 mg q4–6 hours PO prn	2–3 hours
Oxymorphone	2.5–5 mg q4–6 hours PO prn	7–-9 hours
Tapentadol	50 mg q6 hours PO prn	4 hours
Tramadol	25–50 mg q6 hours PO prn	6–9 hours

Disposition

- Refer chronic pain or frequent recurrent pain patients to their primary care provider
- Referral to a Pain Management Clinic is appropriate in many situations
- Short courses of controlled pain medications with limited amount of pills and no refills is encouraged depending on the clinical situation
- Chronic or acute pain aftercare instructions

Notes

REFERENCES:

Hooten WM, Timming R, Belgrade M, Gaul J, Goertz M, Haake B, Myers C, Noonan MP, Owens J, Saeger L, Schweim K, Shteyman G, Walker N. Assessment and management of chronic pain. Bloomington (MN): Institute for Clinical Systems Improvement (ICSI); 2013 Nov. 105

Glazier HS. Potentiation of pain relief with hydroxyzine: A therapeutic myth? Ann Pharmacother 1990;24:484–488

Pain Management In The ED: Prompt, Cost-Effective, State-Of-The-Art Strategies Michael A. Turturro, MD, FACEP

Shah A, Hayes CJ, Martin BC. Factors Influencing Long–Tern Opioid Use Among Opioid naïve Patients: An Examination of Initial Prescription Characteristics and Pain Etiologies. J Pain 2017: 18:1374

Ann Emerg Med. 2019;73:481

DRUG INTERACTIONS

Considerations

- Geriatric patients have a 20–30% hospitalization rate from drug effects or interactions
- Drug interactions diagnosed 25% of the time

QTc Interval Prolongation

Symptoms that may occur *(not very common)*

- Syncope
- Sudden death

QTc Prolongation Medications (among others)

Antipsychotics	Antidepressants	Antiemetics (additive)
Pimozide	Tricyclics	Haldol
Olanzapine	Trazodone	Droperidol
Ziprasidone		Promethazine
	Antibiotics	Zofran (ondansetron)
Antiarrhythmics	Macrolides	Reglan (metoclopramide)
Amiodarone	Fluoroquinolones	
Quinidine		

Digoxin (digitalis) Levels

Increased by

- NSAID's
- Verapamil
- Quinidine
- Amiodarone

CYP2C9 Cytochrome Inhibition Drugs that Increase Warfarin, Sulfonylureas, Dilantin Effects or Levels

- Trimethoprim/sulfamethoxazole
- COX-II inhibitors
- Aspirin; salicylates
- ACE inhibitors
- Macrolides
- Phenobarbital
- Isoniazid
- SSRI's
- Amiodarone
- Prilosec
- Cimetidine

Serotonin Syndrome

- Caused by 1 drug by itself or 2 serotonergic drug interaction

Drugs

- Amitriptyline — Demerol (meperidine) — SSRI's
- Citalopram — Tramadol — Amphetamine
- Anafranil — Effexor — Buspar
- Robitussin — Nardil — Most antidepressants
- Fenfluramine — MAO inhibitors
- Prozac — Zoloft

Signs and symptoms of serotonin syndrome

Cognitive abnormalities	Autonomic dysfunction	Neuro-muscular
Confusion	Hyperthermia	Myoclonus
Agitation	Diaphoresis	Hyperreflexia
Coma	Sinus tachycardia	Rigidity
Anxiety	Hypertension	Tremor
Lethargy	Tachypnea	Hyperactivity
Seizures	Dilated pupils	Ataxia

Evaluation

- CBC
- BMP
- CPK

Treatment

- Discontinue offending drugs
- Periactin 4–8 mg PO initially prn; 4 mg PO qid prn
- Ativan or valium prn

Consult criteria recommendation

- All suspected serotonin syndromes

Notes

REFERENCES:

Important Drug-Drug Interactions For The Emergency Physician, Gerald Maloney, DO, emedhome.com/features

Disease Management

Section Contents

When using any management guideline, always follow the Guidelines of Proper Use (page 12).

Hypertension Management

Definitions (JNC 7)

- In adults ≥ 18 years of age, hypertension classifications are the following with 2 or more averaged seated BP measurements over 2 or more office visits (initial BP may be elevated due to anxiety)
  - Normal
    - SBP < 120 mm Hg
    - DBP < 80 mm Hg
  - Prehypertension
    - SBP 120–139 mm Hg
    - DBP 80–89 mm Hg
    - Some controversy exists if this label should be given to patients without diabetic, cardiac or stroke histories
  - Stage 1 hypertension
    - SBP 140–159 mm Hg
    - DBP 90–99 mm Hg
  - Stage 2 hypertension
    - SBP ≥ 160 mm Hg
    - DBP ≥ 100 mm Hg

Considerations

- SBP > 140 mm Hg in age > 50 years is more important cardiovascular disease (CVD) risk factor than elevated diastolic pressure > 90 mm Hg
- Risk doubles for CVD for each SBP/DBP increase of 20/10 mm Hg starting at 115/75 mm Hg blood pressure (BP)
- Thiazide diuretics should be used initially or in combination with other antihypertensive medications in uncomplicated hypertension
- Most patients will require 2 or more antihypertensive medications to achieve target blood pressure of < 140/90 mm Hg in patients without diabetes or chronic kidney disease
- If blood pressure is > 20/10 mm Hg over target BP, consideration should be given to initiating 2 antihypertensive drugs, one of which should be a thiazide diuretic usually
- Clinician's judgment remains paramount in using guidelines
- Self-measured averaged blood pressures at home > 135/85 mm Hg are considered hypertensive

High risk conditions that have indications for initiation of other antihypertensive medications besides a diuretic

- Heart failure
- Postmyocardial infarction
- High coronary disease risk
- Diabetes
- Chronic kidney disease
- Recurrent stroke prevention in patients with history of stroke

Evaluation

- U/A
- CBC
- CMP
- EKG
- Lipid profile
- Bilateral arm blood pressures
- Optic fundus examination
- Body mass index (BMI) calculation
- Auscultation for carotid, abdominal and femoral bruits
- Thyroid gland palpation
- Heart and lung examination
- Abdominal examination for masses and abdominal aortic pulsation
- Check legs for edema and arterial pulses
- Neurologic examination

JNC 8 Goals of Therapy

- Age < 60 years initiate treatment for a SBP ≥ 140 mm Hg or DBP ≥ 90 mm Hg to achieve a target SBP of < 140 mm Hg and DBP < 90 mm Hg in patients without diabetes or chronic kidney disease
- Age ≥ 60 years treat SBP ≥ 150 mm Hg or DBP ≥ 90 mm Hg to

achieve SBP < 150 mm Hg and DBP < 90 mm Hg

- If SBP < 140 mm Hg is well tolerated and without adverse effects on quality of life, then medications do not need to be adjusted
- Age ≥ 18 years with diabetes or chronic kidney disease (CKD), initiate treatment if SBP ≥ 140 mm Hg DBP ≥ 90 mm Hg to achieve SBP < 140 mm Hg and DBP < 90 mm Hg
- General nonblack population initiate treatment with either a thiazide diuretic, CCB, ACEI or ARB
- General black population
  - Initial therapy with either a thiazide diuretic or CCB
    - More effective than beta–blockers, ACEIs or ARBs
  - ACEI induced angioedema occurs 2–4 times more frequent than in other groups
    - Treat with FFP (fresh frozen plasma) if needed
    - Tranexamic acid 1 gm IV over 10 minutes may be effective (no faster than 100 mg/minute)
- Age ≥ 18 years with CKD, initial or add-on therapy should include an ACEI or ARB
  - Improves kidney outcomes
- If blood pressure goal cannot be achieved in 1 month, increase or add a second drug from the list of thiazide diuretic, CCB, ACEI or ARB. If blood pressure control cannot be achieved with 2 drugs from the above list, add and titrate a third drug. If 3 drugs do not control blood pressure, a drug from another class can be added. Do not use an ACEI with an ARB

American Heart Association (AHA) 2017 Guidelines

- New targets for treatment: These recommend reductions in blood pressure <130/80 mm Hg in most adults (down from 140/90 mm Hg)
- Stage 1 hypertension adults with an average systolic pressure of 130 –139/80–89 mm Hg (these patients would have previously been considered as having "prehypertension").
- Atherosclerotic risk estimation to guide decisions in stage 1 hypertension: For patients at low atherosclerotic risk (10-year risk <10%), lifestyle changes alone are recommended, whereas for patients at high risk (including those with diabetes and kidney disease), lifestyle changes plus drug therapy is advised.
- Stage 2 classification: Patients with average systolic pressure >140 mm Hg or diastolic > 90 mm Hg
  - As before, drug therapy is recommended for all these patients irrespective of atherosclerotic risk
- Older adults have the same treatment target as younger patients, and drug therapy is recommended for all older adults (age > 65 years) with an average systolic pressure of 130 mm Hg or greater
- Most adults with blood pressure sufficiently elevated to warrant drug therapy should be treated initially with two agents, especially patients who are black or have stage 2 hypertension.
- More accurate estimation of blood pressure: Use average of measures taken over several visits, as well as out-of-office measurements

Treatment Options without High Risk Conditions

Prehypertension

- Lifestyle modification with
  - Weight loss diet rich in potassium and calcium (DASH eating plan)
  - 2400 mg sodium diet
  - Increased physical activity
  - Moderation of alcohol consumption

Stage 1 hypertension

- Lifestyle modification
- Thiazide diuretic for most patients
- May also consider
  - Angiotensin converting enzyme inhibitor (ACEI)
  - Angiotensin receptor blocker (ARB)
  - Beta–blocker (BB)
  - Calcium channel blocker (CCB)

OR

- Combination of above medications

Stage 2 hypertension

- Lifestyle modification
- Two drug combination of stage 1 hypertension medications usually (caution if risk of orthostatic hypotension–usually elderly)

Treatment Options with High Risk Conditions

Prehypertension

- Lifestyle modification
- Drugs as applicable in conditions below

Heart failure

- If asymptomatic give ≥ 1 medication
  - Angiotensin converting enzyme inhibitor
  - Beta–blocker
- If symptomatic give ≥ 1 medication with a loop diuretic — Lasix (furosemide) or Bumex (bumetanide)
  - Angiotensin converting enzyme inhibitor
  - Beta–blocker
  - Angiotensin receptor blocker
  - Aldosterone antagonist

Ischemic heart disease (stable angina)

- Beta–blocker

OR

- Long acting calcium channel blocker such as amlodipine

Post myocardial infarction options

- Beta–blocker
- ACEI
- Aldosterone antagonist
- Lipid management
- Low dose aspirin 160–325 mg PO qday

High risk for coronary disease options

- Thiazide diuretic
- Beta–blocker
- ACEI
- CCB
- Lipid management
- Low dose aspirin 160–325 mg PO qday

Diabetic hypertension options

Combination of ≥ 2 drugs usually needed

- Thiazide diuretic
- Beta–blocker
- ACEI or ARB (reduces diabetic nephropathy)
- CCB

Chronic kidney disease options

Definition of chronic kidney disease

- Glomerular filtration rate (GFR) < 60 cc/min
- Creatinine > 1.5 mg/dL in men and creatinine > 1.3 mg/dL in women
- Albuminuria > 300 mg/day or 200 mg of albumin/gm creatinine

Medication options

- ACEI
- ARB
- Loop diuretic such as Lasix (furosemide) may be needed with creatinine > 2.5 mg/dL
- Limited rise of up to 35% of creatinine with ACEI or ARB therapy is acceptable as long

as hyperkalemia does not develop

Recurrent stroke prevention options

- Thiazide diuretic
- ACEI
- Lipid management
- Low dose aspirin (160–325 mg PO qday) if hypertension reasonably controlled

Elderly patients

- Initial lower drug doses may be needed, though standard doses and multiple drugs are needed eventually in the majority to achieve BP control
- They are at risk of postural hypotension due to the frequent use of multiple medications

Follow Up and Achieving Blood Pressure Control

- Monthly follow up till blood pressure control is achieved
- Follow up every 3–6 months when blood control is achieved
- Serum creatinine and potassium should be checked 1–2 times per year
- Heart failure, diabetes and other comorbidities influence frequency of visits and tests needed
- Addition of a second drug should be in a different class if a single drug regimen was started initially and failed to achieve control
- Do not use 2 drugs in the same class at the same time (exception is Maxzide or Dyazide which are combination diuretic drugs)

Consult Criteria

- Unable to achieve target blood pressure reductions over several visits
- Blood pressure ≥ 180/110 mm Hg on 2 or more medications
- Symptomatic high risk conditions or comorbidities (CHF, progressive renal insufficiency, hyperkalemia, angina, stroke, etc.)
- More than 2 drugs needed to control blood pressure

Antihypertensive Medications (refer to PDR or drug databases)

Thiazide diuretics

- Chorothiazide (Diuril) 125–250 mg PO qday-bid
- Chorthalidone 12.5–25 mg PO qday
- Hydrochlorothiazide (HCTZ) 12.5–50 mg PO qday

Loop diuretics

- Lasix (furosemide) 20–40 mg PO bid
- Bumex (bumetanide) 0.5–1 mg PO bid
- Torsemide 2.5–10 mg PO qday

Potassium sparing diuretics

- Triamterene 25–50 mg PO qday-bid
- Amiloride 5 mg PO qday-bid

Aldosterone receptor blockers

- Aldactone 25–50 mg PO qday

Beta–blockers

- Atenolol 25–100 mg PO qday
- Metoprolol 50–100 mg PO qday-bid (NMT 450 mg daily)
    - Metoprolol tartrate is bid dosing and metoprolol succinate is qday dosing
- Corgard (Nadolol) 40–120 mg PO qday
- Toprol XL (metoprolol) 50–100 mg PO qday
- Propranolol 20–80 mg PO bid

Beta-blockers with intrinsic sympathomimetic activity

- Sectral (acebutolol) 200–400 mg PO bid
- Pindolol 5–10 mg PO bid

Combined alpha and beta-blockers

- Coreg (carvedilol) 6.25–25 mg PO bid increase every 1–2 weeks as tolerated and needed up to 25 mg bid

- Labetalol 100–400 mg PO bid

Angiotensin converting enzyme inhibitors (ACEI)

- Lisinopril 5–40 mg PO qday
- Captopril 12.5–50 mg PO bid
- Accupril (quinapril) 10–80 mg PO qday

Angiotensin receptor blockers

- Atacand (candesartan) 8–32 mg PO qday
- Losartan 25–50 mg PO qday-bid
- Diovan (valsartan) 80–320 mg PO qday

Calcium channel blockers—non-Dihydropyridines

- Cardizem CD (diltiazem) 180–420 mg PO qday
- Cardizem LA (diltiazem) 120–540 mg PO qday
- Calan (verapamil) SR 120–240 mg PO qday-bid

Calcium channel blockers—dihydropyridines

- Amlodipine 2.5–10 mg PO qday
- Procardia XL (nifedipine) 30–60 mg PO qday

Alpha-1 blockers (not first line drugs)

- Cardura (doxazosin) 1–16 mg PO qday
- Cardura XL (doxazosin) 4–8 mg PO qday
- Minipres (prazosin) 1–5 mg PO bid-tid
- Caution for orthostatic hypotension — give first dose and any increases at bedtime

Central alpha-2 agonists

- Clonidine 0.1–0.3 mg PO bid-tid
- Catapres –TTS (clonidine) patch 0.1–0.3 mg qweek (NMT 0.6 mg/24 hours)

Combination drugs (some)

- ACEI+CCB (Lotrel) amlodipine and benazepril 2.5/10–10/20 mg PO qday
- ACEI+HCTZ (Zestoretic) Lisinopril and HCTZ 10/12.5–20/25 mg PO qday
- ARBs+diuretic (Diovan-HCT) valsartan and HCTZ 80/12.5–160/50 mg PO qday
- Beta–blocker+diuretic (Tenoretic) atenolol and HCTZ 50/25 to 100/25 PO qday
- Diuretic and diuretic (Aldactazide) 25/25 to 50/50 mg PO qday-bid

Notes

REFERENCES:

nhlbi.nih.gov/guidelines/hypertension/express.pdf

JNC 7 — The Seventh Report of the Joint National Committee on Prevention, Detection, Evaluation and Treatment of High Blood Pressure

Hypertension Treatment & Management
Author: Meena S Madhur, MD, PhD; Chief Editor: David J Maron, MD, FACC, FAHA

2014 Evidence-Based Guideline for the Management of High Blood Pressure in Adults
Report From the Panel Members Appointed to the Eighth Joint National Committee (JNC 8)

New US Hypertension Guidelines: Experts Respond
Sue Hughes December 05, 2017

Coronary Artery Disease Management

Definitions

- Atherosclerotic changes in the walls of coronary arteries resulting in plaque formation and vascular remodeling

Differential diagnosis

- GERD
- Esophageal spasm
- Pulmonary embolism
- Musculoskeletal truncal pain
- Pleurodynia
- Anxiety disorder
- Panic disorder
- Aortic stenosis
- Aortic dissection
- Coronary artery vasospasm
- Cocaine abuse
- Pericarditis
- Myocarditis
- Peptic ulcer disease
- Gastritis
- Hiatal hernia
- Cholecystitis
- Biliary colic

Considerations

- Can cause diminished blood flow to cardiac muscle
- 14 million Americans have coronary artery disease (CAD)
- 1.5 million myocardial infarctions per year
- Greater than 500,000 deaths per year
- All NSAIDs increase the risk of MI and death from CV disease, even with short-term use (7–10 days).
  - Naproxen causes the least amount of CV side effects, and is the preferred NSAID for patients taking prophylactic low-dose aspirin
- Medium-size coronary plaques (30%–40% stenosis) may be vulnerable to cause occlusion because they are less mature, with a large lipid core and a thin cap prone to rupture or erode, exposing the thrombogenic subendothelial components
- Patient education very important

Risk factors

- Smoking
- Male sex
- Age
- Hypertension
- Hyperlipidemia
- Dyslipidemia
- Diabetes mellitus
- Family history
- Sedentary lifestyle
- Obesity
- Metabolic syndrome
- Rheumatoid arthritis/SLE (females > males)

Acute coronary syndrome (unstable angina or AMI)

- Unstable plaque rupture causing thrombus formation obstructing vessel lumen leading to angina and/or AMI
- May have less than 50% blockage of artery by plaque alone
- Decreased incidence with statin and ACE inhibitor treatment
  - ACE inhibitors improve endothelial function
- Decreased incidence with antiplatelet agents

New York Heart Association classification

- Class I — No limitation of physical activity (ordinary physical activity does not cause symptoms)
- Class II — Slight limitation of physical activity (ordinary physical activity does cause symptoms)
- Class III — Moderate limitation of activity (patient is comfortable at rest, but less

than ordinary activities cause symptoms)

- Class IV — Unable to perform any physical activity without discomfort, therefore severe limitation (patient may be symptomatic even at rest)

Unstable angina

- New-onset angina (within 2 mo. of initial presentation) of at least class III severity
- Significant recent increase in frequency and severity of angina
- Angina at rest

Signs and symptoms

- May be asymptomatic
- Chest pain centrally located or can be in various locations
  - May occur at rest, from exertion or from emotional stress
- Arm pain
- Jaw pain
- Shortness of breath
  - Dyspnea on exertion
- Diaphoresis
- Nausea
- Vomiting
- Syncope
- Sudden cardiac arrest or ventricular fibrillation (sudden death)
- Congestive heart failure

Physical Examination

- Usually normal
- S3/S4 heart sounds may be heard during anginal episode
- Levine sign — clenched fist over central chest during chest pain suggestive of angina
- Xanthelasma or xanthoma as hyperlipidemia stigmata
- Carotid or aortic bruit
- Pulmonary rales from heart failure

Evaluation options

Initial tests

- EKG
- CBC
- BMP or CMP
- HbA1c if diabetic or glucose intolerant
- Fasting lipid profile
- Thyroid function tests
- Chest x-ray
- BNP (B-type natriuretic peptide) if heart failure considered
- C-reactive protein
- Urinary albumen to creatinine ratio
- Troponin for prolonged chest pain (≥ 10 minutes) in the past week that has resolved (if angina occurring in office that appears unstable — send to ER)
  - Troponin remains elevated 7–10 days

Imaging or stress testing

- Exercise with EKG monitoring
  - Initial procedure of choice without ST segment baseline resting abnormalities
  - ≥ 1 mm ST segment depression 80 msec from J point most characteristic change with positive test for ischemia
  - Withhold beta-blockers for 48 hours before test if possible
  - Dobutamine, adenosine and dipyridamole stress testing may be performed in patients unable to exercise
- Stress echocardiogram — sensitivity 78% and specificity 86%
  - Localizes ischemia and severity
  - Assists in evaluating left ventricle wall motion, cardiac chamber size and for valvular disease
  - May be technically difficult to get good images
- Myocardial perfusion scintigraphy — sensitivity of 83% and specificity of 77%
- Do not perform exercise stress testing with symptomatic arrhythmias, aortic stenosis or recent AMI

- Stop exercise stress testing with development of
  - Chest pain
  - Drop in systolic blood pressure > 10 mm Hg
  - Severe shortness of breath, fatigue, dizziness or near syncope
  - ST segment depression > 2 mm
  - ST segment elevations > 1 mm without diagnostic Q waves
  - Ventricular tachyarrhythmia
- 64 slice CT angiogram which has nearly 100% negative predictive value
- Coronary angiography

Treatment options

- Treat risk factors (see specific management sections)
- Smoking cessation
- Statins (see Cholesterol Management)
- ACE inhibitors and angiotensin receptor blockers
- Platelet inhibitors
  - Aspirin (ASA) 162–325 mg PO qday
  - Clopidogrel (Plavix) 12 months after ACS episode, then ASA qday
- Beta–blockers
  - Stable or exertional angina
  - Heart failure
- Calcium channel blockers
- Nitrates (may cause hypotension with IHSS/ASH — hypertrophic cardiomyopathy)
- Ranolazine — reserved usually until after standard therapy has failed to control symptoms (not a first–line drug)
- Weight reduction as appropriate
- Increased physical activity as tolerated
- Cardiac rehabilitation

Medication treatment for stable angina

Anginal episode ≤ 1/week

- ASA
- NTG SL prn — may repeat q5minutes x 2 prn

Anginal episode ≥ 2 /week

- ASA
- NTG SL prn — may repeat q5minutes x 2 prn
- Long acting NTG

May add as needed

- Beta-blocker
- ACEI or ARB to a beta-blocker
- Add calcium channel blocker when symptoms persist on beta–blocker or beta–blocker cannot be used (do not use verapamil with beta–blocker)

High risk patient

- ASA or clopidogrel
- ACEI or ARB added to nitrates and beta–blockers

Angina persists or not controlled on 3 medications

- Coronary angiography

Medication selections

Statins

- May causes liver and muscle disease
- Stop if CPK becomes elevated
- Read drug information for adverse reactions, cautions and contraindications
- Avoid in heavy alcohol use
- See Cholesterol Management section

Atorvastatin (Lipitor)

- 10–20 mg PO qday initially
- 10–80 mg PO qday maintenance
- Stop if LFT's > 3 times normal

Pravastatin (Pravachol)

- 10–40 mg PO qday — not to exceed 80 mg/day
- Hepatic and renal impairment — 10 mg PO qday

- Do not use in active liver disease

Simvastatin (Zocor)

- 10–20 mg PO qday in the evening
- If high risk for CAD — 40 mg PO qday in the evening
- Stop if LFT's > 3 times normal or renal failure develops
- Myopathy risk greater at 80 mg PO qday dosing

Rosuvastatin (Crestor)

- 10–20 mg PO qday initially — may titrate but not to exceed 40 mg PO qday
- Caution in liver disease
- Start at 5 mg PO qday in Asians

Lovastatin (Altoprev)

- 10–60 mg PO qhs
- Reduce if creatinine clearance < 30 mL/minute
- Stop if LFT's > 3 times normal, renal failure or myopathy with elevated CPK develops
- Avoid in heavy alcohol use

Fluvastatin (Lescol, Lescol XL)

- Start 20–40 mg PO qhs
- Dose range 20–80 mg PO qday
  - Divide bid if 80 mg used
- Stop if LFT's > 3 times normal, renal failure or myopathy with elevated CPK develops

Nitrates

- Decreases preload, afterload, myocardial work and oxygen consumption
- Dilates coronary arteries
- Long-acting nitrates used continuously throughout the day will develop tolerance in 24–48 hours and lose effectiveness, so a nitrate free period for 8–12 hours each day with no long-acting nitrates is needed, frequently performed during sleep periods

Short-acting nitrates

- NTG 0.3–0.6 SL prn — may repeat x 2 q5minutes prn continued ischemic cardiac pain
- May use before anginal provoking activities
  - Comes in tablets or spray
  - Tablets need refrigeration and last 3–6 months, and should tingle under tongue when used
  - NTG spray lasts 2–3 years

Long-acting nitrates for stable angina

- Timing — taken at time of day that anginal symptoms or anginal equivalent symptoms (i.e., dyspnea) are most prevalent
- NTG 2.5 mg or 6.5 mg PO bid
- Isosorbide mononitrate
  - Standard dose — 20 mg PO bid given 7 hours apart
  - Smaller patients start 5 mg PO bid given 7 hours apart and increase to 10–20 mg PO bid given 7 hours apart over 2–3 days
  - Take on empty stomach 30 minutes prior to a meal or 1 hour after a meal
- Isosorbide mononitrate ER (extended release)
  - 30–120 mg PO qday
- Transdermal nitroglycerin (Nitro-Dur)
  - 0.2–0.4 mg/hr. qday — remove for 10–12 hours each day
  - Max dose 0.4–0.8 mg/hr. qday
  - Starts acting in 30 minutes and lasts 8–14 hours

Nitrate side-effects (some)

- Headache
- Hypotension
- Tachycardia
- Nausea

Nitrate contraindications

- Shock or hypotension

- SBP < 90 m Hg or ≥ 30 mm Hg below baseline SBP in ACS
- Bradycardia < 50 beats per minute
- Tachycardia in absence of heart failure (> 100 beats per minute)
- Acute right ventricular myocardial infarction
    - Caution in inferior myocardial infarction
- Use of erectile dysfunction medications (sildenafil, tadalafil, or vardenafil)
- Severe anemia

Beta-blockers

- Reduce heart rate, blood pressure and cardiac contractility which decreases cardiac work and oxygen needs
- First choice usually in stable angina
- Prolongs survival and decreases second AMI incidence

Selective beta–1 blocker

- Metoprolol tartrate (Lopressor) initially 50 mg PO bid and may be increased to 200 mg PO bid
- Metoprolol succinate (Toprol XL) 100 mg PO qday — NMT 400 mg PO qday
- Atenolol (Tenormin) 50 mg PO qday — NMT 200 mg PO qday

Non-selective beta–blocker

- Propranolol (Inderal) 80–120 mg PO bid — may increase at weekly intervals as needed
- Inderal LA 80–160 mg PO qday
- NMT 320 mg PO qday

Beta–blocker side effects (some)

- Bradycardia
- Hypotension
- Worsening of asthma and COPD
- Depression
- Heart failure
- Exacerbation of angina and hypertension on abrupt withdrawal (Black Box Warning)
- Worsening of peripheral arterial disease symptoms

Contraindications (some)

- Pre-existing sinus bradycardia (< 60 beats/minutes)
- Moderate to severe left ventricle failure and pulmonary edema
- SBP < 100 mm Hg
- Signs of poor peripheral perfusion
- 2nd and 3rd degree heart block
- Asthma and COPD
- Sick sinus syndrome without pacemaker
- Untreated pheochromocytoma

ACE inhibitors

- Reduces death, AMI, stroke, coronary stents revascularization and CABG
- May use in high risk patients even if no hypertension or heart failure present
- Start at low dose and titrate upward as tolerated

Ramipril (Altace)

- 2.5–10 mg PO qday

Lisinopril (Zestril)

- Start at 10 mg PO qday — usual range 20–40 mg PO qday

Quinapril (Accupril)

- Initially 5–10 mg PO qday — maintenance 20–80 mg PO qday

Side effects

- ACE inhibitor induced angioedema (may be treated with fresh frozen plasma or tranexamic acid, and discontinue the ACEI or ARB)
- Renal impairment
- Hyperkalemia
- Hypotension
- Do not use in pregnancy, bilateral renal artery stenosis, hypersensitivity and history of angioedema

Calcium channel blockers

- Dilate vessels, lowers blood pressure and decreases cardiac workload
- Not as effective in decreasing angina frequency as beta–blockers, but similar as beta–blockers in reducing need for NTG and improving exercise tolerance
- Use calcium channel blocker when symptoms persist on beta–blocker or beta–blocker cannot be used (do not use verapamil with beta–blocker)

Amlodipine (Norvasc)

- 5–10 mg PO qday initially
- 10 mg PO qday maintenance
- Elderly 5 mg PO qday
- With hepatic impairment start with 5 mg PO qday

Diltiazem (Cardizem)

- Start 30 mg PO qid and increase every 1–2 days to control angina as needed up to 90 mg PO qid

Diltiazem (Cardizem CD)

- Start 120–180 mg PO qday and increase as needed over 1–2 weeks — NMT 480 mg PO qday

Calcium channel blocker side effects (some)

- Heart failure
- AV block
- Hypotension
- Erythema multiforme
- Peripheral edema
- Headache
- Elevated LFT's

Contraindications (some)

- Pre-existing sinus bradycardia
- 2nd and 3rd degree heart block
- Sick sinus syndrome without pacemaker
- Hypersensitivity

Ranolazine (Renexa)

- Antianginal agent (not first–line treatment)
- May be used in addition to other antianginal medications when angina is uncontrolled
- 500 mg PO bid initially — NMT 1,000 mg PO bid

Cautions and contraindications

- Do not use in hepatic cirrhosis patients
- Contraindicated with strong CYP3A inhibitors or inducers
  - Ketoconazole, itraconazole, clarithromycin, rifampin, carbamazepine, phenytoin, St. John's wort, nelfinavir, ritonavir, indinavir among others
- Not for acute anginal episodes
- Avoid grapefruit products
- Lower dose to 500 mg PO bid with aprepitant, diltiazem, erythromycin, fluconazole, grape-fruit juice or products, verapamil — read literature for all drug interactions

Referral criteria

- Angina not controlled with 2–3 antianginal medications
- Acutely worsening angina

Notes

REFERENCES:

Circulation 2010;122:S787–S817

CHEST October 2011;140(4_MeetingAbstracts):594A-594A. doi:10.1378/chest.1112163

CHEST August 2011;140(2):509–518. doi:10.1378/chest.10–2468

Angina Pectoris Author: Jamshid Alaeddini, MD, FACC, FHRS; Chief Editor: Eric H Yang, MD

emedicine.medscape.com/article/150215

Amsterdam EA, Wenger NK. The 2014 American College of Cardiology ACC/American Heart Association guideline for the management of patients with non-ST-elevation acute coronary syndromes: ten contemporary recommendations to aid clinicians in optimizing patient outcomes. *Clin Cardiol.* 2015 Feb. 38(2):121-3

Acute Coronary Syndrome; Author: David L Coven, MD, PhD; Chief Editor: Eric H Yang, MD emedicine.medscape.com/article/1910735

Circulation 1979 Mar;59(3):585-8; Blood levels after sublingual nitroglycerin. Armstrong PW, Armstrong JA, Marks GS

Age-Adjusted D-Dimer Cutoff Levels to Rule Out Pulmonary Embolism: The ADJUST-PE Study *JAMA.* 2014;311(11):1117-1124. doi:10.1001/jama.2014.2135

JEM, epub, 7/29/16

CCJM;81:233

Heart Failure Management

Definition

- Inability of the heart to pump enough blood to meet the metabolic needs of the body

Differential diagnosis

- COPD
- Pneumonia
- Asthma
- Acute myocardial infarction
- Pulmonary embolism
- Pulmonary fibrosis
- Adult respiratory distress syndrome
- End–stage renal disease

Considerations

- Fastest growing cardiac disease in the U.S.
- Systolic heart failure has decreased left ventricle (LV) pump function (decreased ejection fraction)
- Diastolic heart failure has normal or slightly reduced left ventricle ejection fraction
  - Impaired relaxation and stiffness of the LV causes decreased filling and amount of blood pumped per contraction
  - Has increased LV diastolic filling pressure
  - Associated with lower mortality but high morbidity
- Most common cause of decompensation is decrease in therapy (medical or dietary noncompliance)
- Mortality following hospitalization for heart failure is 10% at 30 days, 20% at 1 year, 42% at 5 years
- Mortality for cardiogenic shock is ~80%
- ACE inhibitors and beta–blockers decrease mortality and are the recommended cornerstone of treatment

B-type natriuretic peptide (BNP)

- < 100 pg/mL – 90% do not have heart failure
- > 500 pg/mL – 90% have heart failure
- Different assays have different cut–off values

Cardiorenal syndrome

- Worsening heart failure
- Decreasing renal function
- Increasing diuretic resistance
- Treatment involves combination diuretics, vasodilators, inotropes and possibly ultrafiltration

  - May be mistaken for the creatinine increase that may occur after initiation of diuretic therapy

Causes of heart failure

- Coronary artery disease
- Hypertension
- Diabetes mellitus
- Valvular heart disease
- Cardiomyopathy
  - Idiopathic
  - Alcoholic
  - Cocaine
  - Chemotherapy
  - Postpartum
  - Myocarditis
- Arrhythmia (i.e., atrial fibrillation)
  - May need cardiac resynchronization therapy
- Congenital heart disease
- NSAID's can worsen heart failure
- Calcium channel blockers and antiarrhythmics (except class III) can worsen heart failure (amiodarone ok)

Signs and symptoms (some or all)

Left or biventricular heart failure

- Tachycardia
- Rales
- S3 gallop
- Nocturnal cough
- Pleural effusion
- Dyspnea at rest or with exertion
- Orthopnea
- Paroxysmal nocturnal dyspnea
- Tachypnea
- Bilateral pitting pedal or pretibial edema
- Jugular venous distension
- Hypotension in late or preterminal stages

Isolated or predominant right heart failure

- Ascites
- Bilateral leg edema or anasarca
- Hepatomegaly
- Nausea
- Constipation
- Absence of pulmonary congestion
- Pleural effusion (increase in death rate when right heart failure causes pleural effusion as compared to right heart failure without pleural effusion)
- S3 gallop

New York Heart Association classification

- Class 1 – no limitations of physical activity
- Class 2 – slight limitation of physical activity
- Class 3 – marked limitation of physical activity
- Class 4 – symptoms at rest and unable to do physical activity without discomfort

Evaluation options

- History and physical examination
- EKG
- Chest x-ray
- CBC (for anemia or infection)
- U/A for proteinuria
- CMP
- NT–ProBNP
- Lipid profile
- TSH and thyroid function tests
- 2–D echocardiogram
- Exercise testing to determine suitability for exercise training
- Coronary angiography or nuclear cardiac stress test for suspected angina

Treatment options

- Patient education
- 2 to 3 gram sodium diet
- Avoid NSAID's, class I antiarrthymia drugs (amiodarone

and dofetilide OK) and calcium channel blockers (if LV function is decreased)

- Fluid restriction to 2 liters/day if serum Na < 130 mEq/dL and if sodium restriction and loop diuretics (furosemide etc.) do not control fluid status
- Acute CHF exacerbation see Congestive Heart Failure Protocol
- Oxygen — avoid high flow oxygen (maintain O_2 saturation ≥ 90–96%)
  - Causes coronary and systemic vasoconstriction
  - Avoid very high O_2 saturations caused by supplemental oxygen

Long term therapy

Stage A patient

- At risk for heart failure without structural heart disease and without symptoms
  - Hypertension
  - Atherosclerotic disease
  - Diabetes
  - Obesity
  - Metabolic syndrome

Treatment

- Hypertension control
- Smoking cessation
- Treat lipid disorders
- Regular exercise
- Discourage alcohol intake
- Control metabolic syndrome
- ACEI or ARB for diabetes or vascular disease

Stage B patient

- Structural heart disease without signs or symptoms of heart failure
  - AMI
  - Left ventricular hypertrophy and low ejection fraction (EF)
  - Asymptomatic valvular disease

Treatment

- Stage A patient treatment

  Plus
- ACEI or ARB as appropriate

  and/or
- Beta–blocker (BB) as appropriate

Stage C patient

- Structural heart disease with existing heart failure or history of heart failure

Treatment

- Routinely used
  - Diuretics for fluid retention
  - ACEI or ARB
  - Beta–blocker
- Selected patients
  - Aldosterone antagonist
  - ARB's
  - Digoxin
  - Hydralazine/nitrates
- Devices in selected patients
  - Biventricular pacing
  - Implantable defibrillator

Stage D patient

- Refractory heart failure despite maximal medical therapy requiring specialized interventions

Treatment

- Stage A, B and C treatments
- Hospice optional
- Extraordinary measures
  - Heart transplant
  - Chronic inotropes
  - Permanent mechanical support
  - Experimental surgery or drugs

Medications

ACE inhibitors (ACEI)

Used as first line therapy to decrease mortality

- Lisinopril (Zestril) 2.5–5 mg PO qday initially — target dose of 20 mg PO qday if needed
- Captopril (Capoten) 6.25 mg PO tid initially — target dose of 50 mg PO tid if needed

- Enalapril (Vasotec) 2.5 mg PO bid initially — target dose of 10 mg PO bid if needed

Angiotensin receptor blockers

May be used as first line therapy for heart failure and LV dysfunction or as add-on therapy

- Losartan (Cozaar) 12.5–254 mg PO qday initially — target dose of 150 mg PO qday if needed
- Valsartan (Diovan) 40 mg PO bid initially — target dose of 160 mg PO bid if needed

Combination neprilysin inhibitor and angiotensin II receptor blocker

- Sacubitril/Valsartan (Entresto)
  - Neprilysin inhibitors work to decrease the degradation of natriuretic peptides thereby increasing natriuresis (urinary sodium excretion)
  - Reduces the risk of cardiovascular death and hospitalization for heart failure in patients with NYHA class II-IV heart failure and reduced ejection fraction

Beta–blockers (BB)

All patients with chronic heart failure and systolic dysfunction unless contraindicated

- When patients are euvolemic and on afterload reduction such as ACEI's/ARB's
- Carvedilol (Coreg) 3.125 mg PO bid initially — target dose of 25 mg PO bid if needed
  - Moderate afterload and slight preload reduction
- Metoprolol succinate (Toprol XL) 12.5–25 mg PO qday initially — target dose of 200 mg PO qday if needed
  - Reduces heart rate and blood pressure
- Beta–blockers may be discontinued or decreased by 50% with acute heart failure exacerbations if needed

Aldosterone antagonists

Recommended for heart failure patients who are hospitalized frequently or have moderate to severe symptoms and are on ACEI's and BB

- Spironolactone (Aldactone) 12.5–25 mg PO qday initially — target dose of 25 mg PO qday if needed (some decrease in hospitalizations)
  - Start at low dose in elderly and in patients with chronic renal insufficiency
  - May cause hyperkalemia — avoid if potassium > 5 mEq/L or creatinine > 2.5 mg/dL
    - Check potassium ≤ 1 week after starting
    - Stop potassium supplements
- Eplerenone (Inspra) 25 mg PO qday for heart failure after MI, may titrate to 50 mg PO qday over 4 weeks as needed

Vasodilators

Reduces afterload — can be used especially for African Americans already on optimal therapy with ACEI's/ARB, BB and diuretics for moderate to severe symptoms

- Hydralazine/isosorbide (Bidil) 37.5 mg hydralazine/20 mg isosorbide PO tid — with double of that as the target dose if needed

- Hydralazine (Apresoline) 37.5 mg PO qid initially with target dose of 75 mg PO qid if needed

Nitrates

Reduces preload and to a lesser extent afterload — may be used as first line agent when hypotension is not present or a concern

- NTG SL prn for acute heart failure exacerbation associated with mild to severe hypertension (immediate onset in 1–3 minutes)
- NTG ointment 1–2 inches for acute heart failure exacerbation depending on degree of hypertension (onset in 1 hour for hemodynamic effects, lasting 3–6 hours)

Loop diuretics

Used for fluid retention prn

- Furosemide (Lasix) 20 mg PO qday up to 40 mg PO tid (NMT 600 mg PO qday)
- Torsemide (Demadex) 10 mg PO qday prn (NMT 200 mg PO qday)

Inotropic agents

Decreases hospitalizations and heart failure symptoms but does not improve survival long term

- Digoxin (Lanoxin) 0.125–0.5 mg PO qday — usual daily dose is 0.125 mg (elderly) to 0.25 mg PO
  - Initial loading dose is 0.375–0.625 mg PO bid x 1 day
  - Therapeutic range is 0.8–2.0 ng/mL
  - Can also be used for atrial fibrillation control in addition to heart failure treatment
  - Monitor digoxin levels 24 hours after starting, then weekly until stable — measure trough or 1 hour before scheduled dose
  - Hypokalemia and hypomagnesemia may potentiate toxicity
  - Can cause AV block, severe bradycardia, PAT with block, ventricular arrhythmias, vomiting, etc. (read literature for cautions and contraindications)

Calcium channel blockers

- Usually not used in heart failure
- Amlodipine 2.5–10 mg PO qday in heart failure with preserved EF (HFpEF)

Soluble guanylate cyclase stimulator

- Smooth muscle relaxation and vasodilation
- Vericiquat (Verquvo) 2.5 mg PO qday, increasing 2.5 mg every 2 weeks up to 10 mg PO qday as tolerated

Sinus node inhibitors

- Ivabradine 2.5–5 mg PO bid, titrated at 2 week intervals to heart rate of 50–60 beats/minute
- For HFrEF patients who need further treatment despite beta–blocker and other maximal guideline therapy and heart rate > 70 beats/minute
- Do not use in acutely decompensated heart or BP < 90/50 or heart rate < 60 initially
- Do not use with SA block, sick sinus syndrome or 3rd degree AV block (unless demand pacemaker present)

Anticoagulation

- Aspirin 162 mg PO qday recommended — especially in ischemic heart disease
- Warfarin
  - Heart failure with atrial fibrillation (INR target is 2.0–3.0)

- Ischemic cardiomyopathy and recent large anterior MI or documented LV thrombus
- Thromboembolic event with or without evidence of an LV thrombus
- Paroxysmal or chronic atrial arrhythmias.
- Can be used as alternative to aspirin

- Clopidogrel (Plavix) 75 mg PO qday
  - Can be used as alternative to aspirin

Implantable cardiac defibrillators

- May be considered in patients with ejection fraction < 35% , NYHA Class 2 and 3 and estimated survival > 1 year
- Consider for patients with NYHA I through III heart failure.
  - ICDs are not indicated for those with refractory end-stage heart failure (nonambulatory patients with NYHA IV heart failure)
- Patient should be receiving optimal medical therapy with an ACEI or an ARB and a β-blocker
- Treatment for sudden cardiac death
- Newly diagnosed nonischemic heart failure
  - Optimize medical therapy and wait at least 3 months
  - Reevaluate the ejection fraction
  - This is to avoid placing an ICD in a patient whose condition will significantly improve with optimal medical therapy

Ultrafiltration

- Hospitalized patients with cardiorenal syndrome

LV assist devices

Consult criteria

- Refractory heart failure
- Heart failure requiring multiple medications
- New York Heart Association class 3 and 4

Notes

REFERENCES:

Cornet AD, et al. *Crit Care* 2013 Apr 18;17:313

emedicine.medscape.com/article/163062

Bermingham M, Shanahan MK, O'Connell E; et al. Aspirin use in heart failure: is low-dose therapy associated with mortality and morbidity benefits in a large community population? Circ Heart Failure. 2014;7:243–250

Pitt B, Pfeffer MA, Assmann SF, Boineau R, Anand IS, Claggett B, et al. Spironolactone for heart failure with preserved ejection fraction. N Engl J Med 2014; 370:1383–92

Heart Failure Society of America. Executive summary: HFSA 2006 Comprehensive Heart Failure Practice Guideline. *J Card Fail.* 2006;12:10–38.

Hunt SA, Abraham WT, Chin MH, et al; American College of Cardiology; American Heart Association Task Force on Practice Guidelines; American College of Chest Physicians; International Society for Heart and Lung Transplantation; Heart Rhythm Society. ACC/AHA 2005 guideline update for the diagnosis and management of chronic heart failure in the adult: summary article: a report of the American College of Cardiology/American Heart Association Task Force on Practice Guidelines (writing committee to update the 2001 guidelines for the evaluation and management of heart failure). *Circulation.* 2005;112:e154–e235

Heart Failure Treatment & Management Updated: May 07, 2018 Author: Ioana Dumitru, MD; Chief Editor: Gyanendra K Sharma, MD, FACC, FASE; emedicine.medscape (updated Mar 2, 2021)

TYPE 1 DIABETES MELLITUS MANAGEMENT

Definition

- Disease process that is dependent on exogenous insulin to sustain life

Classification of diabetes

The classification of diabetes includes four clinical classes:

- Type 1 diabetes (results from β-cell destruction, usually leading to absolute insulin deficiency)
- Type 2 diabetes (results from a progressive insulin secretory defect on the background of insulin resistance)
- Other specific types of diabetes due to other causes, e.g., genetic defects in β-cell function, genetic defects in insulin action, diseases of the exocrine pancreas (such as cystic fibrosis), and drug or chemical-induced (such as in the treatment of HIV/AIDS or after organ transplantation)
- Gestational diabetes mellitus (GDM) — diabetes diagnosed during pregnancy in a patient that is not clearly an overt diabetic

Differential diagnosis for Type 1 diabetes

- Type 2 diabetes mellitus
- Alcoholic ketoacidosis (for DKA)

Considerations

- Insulin levels are very low or absent
- Strong genetic predisposition
- Frequently presents with diabetic ketoacidosis (DKA)
- Increase incidence of infections
- Education is the most important aspect of treatment
  - Requires dietician, nurse, diabetic counselor and medical provider in a team approach
- HbA1c levels reflects the previous 3 months of glycemia
- Fasting C-peptide level greater than 1 mg/dL is associated more with type 2 diabetes mellitus
- For many patients, the HbA1c target should be less than 7%, with a premeal blood glucose level of 80–130 mg/dL
  - Targets should be individualized
  - Individuals with recurrent episodes of severe hypoglycemia, cardiovascular disease, advanced complications, substance abuse, or untreated mental illness may require higher targets
    - HbA1c of less than 8% and pre-prandial glucose levels of 100–150 mg/dL for these patients is acceptable
- Although tight glycemic control is beneficial, an increased risk of severe hypoglycemia accompanies lower blood glucose levels
  - The 2011 AACE guidelines for developing a comprehensive care plan emphasize that hypoglycemia should be avoided

Latent autoimmune diabetes of adults (LADA)

- Commonly confused with type 2 diabetes mellitus
- Islet cell antibodies slowly destroy ß–cell function
- Not insulin requiring for at least the first 6 months of onset
- Most patients will require insulin within 6 years
- Insulin therapy is treatment of choice when diagnosis is made

- Will ultimately require insulin and the treatment is similar to type 1 diabetes mellitus
- May take up to 12 years in some patients to have complete failure of ß–cell function
- 10% of patients over age 35 years and 25% of patients under age 35 years diagnosed with type 2 diabetes mellitus will actually have LADA
- Pancreatic islet cell antibodies testing is used to diagnose and differentiate LADA from type 2 diabetes mellitus as needed

Diagnostic criteria

- Hb1Ac level ≥ 6.5%
  - HbA1c is the diagnostic test of choice for diabetes mellitus
- Fasting serum glucose ≥ 126 mg/dL on 2 occasions
- Random serum glucose ≥ 200 mg/dL and classic diabetic symptoms (polyuria, polydipsia, polyphagia and weight loss)
- 2 hour oral glucose tolerance test (75 gm glucose PO load) — serum glucose ≥ 200 mg/dL at 2 hours post ingestion of glucose load

Symptoms

- Polydipsia
- Polyuria
- Increased appetite
- Weight loss
- Blurred vision
- Yeast infections
- Paresthesias

DKA (See DKA section)

- Polydipsia
- Polyuria
- Blurred vision
- Tachypnea (Kussmaul respirations)
- Tachycardia
- Nausea and vomiting
- Abdominal pain
- Altered mental status
- Metabolic acidosis
- Elevated serum ketones

Long term complications

- Macrovascular complications
  - Coronary arterial disease (CAD)
  - Cerebrovascular disease
  - Peripheral arterial disease (PAD)
- Microvascular disease
  - Renal insufficiency
  - Retinal neovascularization
    - May occur in pre-diabetes
- Neuropathic disease
  - Peripheral neuropathy
  - Autonomic neuropathy
  - Gastroparesis (may respond to erythromycin or metoclopramide)
- Gestational diabetes complicates 4% of pregnancies
- Congestive heart failure

Evaluation

- Physical examination
  - Assess vital signs
  - Funduscopic exam
  - Foot exam for ulcers, impaired circulation and decreased sensation
- Fasting serum glucose
- Random serum glucose
- HbA1c level
  - Screening with Hb1Ac in obese patients with BMI > 25 kg/m^2 or that have cardiovascular risk factors
- CMP
- Creatinine level should be monitored at least yearly
- U/A
  - Evaluate for microalbuminuria which is 30–200 mg/day
  - Ratio of spot urine albumin(mg) to creatinine(gm) ≥ 30 indicates need for a timed collection of urine, either an overnight or 10 hour or 24 hour urine collection
    - Linked to increase in coronary artery disease
    - Microalbuminuria is weaker predictor of future renal

disease in type 2 diabetes mellitus than in type 1 diabetes mellitus

- Autoantibodies to islet cells, insulin and glutamic acid decarboxylase are absent in type 2 diabetes
- Antibodies directed against GAD65 (glutamic acid decarboxylase) can be tested and is present in 70% of Type 1 insulin dependent patients (distinguishes between patients with type 1 and type 2 diabetes)

General treatment

- Dietary counseling
- Appropriate weight loss
- Increased activity regimen
- Hypertension management
- Hyperlipidemia management
  - Statin therapy to reduce cholesterol in males age > 40 years and females age > 45 years by 30–40% with LDL cholesterol target of < 100 mg/dL
  - Younger diabetic patients with risk factors (hypertension, nephropathy, CAD or peripheral arterial disease) or longstanding disease treat with statins
  - Possible target of LDL < 70 mg/dL in diabetic patients with known cardiovascular disease
  - Most diabetics should be on a moderate statin
- Manage vascular complications

Diabetic treatment

- Tight glycemia control decreases long term complications but must be individualized to minimize hypoglycemic reactions
  - Recurrent and chronic hypoglycemia has been linked to cognitive impairment
  - A "honeymoon" period may occur with DM type 1 patients initially where they do not require insulin after initial diagnosis and treatment, only to develop insulin dependence after weeks to months later, sometimes up to 1–2 years

Outpatient patients glycemic targets

- Premeal blood glucose level of 80–130 mg/dL
- Adults HbA1c target < 7.0%
- HbA1c target < 7.5% for children is now recommended
- However, targets should be individualized

Hospitalized patients

- Medical ICU (nonsurgical) patients target blood glucose is 140 – 200 mg/dL
- Surgical critical care (such as after CV surgery) patients should have blood glucose around 150– 180 mg/dL with acute hyperglycemia of illness

Diet per dietician

- Caloric intake
  - 20% at breakfast
  - 35% at lunch
  - 30% at dinner
  - 15% late evening snack
  - Fat intake ≤ 30% of total calories
- Protein 1–1.5 gm/kg/day — and less than that in renal insufficiency or failure

Exercise

- Routine exercise sessions for 30 minutes or more — patient may need to decrease insulin 10–20% or have an extra snack (>150 minutes/week recommended if tolerated)

Insulin therapy initiation

- Calculate based on patient weight
- Usually new diabetics can be started on a total daily insulin dose of 0.2–0.4 units/kg SQ initially, but will ultimately need 0.6–0.7 units/kg SQ as the total daily dose
- ½ dosed before breakfast, ¼ before dinner and ¼ at bedtime
- Adjust dose to maintain pre–prandial serum glucose 80–150 mg/dL

- Dosing is adjusted usually 10% at a time and assessed over a 3 day period before making further adjustments
- Children with moderate hyperglycemia without ketonuria or metabolic acidosis may be started with qday SQ injection of 0.3–0.5 U/kg of intermediate insulin
  - Children with ketonuria without metabolic acidosis or dehydration may be started on 0.5–0.7 U/kg SQ of intermediate insulin qday and 0.1 U/kg SQ at 4–6 hour intervals

Insulin maintenance schedules

- Usually ½ of the daily insulin dose is given as a long acting basal dose
- Multiple injections per day needed to maintain glucose levels in desired range
- ¼ of daily insulin given at bedtime as long acting insulin
- Additional insulin given as rapid-acting or short-acting insulin before meals based on home glucose monitoring

Insulin types administered subcutaneously

- Rapid-acting — onset in 15 minutes, peak in 1–3 hours and lasts 3–5 hours
  - Novolog (insulin aspart)
  - Apidra (insulin glulisine)
  - Humalog (insulin lispro)
- Short-acting — onset in 30–60 minutes, peak in 2–4 hours, and lasts 6–12 hours
  - Humulin R and Novolin R (regular insulin)
- Intermediate-acting — onset in 1–2 hours, peak in 4–14 hours, and lasts 16–24 hours
  - Humulin N, Novolin N (insulin NPH)
- Long-acting — onset 1 hour and lasts 24 hours
  - Lantus (insulin glargine)
  - Levemir (insulin detemir) duration 6 hours with low dose to 24 hours with high dose
- Premixed — rapid–acting mixed with intermediate-acting insulin
  - NovoLog 50/50 and 70/30 (insulin aspart protamine/insulin aspart
  - Humalog 50/50 and 75/25 (insulin lispro protamine/insulin lispro

Other treatment

- Symlin (pramlintide)
  - Delays gastric emptying
  - Decreases glucagon secretion
  - Helps to control appetite
  - May be used with type 1 and 2 diabetes mellitus along with insulin
  - Used to improve control when needed

Hypoglycemia management

- Caused by missed meals, vomiting, exercise, or excess insulin

Symptoms

- Confusion, light-headiness, diaphoresis or headache

Treatment options

- Patient consumes or family gives patient glucose, sugar or candy if alert enough to control oral intake
- D50W 25 ml IV — adults
- D25W 1 ml/kg IV — young children
- Glucagon 1 mg SQ, IM or IV
- Adjust medications as needed

Glucose monitoring

Home monitoring

- Daily before meals and at bedtime
- May need to perform 2 hours after meals prn
- Patients should adjust their insulin according to patient education and glucose levels
- Patients should test every week for several weeks with

initiation of insulin therapy at 0200–0400 in the morning, and as indicated afterward

- Patients should test for urine ketones with dipstick when illness develops or very high blood glucose levels occur
- Continuous glucose monitoring may be used in all persons aged 18 years or older with type 1 DM
    - 2018 edition of the ADA's Standards of Medical Care in Diabetes

Office monitoring

- HbA1c every 3 months

Consult criteria

- HbA1c > 10% after therapy maximization
- Metabolic acidosis
- Progressive renal insufficiency
- Baseline creatinine ≥ 2 mg/dL
- Hypoglycemia complications
- Blood glucose > 450 mg/dL despite therapy
- New diagnosis

American Diabetes Association's Standards of Medical Care in Diabetes-2018

- Align approaches to diabetes management with the Chronic Care Model, emphasizing productive interactions between a prepared, proactive care team and an informed, activated patient
- Providers should assess social factors that can affect patients with diabetes, such as potential food insecurity, housing stability, and financial barriers, and apply that information to treatment decisions
- Provide patients with self-management support from lay health coaches, navigators, or community health workers, when available
- Effective diabetes self-management education and support should be patient centered, may be given in group or individual settings or using technology, and should help guide clinical decisions
- Psychosocial care should be integrated with a collaborative, patient-centered approach and provided to all people with diabetes, with the goal of optimizing health outcomes and health-related quality of life
- A reasonable A_{1C} goal for many nonpregnant adults is below 7% (53 mmol/mol)
- Insulin-treated patients with hypoglycemia unawareness or an episode of clinically significant hypoglycemia should be advised to raise their glycemic targets to strictly avoid hypoglycemia for at least several weeks in order to partially reverse hypoglycemia unawareness and reduce risk of future episodes
- Most people with type 1 diabetes should be treated with a multiple daily injection regimen of prandial insulin and basal insulin or continuous subcutaneous insulin infusion
- Most individuals with type 1 diabetes should use rapid-acting insulin analogs to reduce hypoglycemia risk
- Most patients with diabetes and hypertension should be treated to a systolic blood pressure goal of less than 140 mmHg and a diastolic blood pressure goal of under 90 mmHg
- Patients with a confirmed office-based blood pressure of 140/90 mmHg or above should, in addition to lifestyle therapy, have prompt initiation and timely titration of pharmacologic therapy to achieve blood pressure goals
- Patients with a confirmed office-based blood pressure of 160/100 mmHg or above should, in addition to lifestyle therapy, have prompt initiation and timely titration of two drugs or a single-pill combination of drugs demonstrated to reduce

cardiovascular events in patients with diabetes

- Treatment for hypertension should include drug classes demonstrated to reduce cardiovascular events in patients with diabetes (angiotensin-converting enzyme [ACE] inhibitors, angiotensin receptor blockers [ARBs], thiazide-like diuretics, or dihydropyridine calcium channel blockers)
- Multiple-drug therapy is generally required to achieve blood pressure targets; however, combinations of ACE inhibitors and ARBs and combinations of ACE inhibitors or ARBs with direct renin inhibitors should not be used
- Lifestyle modifications focusing on weight loss (if indicated); the reduction of saturated fat, trans fat, and cholesterol intake; an increase in dietary omega-3 fatty acids, viscous fiber, and plant stanol/sterol intake; and increased physical activity should be recommended to improve the lipid profile in patients with diabetes
- High-intensity statin therapy should be added to lifestyle therapy for patients of all ages with diabetes and atherosclerotic cardiovascular disease (ASCVD)
- For patients aged 40-75 years who have diabetes but do not have ASCVD, use moderate-intensity statin treatment in addition to lifestyle therapy
- For patients with diabetes and ASCVD, if the low-density lipoprotein (LDL) cholesterol level is 70 mg/dL (3.9 mmol/L) or above on maximally tolerated statin dose, consider adding additional LDL-lowering therapy (such as ezetimibe or a proprotein convertase subtilisin/kexin type 9 [PCSK9] inhibitor) after evaluating the potential for further ASCVD risk reduction, drug-specific adverse effects, and patient preferences; ezetimibe may be preferred due to lower cost
- Combination therapy (statin/fibrate) has not been shown to improve ASCVD outcomes and is generally not recommended
- Combination therapy (statin/niacin) has not been shown to provide additional cardiovascular benefit above statin therapy alone, may increase the risk of stroke with additional side effects, and is generally not recommended
- Use aspirin therapy (75-162 mg/day) as a secondary prevention strategy in patients with diabetes and a history of ASCVD
- In asymptomatic patients, routine screening for coronary artery disease is not recommended as it does not improve outcomes as long as ASCVD risk factors are treated
- Optimize glucose control to reduce the risk or slow the progression of diabetic kidney disease
- Optimize blood pressure control to reduce the risk or slow the progression of diabetic kidney disease
- Patients should be referred for evaluation for renal replacement treatment if they have an estimated glomerular filtration rate (eGFR) below 30 mL/min/1.73m^2
- Optimize glycemic control to reduce the risk or slow the progression of diabetic retinopathy
- Optimize blood pressure and serum lipid control to reduce the risk or slow the progression of diabetic retinopathy
- Promptly refer patients with any level of macular edema, severe nonproliferative diabetic retinopathy (a precursor of proliferative diabetic retinopathy), or any proliferative diabetic retinopathy to an ophthalmologist who is knowledgeable and experienced in the management of diabetic retinopathy
- The traditional standard treatment, panretinal laser photocoagulation therapy, is indicated to reduce the risk of vision loss in patients with high-risk proliferative diabetic retinopathy and, in some cases, severe nonproliferative diabetic retinopathy

- Intravitreous injections of the vascular endothelial growth factor inhibitor ranibizumab are not inferior to traditional panretinal laser photocoagulation and are also indicated to reduce the risk of vision loss in patients with proliferative diabetic retinopathy
- Intravitreous injections of vascular endothelial growth factor inhibitor are indicated for central-involved diabetic macular edema, which occurs beneath the foveal center and may threaten reading vision
- The presence of retinopathy is not a contraindication to aspirin therapy for cardioprotection, as aspirin does not increase the risk of retinal hemorrhage
- Either pregabalin or duloxetine is recommended as initial pharmacologic treatment for neuropathic pain in diabetes

ADA: Position statement on type 1 diabetes in children and adolescents 2018

- Consult a pediatric endocrinologist before diagnosing type 1 diabetes when isolated glycosuria or hyperglycemia is discovered in patients with acute illness in the absence of classic symptoms
- Differentiating type 1 diabetes, type 2 diabetes, monogenic diabetes, and other forms of diabetes is based on patient history and characteristics, as well as on laboratory tests, such as an islet autoantibody panel
- The majority of children with type 1 diabetes should be treated with intensive insulin regimens using multiple daily injections of prandial insulin and basal insulin or continuous subcutaneous insulin infusion
- A_{1C} should be measured every 3 months
- Blood glucose levels should be monitored up to 6-10 times daily
- Continuous glucose monitors (CGM) should be considered in all children and adolescents with type 1 diabetes; the benefits of CGM correlate with adherence to ongoing use of the device
- Blood or urine ketone levels should be monitored in children with type 1 diabetes in the presence of prolonged/severe hyperglycemia or acute illness
- Individualized medical nutrition therapy is recommended for children and adolescents
- Exercise is recommended, with a goal of 60 minutes a day of moderate to vigorous aerobic activity, along with vigorous muscle-strengthening and bone-strengthening activities at least 3 days a week
- It is important to frequently monitor glucose before, during, and after exercise (with or without CGM use) to prevent, detect, and treat hypoglycemia and hyperglycemia
- All individuals with type 1 diabetes should have access to an uninterrupted supply of insulin; lack of access and insulin omissions are major causes of diabetic ketoacidosis
- Glucagon should be prescribed for all individuals with type 1 diabetes, and caregivers or family members should be instructed regarding administration
- Once the child has had diabetes for 5 years, annual screening for albuminuria, using a random spot urine sample (morning sample preferred to avoid effects of exercise) to assess the albumin-to-creatinine ratio, should be considered at puberty or at age greater than 10 years, whichever occurs earlier
- Once the youth has had diabetes for 3-5 years, an initial dilated and comprehensive eye examination is recommended at age 10 years or after puberty has started, whichever is earlier, and an annual routine follow-up is generally recommended
- For adolescents who have had type 1 diabetes for 5 years, consider an annual comprehensive foot exam

at the start of puberty or at age 10 years, whichever is earlier

- Blood pressure should be measured at each routine visit; children who have high-normal blood pressure (systolic blood pressure [SBP] or diastolic blood pressure [DBP] at 90th percentile for age, sex, and height) or hypertension (SBP or DBP at 95th percentile for age, sex, and height) should have blood pressure confirmed on 3 separate days
- Initial treatment of high-normal blood pressure (SBP or DBP consistently at the 90th percentile for age, sex, and height) includes dietary modification and increased exercise for weight control; if target blood pressure is not reached within 3-6 months after lifestyle intervention, consider pharmacologic treatment
- ACE inhibitors or ARBs should be considered for the initial pharmacologic treatment of hypertension, following reproductive counseling because of the potential teratogenic effects of both drug classes
- The blood pressure treatment goal is consistently less than the 90th percentile for age, sex, and height
- If low-density lipoprotein (LDL) cholesterol is within an acceptable risk level (< 100 mg/dL [2.6 mmol/L]), a lipid profile every 3-5 years is reasonable
- If lipid levels are abnormal, initial therapy should consist of optimizing glucose control and initiating a Step 2 American Heart Association diet (restricting saturated fat to 7% of total calories and dietary cholesterol to 200 mg/day)
- After age 10 years, consider adding a statin if, despite 6 months of medical nutrition therapy and lifestyle changes, LDL cholesterol remains greater than 160 mg/dL (4.1 mmol/L) or LDL cholesterol remains greater than 130 mg/dL (3.4 mmol/L) with one or more cardiovascular disease (CVD) risk factors present (after reproductive counseling because of the potential teratogenic effects of statins)
- The LDL therapy goal is less than 100 mg/dL (2.6 mmol/L)
- In children with type 1 diabetes, consider testing for antithyroid peroxidase and antithyroglobulin antibodies soon after diagnosis
- In children and adolescents with type 1 diabetes, an A_{1C} target of less than 7.5% should be considered but individualized
- Glucose (15g) is preferred treatment for conscious individuals with hypoglycemia (blood glucose < 70 mg/dL [3.9 mmol/L]), but any form of carbohydrate may be used; treatment should be repeated if self-monitoring blood glucose (SMBG) 15 minutes after treatment shows hypoglycemia is still present; when blood glucose concentration returns to normal, consider a meal or snack and/or reduce insulin to prevent recurrence of hypoglycemia
- In patients with classic symptoms, blood glucose measurement is sufficient to diagnose diabetes (symptoms of hyperglycemia or hyperglycemic crisis and random plasma glucose ≥200 mg/dL [11.1 mmol/L])
- Measure thyroid-stimulating hormone concentrations when the patient is clinically stable or once glycemic control has been established; if normal, suggest rechecking every 1-2 years (or sooner if the patient develops symptoms or signs that suggest thyroid dysfunction, thyromegaly, an abnormal growth rate, or unexplained glycemic variability)
- Screen children for celiac disease by measuring IgA tissue transglutaminase antibodies
- Criteria for diagnosis of diabetes is fasting plasma glucose (FPG) ≥126 mg/dL (7.0 mmol/L)
- In asymptomatic children and adolescents at high risk for diabetes, if FPG ≥126 mg/dL (7 mmol/L), if 2-hr PG ≥200 mg/dL

(11.1 mmol/L), or if A_{1C} ≥6.5%, testing should be repeated on a separate day to confirm the diagnosis

Notes

____

____

____

REFERENCES:

Latent Autoimmune Diabetes in Adults Definition, Prevalence, β-Cell Function, and Treatment
doi: 10.2337/diabetes.54.suppl_2.S68
Diabetes December 2005 vol. 54 no. suppl 2 S68–S72

Standards of Medical Care in Diabetes — 2011
Diabetes Care. Jan 2011; 34(Suppl 1): S11–S61.
doi: 10.2337/dc11–S011

American Association of Clinical Endocrinologists medical guidelines for clinical practice for developing a diabetes mellitus comprehensive care plan

[Guideline] Handelsman Y, Mechanick JI, Blonde L, Grunberger G, Bloomgarden ZT, Bray GA, et al. American Association of Clinical Endocrinologists Medical Guidelines for Clinical Practice for developing a diabetes mellitus comprehensive care plan. *Endocr Pract*. Mar-Apr 2011;17 Suppl 2:1–53

[Guideline] Moghissi ES, Korytkowski MT, DiNardo M, Einhorn D, Hellman R, Hirsch IB, et al. American Association of Clinical Endocrinologists and American Diabetes Association consensus statement on inpatient glycemic control. *Diabetes Care*. 2009 Jun. 32(6):1119-31

[Guideline] Qaseem A, Humphrey LL, Chou R, Snow V, Shekelle P. Use of intensive insulin therapy for the management of glycemic control in hospitalized patients: a clinical practice guideline from the American College of Physicians. *Ann Intern Med*. 2011 Feb 15. 154(4):260-7

Kansagara D, Fu R, Freeman M, Wolf F, Helfand M. Intensive insulin therapy in hospitalized patients: a systematic review. *Ann Intern Med*. 2011 Feb 15. 154(4):268-82

Type 1 Diabetes Mellitus Treatment & Management
Author: Romesh Khardori, MD, PhD, FACP; Chief Editor: George T Griffing, MD
emedicine.medscape.com/article/117739

[Guideline] Chiang JL, Maahs DM, Garvey KC, et al. Type 1 Diabetes in Children and Adolescents: A Position Statement by the American Diabetes Association. *Diabetes Care*. 2018 Sep. 41 (9):2026-44

[Guideline] American Diabetes Association. *Standards of Medical Care in Diabetes-2018*Abridged for Primary Care Providers. *Clin Diabetes*. 2018 Jan. 36 (1):14-37

TYPE 2 DIABETES MELLITUS MANAGEMENT

Definition

- Hyperglycemia disorder resulting from insulin resistance and decreased insulin secretion

Differential diagnosis

- Type 1 diabetes mellitus

Considerations

- Does not require exogenous insulin treatment to sustain life
- Can present with DKA in young adults, Hispanics and African–Americans initially
- Gestational diabetes complicates 4% of pregnancies
- 90% of patients are obese
- Genetic predisposition is common
- Diagnostic criteria
  - Hb1Ac level ≥ 6.5%
    - HbA1c is the diagnostic test of choice for diabetes mellitus
  - Fasting serum glucose ≥ 126 mg/dL on 2 occasions
  - Random serum glucose ≥ 200 mg/dL and classic diabetic symptoms (polyuria, polydipsia, polyphagia and weight loss)
  - 2 hour oral glucose tolerance test (75 gm glucose PO load) serum glucose ≥ 200 mg/dL at 2 hours post ingestion of glucose load
- HbA1c > 6% but < 6.5% commonly need lifestyle modification, nutrition counseling, and increased physical activity
- HbA1c levels reflects previous 3 months of glycemia
- Fasting C-peptide level more than 1 mg/dL is associated more with type 2 diabetes mellitus
- Impaired fasting glucose is a serum glucose of 100–125 mg/dL
- Impaired glucose tolerance
  - Plasma glucose ≥ 140 mg/dL-199 mg/dL 2 hours after 75 gm oral glucose load
- Prognosis strongly influenced by disease control
- Linked to depression
- Tight control yielding HbA1c ≤ 7% is valuable in new onset diabetes mellitus in reducing complications
  - Less beneficial in complication reduction in diabetic patients ≥ 15 years in duration
- Hypertension and hyperlipidemia control important also to decrease vascular complications in diabetes
- Patient education should be intensive and comprehensive with multiple health care professionals involved:
  - Practitioner
  - Nutritionist
  - Diabetes educator
  - May require individual education in certain cases
- At time of diagnosis, patients are estimated to have had diabetes for 4–7 years
- Pre-diabetes
  - Fasting blood glucose 100–125 mg/dL
  - Blood glucose 140–200 mg/dL in a 2 hour oral glucose tolerance test (OGTT)
  - Associated with macrovascular disease and development of frank diabetes
- Metabolic syndrome (Syndrome X) confused with Pre-diabetes
  - 3 out of 5 below
    - Abdominal obesity
    - Low HDL cholesterol
    - Elevated triglyceride level
    - Elevated blood pressure
    - Fasting glucose ≥ 100 mg/dL
- For patients with non-alcoholic steatohepatitis(NASH), consider pioglitazone or GLP-1 agonist.

Long term complications

- Macrovascular complications
  - Coronary arterial disease (CAD)
  - Cerebrovascular disease
  - Peripheral arterial disease (PAD)
- Microvascular disease
  - Renal insufficiency
  - Retinal neovascularization
    - May occur in pre-diabetes
- Neuropathic disease
  - Peripheral neuropathy
  - Autonomic neuropathy
  - Gastroparesis
- Diabetes mellitus is the leading cause of
  - Blindness

- ESRD (End-stage renal disease)
- Lower limb amputations

Symptoms

- Polydipsia
- Polyuria
- Increased appetite
- Weight loss
- Blurred vision
- Yeast infections
- Paresthesia

History

- How long has the patient had diabetes?
- Level of glucose control?
- Are there episodes of hypoglycemia?
- Vascular complications such as renal (elevated creatinine level), cardiac disease, peripheral arterial disease or TIA/CVA?
- Is there home glucose testing and what are the measured levels?
- What was the last HbA1c level?
- Any of the symptoms listed in above section?
- Frequent infections?
- Ulcers or amputations?
- Hyperlipidemia history and treatment?

Evaluation

- Physical examination
  - Assess vital signs
  - Funduscopic exam
  - Foot exam for ulcers, impaired circulation and decreased sensation
- Fasting serum glucose
- Random serum glucose
- HbA1c level
  - Screening with Hb1Ac in obese patients with BMI > 25 kg/m^2 or that have cardiovascular risk factors
- BMP (glucose, electrolytes, creatinine and BUN)
- U/A
  - Evaluate for microalbuminuria which is 30–200 mg/day
  - Ratio of spot urine albumin(mg) to creatinine(gm) ≥ 30 indicates need for a timed collection of urine, either an overnight or 10 hour or 24 hour urine collection
  - Linked to increase in coronary artery disease
  - Microalbuminuria is weaker predictor of future renal disease in type 2 diabetes mellitus than in type 1 diabetes mellitus
- Autoantibodies to islet cells, insulin and glutamic acid decarboxylase are absent in type 2 diabetes

Goals of treatment

- Microvascular (i.e., eye and kidney disease) risk reduction through control of glycemia and blood pressure
- Macrovascular (i.e., coronary, cerebrovascular, peripheral vascular) risk reduction through control of lipids and hypertension, smoking cessation
- Metabolic and neurologic risk reduction through control of glycemia

Recommendations for the treatment of type 2 diabetes mellitus from the European Association for the Study of Diabetes (EASD) and the American Diabetes Association (ADA)

- Place the patient's condition, desires, abilities, and tolerances at the center of the decision–making process

The EASD/ADA position statement contains 7 key points:

- Individualized glycemic targets and glucose-lowering therapies
- Diet, exercise, and education as the foundation of the treatment program
- Use of metformin as the optimal first-line drug unless contraindicated
- After metformin, the use of 1 or 2 additional oral or

injectable agents, with a goal of minimizing adverse effects if possible

- Ultimately, insulin therapy alone or with other agents if needed to maintain blood glucose control
- Where possible, all treatment decisions should involve the patient, with a focus on patient preferences, needs, and values
- A major focus on comprehensive cardiovascular risk reduction

ADA/EASD updated recommendations on hyperglycemia management October 2018

- Providers and health-care systems should prioritize the delivery of patient-centered care
- All people with type 2 diabetes should be offered access to ongoing diabetes self-management education and support (DSMES) programs
- Facilitating medication adherence should be specifically considered when selecting glucose-lowering medications
- Among patients with type 2 diabetes who have established atherosclerotic cardiovascular disease (ASCVD), sodium-glucose cotransporter 2 (SGLT2) inhibitors or glucacon-like peptide 1 (GLP-1) receptor agonists with proven cardiovascular benefit are recommended as part of glycemic management
- Among patients with ASCVD in whom heart failure coexists or is of special concern, SGLT2 inhibitors are recommended
- For patients with type 2 diabetes and chronic kidney disease (CKD), with or without CVD, consider the use of an SGLT2 inhibitor shown to reduce CKD progression or, if contraindicated or not preferred, a GLP-1 receptor agonist shown to reduce CKD progression
- An individualized program of medical nutrition therapy (MNT) should be offered to all patients
- All overweight and obese patients with diabetes should be advised of the health benefits of weight loss and encouraged to engage in a program of intensive lifestyle management, which may include food substitution
- Increased physical activity improves glycemic control and should be encouraged in all people with type 2 diabetes
- Metabolic surgery is a recommended treatment option for adults with type 2 diabetes and 1) a body mass index (BMI) of 40.0 kg/m ^{2} or higher (BMI of 37.5 kg/m ^{2} or higher in people of Asian ancestry) or 2) a BMI of 35.0-39.9 kg/m ^{2} (32.5-37.4 kg/m ^{2} in people of Asian ancestry) who do not achieve durable weight loss and improvement in comorbidities with reasonable nonsurgical methods
- Metformin is the preferred initial glucose-lowering medication for most people with type 2 diabetes
- The stepwise addition of glucose-lowering medication is generally preferred to initial combination therapy
- The selection of medication added to metformin is based on patient preference and clinical characteristics; important clinical characteristics include the presence of established ASCVD and other comorbidities such as heart failure or CKD; the risk for specific adverse medication

effects, particularly hypoglycemia and weight gain; and safety, tolerability, and cost
- Intensification of treatment beyond dual therapy to maintain glycemic targets requires consideration of the impact of medication side effects on comorbidities, as well as the burden of treatment and cost
- In patients who need the greater glucose-lowering effect of an injectable medication, GLP-1 receptor agonists are the preferred choice to insulin; for patients with extreme and symptomatic hyperglycemia, insulin is recommended
- Patients who are unable to maintain glycemic targets on basal insulin in combination with oral medications can have treatment intensified with GLP-1 receptor agonists, SGLT2 inhibitors, or prandial insulin
- Access, treatment cost, and insurance coverage should all be considered when selecting glucose-lowering medications

2013 ADA guidelines for SMBG (self-monitoring of blood glucose) frequency focus on an individual's specific situation rather than quantifying the number of tests that should be done.

- Patients on intensive insulin regimens
  - Perform SMBG at least before meals and snacks
    - As well as occasionally after meals; at bedtime; before exercise and before critical tasks (driving etc.)
    - When hypoglycemia is suspected
    - After treating hypoglycemia until normoglycemia is achieved
- Patients using less frequent insulin injections or noninsulin therapies
  - Use SMBG results to adjust to food intake, activity, or medications to reach specific treatment goals
- Clinicians must not only educate these individuals on how to interpret their SMBG data, but they should also reevaluate the ongoing need for and frequency of SMBG at each routine visit

Approaches to prevention of diabetic complications include the following:

- HbA1c every 3–6 months
- Yearly dilated eye examinations
- Annual microalbumin checks
- Foot examinations at each visit
- Blood pressure < 130/80 mm Hg, lower in diabetic nephropathy
- Statin therapy to reduce low-density lipoprotein cholesterol

Recommendations from Standards of Medical Care in Diabetes 2014

- Perform the A1C test at least two times a year in patients who are meeting treatment goals (and who have stable glycemic control)
- Perform the A1C test quarterly in patients whose therapy has changed or who are not meeting glycemic goals
- Use of POC testing for HbA1C provides the opportunity for more timely treatment changes

Treatment

- Dietary counseling
- Appropriate weight loss

- Increased activity regimen (> 150 minutes/week recommended if tolerated)
- Hypertension management
- Hyperlipidemia management
  - Statin therapy to reduce cholesterol in males age > 40 years and females age > 45 years by 30–40% with LDL cholesterol target of < 100 mg/dL
  - Younger diabetic patients with risk factors or longstanding disease treat with statins
  - Possible target of LDL < 70 mg/dL in diabetic patients with known cardiovascular disease
- Manage vascular complications

Lab monitoring

Type 2 treated with insulin

- HbA1c every 3 months
- Fasting lipid profile yearly
- Creatinine level yearly
- Urine microalbumin yearly
- EKG baseline

Type 2 without insulin treatment

- HbA1c every 3–6 months
- Fasting lipid profile yearly
- Creatinine level yearly
- Urine microalbumin measured yearly
- EKG baseline

Pharmacologic Treatment for Type 2 Adult Diabetes

Obese

Monotherapy

- Metformin 500 mg PO bid with or after meals × 1 week, increase weekly by 500 mg to achieve 1000 mg PO bid
  - Decreases HbA1c approximated 1.5%

Second drug if needed

- Glipizide (Glucotrol) 5 mg PO qday with breakfast (elderly 2.5 mg PO)
  OR
- Consider GLP-1 agonist such as Exenatide (Byetta) 5 mcg SQ bid x 1 month and then may increase as needed to 10 mcg SQ bid
- Give 1 hr. before AM and PM meals

OR

- Consider SLGT2 inhibitor such as Empagliflozin (Jardiance) 10 mg PO daily

Third drug if needed

- Insulin glargine 10 units SQ (or 0.2 units/kg) –adjust by 1 unit/day to achieve fasting glucose < 100 mg/dL

OR

- Sitagliptin (Januvia) 50 or 100 mg qday

Non-obese

Monotherapy

- Metformin 500 mg PO bid with or after meals × 1 week, increase weekly by 500 mg to achieve 1000 mg PO bid

OR

- Glipizide (Glucotrol) 5mg PO qday (elderly 2.5 mg PO)

Second drug if needed

- Metformin 500 mg PO bid with or after meals × 1 week, increase weekly by 500 mg to achieve 1000 mg PO bid

OR

- Glipizide 5mg (Glucotrol) PO qday (elderly 2.5 mg PO)

Third drug if needed

- Consider DLP-1 Agonist such as Exenatide (Byetta) 5 mcg SQ bid x 1 month and then may increase as needed to 10 mcg SQ bid
  - Give 1 hr. before AM and PM meals

OR

- Insulin glargine 10 units SQ – adjust by 1 unit/day to achieve fasting glucose < 100 mg/dL

Elderly

Monotherapy

- Metformin 500 mg bid with or after meals x 1 week, increase weekly by 500 mg to achieve 1000 mg PO bid
- If unable to tolerate metformin, consider repaglinide (Prandin) 0.5–4 mg PO up to qid ac (not to exceed 16 mg daily)

Monotherapy failure

- Consider DPP–4 inhibitor such as Januvia (Sitagliptin) 50 mg PO daily

OR

- Consider switch to long acting insulin 10 units SQ bedtime

Asians

Monotherapy

- Pioglitazone (Actos) 30 mg PO qday — do not use in bladder cancer, history of bladder cancer, moderate or severe hepatic disease or symptomatic heart failure (NYHA class 3 or 4)

Second drug if needed

- Metformin 500 mg PO bid with or after meals × 1 week, increase weekly by 500 mg to achieve 1,000 mg PO bid

Third drug if needed

- Glipizide or glimepiride

OR

- Exenatide (Byetta) 5 mcg SQ bid x 1 month and then may increase as needed to 10 mcg SQ bid (not FDA approved with Actos)
  - Give 1 hr. before AM and PM meals

OR

- Insulin glargine 10 units SQ — adjust by 1 unit/day to achieve fasting glucose < 100 mg/dL

Symptomatic patients

- Repaglinide (Prandin) 0.5–4 mg PO up to qid ac (not to exceed 16 mg qday) or insulin to decrease glucose at start of monotherapy initiation

Diabetic medications, mechanism of actions and clinical effects

Biguanides

- Metformin is the only biguanide in clinical use
- Initial drug of choice
- Decreases hepatic gluconeogenesis production
- Decreases intestinal absorption of glucose
- Improves insulin sensitivity by increasing peripheral glucose uptake and utilization
- Unlike oral sulfonylureas, metformin rarely causes hypoglycemia
- Significant improvements in hemoglobin A1c and lipid profile
- Only oral diabetes drug that reliably facilitates modest weight loss
- Probably improves macrovascular risk
- Lactic acidosis during metformin use is very rare
- Do not use in men if creatinine > 1.5 mg/dL and in women serum creatinine > 1.4 mg/dL
- Do not use within 48 hours of iodinated contrast exam

Sulfonylureas

- Glyburide, glipizide and glimepiride
- Stimulate insulin release from pancreatic beta cells
- Indicated for use as adjuncts to diet and exercise in adult patients with type 2 diabetes mellitus
- Generally well-tolerated, with hypoglycemia the most common side effect
- Glyburide had highest cardiovascular mortality

(7.5%) compared with other sulfonylureas, such as gliclazide and glimepiride (2.7%) and raises question of whether it should be used

Meglitinide derivatives

- Repaglinide and nateglinide
- Much shorter-acting insulin secretagogues (stimulate insulin release) than the sulfonylureas
- Can be used as monotherapy
- If adequate glycemic control is not achieved, then metformin or a thiazolidinedione may be added

Alpha-glucosidase inhibitors

- Acarbose (Precose) and Miglitol (Glyset)
- Delay sugar absorption and help to prevent postprandial glucose surges
- Induction of flatulence greatly limits their use

Thiazolidinediones (TZDs)

- Pioglitazone (Actos) and rosiglitazone (Avandia)
- Insulin sensitizers and require presence of insulin to work
- May be used as monotherapy or in combination with sulfonylurea, metformin, meglitinide, DPP-4 inhibitors, GLP-1 receptor agonists, or insulin
- Only antidiabetic agents that have been shown to slow the progression of diabetes (particularly in early disease)
- Edema (including macular edema) and weight gain may be problematic adverse effects
- May induce or worsen heart failure in patients with left ventricular compromise and occasionally in patients with normal left ventricular function
- Food and Drug Administration (FDA) currently recommends not prescribing pioglitazone for patients with active bladder cancer and using it with caution in patients with a history of bladder cancer
- In women with type 2 diabetes, long-term (i.e., 1 year or longer) use of TZDs doubles the risk of fracture
- Elevated risk of myocardial infarction in patients treated with rosiglitazone (FDA limits to patients already being successfully treated with this agent and to patients whose blood sugar cannot be controlled with other antidiabetic medicines and who do not wish to use pioglitazone)

Glucagonlike peptide–1 (GLP-1) agonists

- Exenatide, liraglutide, albiglutide and dulaglutide
- Stimulate glucose-dependent insulin release
- Reduces glucagon and slows gastric emptying
- GLP-1 in addition to metformin and/or a sulfonylurea may result in modest weight loss

Dipeptidyl peptidase IV (DPP-4) inhibitors

- Sitagliptin, saxagliptin and linagliptin
- Prolongs the action of incretin hormones (stimulate insulin secretion)
- May be added, if inadequate diabetic control, to metformin and sulfonylurea combination improving glycemic control
- Saxagliptin and alogliptin may increase heart failure risk, especially in patients with preexisting heart or renal disease

Selective sodium-glucose transporter-2 (SGLT-2) inhibitors

- Canagliflozin, dapagliflozin (Farxiga) and empagliflozin

- Increased urinary glucose excretion
- Adjunct to diet and exercise to improve glycemic control
- Renal dosing adjustments and warnings
- Dapagliflozin is indicated as monotherapy, as initial therapy with metformin, or as an add-on to other oral glucose-lowering agents, including metformin, pioglitazone, glimepiride, sitagliptin, and insulin
- Empagliflozin (Jardiance) and dapagliflozin (Farxiga) have decreased mortality benefit in patients with heart failure

Insulins

- Many patients with type 2 diabetes mellitus become markedly insulinopenic
- Most patients are insulin resistant
- Small changes in insulin dosage may make no difference in glycemia in some patients
- Therapy must be individualized in each patient
- For lowering postprandial glucose, premixed insulin analogues are more effective than either long-acting insulin analogues alone or premixed neutral protamine Hagedorn (NPH)/regular human insulin 70/30
- For lowering HbA_1c, premixed insulin analogues are as effective as premixed NPH/regular human insulin 70/30 and more effective than long-acting insulin analogues
- The frequency of hypoglycemia reported with premixed insulin analogues is similar to that with premixed human insulin and higher than that with oral antidiabetic agents

Amylinomimetics

- Pramlintide
- Mimics the effects of endogenous amylin, which is secreted by pancreatic beta cells
- Delays gastric emptying, decreases postprandial glucagon release, and modulates appetite

Bile acid sequestrants

- Colesevelam
- Developed as lipid-lowering agents for the treatment of hypercholesterolemia but were subsequently found to have a glucose-lowering effect
- Adjunctive therapy to improve glycemic control
- Favorable, but insignificant, impact on FPG and HbA_1c levels

Dopamine agonists

- Bromocriptine mesylate (Cycloset)
- Adjunct to diet and exercise to improve glycemic control in adults with type 2 diabetes mellitus
- May be considered for obese patients who do not tolerate other diabetes medications or who need only a minimal reduction in HbA_1c to reach their glycemic goal
- Can cause orthostatic hypotension and syncope

Agency for Healthcare Research and Quality

- AHRQ concluded that although the long-term benefits and harms of diabetes medications remain unclear, the evidence supports the use of **metformin** as a first-line agent
- On average, monotherapy with many of the oral diabetes drugs reduces HbA1c levels by 1 percentage point (although metformin has been found to be more efficacious than the DPP-4 inhibitors), and 2-drug combination therapies reduce HbA1c about 1 percentage point more than do monotherapies

Other AHRQ findings included the following:

- Metformin decreased LDL cholesterol levels relative to pioglitazone, sulfonylureas, and DPP-4 inhibitors
- Unfavorable effects on weight were greater with TZDs and sulfonylureas than with metformin (mean difference of +2.6 kg)
- Risk of mild or moderate hypoglycemia was 4-fold higher with sulfonylureas than with metformin alone; this risk was more than 5-fold higher with sulfonylureas plus metformin than with a TZD plus metformin
- Risk of heart failure was higher with TZDs than with sulfonylureas
- Risk of bone fractures was higher with TZDs than with metformin

Consult criteria

- HbA1c > 10% after therapy maximization
- Metabolic acidosis
- Progressive renal insufficiency
- Baseline creatinine ≥ 2 mg/dL
- Hypoglycemia complications
- Blood glucose > 450 mg/dL despite treatment

Notes

____

____

____

REFERENCES:

Latent Autoimmune Diabetes in Adults

Definition, Prevalence, β-Cell Function, and Treatment

doi: 10.2337/diabetes.54.suppl_2.S68 Diabetes December 2005 vol. 54 no. suppl 2 S68–S72

Standards of Medical Care in Diabetes — 2011

Diabetes Care. Jan 2011; 34(Suppl 1): S11–S61.

doi: 10.2337/dc11–S011

American Association of Clinical Endocrinologists medical guidelines for clinical practice for developing a diabetes mellitus comprehensive care plan

[Guideline] Handelsman Y, Mechanick JI, Blonde L, Grunberger G, Bloomgarden ZT, Bray GA, et al. American Association of Clinical Endocrinologists Medical Guidelines for Clinical Practice for developing a diabetes mellitus comprehensive care plan. *Endocr Pract*. Mar-Apr 2011;17 Suppl 2:1–53

Standards of Medical Care in Diabetes — 2014

Diabetes Care Volume 37, Supplement 1, January 2014

Keller DM. New EASD/ADA Position Paper Shifts Diabetes Treatment Goals. Medscape Medical News. Available at medscape.com/viewarticle/771989

Inzucchi SE, Bergenstal RM, Buse JB, Diamant M, Ferrannini E, Nauck M, et al. Management of hyperglycaemia in type 2 diabetes: a patient-centered approach. Position statement of the American Diabetes Association (ADA) and the European Association for the Study of Diabetes (EASD). *Diabetologia*. Jun 2012;55(6):1577–96.

Inzucchi SE, Bergenstal RM, Buse JB, Diamant M, Ferrannini E, Nauck M, et al. Management of hyperglycemia in type 2 diabetes: a patient-centered approach: position statement of the American Diabetes Association (ADA) and the European Association for the Study of Diabetes (EASD). *Diabetes Care*. Jun 2012;35(6):1364–79

Synopsis of the 2016 ADA Standards of Medical Care in Diabetes Clinical

Guidelines Published online 1 March 2016

James J. Chamberlain, MD; Andrew S. Rhinehart, MD; Charles F. Shaefer, Jr., MD; Annie Neuman, PA-C

Type 2 Diabetes Mellitus Author: Romesh Khardori, MD, PhD, FACP; Chief Editor: George T Griffing, MD emedicine.medscape.com/article/117853

Type 2 Diabetes Mellitus Guidelines

Updated: Feb 26, 2019 Author: Romesh Khardori, MD, PhD, FACP; Chief Editor: George T Griffing, MD

Identification of the 64k autoantigen in insulin-dependent diabetes as the GABA-synthesizing enzyme glutamic acid decarbocylase. Baekkeskov S, Aanstoot HJ, Chrsitgau S. Nature 1990; 347: 151

CHOLESTEROL MANAGEMENT

Considerations

- LDL (low density lipoprotein) cholesterol < 100 mg/dL is optimal
- Lowering LDL cholesterol is the primary target of therapy
- "Low HDL" (high density lipoprotein) is < 40 mg/dL
- Lowering triglycerides from levels ≥ 220 recommended
- Diabetes without ASCVD (coronary heart disease) is considered raised to ASCVD risk
- Patients with metabolic syndrome are candidates for lifestyle modification
- Complete lipoprotein profile is recommended as initial screening test
- LDL-C levels of 40 to 60 mg/dL reduces ASCVD

4 Statin benefit groups

- Individuals with clinical ASCVD (atherosclerotic cardiovascular disease) — angina, MI, stroke, TIA or peripheral arterial disease
- Individuals with primary elevations of LDL–C ≥ 190 mg/dL
- Individuals age 40–75 years of age with diabetes and LDL–C 70–189 mg/dL without clinical ASCVD
- Individuals age 40–75 years of age without diabetes or ASCVD with LDL-C 70–189 mg/dL that have an estimated 10 year ASCVD risk ≥ 7.5%

Statin therapy

High–intensity (lowers LDL–C ≥ 50%)

- Atorvastatin 40–80 mg
- Rosuvastatin 20–40 mg

Moderate–intensity (lowers LDL–C 30% to < 50%)

- Atorvastatin 10–20 mg
- Rosuvastatin 20–40 mg
- Simvastatin 20–40 mg
- Pravastatin 40–80 mg
- Lovastatin 40 mg
- Fluvastatin 40 mg bid

Low–intensity (lowers LDL–C < 30%)

- Simvastatin 10 mg
- Pravastatin 10–20 mg
- Lovastatin 20 mg
- Fluvastatin 20–40 mg

Non-statin therapy

- Repatha (evolocumab) SQ q2weeks
  - High cost
  - May be used in statin intolerant patients
  - Lowers LDL-C > 50%
  - Patients who require additional lowering of low density lipoprotein cholesterol

after starting maximal statin treatment

- Alirocumab (Praluent)
  - Adjunct to diet and maximally tolerated statin therapy in adults with heterozygous familial hypercholesterolemia or clinical atherosclerotic cardiovascular disease, who require additional lowering of low density lipoprotein cholesterol
- Zetia (ezetimibe) 10 mg PO qday
  - Inhibits cholesterol absorption in small intestine
- Cholestoff over the counter (plant sterols)
- Coenzyme Q–10 not proven effective in studies

Individuals with clinical ASCVD (atherosclerotic cardiovascular disease)

Age ≤ 75 years of age

- High–intensity statin
  - Moderate–intensity statin if not candidate for high–intensity statin

Age > 75 years of age

- Moderate–intensity statin

Individuals with primary elevations of LDL–C ≥ 190 mg/dL

- High–intensity statin
  - Moderate–intensity statin if not candidate for high–intensity statin

Individuals age 40–75 years of age with diabetes and LDL–C 70–189 mg/dL without clinical ASCVD

- Moderate–intensity statin
  - High–intensity statin if estimated 10 year ASCVD risk ≥ 7.5%

Individuals age 40–75 years of age without diabetes or ASCVD with LDL-C 70–189 mg/dL that have an estimated 10 year ASCVD risk ≥ 7.5%

- Moderate to high intensity statin
- Clincalc.com/Cardiology/ASCVD/PooledCohort.aspx for ASCVD risk calculation

ASCVD prevention benefit of statins may be less clear in other groups

- Primary LDL–C ≥ 160 mg/dL
- Genetic hyperlipidemias
- Family history of premature ASCVD
  - < 55 years of age of first degree male relative
  - < 65 years of age of first degree female relative
- CRP ≥ 2 mg/L
- Ankle–brachial index < 0.9
- Elevated lifetime risk of ASCVD

Major risk factors (excluding LDL cholesterol)

- Cigarette smoking
- Blood pressure ≥ 140–150/90 mm Hg depending on JNC 8 recommendations or on hypertension medications (see hypertension management section)
- HDL cholesterol < 40 mg/dL
- Diabetes (is a risk equivalent)
- Family history of premature ASCVD
  - Male 1st degree relative age < 55 years
  - Female 1st degree relative age < 65 years
- Age
  - Men ≥ 45 years
  - Women ≥ 55 years

Testing for statin therapy initiation

- Fasting lipid profile

- ALT (evaluate unexplained increases 3X normal)
- Hemoglobin A1c (if diabetes status not known)
- CPK if indicated
- Consider evaluation for other secondary causes or conditions that influence statin safety
- Treat secondary of LDL-C ≥ 190 mg/dL

Secondary causes of increased LDL cholesterol

- Diabetes
- Hypothyroidism
- Obstructive liver disease
- Moderate chronic renal failure
- Drugs
  - Progestins
  - Corticosteroids
  - Anabolic steroids

ASCVD risk equivalents

- Peripheral arterial disease
- Aortic aneurysm
- Symptomatic carotid disease
- Diabetes
- Multiple risk factors that confer a 10 year risk of ASCVD or recurrent ASCVD > 20%

Metabolic syndrome

Definition

- Lipid and nonlipid risk factors of metabolic origin which enhances the risk for ASCVD

Risk factors

- Abdominal obesity
  - Men's waist size > 40 inches
  - Women's waist size > 35 inches
- Triglycerides ≥ 150 mg/dL
- HDL cholesterol
  - Men < 40 mg/dL
  - Women < 50 mg/dL
- Blood pressure ≥ 135/≥ 85 mm Hg
- Fasting glucose ≥ 110 mg/dL

Treatment

- Weight reduction as appropriate
- Increased physical activity
  - A fibrate or nicotinic acid is no longer recommended per recent FDA determination

10 year risk estimation for ASCVD to occur (examples)

Men ≥ 20% risk

Age 55–59

Total Cholesterol 200–239

Smoker

SBP ≥ 140 mm Hg

Women ≥ 20% risk

Age 60–64

Total Cholesterol 200–239

Smoker

SBP ≥ 140 mm Hg

Men's and women's risk approximately ≤ 10% with above data if not a smoker

Treatment to achieve goals

- Treat any secondary causes of increased LDL cholesterol
- Weight loss and increased physical activity
- Low (saturated) fat and low cholesterol diet
- High (soluble) fiber diet of 10–25 gms/days

Time table for follow up and treatment

- Recheck in 6 weeks and if target not met
  - Add plant sterols or stanols 2 gms per day (vegetables, fruits, legumes, nuts, and seeds)
  - Increase fiber if possible
- Recheck in 4–12 weeks and if target not met
  - Start an appropriate strength statin as indicated above
- Recheck again in 4–12 weeks and if target not met
  - Intensify statin therapy

- **ASCVD high risk patients**
  - Individuals with clinical ASCVD < 75 years of age
  - Individuals with baseline LDL–C ≥190 mg/dL
  - Individuals 40 to 75 years of age with diabetes mellitus
- Recheck in 4–12 weeks and if target still not met
  - Discuss with physician
- Recheck every 3–12 months to monitor response and adherence to therapy if targets met
- See Statin therapy section above for targets
- Monitor side effects and toxicity (myopathy, etc.)

Also treat or modify ASCVD risk factors

Notes

REFERENCES:

2013 ACC/AHA Guideline on the Treatment of Blood Cholesterol to Reduce Atherosclerotic Cardiovascular Risk in Adults: A Report of the American College of Cardiology/American Heart Association Task Force on Practice Guidelines

www.nhlbi.nih.gov/guidelines/cholesterol/atp3xsum.pdf Third Report of the National Cholesterol Education Program (NCEP) Expert Panel on Detection, Evaluation, and Treatment of High Blood Cholesterol in Adults (Adult Treatment Panel III)

[Docket No. FDA-2016-N-1127] AbbVie Inc. et al; Withdrawal of Approval of Indications Related to the Coadministration With Statins in Applications for Niacin Extended-Release Tablets and Fenofibric Acid Delayed Release Capsules

Consultant. 2016;56(5):S2-S4. Suppl.

STROKE PREVENTION MANAGEMENT

Considerations

- There are 795,000 strokes in the U.S. each year
- 134,000 stroke deaths per year
- Stroke is the third leading cause of death
- Prevention is most effective approach to manage stroke
- Primary prevention is treatment with no prior history of stroke
- Secondary prevention is treatment of patients with history of stroke or TIA
- Common viral infections linked to stroke in children
  - Vaccines decrease this risk

Primary prevention measures include

(In patients with no history of stroke)

- Hypertension treatment
- Platelet inhibitor agents
- Dyslipidemia treatment with statin medications
- Smoking cessation
- Dietary modification
- Weight loss as appropriate
- Exercise

Hypertension

- Most important risk factor to modify
- Target < 140/90 mm Hg
- Diabetic or renal patients the target is < 130/80 mm Hg
- Angiotensin–converting enzyme inhibitor (ACEI) or ARB (angiotensin–receptor blocker) is recommended in

hypertension treatment in diabetic patients

Platelet inhibitor agents

- Aspirin 325 mg PO qday may be useful in patients with high risk for cardiovascular events
  - Not useful in low risk patients
- May be used in atrial fibrillation when warfarin, direct thrombin or factor Xa inhibitors cannot be used

Dyslipidemia

- Statins may be useful in diabetic patients
- Target of LDL ≤ 70 mg/dL in diabetic patients is recommended
- See Cholesterol Management section

Smoking cessation

- Counseling
- Oral smoking cessation medications
  - Bupropion (Zyban) 150 mg PO qday for 3 days then increase to 150 mg PO bid
  - Varenicline (Chantix) 0.5 mg PO for 3 days, then 0.5 mg PO bid for 4 days, then 1 mg PO bid for 11 weeks
- Nicotine replacement

Dietary medication

- Low sodium and high potassium diet
- High fruit and vegetable
- Weight reduction in obese patients with BMI > 25 kg/m^2

Imaging evaluation for TIA and new CVA

- Carotid duplex and transcranial doppler, MRI brain and MRA of head and neck, CT brain scan
- Refer to specialist if abnormal
- Refer new CVA or TIA to specialist
- Send to ER immediately if new CVA/TIA < 7 days old or has associated headache or other concerning symptoms

Atrial fibrillation

- Should be screened for at age > 65 years
- Aspirin 325 mg PO daily may be used for low risk for stroke, CHA_2DS_2VASc score 0–1
- Treatment with warfarin in post–AMI patients with left ventricular thrombus or akinetic segment is reasonable

Anticoagulation recommendations in patients with nonvalvular atrial fibrillation per American Academy of Neurology

- Inform patients of the benefits of anticoagulation vs. the risks of major bleeding
- TIA/CVA patients with atrial fibrillation should be offered anticoagulation therapy if bleeding risks acceptable
- Dabigatran, rivaroxaban or apixaban which have a lower risk of intracranial bleeding than warfarin may be offered to patients who have a higher risk of intracranial bleeding
- Dabigatran, rivaroxaban or apixaban may be used in patients unable to undergo frequent INR testing for warfarin therapy
- Dementia patient families or those that fall occasionally should be informed of the risk–benefit ratio is uncertain

CHA_2DS_2VASc score

- Used to quantify risk of stroke in atrial fibrillation patients
- 2014 AHA/ACC/HRS Guideline for the Management of Patients With Atrial Fibrillation deemphasizes aspirin or use of platelet agents if warfarin (Coumadin), dabigatran (Pradaxa), rivaroxaban (Xarelto) or apixaban (Eliquis) can be safely used and are indicated
- Stands for heart failure, hypertension, age ≥ 75 years , diabetes mellitus and prior

stroke/TIA, vascular disease (MI, PAD or aortic plaque), age ≥ 65 and sex category (female)

- 1 point each for heart failure, hypertension, diabetes mellitus, age ≥ 65 and sex category (female)
- 2 points for prior stroke/TIA and age ≥ 75 years
  - Low risk = 0 points
  - Moderate risk = 1–2 points
  - High risk = 3–6 points
- Long–term anticoagulation for nonvalvular atrial fibrillation recommended with score of ≥ 2, if no significant risk of hemorrhage
  - Warfarin (Coumadin), dabigatran (Pradaxa), rivaroxaban (Xarelto) or apixaban (Eliquis)
- With warfarin determine INR weekly initially, then monthly when stable
- Direct thrombin or factor Xa inhibitor recommended if unable to maintain therapeutic INR
- Evaluate renal function prior to direct thrombin inhibitors or factor Xa inhibitors and annually
- Adjust dosage per creatinine clearance for each specific drug (warfarin adjusted per INR) per PDR or other references

Warfarin prophylaxis

- CHA_2DS_2VASc score ≥ 2
- Age > 75 years
- Target INR 2.0–3.0
  - May be lower (1.8–2) in high risk bleeding patients, or 2.5–3.5 in mechanical artificial valve, rheumatic heart disease, or recurrent stroke patients
- May be used age 65–75 years at discretion of clinician based on underlying disorders such as valvular disease etc.

Dabigatran (Pradaxa)

- CHA_2DS_2VASc score ≥ 2
- 150 mg PO bid for stroke prevention in nonvalvular atrial fibrillation is indicated in patients with CrCl > 30 mL/min
  - 75 mg PO bid CrCl 15–30 mL/min
- Not recommended if CrCl < 15 mL/min
- Less bleeding risk than warfarin
- Read Physician Desk Reference (PDR) drug or database information

Rivaroxaban (Xarelto)

- CHA_2DS_2VASc score ≥ 2
- 20 mg PO qday for stroke prevention in nonvalvular atrial fibrillation/min for CrCl > 50 mL/min
  - 15 mg PO qHS if creatinine clearance (CrCl) 15–50 mL/minute
  - Not recommended for CrCl ≤ 15
- Less bleeding risk than warfarin
- Read Physician Desk Reference (PDR) drug or database information

Apixaban (Eliquis)

- CHA_2DS_2VASc score ≥ 2
- 5 mg PO bid for CrCl ≥ 30 mL/min
  - 2.5 mg PO for age > 80 years, weight < 60 kg, creatinine ≥ 1.5 mg/dL
  - Not recommended in severe liver disease
- Less bleeding risk than warfarin
- Read Physician Desk Reference (PDR) drug or database information

Dabigatran, rivaroxaban, apixaban or warfarin should not be used in the following patients — aspirin safer

- Poor compliance

- Uncontrollable hypertension
- Aortic dissection
- Bacterial endocarditis
- Alcohol dependency
- Liver disease
- Bleeding lesions
- Malignant tumor
- Retinopathy with bleeding risk
- Advanced microvascular changes in the brain
- Known aneurysm of a cerebral artery
- Previous spontaneous cerebral hemorrhage
- Bleeding diathesis (e.g., coagulopathies, thrombocytopenia)

HEMORR$_2$ HAGES risk model is for 100 patient years of warfarin

Bleeding risk with warfarin (2 points for history of bleeding, 1 point for the rest) hepatic or renal disease

- Ethanol abuse
- Malignancy
- Old age (>75 y)
- History of bleeding
- Low platelet counts or platelet dysfunction
- Hypertension that is uncontrolled
- Anemia
- Genetic factors
- Elevated fall risk
- Stroke

HEMORR$_2$ HAGES score Bleeding risk 100 pt./yr.

- 0 1.9
- 1 2.5
- 2 5.3
- 3 8.4
- 4 10.4
- >5 12.3
- Any score 4.9%

Monitor routinely for bleeding

Sickle cell disease

- Risk of stroke in children is 1% per year
- Prevalence of stroke by age 20 years is 11%
- Screen with transcranial Doppler ultrasound in children every 2 years
- Children with cerebral blood flow > 200 cm/second by transcranial Doppler ultrasound have stroke rate > 10% per year
  - Red cell long–term transfusion is only therapy in clinical trials shown to prevent stroke

Cardiac conditions associated with an increased risk of stroke

- Atrial arrhythmias
- Cardiac tumors
- Valvular disease
- Prosthetic valves
- Dilated cardiomyopathy
- Coronary artery disease
- Endocarditis
- Congenital cardiac anomalies
- Low left ventricular ejection fraction

Secondary prevention

(Patients with history of stroke or TIA)

Measures include

- Hypertension treatment SBP < 140 mm Hg
- Statins
- Lifestyle changes
- Obesity management
- Smoking cessation
- Alcohol cessation
- Sleep apnea treatment
- Carotid endarterectomy (CEA) for 70–99% ipsilateral carotid stenotic lesion and CEA mortality risk <6% (Class 1, Level of evidence A)
- Carotid endarterectomy (CEA) for 50–69% ipsilateral carotid

stenotic lesion and CEA mortality risk <6% (Class 1, Level of evidence B)

- ASA 325 mg PO qday (may add clopidogrel 75 mg PO qday) for intracranial atherosclerosis 50–99%
  - Maintain SBP < 140 mm Hg with coadministration of statin

Consult criteria

- Consult with physician for new anticoagulation therapy
- New CVA or TIA
- New onset atrial fibrillation
- Difficult anticoagulation management or high risk bleeding concerns
- Actual bleeding

Notes

____

____

____

REFERENCES:

Guidelines for the Primary Prevention of Stroke

A Guideline for Healthcare Professionals from the American Heart Association/American Stroke Association

ACC/AHA/ESC Practice Guidelines

ACC/AHA/ESC 2006 Guideline for the Management of Patients with Atrial Fibrillation

2014 AHA/ACC/HRS Guideline for the Management of Patients with Atrial Fibrillation

Stroke Anticoagulation and Prophylaxis Author: Salvador Cruz-Flores, MD, MPH, FAHA, FCCM; Chief Editor: Helmi L Lutsep, MD

Stroke Prevention Updated: Feb 15, 2018

Author: Brian Silver, MD, FRCPC, FAHA, FAAN, FANA; Chief Editor: Stephen Kishner, MD, MHA

Emedicine.medscape.com

OBESITY MANAGEMENT

Definition

Obesity

- Males with body fat > 25% of body weight
- Females with body fat > 33% of body weight

Overweight classifications

Grade 1 overweight ("overweight")

- BMI (body mass index) 25–29.9 kg/m^2

Grade 2 overweight ("obesity")

- BMI 30–39.9 kg/m^2

Grade 3 overweight ("morbid obesity")

- BMI ≥ 40 kg/m^2

Children

- BMI > 85th percentile for age are "overweight"
- BMI > 95th percentile for age are "obese"

Differential diagnosis

- Hypothyroidism
- Cushing syndrome
- Acromegaly
- Bulimia
- Cardiomyopathy
- Nephrotic syndrome
- Polycystic ovarian syndrome
- Diabetes mellitus
- Medication related obesity — antidepressants, antipsychotics,

diabetes treatment with insulin or oral agents, corticosteroids
- Growth hormone deficiency
- Oral contraceptives

Considerations

- A diagnosis of being overweight told to the patient increases the chance of positive behavioral changes with diet and/or activity
- Leptins (an endogenous protein) is involved in weight regulation — leptin resistance with high levels is present in overweight/obese patients
- BMI ≥ 40 kg/m² is associated with decreased life expectancy of 20 years in men and 5 years in women
- 90–95% of weight loss patients regain their weight in 5 years
- 22 kcal/kg per day is needed to sustain patient's present weight
- Clinical judgment should be used in evaluating BMI — for example muscular individuals with high BMI may be healthy
- Weight loss is not necessarily recommended for those with a BMI of 25–29.9 kg/m² or a high waist circumference, unless they have two or more comorbidities
- Diet beverages with artificial sweeteners increase weight in studies

Conditions associated with being overweight

- Coronary artery disease
- Diabetes mellitus
- Stroke
- Hypertension
- Obstructive sleep apnea
- Asthma
- Malignancy (uterine, prostate, breast, gallbladder)
- Increased intracranial pressure
- Meralgia paresthetica
- Urinary (bladder) stress incontinence
- Depression
- Osteoarthritis (DJD — degenerative joint disease)
- Back pain
- Venous stasis disease with edema in legs
- Increased post-surgical complications — pneumonia, wound infections, DVT/PE, and increased surgical risk
- Fatty liver with potential risk for development of cirrhosis

American Association of Clinical Endocrinologists and American College of Endocrinology Clinical Practice Guidelines For Comprehensive Medical Care of Patients with Obesity – Executive Summary 2016 (selected)

- Medication-assisted weight loss employing phentermine/topiramate ER, liraglutide 3 mg, or orlistat should be considered in patients at risk for future type 2 diabetes and should be used when needed to achieve 10% weight loss in conjunction with lifestyle therapy
- Obesity is estimated to add $3,559 annually (adjusted to 2012 dollars) to per-patient medical expenditures
- Patients with a BMI of ≥ 40 kg/m2 without coexisting medical problems and for whom the procedure would not be associated with excessive risk should be eligible for bariatric surgery
    - Bariatric surgery with overweight comorbidities can be considered with BMI of ≥ 30–35 kg/m2
- Weight loss is effective to treat diabetes risk (i.e., prediabetes, metabolic syndrome) and prevent progression to type 2 diabetes
    - Weight loss goal is 10%

Screening or evaluation of obese patients for these conditions

- Obstructive sleep apnea
  - Patients with overweight or obesity and obstructive sleep apnea should be treated with weight-loss therapy including lifestyle interventions and additional modalities as needed, including phentermine/topiramate ER or bariatric surgery;
  - Weight-loss goal should be at least 7% to 11% or more
- Asthma and reactive airway disease
  - Weight-loss goal should be at least 7% to 8%
- Diabetes risk, metabolic syndrome, and prediabetes
- Type 2 diabetes
  - Weight loss of >5% to 15%
- Dyslipidemia
  - Weight loss of 5% to 10% weight loss or more as needed to achieve therapeutic targets
- Hypertension
  - Weight loss of >5% to 15%
- Cardiovascular disease
- Nonalcoholic fatty liver disease and nonalcoholic steatohepatitis
  - Weight loss as high as 10% to 40% may be required
- Polycystic ovary syndrome (PCOS)
  - Weight loss of >5% to 15%
- Female infertility
- Male hypogonadism
  - Weight loss of more than 5% to 10% is needed for significant improvement in serum testosterone
- Osteoarthritis
  - Weight loss of 5% to 10%
- Urinary stress incontinence
  - Weight loss of 5% to 10%
- Gastroesophageal reflux disease (GERD)
  - Weight loss of 10% or greater
- Depression

Exclusion from weight loss programs

- Pregnant or breast feeding patients
- Serious and uncontrolled psychiatric illness
- Eating disorder
- Patients with a serious medical condition that may worsen with caloric restriction

High waist circumference and BMI 25–34.9 kg/m²

- Increases cardiovascular disease, diabetes mellitus, hypertension and dyslipidemia risk

Men

- Waist circumference > 94 cm
- Waist to hip ratio > 0.95
  - Severe potential risk with waist circumference > 104 cm

Women

- Waist circumference > 80 cm
- Waist to hip ratio > 0.8
  - Severe potential risk with waist circumference > 88 cm

Elderly

- Patients with a BMI 25–29.9 kg/m² appear to not be at greater risk of death from all causes

Evaluation

- Lipid panel
- Liver function tests
- Thyroid function tests
- 24 hour urinary free cortisol

- Caliper measured skin thickness and other measurements of waist, hips etc.

Treatment

Preinclusion screening

- Determine patient's expectations
- Determine patient's motivation
- Unrealistic expectations need to be changed prior to starting a weight loss program
- Evaluate for an eating or psychiatric disorder
- Informed consent and written expectations
- Manage co–morbidities

Weight loss program

- Weight loss of 0.9–1.5 kg/week is a reasonable goal
- Weight loss goal must be individualized
- There needs to be a team approach with a motivated patient, with a medical provider, dietician, exercise therapist and psychiatric or behavioral therapy as needed based on the individual needs
- Loss of 10% of body weight in overweight patients with BMI < 40 kg/m^2 is associated with significant benefits and further weight loss may not be needed and may be difficult to sustain

Diet

- Water consumption (500 ml in adults and 10 ml/kg in children) before meals increases weight loss up to 44% more than without water consumption — increases basal metabolic rate
- Diets of ≤ 800 kcal/day are not recommended
- Balanced conventional diets are recommended
  - Reduction of 500–1,000 kcal/day produces 1–2 pounds of weight loss/week
- Reasonable women's diet would be 1,000–1,500 kcal/day depending on activity and BMI (higher BMI and/or activity may have higher caloric intake needs and may change over time) — refer to diet counselor
- Reasonable men's diet would be 1,500–2,400 kcal/day depending on activity and BMI (higher BMI and/or activity may have higher caloric intake needs and may change over time) — refer to diet counselor

Exercise

- Aerobic and resistance exercise is important in building muscle mass and increasing metabolic rate
- Decreases muscle mass loss that occurs with dieting
- Patients should be evaluated for underlying cardiac or respiratory conditions before the exercise program is started to determine its risk

Moderate activity examples

- 45–50 minutes of washing or waxing a car, washing windows, gardening
- Walking 2 miles in 30 minutes
- Swimming laps for 20 minutes
- Fast social dancing for 30 minutes
- Running 1.5 miles in 15 minutes
- Bicycling 5 miles in 30 minutes

Behavioral therapy

- Personal weight monitoring
- Stress management
- Stimulus control
- Cognitive therapy
- Social support

Medications

- For BMI ≥ 27 with comorbidities or BMI ≥ 30
  - Orlistat 120 mg PO tid with or < 1 hour after a fatty meal
  - Selective serotonin reuptake inhibitors (SSRI's) have been used as an adjunct (fluoxetine, paroxetine)

Weight loss surgery

- Highly motivated individuals

- BMI ≥ 40 kg/m² may warrant surgical treatment
  - BMI ≥ 35 kg/m² with severe comorbidities may warrant surgical treatment

Pediatric obesity treatment

- Increase activity
- Adjust diet
- Decrease sedentary activity
- Orlistat 120 mg PO tid with or < 1 hour after a fatty meal only for age 12–16 years

Long term monitoring

- Regular clinic visits
- Group meetings
- Encouragement by email or telephone

Notes

REFERENCES:

NHLBI Obesity Education Initiative Expert Panel on the Identification, Evaluation and Treatment of Overweight and Obesity in Adults

American Association of Clinical Endocrinologists and American College of Endocrinology Clinical Practice Guidelines For Comprehensive Medical Care of Patients with Obesity – Executive Summary 2016

Asthma Management

Definition

- A disorder of variable and recurring symptoms, airflow obstruction, and bronchial hyper-responsiveness with an underlying bronchial inflammation

Differential diagnosis

- Bronchiolitis
- Bronchitis
- COPD
- Airway foreign body
- Vocal cord dysfunction
- Heart failure
- URI
- Pulmonary embolism
- Cystic fibrosis
- Bronchopulmonary dysplasia (premature birth history)

Considerations

- Reversible airway constriction
  - May not be completely reversible over time
- Persistent changes in airways occur
- May be seasonal or perennial
- GERD, OSA (obstructive sleep apnea) and sinusitis may exacerbate asthma

Causes

- Innate immunity changes
- Genetic predisposition
- Environmental factors
  - Allergens and infectious causes (viral URI most common infectious cause)

Signs and symptoms

- Cough (worse at night) — may be only symptom in children
- Wheezing
- Dyspnea
- Chest tightness
- Sputum production

Principles of asthma management

- Assess severity initially
- Assess control of symptoms with treatment to adjust therapy
- Assess severity once control with treatment is achieved
- Identify precipitating factors

- Identify comorbid conditions such as GERD, OSA (obstructive sleep apnea), sinusitis, obesity, emotional stress etc.
- Assess patient's knowledge and ability to self-manage
- Patient instruction for self-monitoring
- Periodic clinic visits to monitor asthma
  - Every 2–6 weeks at start of therapy
  - Every 1–6 months after control is achieved to monitor therapy
- Spirometry — initially, and then after therapy has started, and during periods of exacerbation and every 1–2 years otherwise
- Provide a written asthma plan to patient
- Patient education

Classification of asthma severity

Well controlled

- Symptoms ≤ 2 days/week
- Nighttime awakening ≤ 2 times/month
- No interference with activity
- Short-acting beta–agonist (SABA) use ≤ 2 days/week (excludes exercise-induced asthma)
- FEV1 or peak flow > 80% of predicted or personal best

Not well controlled

- Symptoms > 2 days/week
- Nighttime awakening 1–3 times/week
- Some limitation of normal activity
- SABA use > 2 days/week (excludes exercise-induced asthma)
- FEV1 or peak flow 60–80% of predicted or personal best

Very poorly controlled

- Symptoms throughout the day
- Nighttime awakenings ≥ 4 times/week
- Extremely limited activity
- SABA use several times a day (excludes exercise-induced asthma)
- FEV1 or peak flow < 60% of predicted or personal best

Severe exacerbation

- Dyspnea at rest and interferes with conversation
- Peak expiratory flow (PEF) < 40% of predicted or personal best

Acute treatment of severe exacerbation

- Inhaled short-acting beta–agonist (albuterol) and ipratropium (if available) — repeat q15minutes × 3 prn or continuous nebulizer awaiting EMS
- Send to emergency department (by ambulance preferentially)

Life threatening exacerbation

- Too dyspneic to speak; diaphoretic
- PEF < 25% of predicted or personal best

Treatment

- See Asthma Protocol
- Inhaled short-acting beta–agonist (albuterol) and ipratropium (if available) — repeat q15minutes × 3 prn or continuous nebulizer awaiting EMS
- Epinephrine 0.3 mg (adults) or terbutaline 2.5 – 5 mg SQ (adults)
  - Caution in CAD patients
- Epinephrine 0.01 mg/kg in children not to exceed adult dose
- Send by ambulance to emergency department and call emergency department with report

Stepwise approach to asthma management ≥ 12 years of age

- To assist but not replace clinical decision making on individual patients

Step-up as needed

- First check medication adherence, environmental control and comorbid conditions
- Assess control
- Step down when possible and when asthma is controlled for 3 months
- Step up treatment when SABA used > 2 days/week
- Short course oral corticosteroid may be needed for exacerbations up to 10 days (no taper) — dexamethasone preferred (dexamethasone 6 mg = prednisone 40 mg)

Intermittent asthma

Step 1

Preferred:

- Inhaled short-acting beta–agonist (SABA) prn therapy

Persistent asthma: Daily medication

- Consider SQ immunotherapy for Step 2–4 in patients with allergic asthma

Step 2

- SABA prn

Preferred:

- Low-dose inhaled corticosteroid (ICS)

Alternatives to ICS

- Leukotriene receptor antagonist (LTRA)
- Theophylline

Step 3

- SABA prn

Preferred:

- Low-dose ICS + long-acting inhaled beta–agonist (LABA)

OR

- Medium-dose ICS

Alternatives:

- Low-dose ICS + either LTRA, theophylline or zileuton (expensive)

Step 4 (consult specialist)

- SABA prn

Preferred:

- Medium-dose ICS + LABA

Alternative:

- Medium-dose ICS + either LTRA, theophylline or zileuton

Step 5 (consult specialist)

- SABA prn

Preferred:

- High-dose ICS + LABA

AND

- Consider omalizumab in allergic asthma patients

Step 6 (consult specialist)

- SABA prn

Preferred:

- High-dose ICS + LABA + oral steroid
- AND
- Consider omalizumab in allergic asthma patients

Stepwise approach to asthma management age 0–4 years of age

- To assist but not replace clinical decision making on individual patients

Step-up as needed

- First check medication adherence, environmental control and comorbid conditions
- Assess control
- Step down when possible and when asthma is controlled for 3 months
- Step up treatment when SABA used > 2 days/week
- Short course oral corticosteroid may be needed for exacerbations up to 10 days (no taper) — dexamethasone

preferred (0.15–0.3 mg/kg) not to exceed 6 mg daily

Intermittent asthma

Step 1

Preferred:

- Inhaled short-acting beta–agonist (SABA) prn therapy

Persistent asthma: Daily medication

Step 2 (consider consultation with specialist)

- SABA prn

Preferred:

- Low-dose inhaled corticosteroid (ICS)

Alternatives to ICS

- Montelukast (Singulair)

Step 3 (consult specialist)

- SABA prn

Preferred:

- Medium-dose ICS

Step 4 (consult specialist)

- SABA prn

Preferred:

- Medium-dose ICS + LABA or montelukast (Singulair)

Step 5 (consult specialist)

- SABA prn

Preferred:

- High-dose ICS + LABA or montelukast (Singulair)

Step 6 (consult specialist)

- SABA prn

Preferred:

- High-dose ICS + LABA or montelukast (Singulair) + oral corticosteroid and ICS

Stepwise approach to asthma management age 5–11 years of age

- To assist but not replace clinical decision making on individual patients

Step-up as needed

- First check medication adherence, environmental control and comorbid conditions
- Assess control
- Step down when possible and when asthma is controlled for 3 months
- Step up treatment when SABA used > 2 days/week
- Short course oral corticosteroid may be needed for exacerbations up to 10 days (no taper) — dexamethasone preferred (0.15–0.3 mg/kg) not to exceed 6 mg daily

Intermittent asthma

Step 1

Preferred:

- Inhaled short-acting beta–agonist (SABA) prn therapy

Persistent asthma: Daily medication

- Consider SQ immunotherapy for Step 2–4 in patients with allergic asthma

Step 2

- SABA prn

Preferred:

- Low-dose inhaled corticosteroid (ICS)

Alternatives to ICS

- LTRA or theophylline

Step 3 (consider consultation with specialist)

- SABA prn

Preferred:

- Low-dose ICS + LABA, LTRA or theophylline

OR

- Medium-dose ICS

Step 4 (consult specialist)

- SABA prn

Preferred:

- Medium-dose ICS + LABA

Alternative:

- Medium-dose ICS + LTRA or theophylline

Step 5 (consult specialist)

- SABA prn

Preferred:

- High-dose ICS + LABA

Alternative:

- High-dose ICS + LTRA or theophylline

Step 6 (consult specialist)

- SABA prn

Preferred:

- High-dose ICS + LABA + oral corticosteroid

Alternative:

- High-dose ICS + LTRA or theophylline + oral corticosteroids

Medications

Short-acting beta–agonist (SABA)

Albuterol HFA inhaler

All ages

- 2 puffs q4–6hr prn
  - Separate the puffs by 1 minute
- Spacer recommended

Nebulized albuterol

Age < 5 years

- 0.63–2.5 mg in 3 ml NS q4–8hr prn

Age ≥ 5 years

- 1.25–5 mg in 3 ml NS q4–6hr prn

Inhaled corticosteroid (ICS)

Fluticasone HFA/MDI (Flovent)

Low daily dose

Age < 5 years

- 176 mcg

Age ≥ 5 years

- 88–176 mcg

Medium daily dose

0–11 years

- > 176–352 mcg

Age ≥ 12 years

- > 264–440 mcg

High daily dose

Age ≤ 11 years

- > 352 mcg

Age ≥ 12 years

- > 440 mcg

Short term oral corticosteroids

- Course 3–10 days (no taper needed)

Dexamethasone preferred

Age ≤ 11 years

- 0.15–0.3 mg/kg PO qday (NMT 6 mg)

Age ≥ 12 years

- 4–6 mg PO qday

Long-acting beta–agonists (LABA)

Salmeterol DFI 50 mcg/blister

Age ≥ 5 years

- 1 blister q12hr

Formoterol

Age ≥ 5 years

- 1 capsule q12hr

Combination ICS/LABA

Budesonide/formoterol HFA/MDI (Symbicort)

Age ≥ 5 years

- 2 puffs bid (depends on level of control)

Leukotriene receptor antagonist (LTRA)

Montelukast (Singulair) chewable tablet

Age 1–5 years

- 4 mg qhs

Age 6–14 years

- 5 mg qhs

Age ≥ 15 years

- 10 mg qhs

Zileuton 600 mg tablet

Age ≥ 12 years

- 600 mg qid

Theophylline

Age < 1 year

- Starting dose 10 mg/kg/day
- Usual maximum dose 0.2 × age in weeks + 5 = mg/kg/day — full term up to 26 weeks divided q8hr and divided q6hr for age 26–52 weeks

Age 1–11 year

- Starting dose 10 mg/kg/day
- Usual maximum 16 mg/kg/day

Age ≥12 years

- Starting dose 10 mg/kg/day up to 300 mg/day
- Usual maximum 800 mg/day

Immunotherapy medications

- Monoclonal antibody therapy
  - Omalizumab
    - Moderate-to-severe persistent asthma who have a positive skin test result or in vitro reactivity to a perennial aeroallergen and whose symptoms are inadequately controlled with inhaled corticosteroids
    - Patients should have IgE levels between 30 and 700 IU and should not weigh more than 150 kg
  - Mepolizumab or Reslizumab

Allergen immunotherapy

- A relationship is clear between symptoms and exposure to an unavoidable allergen to which the patient is sensitive
- Symptoms occur all year or during a major portion of the year
- Symptoms are difficult to control with pharmacologic management because the medication is ineffective, multiple medications are required, or the patient is not accepting of medication

Consult criteria

- As noted in the Stepwise approach above
- Usually Step 3 or higher
- Consider consultation for subspecialty evaluation for:
  - Life-threatening asthma exacerbations or intubation
  - Recurrent hospitalizations or ED visits in patients felt to be adherent to the written action plan — i.e., unresponsive to therapy
  - Atypical features to the patient presentation raising questions as to other problems that mimic asthma such as vocal cord dysfunction syndrome, allergic bronchopulmonary aspergillosis, etc.
  - Immunotherapy

Notes

REFERENCES:

Expert Panel Report 3 (EPR-3): Guidelines for the Diagnosis and Management of Asthma - Summary Report 2007

Abramson MJ, Puy RM, Weiner JM. Allergen immunotherapy for asthma. *Cochrane Database Syst Rev*. 2003. CD001186

Asthma Author: Michael J Morris, MD, FACP, FCCP; Chief Editor: Zab Mosenifar, MD, FACP, FCCP emedicine.medscape.com/article/296301

Asthma Guidelines

Updated: Jan 07, 2019 Author: Michael J Morris, MD, FACP, FCCP; Chief Editor: Zab Mosenifar, MD, FACP, FCCP

COPD MANAGEMENT

Definition

- Disease state with chronic airflow obstruction that is not fully reversible, and is progressive — and includes chronic bronchitis and/or emphysema and/or fixed asthmatic bronchitis and many patients will have substantial overlapping conditions

Differential diagnosis

- Acute bronchitis
- Pulmonary embolism
- Heart failure with bronchospasm
- Bronchiectasis
- Pneumonia
- Chronic asthma

Considerations

- 4th leading cause of death in the U.S.
- Chronic bronchitis defined as 3 months of chronic productive cough each of the past 2 years (other causes of cough excluded)
- Emphysema has permanent enlargement of the airways distal to the terminal bronchioles
- Asthma — see Asthma Management
- Cigarette smoking is leading cause of COPD
- Increase in lung volume occurs

2018 clinical practice guidelines from the GOLD report on COPD

- COPD should be considered in any patient with dyspnea, chronic cough or sputum production, and/or a history of exposure to risk factors
- Spirometry is required to make the diagnosis; a post bronchodilator FEV1/FVC ratio of less than 0.70 confirms the presence of persistent airflow limitation
- COPD assessment goals are to determine the level of airflow limitation, the impact of disease on the patient's health status, and the risk of future events (e.g., exacerbations, hospital admissions, death) to guide therapy
- Concomitant chronic diseases occur frequently in COPD patients and should be treated because they can independently affect mortality and hospitalizations

Signs and symptoms

- Productive cough
- Acute chest illness
- Wheezing
- Rhonchi
- Inspiratory crackles
- Dyspnea
- Use of respiratory accessory muscles
- Cor pulmonale (right heart failure and edema)
- Occasional left heart failure
- Barrel chest (emphysema)
- Heart tones distant
- Obesity (more in chronic bronchitis patients)
- Prolonged expiration
- pCO_2 retention
- Metabolic alkalosis compensating for chronic respiratory acidosis
- Respiratory failure (end-stage)

Evaluation options

- History and physical examination
- Chest x-ray
- CBC
- Spirometry
    - Forced expiratory volume in 1 second over forced vital capacity (FEV_1/FVC) is less than 70% of predicted commonly

- ABG (pH should be normal; less than 7.30 indicates significant respiratory compromise
  - Any decrease in pH below normal (7.35) from increasing pCO_2 is important and needs immediate evaluation and treatment
- Sputum evaluation for acute exacerbations prn
  - Streptococcal pneumonia, hemophilus influenza and moraxella catarrhalis most common bacterial organisms
  - Pseudomonas aeruginosa and enterobacteriaceae may occur in severe obstruction
- CT chest scan prn
- Pulse oximetry

Treatment

- Smoking cessation
- Patient education
- Proton pump inhibitor for GERD
- Long term oxygen for pO_2 < 55 mm Hg; or < 59 mm Hg for cor pulmonale or polycythemia
- Use titrated oxygen instead of high flow oxygen
  - Mortality is significantly lower with titrated oxygen

Stage 1 (mild obstruction) - FEV_1 80% or greater of predicted

- Influenza vaccine
- Short-acting bronchodilator prn

Stage 2 (moderate obstruction) - FEV_1 50-79% of predicted

- Influenza vaccine
- Short-acting beta–agonist (SABA) prn
- Long-acting bronchodilator
- Cardiopulmonary rehabilitation

Stage 3 (severe obstruction) - FEV_1 30-49% of predicted

- Stage 2 treatment plus inhaled corticosteroids (ICS) for repeated exacerbations
- Consider subspecialty consultation

Stage 4 (very severe obstruction) - FEV_1 less than 30% of predicted

- Stage 3 plus oxygen prn
- Surgery options
- Consider subspecialty consultation

Medication options

Short-acting beta–agonist (SABA)

Albuterol HFA inhaler

- 2 puffs q4–6h prn
- Spacer recommended

Long-acting beta–agonists (LABA)

Salmeterol DFI 50 mcg/blister

- 1 blister q12hr

Formoterol

- 1 capsule q12hr

Anticholinergic agents

Ipratropium (Atrovent)

- 2 puffs qid (NMT 12 puffs qday)

Tiotropium (Spiriva)

- 2 inhalations of 1 capsule qday

Inhaled corticosteroid (ICS)

Fluticasone (Flovent)

Low daily dose

- 88–176 mcg

Medium daily dose

- > 264–440 mcg

High daily dose

- > 440 mcg

Short term oral corticosteroids for acute exacerbations

- Course 5–10 days (no taper needed) — evidence B

Dexamethasone

- 6 mg PO qday (= prednisone 40 mg)

OR

Methylprednisolone, prednisolone and prednisone

- 40 mg PO qday

Combination albuterol/ipratropium (Combivent)

MDI

- 2 puffs qid prn (NMT 12 puffs qday)

Combination SABA/ICS

Budesonide/formoterol 160 mcg/4.5 mcg (Symbicort)

- 2 inhalations bid

Fluticasone/salmeterol (Advair diskus) 50 mcg/250 mcg

- 1 inhalation bid

Antibiotic choices for exacerbations

Aged 40 years who are smokers or have a history of smoking

- Azithromycin (Z-pak)
- Doxycycline 100 mg PO bid for 10 days
- Amoxicillin 500 mg PO tid for 10 days
- Septra DS PO bid for 10 days
- Cefuroxime (Zinacef) 250–500 mg PO BID for 10 days

Pulmonary rehabilitation

Goals

- Lessen airflow limitation
- Prevent and treat secondary medical complications (e.g., hypoxemia, infection)
- Decrease respiratory symptoms and improve quality of life

Program

- Patient and family education
- Smoking cessation
- Medical management (including oxygen and immunization)
- Respiratory and chest physiotherapy
- Physical therapy with bronchopulmonary hygiene, exercise, and vocational rehabilitation
- Psychosocial support

Smoking cessation

- Nicorette
- Zyban
- Chantix

Consult criteria

- Uncontrolled COPD despite maximal medication therapy
- Home oxygen needed
- Respiratory acidosis with a pH < 7.35 (send to emergency department)
- Respiratory fatigue (send to emergency department)
- Progressive weight loss
- Fever ≥ 101.5° F (38.6° C) — remember to evaluate for other causes of fever — UTI, prostatitis, viral syndromes (influenza), etc.

Notes

____

____

____

REFERENCES:

Austin MA, et al. *BMJ* 2010, 341:c5462

Chronic Obstructive Pulmonary Disease Author: Zab Mosenifar, MD; Chief Editor: Zab Mosenifar, MD emedicine.medscape.com/article/297664

Vestbo J, et al. *Am J Respir Crit Care Med* 2013;187(4):347–65

[Guideline] Global Initiative for Chronic Obstructive Lung Disease. Global Strategy for the Diagnosis, Management, and Prevention of Chronic Obstructive Pulmonary Disease 2018 Report. Goldcopd.org

[Guideline] Criner GJ, Bourbeau J, Diekemper RL, et al. Prevention of acute exacerbations of COPD: American College of Chest Physicians and Canadian Thoracic Society Guideline. Chest. 2015 Apr. 147 (4):894-942

Chronic Obstructive Pulmonary Disease (COPD)

Updated: Apr 05, 2019

Author: Zab Mosenifar, MD, FACP, FCCP; Chief Editor: John J Oppenheimer, M

Emedicine.medscape.com

Ventilator Management

For clinical settings that permit the practitioner to perform ventilator management and they are trained and experienced to perform those duties Use (page 12).

Considerations

- Mechanical ventilation after intubation is a common lifesaving therapy in critically ill patients
- Potential benefits of mechanical ventilation
- Improved oxygenation with increased FiO_2 and the application of positive end-expiratory pressure (PEEP)
- Improved ventilation through manipulation of the tidal volume and respiratory rate
- Decreased work of breathing
- Optimization of ventilation parameters may decrease complications and hospital length of stay
- Low tidal volume ventilation (6 mL/kg ideal body weight) decreases barotrauma
- Weaning FiO_2 to target an O_2 saturation of 90–93 percent. Prolonged hyperoxia promotes inflammation and contributes to tissue injury
- Checking an ABG 30 minutes after ventilator adjustments may help the clinician assess the adequacy of oxygenation and ventilation
- A reliable pulse oximeter waveform is generally as useful as checking serial ABGs to monitor oxygenation.
- Manipulate one parameter at a time when changes are needed (respiratory rate, tidal volume, PEEP, FiO_2 etc.)
- If the practitioner feels that intubation is needed, then it most likely is needed
- No absolute contraindications to intubation exist
  - Extreme caution is needed in cervical spine injuries or with cervical spine rheumatoid arthritis or ankylosing spondylitis
  - Clinicians should anticipate precipitous drops in BP in hypotensive patients at the time of intubation, and medications (vasopressors) and IVFs should be available for administration

Common disease processes requiring intubation when severe

- Asthma
- Heart failure
- COPD exacerbation
- Sepsis
- ARDS
- Pneumonia
- Trauma
- Neuromuscular disorders
- Drug overdose

Complications

Pulmonary

Barotrauma – high peak pressures > 40 cm H20

- Pneumothorax
- Pneumomediastinum
- Development of bronchopleural fistula
- Interstitial emphysema

High oxygen concentration

- Free radical cellular damage
- Absorption atelectasis from nitrogen washout

Other

- Nosocomial pneumonia

Cardiovascular effects

- From high PEEP (high intrathoracic pressures)
  - Decreased venous preload and cardiac output
  - Right ventricular dysfunction
- Decreased cardiac output effects
  - Decreased renal, hepatic, and other end-organ blood flow leading to impaired functioning

Rapid sequence intubation (RSI)

- Preoxygenate with 100% FiO_2 with mask for 5 minutes if possible
- 8 vital capacity breaths of 100% FiO_2 if time limited
- Children (age ≥1 year) uncuffed ET tube size: internal diameter mm = age/4 + 4 (round down if needed due to fraction) — can use Broselow tape
  - 3.5 mm for infants up to 1 year of age
- Children cuffed ET tube internal diameter = age/4+3 — can use Broselow tape
  - 3.0 mm may be used for infants more than 3.5 kg. and <1 year
- ET tube size: adult female 6.5–8.0 mm; adult male 7.0–8.0 mm
- ET tube depth
  - ETT depth = 0.1[height in cm] + 4
  - Average sized female ET tube depth at lips of 21 cm (adjust per exam and x–ray)
  - Average sized male ET tube depth at lips 23 cm (adjust per exam and x–ray)
- 3-3-2 rule to determine chance of success
  - Patient is able to insert 3 of his or her own fingers between the teeth
  - 3 finger breadths between the hyoid bone and the mentum
  - 2 finger breadths between the hyoid bone and the thyroid cartilage
- Visualize the ET tube passing through the vocal cords

Induction agents to choose from

- Etomidate 0.3 mg/kg IV
  - Onset 15–45 seconds
  - Duration 3–12 minutes
  - Minimal hemodynamic instability
  - Cerebroprotective
- Propofol 2–3 mg/kg IV (use ~1.5 mg/kg IV in debilitated patients
  - Onset 15–45 seconds
  - Duration 5–10 minutes
  - Cerebroprotective
  - Amnesia
  - May cause hypotension, bradycardia (not an analgesic)
- Ketamine 2 mg/kg IV or 4 mg/kg IM
  - Onset 45–60 seconds
  - Duration 10–20 minutes
  - Bronchodilator , amnesia, analgesia (useful in bronchospasm)
  - Preserves respiratory drive (consider in difficult airway patients)
  - Increase blood pressure
- Midazolam 0.2–0.3 mg/kg IV
  - Onset 60–90 seconds
  - Duration 15–30 minutes
  - Amnestic
  - Anticonvulsant
  - Significant respiratory depression

Neuromuscular blocking agents to choose from

- Succinylcholine 2 mg/kg IV based on actual body weight (depolarizing agent)
  - Onset 45–60 seconds
  - Duration 6–10 minutes
  - Fast onset and short duration
  - Do not use with personal or family history of malignant hyperthermia, neuromuscular disease, muscular dystrophy, rhabdomyolysis, hyperkalemia with EKG changes, spinal cord injury, stroke >48 hours and < 6 months old, or burns/crush injuries
  - Transient rise of potassium of 0.5 mEq/L
- Rocuronium 0.6–1.2 mg/kg IV (non–depolarizing agent
  - Onset 45–60 seconds (depending on dose)
  - Duration 40–60 minutes (depending on dose)
  - Reversible
- Vecuronium 0.1–0.3 mg/kg IV
  - Onset 2–3 minutes with 0.1 mg/kg IV (low dose)
  - Onset 75–90 seconds with 0.3 mg/kg IV (high dose)
  - Duration 30 minutes with low dose
  - Duration 90 minutes with high dose
  - Slowest onset and longest duration of paralytics

Indications for mechanical ventilation

Clinical indications

- Bradypnea or apnea
- Severe or advanced respiratory fatigue
- Coma
- Obtundation
- Loss of protective airway reflexes (cough and gag reflexes)
- Acute lung injury or ARDS with inability to oxygenate or ventilate by non-invasive means
- Shock, particularly with metabolic acidosis and inadequate respiratory compensation

Clinical conditions

Hypercapneic respiratory failure

- COPD
- Status asthmaticus
- Neuromuscular disease
- Severe chest wall trauma (flail chest)

Hypoxemic respiratory failure

- Pneumonia
- Non-cardiogenic pulmonary edema (ARDS, neurogenic pulmonary edema, other conditions)
- Cardiogenic pulmonary edema
- Diffuse lung disease
  - Interstitial fibrosis or inflammation
  - Pulmonary hemorrhage
- Extreme work of breathing with developing respiratory fatigue
- Protect or ensure patency of airway and control secretions with impaired cough reflex
  - CVA
  - Drug overdose
  - Cervical spine injury
  - Anaphylaxis or other causes of airway edema

Laboratory indications

- $PaCO_2$ > 50 mm Hg with a pH < 7.25
- PaO_2 < 55 mm Hg on maximal supplementary oxygen (usually either a 100 percent non-rebreather, CPAP, or BiPAP)

Pulmonary function test abnormalities which suggest impending respiratory failure

- Vital capacity < 15mL/kg in adults
- Vital capacity < 10 mL/kg in children

- Negative inspiratory force < -20 cm H20 (normal -65 to -75 cm H20
- Forced expiratory volume (FEV1) < 5 mL/kg

Basic modes of mechanical ventilation

Volume-cycled

- Delivers a set tidal volume during a specified time (which is determined by the respiratory rate)
- Delivers constant inspiratory flow rate
- Airway pressures vary with changes in pulmonary compliance and resistance
- When paired with a set respiratory rate, volume-cycled modes guarantee a minimum minute ventilation
- High airway pressures can occur in non-compliant lungs resulting in barotrauma and potentially pneumothorax. This can be seen with:
    - ARDS or other diffuse lung disease with decreased lung compliance
    - Right mainstem intubation
    - Increased intra-abdominal pressure
    - Chest wall rigidity
    - "Fighting the ventilator" due to patient agitation

Pressure-cycled

- Delivers a set pressure until a specified time (pressure control) or flow (pressure support) is met
- Useful in situations with non-compliant lungs (ARDS) because they guarantee a set peak pressure will not be exceeded; however this may be at the expense of the tidal volume
- Changes in lung compliance may result in varying tidal volumes which is a disadvantage and requires close monitoring
- Some ventilators allow for volume assured pressure-cycled ventilation with breath-to-breath adjustments in pressure as needed to deliver a desired tidal volumes

Specific modes of mechanical ventilation

There are many modes of mechanical ventilation, some of which are quite complex. It should be noted that no mode has been proven to be superior to another mode in the general population of mechanically ventilated patients.

Assist-controlled ventilation

- Patient is guaranteed to get a preset tidal volume (volume-cycled) or pressure (pressure-cycled) at a set respiratory rate. Ventilator cycles with patient respiratory effort above the set rate and will deliver additional tidal volumes or pressure for extra breaths.
- Tachypnea can lead to breath stacking and air trapping, particularly in patients with COPD.

Synchronous intermittent mandatory ventilation

- Patient is guaranteed to get a preset tidal volume or pressure at a set respiratory rate. Additional patient respirations are allowed but not supported.
- Typically, additional breaths above the set respiratory rate are pressure supported.

Airway pressure release ventilation and Bivent

- A type of pressure control ventilation delivering a high pressure (P_{high}) for a longer interval (T_{high}) and low pressure (P_{low}) for a shorter interval (T_{low}). This contrasts other modes where the inspiratory phase is shorter than the expiratory phase.
- Improves oxygenation by maximizing mean airway pressures

- Ventilation can worsen in some patients and the pH and PCO_2 must be monitored carefully
- Most commonly employed in patients with ARDS
- Clinician should be trained in the use of this complex mode of ventilation

Pressure support ventilation

- For spontaneously breathing patients
- Level of pressure support is set to assist spontaneous respirations
- Can be useful in determining readiness for extubation
- May improve patient comfort

Noninvasive ventilation

- Positive pressure ventilation through a mask
- Useful in specific types of respiratory failure
- Good evidence for decreased mortality and decreased hospital length of stay in patients with COPD exacerbations, cardiogenic pulmonary edema, and in immunocompromised patients with acute respiratory failure
- Also may benefit patients with severe asthma exacerbations, neuromuscular disease, and post-extubation for patients with COPD
- Conflicting evidence for benefit in other causes of hypoxic respiratory failure
- Generally, patients must be able to follow commands and protect their airway to attempt non-invasive positive pressure ventilation
- Full mask preferred in acute settings
- Complications
  - Barotrauma (rare)
  - Pressure necrosis of facial tissues
  - Gastric dilation, vomiting, and aspiration
  - Patient intolerance

Continuous positive airway pressure (CPAP)

- Most commonly used in the setting of cardiogenic pulmonary edema in conjunction with diuresis
- Initial settings
  - CPAP pressure 4–12 cm H_2O

Bilevel positive airway pressure (BPAP)

- Similar to CPAP but BPAP may improve ventilation and is therefore most useful to treat COPD with acute hypercapneic respiratory acidosis
- Initial settings:
  - Inspiratory pressure (IPAP) 8–12 cm H_2O
  - Expiratory pressure (EPAP) 3–5 cm H_2O

Commonly used ventilation parameters

- **Tidal volume** (TV)
  - Amount of air delivered in a single breath, typically 4–12 mL/kg
  - Mortality benefit with low tidal volumes (6 mL/kg) in patients with ARDS, and this ventilation strategy is generally applied to most ventilated patients with respiratory failure
- **Respiratory rate** (RR)
- Generally set at 8–24 breaths per minute
- Respiratory rates that are too fast rate can cause air trapping (auto–PEEP) in patients with obstructive lung disease
- **Minute ventilation** is amount of air delivered in a minute, and this equals the TV x RR (5–10 L/min)
- **Peak inspiratory pressure** (PIP)
  - Highest level of pressure applied by the ventilator, which is only partially transmitted to the distal airways
  - In a volume cycled mode, this depends on the size of the tidal volume and on airway resistance.

This is specified in a pressure cycled mode.

- Barotrauma can occur at higher pressures
- Generally aim to keep PIP < 35 cm H_2O

- **Plateau pressure**
  - The pressure applied to the small airways and alveoli. This is a function of lung compliance.
  - Checked by performing an inspiratory hold maneuver
  - Plateau pressure > 30 cm H_20 may lead to increased barotrauma
- **Positive end expiratory pressure** (PEEP)
  - Usually set between 5–15 cm H_2O
  - Can improve oxygenation by recruitment of alveoli to participate in gas exchange
  - High levels of PEEP can have complex effects on the cardiovascular system through decreased RV and LV preload, increased RV afterload, and decreased LV afterload. The cardiac output is typically increased in hypervolemic patients and decreased in euvolemic and hypovolemic patients
  - Generally wean PEEP along with FiO_2 to lowest tolerated levels
- **Fraction of inspired oxygen** (FiO_2)
  - Start at 100 percent, and titrate down to maintain a p_aO_2 > 60 mm Hg or an O_2 saturation > 90 percent
  - Prolonged use of an FiO_2 > 60 percent may be harmful
- **Inspiratory:expiratory ratio** (I:E ratio)
  - Most patients are set at 1:1.5 – 1:4
  - Inadequate expiratory time may lead to air trapping (auto-PEEP)
- **Inspiratory flow rate**
  - The amount of gas given during inspiration (40–100 L/minute)
  - Adjusting the flow rate will affect the I:E ratio

Suggested Initial Ventilator Settings

Volume-cycled assist control – "Volume control"

- Respiratory rate 10–12/minute
- A low RR allows the patient to breathe above the set rate and therefore determine their own respiratory rate, which is generally ideal
- A higher RR might be needed in paralyzed patients who cannot breath spontaneously
- Tidal volume 6–8 mL/kg ideal body weight
- Goal should be 6 mL/kg in ARDS
- PEEP 5–10 cm H_2O
- Severely hypoxic patients will need more PEEP
- FiO_2 — start at 100 percent
- Decrease as permitted to maintain pO_2 > 60 or an O_2 saturation > 90 percent)
- I:E ratio 1:2

Monitoring ventilator support

- Obtaining ABGs after a ventilator parameter change can be helpful, particularly for patients who are not breathing above the set RR. If a patient has a functioning pulse oximeter and they are breathing above the set RR, frequent ABGs are less like to be useful.
  - Maintain pH > 7.3 and < 7.45
    - pH > 7.45 decrease ventilator rate
    - pH 7.15–7.30 increase ventilator rate
    - In patients with ARDS, we tolerate lower tidal volumes, and therefore less minute ventilation and a lower pH/higher pCO_2 (pH as low as 7.20), to minimize barotrauma. This is termed "permissive hypercapnia."
  - Maintain pO_2 60–90 mm Hg

- Maintain pCO_2 35–45 mm Hg unless pH indicates patient is a chronic pCO_2 retainer
  - For example a pH > 7.45 with pCO_2 35–45 mm Hg indicates that the patient may normally have a higher resting pCO_2 from COPD or another condition causing chronic ventilatory impairment
- Cardiac monitoring
- Blood pressure monitoring
- Pulse oximetry (maintain O_2 saturation > 90%)
- Peak pressures < 40 cm H_2O
- Plateau pressures < 30 cm H_2O
- Increase PEEP in 2 cm H_2O increments as needed for hypoxia with assessing vital signs for several minutes afterward

High pO_2 with high FiO_2

- Decrease FiO_2 in 5–10% increments
- Once the FiO_2 < 60%, lower PEEP by 2cm H20 increments
- After each change, allow 5–10 minutes for equilibration to occur
- A stepwise weaning protocol has been developed by the ARDS network investigators (see reference)

High or low pCO_2

- Must be interpreted in the context of the pH
- A high pCO_2 and a near normal pH suggests a chronic respiratory acidosis and no adjustment may be needed
- A high pCO_2 and a low pH indicates increased ventilation is necessary, and the RR or TV should be increased
- With metabolic acidosis, the pH will be low and the pCO_2 should be < 40 to compensate for the primary metabolic process. If the pCO_2 is > 40, the RR or TV should be increased

Reducing risk of ventilator-associated pneumonia

- Shorten the duration of mechanical ventilation
- Protocolized daily spontaneous breathing and spontaneous awakening trials have been shown to result in fewer days on the ventilator
- Chlorhexidine oral rinse
- Diligent hand hygiene
- Elevating head of bed 30–45° when possible
- Note: Stress ulcer prophylaxis is recommended in patients on mechanical ventilation > 48 hr. However, agents that increase pH (PPIs and H2 receptor antagonists) may increase the risk of ventilator associated pneumonia.

Sedation

- Most patients need sedation and/or analgesia by continuous infusion or scheduled dosing
- Daily interruption of sedation allows for less days of mechanical ventilation
- Most patients should be started on a propofol or fentanyl infusion with a RASS (Richmond Agitation Sedation Scale) goal of 0 to -1
- For a comprehensive and up to date approach to sedation in mechanically ventilated patients, please review the information at www.icudelirium.org

Troubleshooting

Sudden respiratory distress

- Disconnect patient from ventilator
- Manually ventilate with an bag valve mask
- Suction the patient to remove secretions that could be obstructing the airway
- If no improvement, check to see if the patient is adequately sedated (tube biting, ventilator dyssynchrony, etc.)
- Obtain a CXR and have the respiratory therapist evaluate the patient

Ventilator problems

- Should improve with manual bagging

- Check tubing for obstruction
- Check for circuit disconnect
- Perform an inspiratory hold to evaluate for a resistance or compliance issue
- Check an expiratory hold to evaluate for auto-PEEP

Endotracheal tube problems

Low resistance check for:

- Endotracheal tube (ET) placement
    - Esophageal location
- Cuff leak if low resistance or low peak inspiratory pressure develops
- Internal tube leak if low resistance or low peak inspiratory pressure develops

High resistance (high peak pressures)

- Right mainstem intubation
- Pneumothorax
- Patient biting ET
- Check tubing for obstruction (suction tube)
- Kinked ET tube
- Anything causing reduced lung compliance – ARDS, pneumonia, pulmonary edema, alveolar hemorrhage, etc.

Hypotension treatment options

- IV fluid bolus if pulmonary edema absent
- Think about auto-PEEP. Disconnect ventilator circuit if high levels of auto-PEEP are present on expiratory hold maneuver. Then resume ventilation with a lower RR or lengthen the expiratory time.
- Decrease PEEP as high levels of PEEP may impair cardiac output
- Consider evaluating for pneumothorax or pulmonary embolism

Liberation from mechanical ventilation

- Evaluate patients daily to determine candidacy for a spontaneous breathing trial

Criteria for extubation

- Can patient oxygenate and ventilate independent of mechanical ventilation?
- O_2 saturation > 90 percent and PaO_2 > 60 mm Hg on FiO_2 < 40% and PEEP < 5 cm H_2O
- Patient breathing spontaneously
- Mental status and ability to protect airway
- Patient should be able to follow commands and have strong cough and gag reflexes
- Hemodynamic stability
- Should be on no or minimal dose vasopressors
- Acid-base and electrolyte balance
- pH > 7.25.
- Thyroid and adrenal function sufficient

Spontaneous breathing trial (SBT)

- Place on pressure support (PS) mode with a PS above PEEP at 5, PEEP 5, and FiO_2 40 percent
- Observe patient for 30–120 minutes
- Assess respiratory rate/tidal volume ratio (RSBI)
- RSBI < 105 is predictive of successful extubation
- Age > 70 years with RSBI < 130 may be acceptable
- If patient fails SBT, resume mandatory ventilation for the next 24 hours
- Another option for an SBT is to disconnect the patient from the ventilator and utilize a T-piece. Patient is monitored in a similar fashion and assessed for readiness to extubate at 30–120 minutes.

Consult criteria

- Management under physician's direction
- Requiring mechanical ventilation > 24 hours
- More complicated ventilator or oxygenation problem
- Complex critical illness

Notes

REFERENCES:

Clinical practice guidelines for the use of noninvasive positive-pressure ventilation and noninvasive continuous positive airway pressure in the acute care setting. *CMAJ February 22, 2011 vol. 183 no. 3* First published February 14, 2011, doi: 10.1503/cmaj.100071

Ventilator Management
Author: Allon Amitai, MD; Chief Editor: Zab Mosenifar, MD
emedicine
medscape.com/article/810126

Non-invasive positive pressure ventilation for treatment of respiratory failure due to exacerbations of chronic obstructive pulmonary disease.. Cochrane Database Syst Rev. 2004; (3):CD004104.

Noninvasive ventilation in acute cardiogenic pulmonary edema: systematic review and meta-analysis. Masip J et al. JAMA. 2005; 294(24):3124–30

Ventilation with Lower Tidal Volumes as Compared with Traditional Tidal Volumes for Acute Lung Injury and the Acute Respiratory Distress Syndrome. ARDSNet Investigators. N Engl J Med 2000; 342:1301–1308

Marini, John J., and Arthur P. Wheeler. *Critical Care Medicine: The Essentials*. Philadelphia: Lippincott Williams & Wilkins, 2009. Print.

"ARDSNet." *NHLBI ARDS Network*. Web. 16 June 2014. www.ardsnet.org

"ABCDEFs of Prevention and Safety." *ICU Delirium and Cognitive Impairment Study Group*. Web. 16 June 2014. <http://www.icudelirium.org/>.

Efficacy and safety of a paired sedation and ventilator weaning protocol for mechanically ventilated patients in intensive care (Awakening and Breathing Controlled trial): a randomised controlled trial. Girard TD et al. Lancet. 2008; 371:126–34

REFERENCES:

Clinical practice guidelines for the use of noninvasive positive-pressure ventilation and noninvasive continuous positive airway pressure in the acute care setting. *CMAJ February 22, 2011 vol. 183 no. 3* First published February 14, 2011, doi: 10.1503/cmaj.100071

Ventilator Management
Author: Allon Amitai, MD; Chief Editor: Zab Mosenifar, MD
emedicine
medscape.com/article/810126

Non-invasive positive pressure ventilation for treatment of respiratory failure due to exacerbations of chronic obstructive pulmonary disease.. Cochrane Database Syst Rev. 2004; (3):CD004104.

Noninvasive ventilation in acute cardiogenic pulmonary edema: systematic review and meta-analysis. Masip J et al. JAMA. 2005; 294(24):3124–30

Ventilation with Lower Tidal Volumes as Compared with Traditional Tidal Volumes for Acute Lung Injury and the Acute Respiratory Distress Syndrome. ARDSNet Investigators. N Engl J Med 2000; 342:1301–1308

Marini, John J., and Arthur P. Wheeler. *Critical Care Medicine: The Essentials*. Philadelphia: Lippincott Williams & Wilkins, 2009. Print.

"ARDSNet." *NHLBI ARDS Network*. Web. 16 June 2014. www.ardsnet.org

"ABCDEFs of Prevention and Safety." *ICU Delirium and Cognitive Impairment Study Group*. Web. 16 June 2014. <http://www.icudelirium.org/>.

Efficacy and safety of a paired sedation and ventilator weaning protocol for mechanically ventilated patients in intensive care (Awakening and Breathing Controlled trial): a randomised controlled trial. Girard TD et al. Lancet. 2008; 371:126–34

DEPRESSION MANAGEMENT

Definition

- A state of emotional sadness and withdrawal greater and more prolonged than warranted by objective reasons

Differential diagnosis

- Anxiety disorder
- Bipolar affective disorder
- Dementia
- Hypothyroidism
- Hyperthyroidism
- Cushing syndrome
- Addison disease
- Alcoholism
- Drug abuse
- Chronic fatigue syndrome
- Schizophrenia
- Personality disorders
- Sleep apnea
- Adjustment disorder
- Posttraumatic stress disorder
- Premenstrual dysphoric disorder
- Lyme disease
- Syphilis
- Autoimmune diseases
- B-12 deficiency (pernicious anemia)

Considerations

- Lifetime depression incidence is 12% in men and 20% in women
- Most patients with depression do not realize they have a treatable disease
- Antidepressant medication takes 2–6 weeks to achieve therapeutic effect if there is a benefit to be realized
- Antidepressant medication may worsen the depression potentially leading to suicide – close monitoring of treatment needed
- Most antidepressants need to be tapered when discontinued
- Serotonin levels are thought to be an important factor
- Major depressant disorder is multifactorial
- Genetic link for depression exists in some individuals
- Stressors, chronic medical conditions and chronic pain predispose to depression
- Childhood abuse and neglect increases depression incidence in childhood and later in life
- Major depressive disorder has significant morbidity and mortality
- Treatment can help 70–80% of patients, though 50% may not initially respond to treatment
- Males successfully complete suicides 4.5 times as much as females
- 80% of women develop postpartum mood disturbance that is usually self–limited and of short duration lasting 2 weeks

- Postpartum depression develops over 3 months usually
- Untreated postpartum depression may cause child development and behavior problems
- Seasonal affective disorder — 2 episodes of a mood disorder in 2 years related to a particular season and outnumbers the nonseasonable episodes
- Severe major depression with psychosis is dangerous and often requires psychiatric admission
- Patient education is very important in depression treatment

Presenting complaints

- Somatic complaints such as fatigue, headache, GI complaints and weight changes
- Elderly may present with confusion
- Irritability
- Social withdrawal
- Dysphoric mood and negative attitude
- Psychosis

Major depressive episode

5 of the following in a 2 week period

- Depressed mood (typically over a 3 month period)
- Anhedonia — diminished interest and pleasure in most activities
- Appetite disturbance or weight change
- Fatigue
- Feelings of worthlessness
- Sleep disturbance
- Decreased concentration ability
- Recurrent thoughts of death or suicide
- Interpersonal rejection or suicide attempts/plans

Caveats

- Must have depressed mood or loss of interest/pleasure
- Symptoms must cause significant distress or impairment of social, occupational or interpersonal relationships
- Symptoms not precipitated by substances or medical conditions
- Symptoms do not meet criteria for bipolar illness
- Symptoms are not accounted for by bereavement
- Should not be coexistent with schizophrenia or other psychotic disorders

Evaluation

- Assess for medical conditions or medications that may cause depression — see Differential diagnosis
- Ask about suicidal or homicidal thoughts/plans

Mental status examination

OMI HAT (OMI = organic disease; HAT = psychiatric or functional)

- O – Orientation
- M – Memory
- I – Intellect
- H – Hallucinations
- A – Affect disorder
- T – Thought disorder
- Cognitive impairment evaluated by using Mini–Mental Status Examination

Treatment

- Psychotherapy
- Cognitive behavior therapy
- Medications
    - Combining medications and psychotherapy most effective and sustained approach
- Electroconvulsive therapy for failure of drug therapy and high risk of suicide

Medications

Selective serotonin reuptake inhibitors (SSRI's)

- Ease of dosing and low toxicity

- Preferred in children, adolescents and late onset depression
  - Studies have indicated an increase in suicidal thoughts on SSRI's, but decreased suicidal attempts
- Common side effects are GI upset, sexual dysfunction and fatigue/restlessness

Citalopram (Celexa)

- Initially 10–20 mg PO qday — may adjust every 2–4 weeks as needed — NMT 40 mg PO qday
- NMT 20 mg PO qday if taking cimetidine, omeprazole, fluconazole or other inhibitors of CYP2C19

Escitalopram (Lexapro)

- Depression
  - 10 mg PO qday — may increase to 20 mg PO qday after 2–4 weeks as needed
- Generalized anxiety disorder and depression in elderly
  - 10 mg PO qday for elderly

Paroxetine (Paxil)

- Depression
  - Initially 10–20 mg PO qday — may increase 10 mg/day q2–4weeks up to 50 mg PO qday as needed
  - Paxil CR: initial 12.5–25 mg PO qday — may increase 12.5 mg PO q2–4 weeks as needed — NMT 62.5 mg PO qday
- Obsessive compulsive disorder
  - Initially 20 mg PO qday — may increase 10 mg/day q2–4weeks up to 60 mg PO qday as needed
- Panic disorder
  - Initially 10–20 mg PO qday — may increase 10 mg/day q2–4weeks up to 60 mg PO qday as needed
  - Paxil CR: initial 12.5–25 mg PO qday — may increase 12.5 mg PO q2–4 weeks — NMT 75 mg PO qday

Vilazodone (Viibryd)

- Initially 10 mg PO qday x 7 days, then 20 mg PO qday x 2–4 weeks, then may increase to 40 mg PO qday as needed
- NMT 20 mg PO qday if taking ketoconazole or other CYP3A4 inhibitors

Other SSRI's

- Fluoxetine (Prozac)
- Sertraline (Zoloft)

Selective serotonin/norepinephrine reuptake inhibitors (SNRI's)

Venlafaxine (Effexor)

- Extended–release: 37.5–75 mg PO qday — may increase 75 mg PO qday every 2–4 weeks — NMT 225 mg PO qday

Desvenlafaxine (Pristiq)

- 50 mg PO qday and may increase as needed to 100 mg PO qday in 2–4 weeks

Duloxetine (Cymbalta)

- 30–60 mg PO qday — NMT 60 mg PO qday
- May be used for diabetic peripheral neuropathy, fibromyalgia and generalized anxiety disorder
- Taper gradually

Atypical antidepressants

Bupropion (Wellbutrin)

- Intermediate–release: 100 mg PO bid — may increase to 100 mg PO tid after 2–4 weeks as needed (NMT 150 mg PO tid)
- Sustained–release (SR): Initially 100 mg PO bid — may increase to 150 mg PO

bid after 2–4 weeks — NMT 200 mg PO bid
- Extended–release (XL): 150 mg PO qAM — may increase to 300 mg PO qday after 2–4 weeks (NMT 450 mg PO qday after 4 weeks)

N-methyl-D-aspartate antagonists

- Esketamine nasal spray (Spravato) was approved by the FDA in March 2019 for treatment-resistant depression in conjunction with an oral antidepressant
- **Restricted distribution**

St. John's Wort

Depression, Mild-moderate

- Hypericin 0.2% standardized extract: 250 mg PO BID
- Hyperforin 5% standardized extract: 300 mg PO TID
- Crude: 2-4 g PO qday-TID

Obsessive-compulsive Disorder

- Hypericin 0.3% standardized extract (XR): 450 mg PO BID

Premenstrual Syndrome

- Hypericin 0.3% standardized extract: 300 mg PO qday

Consult criteria

- Depression with psychosis — schizophrenia or bipolar affective disorder
- Refer patients with suicidal or homicidal ideation for immediate evaluation in emergency department or psychiatric facility
- Severe depression refractory to treatment

Notes

REFERENCES:

Depression Author: Jerry L Halverson, MD; Chief Editor: David Bienenfeld, MD emedicine.medscape.com article 286759

Depression Updated: Mar 28, 2019 Author: Jerry L Halverson, MD; Chief Editor: David Bienenfeld, MD Emedicine.medscape.com

HEADACHE MANAGEMENT

Definition

- Cephalic pain disorder

Differential Diagnosis

- Tension headache
- Migraine headache
- Cluster headache
- Sinusitis
- Otitis media
- Trigeminal neuralgia
- Brain tumor
- Subarachnoid hemorrhage
- Subdural hematoma
- Epidural hematoma
- Temporal arteritis
- Chronic daily headache
- Thunderclap headache
- Analgesic rebound headache
- CVA
- Meningitis
- Encephalitis
- Central vein thrombosis
- Normal pressure hydrocephalus
- Pseudotumor cerebri
- Ventricular peritoneal shunt malfunction
- Temporal mandibular joint disorder
- Lyme disease

Considerations

- History is one of the more important tools in headache evaluation
- New headache type in the elderly is suggestive of a higher risk process
- Do not use response to therapy as a judge of the seriousness of the headache

"Functional" or "Primary" headache

- No detectable cause (not uncommon)
- Migraine
- Cluster
- Tension–type headache

"Organic" or "Secondary" headache

From pain sensitive structures; vessels; periosteum

- Postconcussion headaches
- Spinal tap headaches
- Temporal arteritis
- Subarachnoid hemorrhage
- Subdural hematoma
- CVA
- Meningitis
- Encephalitis

Historical red flags

- Sudden onset or onset with exertion
- New, progressive, frequent headaches
- Trauma
- Cancer history
- Immunosuppression/HIV
- Clotting disorders
- First headache
- Worst headache of life
- Fever

Evaluation

- Complete history and physical exam
- Check gait, motor and sensory exam
- Funduscopic exam

Lab (usually not needed in most headaches)

- CBC
- ESR/CRP (age > 50 years: temporal arteritis) — usually not needed with no changes in chronic headache pattern
- UCG prn

Tension- type headache

- Pressing or tightening (nonpulsatile quality)
- Frontal-occipital location
- Bilateral: mild/moderate intensity
- Not aggravated by physical activity
- May have trigger points on scalp or cervical muscles

Causes

- Psychological stress
- Sleep deprivation
- Uncomfortable position or bad posture
- Eyestrain
- Irregular meals

Episodic tension–type headache

- Headaches lasting 30 minutes to 7 days
- Less than 15/month
- Pressure or tightening quality — nonpulsatile
- Mild to moderate intensity — may inhibit but not prohibit daily activities
- Bilateral in location
- Not exacerbated by physical activities
- No nausea or vomiting
- Photophobia or phonophonia — absent or one present
- Secondary type headaches not suspected or confirmed

Chronic tension–type headache

- More than 15 per month for more than 6 months
- Same as episodic tension–type headaches above otherwise

Evaluation

- History and physical exam
- Brain MRI if headache is atypical or concerning, or if the patient has a focal neurological exam — CT brain less useful than MRI

Treatment

- Tailored to individual patient
- Regular exercise and meals
- Proper sleep hygiene
- Trigger point injections prn
- Botulinum toxin is not effective

Episodic tension–type headache

- Physical therapy prn
- Hot and cold applications
- Stretching
- Massage
- Ultrasound therapy
- TENS
- Psychophysiological therapy prn
- Stress management
- Biofeedback techniques
- NSAID's PO prn
- Tylenol prn
- Fiorinal 1–2 PO q4hr prn not to exceed 6 per 24 hour period
- Midrin 1–2 caps qid PO prn

Chronic tension–type headache or > 2 headaches/week or are > 3 hours or severe enough to disrupt daily activities

Tricyclic antidepressants

- Amitriptyline (Elavil) 10 mg-150 mg PO qday — may give bid-tid
  - Taper gradually when discontinuing
- Nortriptyline (Pamelor) 25–100 mg PO qday — may give bid-tid
  - Taper gradually when discontinuing

Selective serotonin reuptake inhibitors (SSRI)

- Less anticholinergic and cardiovascular side effects than tricyclic antidepressants (taper gradually when discontinuing)
- Fluoxetine (Prozac) 20–40 mg PO qday — NMT 60 mg qday
- Sertraline (Zoloft) 50 mg PO qday (may increase 25 mg qweek as needed) — NMT 200 mg qday
- Paroxetine (Paxil) 20 mg PO qday (may increase 10 mg qweek as needed) — NMT 50 mg qday

Migraine headache

Considerations

- 30 million persons in U.S. have at least 1 migraine per year
- Familial prevalence
- Causes are not fully defined
- Chronic migraines may occur with 8 days of opiates per month (more pronounced in males) and barbiturates 5 days per month (more pronounced in females)
- Increased CVA and AMI incidence
- Usually lasts 4–72 hours
- Postdromal symptoms may include tired or refreshed feeling, increased appetite, muscle weakness or myalgias
- May be associated with seizures
- The unilateral motor weakness associated with a hemiplegic migraine typically lasts from 5 minutes to 72 hours

Migraine variants

- Hemiplegic migraine — unilateral weakness or paralysis
- Basilar migraine — aphasia, syncope or ataxia
- Ophthalmoplegic migraine — third cranial nerve palsy or visual field cut/monocular blindness

- Chronic migraine — 15 days per month for 3 months

Associated with

- Photophobia
- Phonophobia
- Nausea and vomiting
- May be unilateral or bilateral
- Aura occurs 20%
  - Scotoma (blind spots)
  - Fortification (zigzag patterns)
  - Scintilla (flashing lights)
  - Unilateral paresthesia/weakness
  - Hallucinations
  - Hemianopsia

Precipitants

- Stress
- Sleep disorders
- Vasodilators
- Oral contraceptives
- Menstruation or ovulation
- Smoking
- Strong odors
- Tyramine containing foods — yogurt, soy sauce, sour cream etc.

Evaluation

- Exclude other causes of headaches
- ESR and C-reactive protein in older patients to rule out temporal arteritis
- See CT brain headache criteria later in section

Lumbar puncture considered for

- First or worse headache of life
- Progressive headache
- Rapid onset severe headache
- Unusual chronic intractable headache
- Fever
- Papilledema only after mass lesion is ruled out by neuroimaging.

Acute treatment

- Compazine (prochlorperazine) 5–10 mg IV or IM (if available)
- Thorazine (chlorpromazine) 75 mg with Benadryl (diphenhydramine) 25 mg IM
- Ergots DHE 1 mg IV or IM (premedicate with an antiemetic)
- Reglan (metoclopramide) 10 mg IV or IM
- Valproic acid 1 gm IV
- Sumatriptan 6 mg SQ (do not use with history of coronary artery disease) — read drug information
- Maxalt (rizatriptan) 5–10 mg PO q2h prn for headache not to exceed 30 mg/day (do not use with history of coronary artery disease) — read drug information
- Other triptans
- Nurtec ODT (rimegepant) 75 mg PO qday prn migraine
- Ubrelvy (ubrogepant) 50–100 mg PO x 1, may repeat in ≥ 2 hours if needed (NMT 200 mg per day)
- Midrin 2 caps PO initially then 1 cap PO q1hr prn not to exceed 5 caps/day
- Toradol (ketorolac) 30–60 mg IM (do not use if creatinine is elevated)
- Compazine suppository (prochlorperazine) 25 mg PR bid prn (may cause extrapyramidal reaction)
- Acetaminophen
- Aspirin
- Narcotic prn (not preferred)
- Uninterrupted sleep may resolve episode

Prophylactic treatment

- Remove migraine triggers
- Biofeedback and/or cognitive behavior therapy prn
- Naproxen 250 mg PO tid or 500 mg PO bid
- Topiramate (Topamax) 50 mg bid — start at 25mg/day and titrate up over 2 weeks
- Valproic acid (Depakote) start at 500 mg PO qday for 1 week, then increase to 500–1,000 mg

PO divided into a daily or BID dosing — NMT 1,000 mg daily

- Valproic acid adverse reactions
  - Hepatic failure (monitor liver function tests especially in first 6 months of therapy)
  - Pancreatitis
  - Pregnancy fetal risks - should not be used in pregnancy
- Amitriptyline (Elavil) 10 mg-150 mg PO qday — may give bid-tid
  - Taper gradually when discontinuing
- Propranolol 20 mg PO qid may progress up to 80 mg PO tid
- Fluoxetine (Prozac) 20–40 mg PO qday — NMT 60 mg qday
- Sertraline (Zoloft) 50 mg PO qday (may increase 25 mg qweek as needed) — NMT 200 mg qday
- Paroxetine (Paxil) 20 mg PO qday (may increase 10 mg qweek as needed) — NMT 50 mg qday
- Ajovy (fremanezumab–vfrm) 225 mg SQ autoinjector qmonth

Cluster headaches

- More common in males
- Lancinating and severe
- Sudden onset — peaks in 10–15 minutes
- Unilateral facial location
- Duration: 10 minutes to 3 hours per episode
- Character: boring and lancinating to eye
- Distribution: first and second divisions of the trigeminal nerve (approximately 18–20% of patients complain of pain in extratrigeminal regions)
- Autonomic symptoms such as ptosis, conjunctival injection, rhinorrhea, nasal congestion and lacrimation that are ipsilateral to the pain
- Frequency: may occur several times a day for 1–4 months (often nocturnal)
- Patients are very restless (unlike migraine)
- Periodicity: circadian regularity in 47% of patients
- Remission: long symptom-free intervals occur in some patients for 2 months to 20 years

Treatment options

- O_2 8 LPM face mask or 100% nonrebreather mask
- Sumatriptan 6 mg SQ (do not use with history of coronary artery disease) — read drug information
- Lidocaine 1 cc of a 10% solution placed on a swab in each nostril for 5 minutes is potentially helpful
- Capsaicin applied intranasally (has a burning sensation side effect)
- Verapamil 240 mg-480 mg daily for preventative therapy

Trigeminal neuralgia

- Commonly idiopathic
- Shock like severe pains in the distribution of trigeminal nerve
- Onset usually around age 60–70 years of age
- If it occurs at a younger age, work-up including MRI of the brain is warranted
- Pains last seconds to less than 2 minutes
- Can be triggered by specific activities such as eating, talking, brushing teeth, etc.
- No associated neurologic deficits

Glossopharyngeal neuralgia

- Pain is over the distribution of glossopharyngeal nerve triggered by coughing, yawning, swallowing cold liquids

Occipital neuralgia

- Pain is in the posterior scalp region

Treatment options of cranial neuralgias

- Carbamazepine 200 mg PO bid to start (DOC)
  - Titrate increasing dose every 3 days by 200 mg
  - Effective dose is usually 600–1200 mg qday
  - Instruct patient they will need monitoring for aplastic anemia and severe leucopenia
  - Trileptal 150–600 mg bid
  - Lyrica 50–300 mg often divided into bid dosages
- Dilantin (phenytoin) for carbamazepine failures (lower rate of success in treating neuralgia)
  - Dose of 300–600 mg PO qday (levels need monitoring)
  - Cerebyx (fosphenytoin) 250 mg IV for severe attack
- Lamictal (lamotrigine) 100–400 mg PO qday (NMT 250 mg PO qday in children) — read drug information
- Treatment includes occipital nerve blocks

Discharge instructions

- Trigeminal neuralgia aftercare instructions

Consult criteria

- Complicated cranial neuralgias

Temporal arteritis

- True emergency of the elderly
  - Age of onset 50–70 years of age
  - Six times more common in females than in males
- Headache localized over eye or to scalp
- Fever, malaise and weight loss are associated symptoms
- Jaw claudication is an important associated symptom
- Frequently associated with polymyalgia rheumatica (joint and muscles aches)
- ESR 50–100
  - ESR may be normal in 15% of temporal arteritis patients
- C-reactive protein elevated usually
- Vision loss can occur early in course of disease

Treatment

- Prednisone 40–80 mg PO qday or divided bid for several months to one year
  - In suspected temporal arteritis with normal ESR, treat with steroids

Discharge criteria

- Minimal symptoms
- Severe symptoms or question of eye involvement should be admitted with IV high dose steroid treatment and ophthalmology consultation obtained

Discharge instructions

- Temporal arteritis aftercare instructions
- Follow up within 1 day
- Return for visual changes

Consult criteria

- Discuss all temporal arteritis cases with a physician

Subarachnoid hemorrhage (SAH)

- "Thunderclap" headache
- Sudden onset and reaching maximal intensity in seconds to minutes
- 1/3 not exertional
- May awake with SAH
- Sentinel leak in SAH headache may improve over time
- May cause EKG abnormalities

Evaluation

- CT brain scan (3rd generation scanner)
  - Nearly 100% accurate in the first 6 hours
  - Sensitivity (true positives) 93% at 24 hours after onset, 83% at 3 days and 50% at 1 week
  - False negative may occur with severe anemia or small hemorrhage

- Lumbar puncture
  - If CT brain scan negative and SAH suspected as possible cause of headache
  - May be falsely negative within 2 hours of SAH onset
  - Xanthochromia will appears 2–4 hours after bleed and remain for 2 weeks at least, up to 4 weeks in 40% of patients
  - May be negative in 10–15% of patients
- Cerebral angiography
  - If CT brain and lumbar puncture nondiagnostic and diagnostic uncertainly persists
- CT angiography — sensitivity and specificity comparable to cerebral angiography
- MRI brain may be used, but not as accurate as above imaging
- Monitor for acute hydrocephalus in SAH involving the CSF spaces

Headaches Prompting CT Brain Scan Consideration

- Worst headache of life — consider lumbar puncture if CT negative
- Change in headache from previous headache symptoms/patterns
- Focal deficits
- Acute neurologic complaints
- New onset seizure with headache
- Complaints of altered mental status
- Migraine aura that is sensory or motor
- Change in migraine aura
- Headache > 24 hours
- Thunderclap headache
- Headache in elderly
- Historical "Red Flag" headaches
- Minor head trauma on anticoagulation
- Anticoagulation patient with new headache symptoms
- Neuroimaging is not warranted in patients with episodic stable headache pattern with a normal neurological examination

Consider "Don't Miss Diagnoses"

(Perform testing for possible diagnoses when suspected)

- Subarachnoid hemorrhage
- Meningitis and encephalitis
- Temporal arteritis
- Acute narrow angle closure glaucoma
- Hypertensive emergencies
- Carbon monoxide poisoning
- Cerebral venous sinus thrombosis (seen, for example, with OCP use or with patients with coagulopathy)
- Pseudotumor cerebri
- Acute strokes
- Mass lesions

Consult Criteria

- Headaches refractory to treatment
- Headache with fever unless consistent with a benign process
- Acute neurologic complaints or findings
- Above diagnosis suspected in the "Don't miss diagnosis" section
- Questionable diagnosis
- Status migrainosus (> 24 hours; dehydration)
- "Historical Red Flag" headache

Notes

REFERENCES:

Brennan KC, Farrell CP, Deough GP, Baggaley S, Pippitt K, Pohl SP, et al. Symptom codes and opioids: disconcerting headache practice patterns in academic primary care. Presented on April 30, 2014 at the Annual Meeting of the American Academy of Neurology, 2014.

Baden EY, et al. Intravenous dexamethasone to prevent the

recurrence of benign headache after discharge from the emergency department: a randomized, double-blind, placebo-controlled clinical trial *Can J Emerg Med* 2006;8(6):393–400

Migraine Headache Author: Jasvinder Chawla, MD, MBA; Chief Editor: Helmi L Lutsep, MD emedicine.medscape.com/article/1142556

Loder E, Weizenbaum E, Frishberg B, Silberstein S; the American Headache Society Choosing Wisely Task Force. Choosing Wisely in Headache Medicine: The American Headache Society's List of Five Things Physicians and Patients Should Question. Headache. Available at: onlinelibrary.wiley.com/doi/10.1111/head.12233/abstract

Top Magn Reson Imaging, 2015;24:291

Ann of EM, Vol.655:622

Seizure Management

Definition

- Focal or generalized electrical depolarization's of the brain resulting in focal or generalized neurologic and motor findings with or without loss of consciousness
- Epilepsy is defined as 2 of more seizures not provoked by other illness or causations, or a first time seizure that has a predisposition to recur

Differential Diagnosis

- Pseudoseizures
- Migraines
- Encephalitis
- Meningitis
- Transient global amnesia (TGA)
- Psychogenic unresponsiveness
- TIA (rare TIA's can present with focal motor activity or unresponsiveness)
- Cardiogenic syncope
- Hypoglycemia
- Conversion reaction

Considerations

Generalized seizures (most common)

Classic tonic-clonic ("grand mal")

- Sustained generalized muscle contractions followed by loss of consciousness

Absence seizures ("petit mal")

- Brief episodes of sudden immobility and blank stares

Partial seizures

Simple

- Brief sensory or motor symptoms without loss of consciousness
  - Focal motor seizures is an example

Complex

- Mental or psychiatric symptoms
- Affect changes
- Confusion
- Automatisms
- Hallucinations
- Impaired consciousness

Status epilepticus (SE)

- Newly defined as seizure > 5 minutes or 2 or more seizures in which patient does not recover consciousness
- Older definition > 30 minutes or 2 or more seizures in which patient does not recover consciousness (controversy exists about definition)
- Mortality of 10–12%
- Failure to recognize nonconvulsive SE increases poor outcomes

- Prolonged SE leads to electromechanical dissociation
  - Exhibits minor movements: twitching of eyes, face, hands, feet;
  - Coma

Prolactin level

- Helpful if drawn within 10–20 minutes of seizure and elevated 2 times normal (typically elevated 3 or 4-fold with generalized tonic-clonic seizures than with other seizure types)
  - Syncope can also elevate prolactin levels
- Normal prolactin level favors pseudoseizure but cannot differentiate seizure from syncope
- Normal prolactin does not rule out seizure
- Considerable variability of prolactin levels has precluded their routine clinical use

Pseudoseizures

- Closed eyes during seizure: 96% sensitive; 98% specific in indicating pseudoseizure
- Open eyes during seizure: 98% sensitive; 96% specific in indicating true seizure
- Can also occur 10–20% of the time in patients with epilepsy

First–time seizure recurrence risk depends on

- Brain MRI abnormality
- Abnormal EEG
- Partial–onset seizure/focal neurological exam

30–50% recurrence if 1 present

80% recurrence if all 3 present

15% recurrence if none present – may withhold anticonvulsant therapy

- Anticonvulsant treatment decreases the recurrence of first–time grand mal seizure

Causes

- Idiopathic
- Genetic/congenital malformations
- Hypoglycemia or hyperglycemia
- Hypernatremia and hyponatremia
- CVA
- Cerebral mass
- Intracranial hemorrhage — especially subarachnoid or intraparenchymal
- Traumatic brain injury
- Cocaine
- Meningitis
- Encephalitis
- Eclampsia
- Fever
- Prescribed drugs (lowered seizure threshold especially with some antibiotics and analgesics)
- Withdrawal syndromes (drugs and alcohol)

Evaluation

Seizure history

- Any warning before the seizure ("spell") occurred?
- What did patient do during seizure?
- How long did the seizure last?
- Was patient relating to environment during seizure?
- Does the patient recall the seizure?
- How long did it take till the patient was "back to normal" after the seizure (spell) occurred and how did the patient feel after the seizure or spell?
- How frequent do the "spells" or seizures occur?
- Any precipitating events or actions associated with the seizure?
- Any treatment response of seizure disorder?

- Obtain history of associated symptoms
- Drug abuse history

Patients baseline lab

- CMP

- Seizure drug levels if measurable
- U/A
- Pregnancy test of women of child bearing age

Seizure patients with comorbid considerations and new onset seizures

- CMP, Mg^{++} in select patients
- Pregnancy test in childbearing age women
- Consider lumbar puncture (LP) in immunocompromised patient or with meningitis signs
- Consider LP in patients with seizure and fever
- CBC; U/A; chest x-ray as indicated by associated symptoms or findings
- Blood alcohol and drug screen as indicated
- Serum anticonvulsant levels if measurable

Monitoring anticonvulsant levels

- Determine anticonvulsant level that achieves seizure control
- Determine maximal amount of anticonvulsant the patient can tolerate without toxic side effects
- Determine if patient's anticonvulsant levels are therapeutic before accepting medication failure
- Around 30% of patients miss at least 1 dose of anticonvulsant medication per month
- Pharmacokinetic changes may occur with hepatic metabolism over several weeks resulting in decreased anticonvulsant levels
- Some patients are controlled at subtherapeutic anticonvulsant levels

Neuroimaging for new onset seizure or change in seizure

- Brain magnetic resonance imaging) with and without contrast (MRI) is the preferred imaging modality
- CT brain scanning may be ordered if MRI not performed
- CT brain scan on elderly or patients taking Coumadin (warfarin) or DOAC's
- CT brain scan for head trauma
- CT brain scan should usually be performed for new onset seizure

Electroencephalography (EEG)

- Strengthens diagnosis
- Assists with determining prognosis

Treatment

- Goal is to achieve seizure free state without adverse medication effects
  - Achieved in 60% of patients
- Monotherapy is preferred to decrease adverse side–effects and cost, and increase compliance
- Vocational and social rehabilitation may be needed

Precautions

Driving motor vehicles

- Check state laws
- More restricted for commercial vehicle drivers — 5 year seizure–free period usually required
- Usually need to have a State specified seizure–free interval

Water activities

- Do not swim alone
- Wear life preserver
- Be monitored taking baths

Heights and power tools

- Should be avoided

Anticonvulsant medications

(Read adverse reactions and contraindications)

Drug induced seizures

- Benzodiazepines are generally accepted as the first-line anticonvulsant therapy for drug-induced seizures
- Do not give phenytoin (Dilantin)

Generalized seizures

Valproic acid (Depakote, Depacon)

- 125 mg PO tid — increase every 3–7 days by 125 mg a day (usual daily dose 750–4,000 mg total) — NMT 60mg/kg/day
- Therapeutic range 50–100 mcg/mL
- Adverse reactions
    - Hepatic failure (monitor liver function tests especially in first 6 months of therapy)
    - Pancreatitis
    - Pregnancy fetal risks — especially in first trimester

Phenytoin (Dilantin)

- 100 mg PO bid–qid (may dose qday)
- Therapeutic range 10–20 mcg/mL
- Second–line drug
- Should not be used in pregnancy
- Watch for changes in gums
- Calcium and vitamin D replacement with long term usage

Carbamazepine (Tegretol)

- 200 mg PO bid — may increase qweek by 200 mg total daily dose split tid–qid
- NMT 1600 mg PO qday total dose usually needed
- Therapeutic range 5–12 mcg/mL
- Second–line drug

Levetiracetam (Keppra)

- 500 mg PO bid — may increase 1,000 mg daily q2weeks to achieve control
- NMT 1,500 mg PO bid

Lamotrigine (Lamictal)

- Dose varies depending on co–existent anticonvulsant treatment — read drug insert or reference information
- Watch for a new skin rash

Absence seizures

Ethosuximide (Zarontin)

- 500 mg PO qday — increase 250 mg q4–7 days to achieve therapeutic range
- NMT 1,500 mg qday
- Therapeutic range 40–100mcg/mL

Valproic acid (Depakote, Depacon)

- 15mg/kg/day — increase 5–10 mg/kg/day to achieve control (usually < 60 mg/kg/day needed)
- Therapeutic range 50–100 mcg/mL
- Second line drug — for atypical absence seizures

Focal seizures

Carbamazepine (Tegretol)

- 200 mg PO bid — may increase qweek by 200 mg total daily dose split tid–qid
- NMT 1600 mg PO qday total dose usually needed
- Therapeutic range 4–12 mcg/mL
- First–line drug

Phenytoin (Dilantin)

- 100 mg PO bid–qid (may dose qday)
- Therapeutic range 10–20 mcg/mL
- Second–line drug

Oxcarbazepine (Trileptal)

- Adjunct or monotherapy
- Dose varies depending on co-existent anticonvulsant treatment — read drug insert or reference information

Levetiracetam (Keppra)

- 500 mg PO bid — may increase 1,000 mg daily q2weeks
- NMT 1,500 mg PO bid
- Adjunctive therapy when first–line treatment failure

Zonisamide (Zonegran)

- 100 mg/day — increase to 200mg/day after 2 weeks
  - Can increase to 400mg/day with at least 2 weeks between each 100mg increase
- Adjunct therapy

Switching anticonvulsant medications

- Requires a period of overlap
- Give patient a written schedule of the taper to discontinue the medication day–by–day or week–by–week

ACEP Clinical Policy: Critical Issues in the Evaluation and Management of Adult Patients Presenting to the Emergency Department with seizures (January 2014)

- Intended for emergency departments
- Adult patients ≥ 18 years with generalized convulsive seizure
- Not intended for pediatric patients, complex partial seizures, acute head or multisystem trauma, or brain tumor, immunocompromised or eclamptic patients

Level A recommendations

- Emergency providers should administer an additional antiepileptic medication in emergency department patients with refractory status epilepticus who have failed treatment with benzodiazepines

Level B recommendations

- Emergency providers may administer intravenous phenytoin, fosphenytoin, or valproate in emergency department patients with refractory status epilepticus who have failed treatment with benzodiazepines.

Level C recommendations

- Emergency providers need not initiate antiepileptic medication in the emergency department for patients who have had a first provoked seizure
- Precipitating medical conditions should be identified and treated
- Emergency providers need not initiate antiepileptic medication in the emergency department for patients who have had a first unprovoked seizure without evidence of brain disease or injury
- Emergency providers may initiate antiepileptic medication in the emergency department, or defer in coordination with other providers, for patients who experienced a first unprovoked seizure with a remote history of brain disease or injury

Level C recommendations

- Emergency providers need not admit patients with a first unprovoked seizure who have returned to their clinical baseline in the emergency department

Level C recommendations

- Emergency providers may administer intravenous levetiracetam, propofol, or barbiturates in emergency department patients with refractory status epilepticus who have failed treatment with benzodiazepines

Level C recommendations

- When resuming antiseizure medication in the emergency department is advisable, IV or oral route is acceptable at the Providers discretion

Consult criteria

- Intractable seizures

- When surgery contemplated for seizure management
- Discontinuing anticonvulsant therapy
- Patient on multiple anticonvulsants

Notes

REFERENCES:

Seizure Assessment in the Emergency Department
Author: M Tyson Pillow, MD, MEd; Chief Editor: Rick Kulkarni, MD
emedicine.medscape.com/article/1609294

American College of Emergency Physicians Clinical Policy: Critical Issues in the Evaluation and Management of Adult Patients Presenting to the Emergency Department With Seizures (January 2014)

Epilepsy and Seizures Updated: Oct 05, 2018
Author: David Y Ko, MD; Chief Editor: Selim R Benbadis, MD
Emedicine.medscape.com

ARTHRITIS MANAGEMENT

Osteoarthritis (OA)

Definition

- Focal degeneration of the articular cartilage often with bony hypertrophy characterized by:
  - Morning stiffness
  - Joint stiffness after prolonged rest
  - Joint pain with activity relieved by rest
  - Joint range of motion often reduced
  - Gradual onset progressing over years
  - Often leads to disuse muscle atrophy and a feeling of joint instability
  - Joint effusions may occur, but are non–inflammatory with less than 2,000 WBC's/ml

Differential diagnosis

- Rheumatoid arthritis
- Psoriatic arthritis
- Avascular necrosis
- Ankylosing spondylitis
- Bursitis/tendonitis/muscle pain
- Gout or pseudogout
- Referred pain — especially with knee and hip pain
- Septic arthritis
- Hemochromatosis

Considerations

- Prevalence of 15% in the US population — most common in ages > 65 years
- Affects over 20 million in the U.S.
- Most common arthritic problem > 50 years of age
- Progression is slow, occurring over years to decades
- Predominantly a non-inflammatory condition arising from degenerative changes and progressive loss of cartilage with subsequent hypertrophic bone changes
- Mostly primary and idiopathic — secondary causes include trauma, obesity, inflammatory arthropathy and severe neuropathy
- There is an inverse relationship between OA and bone mass
- From age related "wear and tear" or injury with loss or damage to cartilage and synovial membrane allowing bones to come into contact

- Therapy, both medical and physical, is directed at symptom relief and slowing down the disease progression
- Incidence increases with age
- More common in females over males by 2–3 to 1

Risk factors (* = most common)

- Age*
- Female gender
- Joint instability/muscle weakness
- Heredity*
- Obesity*
- Overuse
- Peripheral neuropathy
- Trauma
- Joint infection
- Hypermobility

Evaluation

History

Keys to diagnosis — 2 primary patterns are seen:

- Patients with Heberden and Bouchard nodes with involvement of first CMC joint
- Patients with a noninflammatory asymmetric oligo or monoarthritis affecting the hip, knee, MTP joints or spine

- Most commonly involved joints are knee (medial > lateral), hips, hands, spine, and 1st MTP joint of foot
  - Involved hand joints are distal interphalangeal (DIP) and proximal interphalangeal (PIP) and carpometacarpal (CMC)

Physical examination

- Look for bony overgrowth around the joint, crepitus, and reduced ROM

Plain x–rays (preferred imaging modality)

- Look for non–uniform joint space narrowing, bone sclerosis and osteophytes
- Look for calcium deposits (chrondrocalcinosis), erosions (rheumatoid arthritis and psoriatic arthritis), and fractures (trauma)
- Check for patellofemoral joint space narrowing
- X–ray changes of OA correlate poorly with the degree of disability or pain

Other imaging as needed

- MRI for in–depth evaluation of cartilage or ligament damage
- Bone scans to differentiate osteoarthritis from other diseases as indicated

Labs

- Used to rule out other diseases or infections
- CBC
- ESR/C–reactive protein
- Uric acid
- Creatinine
- If needed to further clarify the arthritic process — rheumatoid factor/ACPA (positive anticitrullinated peptide antibody), ANA, T4, and joint aspiration

- Arthrocentesis if needed to differentiate from septic, inflammatory and crystal arthritis — synovial fluid is usually amber, clear, with normal viscosity and less than 2000 WBCs/ml (see synovial fluid analysis)

Treatment — directed at symptomatic relief and slowing down disease progression

- Patient education in joint protection
- Muscle strengthening and stretching exercises

- Physical and occupational therapy prn
- Weight reduction to ideal body weight
- Adaptive aids — canes, braces, splints
- Acetaminophen or NSAID's to maximum dose (caution in renal disease with NSAID's)
    - Try 3 or 4 different NSAID's before giving up on this type of medication — a patient may respond to one NSAID but not another
    - Glucosamine chondroitin PO — benefits unclear
    - Intra–articular corticosteroid injections when effusion present — NMT 3 per year (relief lasts up to 4–6 weeks)
    - Sodium hyaluronate (Synvisc) knee injections
    - Topical agents (Aspercreme or capsaicin or diclofenac)
    - Tramadol for mild to moderate OA pain
    - Arthroplasty (joint replacement) for disabling disease

Consult criteria

- Failure to respond to medical therapy
- If OA pain severe enough to require narcotics, refer to a physician or rheumatologist for a consult or approval
- Septic arthritis found or suspected — consult immediately
- Joint effusion in a prosthetic joint
- Symptoms/pain out of proportion to findings

Psoriatic arthritis

Definition

- Chronic inflammatory arthritis that usually occurs with established cutaneous psoriasis, with or without nail changes

Differential diagnosis

- Erosive osteoarthritis
- Gout
- Rheumatoid arthritis
- Ankylosing spondylitis
- Reactive arthritis
- Septic arthritis
- Secondary syphilis
- Systemic lupus erythematosus
- Pauciarticular juvenile arthritis

Considerations

- Psoriasis occurs in 1–2% of the population with psoriatic arthritis found in 5–20% of them
- Psoriasis occurs before arthritis in 75% of patients
- Psoriasis occurs after arthritis in 13–15% of patients
- Psoriasis occurs simultaneously in 8–10% of patients
- Genetic association with HLA B27 leukocyte antigen with spondylitis–type
- Accounts for 2–20% of childhood arthritis and is monoarticular with onset
- DIP joints are affected as opposed to MCP/PIP joints in rheumatoid arthritis
- Distal interphalangeal joints are asymmetrically affected as opposed to symmetrical involvement with rheumatoid arthritis
- Increased risk of arthritis with psoriatic nail involvement or widespread skin rash

Presentations — five variants of psoriatic arthritis have been described:

- Asymmetric oligoarthritis of large or small joints is seen in 30–40 % of patients
- DIP arthritis is seen in 10–15% of patients usually in association with nail pitting
- RA-like symmetrical polyarthritis in 25–50% patients
- Psoriatic spondylitis in 20% of patients — 50% of whom are HLA-B27 positive
- Arthritis mutilans in less than 5% of patients

Associated extra–articular manifestations

- Conjunctivitis 20%
- Iritis/uveitis 7%
  - Approximately 40% of iritis patients will have sacroiliitis
- Dactylitis of finger or toe is common

Evaluation

- History and physical examination
- X–rays may reveal asymmetric erosive changes in small joints of feet and hands
- Lab tests are not very helpful
  - ESR may be best guide to disease activity
  - Hyperuricemia may be found in patients with extensive skin disease

X–ray changes

- Asymmetric soft tissue swelling
- Periostitis
- Bony fusion of DIP/PIP joints
- Bony erosions
- Severe joint space narrowing

Treatment

- Treatment should be aimed at reducing symptoms of inflammation, preserving joint function by halting disease progression
- Therapeutic principles should include patient education, joint protection, physical therapy and vocational counseling
- Cold and heat treatments

Mild disease

- NSAID's to maximum dose (caution in renal disease with NSAID's)
  - Acetaminophen can be added to NSAID prn (more effective than hydrocodone 5 mg)
- Judicious use intra–articular corticosteroid injections for inflamed joint avoiding psoriatic plaques

Moderate or severe disease

Disease–modifying antirheumatic drugs (DMARD's) — initiated if NSAID's and joint intra–articular corticosteroids failure to control arthritis

Caveats

- **Specialists work in tandem with referring clinics**
- Read drug information in literature and be familiar with effects and side effects of medications as listed in the literature and/or Physician Desk Reference (PDR)
- Joint surgery referral only for advanced disabling disease in an attempt to regain some function

Considerations

- Check CBC, creatinine, LFT's and investigate abnormalities before DMARD or Biologics medications are used
- Document negative pregnancy test and discussion of contraception in fertile females before treatment
- Consider pneumovax vaccination
- Document PPD results before Biologics therapy

DMARD's

Considerations

- Use lowest effective dose
- Monitor for myelosuppression, immunodeficiency, infections, hepatic disease — read drug information in literature
- Contraindicated in pregnancy
- Check blood tests q4–6weeks — and more frequent testing when initiated

Medications

- **Sulfasalazine (Azulfidine)**
  - CBC with differential and LFT's 2 weeks for 3 months then qmonth for 3 month, then q3months
  - U/A
- **Methotrexate**
  - Avoid in sulfa allergic patients
  - Agranulocytosis in 1% of patients
  - Check for G6PD deficiency before treatment
  - Monitor LFT's and CBC
    - LFT's q1month initially, then every 1-2 months after that, and with dose change
    - CBC q1month
    - Pregnancy test if fertile female prior to therapy (fetal toxicity)
    - Chest x-ray prior to therapy
    - PFT's
    - Check serum albumin
- Leflunamide
  - GI side effects most common
  - If AST or ALT > 2 times normal of upper limit of normal (ULN) then reduce drug
  - If AST or ALT > 3 times normal of upper limit of normal (ULN) then stop drug
  - Monitor for hypertension
  - Monitor for renal dysfunction
- Cyclosporine and/or etretinate may also be used in conjunction with a physician for treatment of psoriasis/psoriatic arthritis
- Plaquenil use contraindicated because it may precipitate skin disease flares

Biologics (tumor necrosis factor inhibitors) for failure to respond to DMARD's (methotrexate at a minimum)

- Anti-TNFs are noted for dramatic improvement in skin and articular manifestations of the disease

Caveats

- **Specialists work in tandem with referring clinics**
- Read drug information in literature and be familiar with effects and side effects of medications as listed in the literature and/or Physician Desk Reference (PDR)

Cautions

- Severe infection risk exists
- Stop all DMARDs and Biologics if infection identified or suspected until treated and resolved
- Malignancy risks may be increased
- Do not use in optic neuritis or multiple sclerosis patients or in a first degree relative of these patients
- Do not use in patients with significant heart failure
- Avoid live vaccines
- Biologics may be used with or without DMARDs

Biologic medications

- Etanercept (Enbrel)
- Inflximab (Remicade)
- Adalimumab (Humira)
- Golimumab (Simponi)

Phosphodiesterase-4 inhibitor

- Apremilast (Otezla)

Interleukin Inhibitors (monoclonal antibody)

- Secukinumab (Cosentyx)
- Ixekizumab (Taltz)

- Brodalumab (Siliq)
- Ustekinumab (Skyrizi)
- And other monoclonal antibodies

Rheumatology referral criteria

- Evaluation and initiation of DMARDs or Biologic therapy
- Failure to respond to treatment
- Pregnancy despite previous warnings
- Surgery referral contemplated
- Psoriatic arthritis refractory to treatment
- Significant side effects of therapy or other unexpected complications

Rheumatoid arthritis (RA)

Definition

- Chronic systemic inflammatory process of unknown etiology primarily involving the peripheral joints characterized by:
  - Symmetrical joint swelling/pain
  - Morning stiffness > 60 minutes
  - Symptoms present > 6 weeks
  - Polyarthritis (> 4 joints) more so than an oligoarthritis (1–4 joints)
  - Positive anticitrullinated peptide antibody (ACPA)

Differential diagnosis

Acutely:

- Reactive arthritis
- Infections (Parvovirus B19, EBV, Lyme disease)
- Systemic lupus erythematosus
- Early scleroderma

Chronic:

- Systemic lupus erythematosus
- Psoriatic arthritis
- Lyme disease
- Reactive arthritis
- Erosive OA
- Polyarticular gout
- Polymyalgia rheumatica
- Sarcoidosis

Considerations

- Common initial site of onset — hands (MCP/PIP/wrist), foot (MTP), knee but may involve any joint with a synovial membrane
- Cervical vertebrae 1 and 2 most common spine involvement — may cause neurologic deficits/symptoms (caution with endotracheal intubation)
- Persistent synovitis weakens the periarticular support structures leading to subluxations and joint deformities, i.e., Boutonniere and Swan neck deformities of the hands
- Genetics account for 50% of occurrence
- Peak onset typically 20–40 years of age, with a female to male prevalence of 3:1, and a second peak at 60 years of age, with prevalence of female: male of 1:1
- Juvenile rheumatoid arthritis is the most common cause of arthritis in children
- Mortality increased 2–3 times over background due to immunosuppression, infection, disability, heart and lung disease, steroids and malignancy
  - Cardiovascular causes are followed in order by infection, respiratory disease and malignancy

Findings and symptoms

Constitutional

- Generalized morning stiffness, malaise

Joint findings

- Soft tissue swelling/pain in the typical joints
- Joint deformities, i.e., subluxations of joints and reduced ROM
- Tendon rupture may occur
- Joint effusion, especially in the knee — look for Baker's cyst

Extra–articular findings

- Pleuritis and pleural effusions
- Interstitial pulmonary fibrosis
- Vasculitis
- Pericarditis/pericardial effusion
- Rheumatoid (subcutaneous) nodules usually found on extensor surfaces and fingers/toes
- Anemia of chronic disease — hemoglobin typically ~ 10 gm/dL (if less then check for iron deficiency anemia and/or blood loss)
- Felty's syndrome (granulocytopenia and splenomegaly) in patients with long standing rheumatoid arthritis
- Eye symptoms — episcleritis, scleritis and keratoconjunctivitis sicca
- Fever (juvenile rheumatoid arthritis)

Rheumatoid arthritis 2010 classification criteria

A score of ≥ 6 out of 10 meets criteria

- 1 large joint — no points
- 2–10 large joints — 1 point
- 1–3 small joints — 2 points
- 4–10 small joints — 3 points
- Greater than 10 small (with 1 small joint) — 5 points
- Negative rheumatoid factor (RF) and anti-citrullinated peptide antibody (ACPA) — 0 points
- Low positive RF or ACPA — 2 points
- High positive RF or ACPA — 3 points
- Normal C–reactive protein (CRP) and erythrocyte sedimentation rate (ESR) — no points
- Elevated CRP or ESR — 1 point
- Symptoms < 6 weeks — no points
- Symptoms ≥ 6 weeks — 1 point

History and physical examination

- Evaluate the whole patient and the effect of joint symptoms on life, work and activity

Labs

- CBC
- Creatinine level
- LFTs
- CRP or ESR
- ACPA and rheumatoid factor (RF)

Lab considerations

- ANA may be positive in ~ 10–30% of RA patients usually in low titer with negative double–stranded DNA (dsDNA)
- RF positive in ~75–80% of patients with RA
- ACPA positive in 100% of RA patients (false positive rate 5–6%)
- CRP/ESR correlate with inflammation and can be used as a crude guide for response to treatment, but RA patients may have inflammation due to other causes that is partially suppressed by RA treatment with DMARD's or Biologics

X–rays

- Look for soft tissue swelling and osteopenia around the joints, bone erosions and joint space narrowing
- Earliest bone erosions often seen on 2nd or 3rd MCP heads, 3rd finger PIP joint or 5th MTP joint
- MRI if C1–2 needs evaluation

Treatment

- Treatment should be aimed at reducing symptoms of inflammation and preserving joint function by halting disease progression
- Therapeutic principles should include patient education, joint protection, physical therapy and vocational counseling
- Occupational therapy for orthotics and splints

- Cold and heat treatments
- Patient education

Early disease

- NSAID's — these may improve symptoms but they do not suppress disease progression (caution with renal disease)
- Judicious use of intra–articular (IA) steroids — infrequently used
- Systemic steroids should be reserved for severe uncontrolled arthritis or corticosteroid bridging therapy till DMARD's take effect
- Analgesics prn besides NSAID's
- Do not use both oral and IA steroids

See DMARDs under Psoriatic Arthritis section for considerations and monitoring

- Treatment with DMARDs and Biologics require periodic toxicity checks
- Specialists work in tandem with referring clinics — earliest possible referral to a rheumatologist is preferable
- Methotrexate — preferred first line agent
- Sulfasalazine (Azulfidine)
- Cyclosporine
  - May be used by a rheumatologist
- Leflunamide
- Minocycline 100 mg PO bid
- Plaquenil

See Biologics (tumor necrosis factor inhibitors) for failure to respond to DMARD's under Psoriatic Arthritis section

- Etanercept (Enbrel)
- Infliximab (Remicade)
  - May use with methotrexate
- Adalimumab (Humira)
- Golimumab (Simponi)

Rheumatology referral criteria

- Evaluation and initiation of DMARDs or Biologic therapy
- Failure to respond to treatment
- Pregnancy despite previous warnings
- Surgery referral contemplated
- Rheumatoid arthritis refractory to treatment
- Significant side effects of therapy or other unexpected complications

Notes

REFERENCES:

Arthritis and Rheumatism

Vol. 62, No. 9, September 2010, pp 2569 - 2581

DOI 10.1002/art.27584 c 2010, American College of Rheumatology

Osteoarthritis Updated: Mar 19, 2019

Author: Carlos J Lozada, MD; Chief Editor: Herbert S Diamond, MD

Emedicine.medscape.com

Glossary

ABG — arterial blood gas

ABI — ankle brachial index

AC — acromioclavicular

ACEI — angiotensin converting enzyme inhibitor

ADT — adult diphtheria tetanus

Anaphylaxis — IgE antibody release of various mediators such as histamine causing varying degrees of symptoms such as rash, pruritus, bronchospasm, GI symptoms, hypoxia, upper airway compromise, hypotension and potentially death

Angina — cardiac chest discomfort, or other discomfort or symptoms, from deficit of blood flow and oxygen delivery to the heart

Anion gap — sodium minus chloride and CO_2 (serum bicarbonate)

Anti-HBS — antibody to hepatitis B surface antigen

Aortic dissection — tearing of the wall of the aorta

ARB — Angiotensin receptor blocker

ASA — aspirin

Asthma — reversible constriction of pulmonary small airways

Asymptomatic hypertension — elevated blood pressure with no acute end-organ compromise of function

Bandemia — increased white blood cell bands from stress, infection, or inflammation

BB — beta-blocker

B-HCG — beta human chorionic gonadotropin

BID (bid) — twice a day

BMI — body mass index

BMP — basic metabolic profile including sodium, potassium, chloride, carbon dioxide (CO_2), glucose, creatinine and BUN (blood urea nitrogen)

BNP — B-type natriuretic peptide, determined by stretch of cardiac muscle from CHF. Elevated in many other conditions that cause strain on the heart in addition to CHF. NT–proBNP distinguishes systolic dysfunction vs. other causes of dyspnea

Bronchitis — reversible constriction of pulmonary small airways from an infection in the lungs

BSA — body surface area

Burst fracture — fracture through entire vertebral body (unstable)

CBC — complete blood count

CCB — calcium channel blocker

CHD — coronary heart disease

CHF — Congestive heart failure. Cardiac dysfunction secondary to decreased ability of the left ventricle (LV) to eject or fill with blood

COPD — chronic obstructive pulmonary disease, usually chronic bronchitis or emphysema, or mixture of both

CPK — creatine phosphokinase (a muscle enzyme)

C-RP — C reactive protein (nonspecific marker of inflammation)

CSF — cerebral spinal fluid

C-spine — cervical spine

CXR — chest x-ray

CVA — brain neuronal death from a deficit of cerebral perfusion resulting in lack of oxygen to parts of the brain

DBP — diastolic blood pressure

D-dimer — a measurable byproduct of fibrinogen pathway indicating some level of blood clot formation

DIC — disseminated intravascular coagulation

DIP — distal interphalangeal joint

DJD — degenerative joint disease (osteoarthritis)

DKA — diabetic ketoacidosis (a metabolic acidotic diabetic condition resulting from insulin resistance or severe deficit of insulin, and fatty acids metabolism for energy needs, that is associated with potential mortality)

DOAC — direct oral anticoagulant
DOC — drug of choice

DUB — dysfunctional uterine bleeding

DVT — deep vein thrombosis

Dyspnea — shortness of breath

EBV — Epstein-Barr virus

Emergency hypertension — acute end-organ injury secondary to elevated blood pressure

Epley maneuver — treatment of BPV (moves otoliths out of semicircular canals). Avoid with recent neck fracture, instability or surgery, carotid disease or recent retinal detachment

ESR — erythrocyte sedimentation rate (nonspecific marker of inflammation)

ESRD — end stage renal disease

FFP — fresh frozen plasma

GC — gonococcal or gonococcus

GERD — gastroesophageal reflux

GI — gastrointestinal

gm(s) — gram or grams

gtt — drop

HAART — highly active antiretroviral therapy with 2 NRTIs and either a protease inhibitor or NNRTI

Hallpike maneuver — patient going from sitting position to supine position rapidly with head below horizontal plane of body and head rotated quickly and carefully to the left or right. Any nystagmus and symptoms induced represent a positive test.

HBIG — hepatitis B immune globulin

HHS — hyperglycemic hyperosmolar syndrome

HIV — human immunodeficiency virus

HR — heart rate

HSV — herpes simplex virus

IBS — irritable bowel syndrome

IG — immune globulin

IM — intramuscular

INR — international normalized ratio (measures warfarin therapy)

IOP — intraocular pressure

IUP — intrauterine pregnancy

IV — intravenous

Jugular venous distension — distension of the external jugular vein in the neck due to increased pressure in the right side of the heart or in the lungs (pulmonary hypertension, COPD, CHF) or mass effect obstructing flow

KUB — kidney, ureter and bladder plain x-ray

LES — lower esophageal sphincter

LFT's — liver function tests

LP — lumbar puncture

LOC — loss of consciousness

MDI — metered dose inhaler

Metabolic acidosis — decreased serum bicarbonate

mmol/L = mEq/L on serum test levels

MP — metacarpophalangeal

MRSA — methicillin resistance staphylococcus aureus

$NaHCO_3^-$ — sodium bicarbonate

NMT — no more than

Nonspecific chest pain — chest pain without evident specific cause

NNRTI — non-nucleoside reverse transcriptase inhibitor

NRTI — nucleoside reverse transcriptase inhibitor

NS — normal saline

NSAID's — nonsteroidal anti-inflammatory drugs

Nystagmus — rhythmic involuntary eye movements named for the quick component

O_2 saturation — percent of hemoglobin carrying oxygen

ORT — oral rehydration therapy

Osmolol gap — the difference between calculated and measured osmolality in the blood, usually less than 10

PAD — peripheral arterial disease

Panic disorder — state of hyperventilation causing decreased pCO_2 measurement on blood gas (respiratory alkalosis), elevated pH, resulting in feeling short of breath, acute calcium shifts into cells (can cause carpospasm), hypokalemia, paresthesias, and a sense of impending doom when more severe

PCP — primary care provider

PCR — polymerase chain reaction

PE — physical examination or pulmonary embolism (use context)

PEP — postexposure prophylaxis

PERC — pulmonary embolism rule out criteria

PID — pelvic inflammatory disease

PIP — proximal interphalangeal

PMN — polymorphonuclear neutrophil

PN — peripheral neuropathy

PO — per oral

POC — products of conception

PPI — proton pump inhibitor

PR — per rectum

PRBC — packed red blood cells

Presyncope or near syncope — state of feeling that a fainting or syncopal episode will occur

prn — as needed

Pseudoaddiction — a condition caused by under-treatment of pain where the patient engages in an active and often repetitive search for pain medications

Pseudoseizures — seizure-like activity caused by psychiatric or functional considerations that is not a true seizure

PSVT — paroxysmal supraventricular tachycardia

Pulmonary embolism — blood clot(s) located in the lung's blood vessels that originated elsewhere, usually from veins in pelvis or proximal legs

Q or **q** — every

QID (qid) — four times a day

RCT — rotator cuff tear

Respiratory acidosis — increased pCO_2 on blood gas measurement

Respiratory alkalosis — decreased pCO_2 and elevated pH on blood gas from increased minute ventilation or hyperventilation

Respiratory failure — increasing blood gas pCO_2 and respiratory fatigue with decreasing pH, resulting in increasing somnolence, altered mental status and hypoxemia

RSV — respiratory syncytial virus

SBO — small bowel obstruction

SBP — systolic blood pressure

Sepsis — usually a bacterial infection frequently used to mean invasion of the blood stream

SLR — straight leg raise

SQ — subcutaneous

SS disease — sickle cell homozygous disease

SSRI — selective serotonin reuptake inhibitor

STD — sexual transmitted disease

SVT — supraventricular tachycardia

Syncope — loss of consciousness from decreased cerebral perfusion

TBSA — total body surface area

TC — total cholesterol

Tdap — tetanus, diphtheria and acellular pertussis vaccine

TGA — transient global amnesia

Thrombocytopenia — low platelet count

TIA — transient ischemic attack

TID (tid) — three times a day

TM — tympanic membrane

Troponin — breakdown cardiac muscle component indicating injury or death to cardiac muscle depending on level

TSH — thyroid stimulating hormone most commonly elevated in primary hypothyroidism

U/A — urine analysis

UCG — urine pregnancy test (urinary chorionic gonadotropin)

UDS — urine drug screen

UGI — upper gastrointestinal

UTI — urinary tract infection

Valsalva — straining of abdomen causing increase in intracranial and intraocular pressure

WBC — white blood count

Well's criteria — criteria developed to assess level of probability of VTE (venous thromboembolic) disease either in extremities or lungs (pulmonary embolism)

Whole bowel irrigation — giving polyethylene glycol (MiraLax or Go-lytely) to flush out the intestines

Index

A

B

C

D

E

F

G

H

I

J

K

L

M

N

O

P

Q

R

S

T

U

V

W

Z

www.ingramcontent.com/pod-product-compliance
Lightning Source LLC
Chambersburg PA
CBHW060418220326
41598CB00021BA/2210

* 9 7 8 1 7 3 7 7 3 8 9 4 7 *